T0200190

KAPLAN & SADOCK'S POCKET HANDBOOK OF CLINICAL PSYCHIATRY

Sixth Edition

KAPLAN & SADOCK'S POCKET HANDBOOK OF **CLINICAL PSYCHIATRY**

Sixth Edition

BENJAMIN J. SADOCK, M.D.

Menas S. Gregory Professor of Psychiatry
Department of Psychiatry
New York University School of Medicine
Attending Psychiatrist, Tisch Hospital
Attending Psychiatrist, Bellevue Hospital Center
New York, New York

SAMOON AHMAD, M.D.

Associate Professor of Psychiatry
Department of Psychiatry
New York University School of Medicine
Attending Physician and Unit Chief Inpatient Psychiatry
Bellevue Hospital Center
New York, New York

VIRGINIA A. SADOCK, M.D.

Professor of Psychiatry
Department of Psychiatry
New York University School of Medicine
Attending Psychiatrist, Tisch Hospital
Attending Psychiatrist, Bellevue Hospital Center
New York, New York

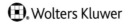
Wolters Kluwer

Philadelphia · Baltimore · New York · London
Buenos Aires · Hong Kong · Sydney · Tokyo

Acquisitions Editor: Chris Teja
Development Editor: Ashley Fischer
Editorial Coordinator: Alexis Pozonsky
Marketing Manager: Rachel Mante Leung
Production Project Manager: Bridgett Dougherty
Design Coordinator: Holly McLaughlin
Manufacturing Coordinator: Beth Welsh
Prepress Vendor: Aptara, Inc.

6th edition

9 8 7 6 5 4

Printed in The United States of America

Library of Congress Cataloging-in-Publication Data

Names: Sadock, Benjamin J., author. | Ahmad, Samoon, author. | Sadock,
  Virginia A., author.
Title: Kaplan & Sadock's pocket handbook of clinical psychiatry / Benjamin J. Sadock,
  Samoon Ahmad, Virginia A. Sadock.
Other titles: Kaplan and Sadock's pocket handbook of clinical psychiatry |
  Pocket handbook of clinical psychiatry | Complemented by (expression):
  Kaplan & Sadock's comprehensive textbook of psychiatry. 10th ed.
Description: Sixth edition. | Philadelphia : Wolters Kluwer, [2019] |
  Complemented by: Kaplan & Sadock's comprehensive textbook of psychiatry /
  editors, Benjamin J. Sadock, Virginia A. Sadock, Pedro Ruiz. 10th ed.
  2017. | Includes bibliographical references and index.
Identifiers: LCCN 2017044540 | ISBN 9781496386939 (alk. paper)
Subjects: | MESH: Mental Disorders | Psychiatry | Handbooks
Classification: LCC RC454 | NLM WM 34 | DDC 616.89—dc23
LC record available at https://lccn.loc.gov/2017044540

LWW.com

Dedicated
to our children
James and Victoria
and to our grandchildren
Celia, Emily, Oliver and Joel
B.J.S
V.A.S

Dedicated
to my parents
Riffat and Naseem
and my son
Daniel
S.A

Preface

Psychiatry underwent a sea change since the last edition of this book was published: A new classification of mental disorders was developed and codified in a fifth edition of the *Diagnostic and Statistical Manual of Mental Disorders* (DSM-5) published by the American Psychiatric Association. The reader will find all of those changes incorporated into this new, sixth edition of the *Pocket Handbook of Clinical Psychiatry*. Every section in this book has been updated and revised and all the diagnoses of mental disorder conform to the criteria listed in DSM-5.

Each disorder is described using the specific parameters of diagnosis, epidemiology, etiology, clinical signs and symptoms, differential diagnosis, and treatment. This book serves as a ready reference to diagnose and treat the full range of mental disorders in both adults and children. Over the years, psychiatrists and nonpsychiatric physicians have found it to be a useful guide as have medical students, especially during their rotations through psychiatry. It is also used by psychologists, social workers, psychiatric nurses, and many other mental health professionals.

The Pocket Handbook is a minicompanion to the recently published encyclopedic tenth edition of *Kaplan & Sadock's Comprehensive Textbook of Psychiatry* (CTP-X) and each chapter in this book ends with references to the more detailed relevant sections in that textbook.

The authors, Benjamin Sadock, M.D. and Virginia Sadock, M.D. are particularly pleased that Samoon Ahmad, M.D., a close friend and professional associate has joined them as a full author. He is a distinguished psychiatrist with a national and international reputation as both an educator and clinician. His participation has immeasurably helped and enhanced the preparation of this book.

We wish to thank several persons who have helped. We want to acknowledge Norman Sussman, M.D. who has collaborated with us as consulting and contributing editor in many Kaplan & Sadock books. We also thank James Sadock, M.D. and Victoria Sadock Gregg, M.D., experts in adult and child emergency medicine respectively, for their help. Our assistant, Heidiann Grech was crucial in the preparation of this book for which we are most grateful. As always, our publishers continue to maintain their high standards for which we are most appreciative. At Wolters Kluwer, we especially want to thank Lexi Pozonsky for her help.

Finally, the authors wish to thank Charles Marmar, M.D., Lucius R. Littauer Professor and Chair of the Department of Psychiatry at New York University School of Medicine. Dr. Marmar has developed one of this country's premier psychiatric centers and has recruited outstanding clinicians, educators, and researchers who work in an academic environment conducive to outstanding productivity. He has been most supportive of our work for which we are most grateful.

We hope this book continues to fulfill the expectations of all those for whom it is intended—the busy doctor-in-training, the clinical practitioner, and all those who work with and care for the mentally ill.

Benjamin J. Sadock, M.D.
Samoon Ahmad, M.D.
Virginia A. Sadock, M.D.

New York University Medical Center
New York, New York

Contents

Classification in Psychiatry

Systems of classification for psychiatric diagnoses have several purposes: to distinguish one psychiatric diagnosis from another, so that clinicians can offer the most effective treatment; to provide a common language among health care professionals; and to explore the still unknown causes of many mental disorders. The two most important psychiatric classifications are the *Diagnostic and Statistical Manual of Mental Disorders* (DSM-5) developed by the American Psychiatric Association in collaboration with other groups of mental health professionals, and the *International Classification of Diseases* (ICD), developed by the World Health Organization.

DSM-5 Classification

The DSM-5 lists 22 major categories of mental disorders, comprising more than 150 discrete illnesses. All of the disorders listed in DSM-5 are described in detail in the sections of the book that follow and cover epidemiology, etiology, diagnosis, differential diagnoses, clinical features, and treatment of each disorder. In this section, only a brief description of the disorders is provided to give the reader an overview of psychiatric classification including some of the changes made from DSM-IV to DSM-5. A complete discussion of each disorder will be found in the chapters that follow.

Neurodevelopmental Disorders

These disorders are usually first diagnosed in infancy, childhood, or adolescence.

Intellectual Disability or Intellectual Developmental Disorder (previously called Mental Retardation in DSM-IV). Intellectual disability (ID) is characterized by significant, below average intelligence and impairment in adaptive functioning. Adaptive functioning refers to how effective individuals are in achieving age-appropriate common demands of life in areas such as communication, self-care, and interpersonal skills. In DSM-5, ID is classified as mild, moderate, severe, or profound based on overall functioning; in DSM-IV, it was classified according to intelligence quotient (IQ) as mild (50–55 to 70), moderate (35–40 to 50–55), severe (20–25 to 35–40), or profound (below 20–25). A variation of ID called *Global Developmental Delay* is for children under 5 years with severe defects exceeding those above. *Borderline Intellectual Functioning* is used in DSM-5 but is not clearly differentiated from mild ID. In DSM-IV it meant an IQ of about 70, whereas in DSM-5 it is categorized as a condition that may be the focus of clinical attention but no criteria are given.

Communication Disorders. There are four types of communication disorders that are diagnosed when problems in communication cause significant impairment in functioning: (1) *Language Disorder* is characterized by a developmental impairment in vocabulary resulting in difficulty producing age-appropriate sentences; (2) *Speech Sound Disorder* is marked by difficulty in articulation; (3) *Childhood-Onset Fluency Disorder or Stuttering* is characterized by difficulty in fluency, rate and rhythm of speech; and (4) *Social or Pragmatic Communication Disorder* is profound difficulty in social interaction and communication with peers.

Autism Spectrum Disorder. The autistic spectrum includes a range of behaviors characterized by severe difficulties in multiple developmental areas, including social relatedness, communication, and range of activity and repetitive and stereotypical patterns of behavior, including speech. They are divided into three levels: Level 1 is characterized by the ability to speak with reduced social interaction (this level resembles Asperger's disorder which is no longer part of DSM-5); Level 2 which is characterized by minimal speech and minimal social interaction (diagnosed as Rett's disorder in DSM-IV, but not part of DSM-5); and Level 3, marked by a total lack of speech and no social interaction.

Attention-Deficit/Hyperactivity Disorder (ADHD). Since the 1990s, ADHD has been one of the most frequently discussed psychiatric disorders in the lay media because of the sometimes unclear line between age-appropriate normal and disordered behavior and because of the concern that children without the disorder are being misdiagnosed and treated with medication. The central features of the disorder are persistent inattention, or hyperactivity and impulsivity, or both, that cause clinically significant impairment in functioning. It is found in both children and adults.

Specific Learning Disorders. These are maturational deficits in development that are associated with difficulty in acquiring specific skills in *reading* (also known as dyslexia); in *written expression*; or in *mathematics* (also known as dyscalculia).

Motor Disorders. Analogous to learning disorders, motor disorders are diagnosed when motor coordination is substantially below expectations based on age and intelligence, and when coordination problems significantly interfere with functioning. There are three major types of motor disorders: (1) *Developmental Coordination Disorder* is an impairment in the development of motor coordination, for example, delays in crawling or walking, dropping things, or poor sports performance; (2) *Stereotypic Movement Disorder* consists of repetitive motion activity, for example, head banging and body rocking; and (3) *Tic Disorder* is characterized by sudden involuntary, recurrent, and stereotyped movement or vocal sounds. There are two types of tic disorders: the first is *Tourette's Disorder*, characterized by motor and vocal tics including coprolalia, and the second is *Persistent Chronic Motor or Vocal Tic Disorders* marked by a single motor or vocal tic.

Schizophrenia Spectrum and Other Psychotic Disorders

The section on schizophrenia and other psychotic disorders includes eight specific disorders (schizophrenia, schizophreniform disorder, schizoaffective disorder, delusional disorder, brief psychotic disorder, substance/medication-induced psychotic disorder, psychotic disorder due to another medical condition, and catatonia) in which psychotic symptoms are prominent features of the clinical picture. The grouping of disorders in DSM-5 under this heading includes schizotypal personality disorder which is not a psychotic disorder; but which sometimes precedes full blown schizophrenia. In this book schizotypal disorder is *discussed under personality disorders* (see Chapter 17).

Schizophrenia. Schizophrenia is a chronic disorder in which prominent hallucinations or delusions are usually present. The individual must be ill for at least 6 months, although he or she need not be actively psychotic during all of that time. Three phases of the disorder are recognized by clinicians although they are not included in DSM-5 as discrete phases. The *prodrome phase* refers to deterioration in function before the onset of the active psychotic phase. The *active phase* symptoms (delusions, hallucinations, disorganized speech, grossly disorganized behavior, or negative symptoms such as flat affect, avolition, and alogia) must be present for at least 1 month. The *residual phase* follows the active phase. The features of the residual and prodromal phases include functional impairment and abnormalities of affect, cognition, and communication. In DSM-IV, schizophrenia was subtyped according to the most prominent symptoms present at the time of the evaluation (paranoid, disorganized, catatonic, undifferentiated, and residual types); however, those subtypes are no longer part of the official DSM-5 nomenclature.

Nevertheless, they are phenomenologically accurate and are included in ICD-10. The subtypes remain useful descriptions that clinicians will still find helpful when communicating with one another.

Delusional Disorder. Delusional disorder is characterized by persistent delusions, for example, erotomanic, grandiose, jealous, persecutory, somatic, mixed, unspecified. In general, the delusions are about situations that could occur in real life such as infidelity, being followed, or having an illness, which are categorized as nonbizarre beliefs. Within this category one finds what was termed in DSM-IV *shared delusional disorder* (also known as *folie a deux*) but which has been renamed *Delusional Symptoms in Partner with Delusional Disorder* in DSM-5 and is characterized by a delusional belief that develops in a person who has a close relationship with another person with the delusion, the content of which is similar. *Paranoia* (a term not included in DSM-5) is a rare condition characterized by the gradual development of an elaborate delusional system, usually with grandiose ideas; it has a chronic course and the rest of the personality remains intact.

Brief Psychotic Disorder. Brief psychotic disorder requires the presence of delusions, hallucinations, disorganized speech, grossly disorganized behavior, or catatonic behavior for at least 1 day but less than 1 month. It may be precipitated by an external life stress. After the episodes the individual returns to his or her usual level of functioning.

Schizophreniform Disorder. Schizophreniform disorder is characterized by the same active phase symptoms of schizophrenia (delusions, hallucinations, disorganized speech, grossly disorganized behavior, or negative symptoms), but it lasts between 1 and 6 months and has no prodromal or residual phase features of social or occupational impairment.

Schizoaffective Disorder. Schizoaffective disorder is also characterized by the same active phase symptoms of schizophrenia (delusions, hallucinations, disorganized speech, grossly disorganized behavior, or negative symptoms), as well as the presence of a manic or depressive syndrome that is not brief relative to the duration of the psychosis. Individuals with schizoaffective disorder, in contrast to a mood disorder with psychotic features, have delusions or hallucinations for at least 2 weeks without coexisting prominent mood symptoms.

Substance/Medication-Induced Psychotic Disorder. These are disorders with symptoms of psychosis caused by psychoactive or other substances, for example, hallucinogens, cocaine.

Psychotic Disorder Due to Another Medical Condition. This disorder is characterized by hallucinations or delusions that result from a medical illness, for example, temporal lobe epilepsy, avitaminosis, meningitis.

Catatonia. Catatonia is characterized by motor abnormalities such as catalepsy (waxy flexibility), mutism, posturing, and negativism. It can be associated with *Another Mental Disorder,* for example, schizophrenia or bipolar disorder or *Due to Another Medical Condition,* for example, neoplasm, head trauma, hepatic encephalopathy.

Bipolar and Related Disorders

Bipolar disorder is characterized by severe mood swings between depression and elation and by remission and recurrence. There are four variants: bipolar I disorder, bipolar II disorder, cyclothymic disorder, and bipolar disorder due to substance/medication or another medical condition.

Bipolar I Disorder. The necessary feature of bipolar I disorder is a history of a manic or mixed manic and depressive episode. Bipolar I disorder is subtyped in many ways: type of current episode (manic, hypomanic depressed, or mixed), severity and remission status (mild, moderate, severe without psychosis, severe with psychotic features, partial remission, or full remission), and whether the recent course is characterized by rapid cycling (at least four episodes in 12 months).

Bipolar II Disorder. Bipolar II disorder is characterized by a history of hypomanic and major depressive episodes. The symptom criteria for a hypomanic episode are the same as those for a manic episode, although hypomania only requires a minimal duration of 4 days. The major difference between mania and hypomania is the severity of the impairment associated with the syndrome.

Cyclothymic Disorder. This is the bipolar equivalent of dysthymic disorder (see below). Cyclothymic disorder is a mild, chronic mood disorder with numerous depressive and hypomanic episodes over the course of at least 2 years.

Bipolar Disorder Due to Another Medical Condition. Bipolar disorder caused by a general medical condition is diagnosed when evidence indicates that a significant mood disturbance is the direct consequence of a general medical condition, for example, frontal lobe tumor.

Substance/Medication-Induced Bipolar Disorder. Substance-induced mood disorder is diagnosed when the cause of the mood disturbance is substance intoxication, withdrawal, or medication, for example, amphetamine.

Depressive Disorders

Depressive disorders are characterized by depression, sadness, irritability, psychomotor retardation and, in severe cases, suicidal ideation. They include a number of conditions described below.

Major Depressive Disorder. The necessary feature of major depressive disorder is depressed mood or loss of interest or pleasure in usual activities. All symptoms must be present nearly every day, except suicidal ideation or thoughts of death, which need only be recurrent. The diagnosis is excluded if the symptoms are the result of a normal bereavement and if psychotic symptoms are present in the absence of mood symptoms.

Persistent Depressive Disorder or Dysthymia. Dysthymia is a mild, chronic form of depression that lasts at least 2 years, during which, on most days, the individual experiences depressed mood for most of the day and at least two other symptoms of depression.

Premenstrual Dysphoric Disorder. Premenstrual dysphoric disorder occurs about 1 week before the menses and is characterized by irritability, emotional lability, headache and anxiety or depression that remits after the menstrual cycle is over.

Substance/Medication-Induced Depressive Disorder. This disorder is characterized by a depressed mood that is due to a substance, for example, alcohol or medication, for example, barbiturate.

Depressive Disorder Due to Another Medical Condition. This condition is a state of depression secondary to a medical disorder, for example, hypothyroidism, Cushing's syndrome.

Other Specified Depressive Disorder. This diagnostic category includes two subtypes: (1) *Recurrent Depressive Episode* which is a depression that lasts between 2 and 13 days and that occurs at least once a month; and (2) *Short-Duration Depressive Episode* which is a depressed mood lasting from 4 to 14 days and which is nonrecurrent.

Unspecified Depressive Disorder. This diagnostic category includes four major subtypes: (1) *Melancholia* which is a severe form of major depression characterized by hopelessness, anhedonia, psychomotor retardation, and which also carries with it a high risk of suicide; (2) *Atypical Depression* which is marked by a depressed mood that is associated with weight gain instead of weight loss and with hypersomnia instead of insomnia; (3) *Peripartum Depression* is a depression that occurs around parturition, or within 1 month after giving birth (called postpartum depression in DSM-IV); and (4) *Seasonal Pattern* which is a depressed mood that occurs at a particular time of the year, usually winter (also known as seasonal affective disorder [SAD]).

Disruptive Mood Dysregulation Disorder. This is a new diagnosis listed as a depressive disorder which is diagnosed in children over age 6 and under age 18 and is characterized by severe temper tantrums, chronic irritability, and angry mood.

Anxiety Disorders

The section on anxiety disorders includes nine specific disorders (panic disorder, agoraphobia, specific phobia, social anxiety disorder or social phobia, generalized anxiety disorder, anxiety disorder caused by a general medical condition, and substance-induced anxiety disorder) in which anxious symptoms are a prominent feature of the clinical picture. Because separation anxiety disorder and selective mutism occur in childhood, they are discussed in the childhood disorders section of this book.

Panic Disorder. A panic attack is characterized by feelings of intense fear or terror that come on suddenly in situations where there is nothing to fear. It is accompanied by heart racing or pounding, chest pain, shortness of breath or choking, dizziness, trembling or shaking, feeling faint or lightheaded, sweating, and nausea.

Agoraphobia. Agoraphobia is a frequent consequence of panic disorder, although it can occur in the absence of panic attacks. Persons with agoraphobia avoid (or try to avoid) situations that they think might trigger a panic attack (or panic-like symptoms) or situations from which they think escape might be difficult if they have a panic attack.

Specific Phobia. Specific phobia is characterized by an excessive, unreasonable fear of specific objects or situations that almost always occurs on exposure to the feared stimulus. The phobic stimulus is avoided, or, when not avoided, the individual feels severely anxious or uncomfortable.

Social Anxiety Disorder or Social Phobia. Social phobia is characterized by the fear of being embarrassed or humiliated in front of others. Similar to specific phobia, the phobic stimuli are avoided, or, when not avoided, the individual feels severely anxious and uncomfortable. When the phobic stimuli include most social situations, then it is specified as *generalized social phobia.*

Generalized Anxiety Disorder. Generalized anxiety disorder is characterized by chronic excessive worry that occurs more days than not and is difficult to control. The worry is associated with symptoms, such as concentration problems, insomnia, muscle tension, irritability, and physical restlessness, and causes clinically significant distress or impairment.

Anxiety Disorder Due to Another Medical Condition. Anxiety disorder caused by a general medical condition is diagnosed when evidence indicates that significant anxiety is the direct consequence of a general medical condition, for example, hyperthyroidism.

Substance/Medication-Induced Anxiety Disorder. Substance-induced anxiety disorder is diagnosed when the cause of the anxiety is a substance, for example, cocaine, or is the result of a medication, for example, cortisol.

Separation Anxiety Disorder. Separation anxiety disorder occurs in children and is characterized by excessive anxiety about separating from home or attachment figures beyond that expected for the child's developmental level.

Selective Mutism. Selective mutism is characterized by persistent refusal to speak in specific situations despite the demonstration of speaking ability in other situations.

Obsessive-Compulsive and Related Disorders

There are eight categories of disorders listed in this section, all of which have associated obsessions (repeated thoughts) or compulsions (repeated activities).

Obsessive Compulsive Disorder (OCD). OCD is characterized by repetitive and intrusive thoughts or images that are unwelcome (obsessions) or repetitive behaviors that the person feels compelled to do (compulsions), or both. Most often, the compulsions are done to reduce the anxiety associated with the obsessive thought.

Body Dysmorphic Disorder. Body dysmorphic disorder is characterized by a distressing and impairing preoccupation with an imagined or slight defect in appearance. If the belief is held with delusional intensity, then delusional disorder, somatic type, might be diagnosed.

Hoarding Disorder. Hoarding disorder is a behavioral pattern of accumulating items in a compulsive manner that may or may not have any utility to the person. The person is unable to get rid of those items even though they may create hazardous situations in the home such as risk of fire.

Trichotillomania or Hair-Pulling Disorder. Trichotillomania is characterized by repeated hair pulling causing noticeable hair loss. It may occur anywhere on the body, for example, head, eyebrows, pubic area.

Excoriation or Skin-Picking Disorder. Skin-picking disorder is marked by the compulsive need to pick at one's skin to the point of doing physical damage.

Substance/Medication-Induced Obsessive-Compulsive Disorder. This disorder is characterized by obsessive or compulsive behavior that is secondary to the use of a medication or a substance such as abuse of cocaine which can cause compulsive skin-picking (called formication).

Obsessive-Compulsive Disorder Due to Another Medical Condition. The cause of either obsessive or compulsive behavior is due to a medical condition, as sometimes may occur after a streptococcal infection.

Other Specified Obsessive-Compulsive and Related Disorder. This category includes a group of disorders such as *obsessional jealousy* in which one person has repeated thoughts about infidelity in the spouse or partner. It must be distinguished from a delusional belief such as *Koro*, which is a disorder found in South and East Asia in which the person believes the genitalia are shrinking and disappearing into the body; and *Body-Focused Repetitive Behavior Disorder* in which the person engages in a compulsive behavioral pattern such as nail-biting or lip-chewing.

Trauma or Stressor-Related Disorder

This group of disorders is caused by exposure to a natural or man-made disaster or to a significant life stressor such as experiencing abuse. There are six conditions that fall under this category in DSM-5.

Reactive Attachment Disorder. This disorder appears in infancy or early childhood and is characterized by a severe impairment in the ability to relate because of grossly pathologic caregiving.

Disinhibited Social Engagement Disorder. This is a condition in which the child or adolescent has a deep seated fear of interacting with strangers, especially adults, usually as a result of traumatic upbringing.

Post-Traumatic Stress Disorder. Post-traumatic stress disorder (PTSD) occurs after a traumatic event in which the individual believes that he or she is in physical danger or that his or her life is in jeopardy. PTSD can also occur after witnessing a violent or life-threatening event happening to someone else. The symptoms of PTSD usually occur soon after the traumatic event, although, in some cases, the symptoms develop months or even years after the trauma. PTSD is diagnosed when a person reacts to the traumatic event with fear and re-experiences symptoms over time or has symptoms of avoidance and hyperarousal. The symptoms persist for at least 1 month and cause clinically significant impairment in functioning or distress.

Acute Stress Disorder. Acute stress disorder occurs after the same type of stressors that precipitate PTSD, however acute stress disorder is not diagnosed if the symptoms last beyond 1 month.

Adjustment Disorders. Adjustment disorders are maladaptive reactions to clearly defined life stress. They are divided into subtypes depending on symptoms—with *anxiety*, with *depressed mood,* with *mixed anxiety and depressed mood*, *disturbance of conduct*, and *mixed disturbance of emotions and conduct.*

Persistent Complex Bereavement Disorder. Chronic and persistent grief that is characterized by bitterness, anger, or ambivalent feelings toward the dead accompanied by intense and prolonged withdrawal characterizes persistent complex bereavement disorder (also known as complicated grief or complicated bereavement). This must be distinguished from normal grief or bereavement.

Dissociative Disorders

The section on dissociative disorders includes four specific disorders (dissociative amnesia, dissociative fugue, dissociative identity disorder, and depersonalization/derealization disorder) characterized by a disruption in the usually integrated functions of consciousness, memory, identity, or perception.

Dissociative Amnesia. Dissociative amnesia is characterized by memory loss of important personal information that is usually traumatic in nature.

Dissociative Fugue. Dissociative fugue is characterized by sudden travel away from home associated with partial or complete memory loss about one's identity.

Dissociative Identity Disorder. Formerly called multiple personality disorder, the essential feature of dissociative identity disorder is the presence of two or more distinct identities that assume control of the individual's behavior.

Depersonalization/Derealization Disorder. The essential feature of depersonalization/derealization disorder is persistent or recurrent episodes of depersonalization (an altered sense of one's physical being, including feeling that one is outside of one's body, physically cut off or distanced from people, floating, observing oneself from a distance, as though in a dream), or derealization (experiencing the environment as unreal or distorted).

Somatic Symptom and Related Disorders (previously called Somatoform Disorders in DSM-IV)

This group of disorders is characterized by marked preoccupation with the body and fears of disease or consequences of disease, for example, death.

Somatic Symptom Disorder. Somatic symptom disorder is characterized by high levels of anxiety and persistent worry about somatic signs and symptoms that are misinterpreted as having a known medical disorder. Also known as hypochondriasis.

Illness Anxiety Disorder. Illness anxiety disorder is the fear of being sick with few or no somatic symptoms. A new diagnosis in DSM-5.

Functional Neurologic Symptom Disorder. Formerly known as conversion disorder in DSM-IV, this condition is characterized by unexplained voluntary or motor sensory deficits that suggest the presence of a neurologic or other general medical condition. Psychological conflict is determined to be responsible for the symptoms.

Psychological Factors Affecting Other Medical Conditions. This category is for psychological problems that negatively affect a medical condition by increasing the risk of an adverse outcome.

Factitious Disorder. Factitious disorder, also called Munchausen syndrome, refers to the deliberate feigning of physical or psychological symptoms to assume the sick role. *Factitious Disorder Imposed on Another* (previously called Factitious Disorder by Proxy) is when one person presents the other person as ill, most often mother and child. Factitious disorder is distinguished from malingering in which symptoms are also falsely reported; however, the motivation in malingering is external incentives, such as avoidance of responsibility, obtaining financial compensation, or obtaining substances.

Other Specified Somatic Symptom and Related Disorder. This category is for disorders that are not classified above. One such disorder is *Pseudocyesis* in which a person believes falsely that she (or he in rare instances) is pregnant.

Feeding and Eating Disorders

Feeding and eating disorders are characterized by a marked disturbance in eating behavior.

Anorexia Nervosa. Anorexia nervosa is an eating disorder characterized by loss of body weight and refusal to eat. Appetite is usually intact.

Bulimia Nervosa. Bulimia Nervosa is an eating disorder characterized by recurrent and frequent binge eating with or without vomiting.

Binge Eating Disorder. Binge eating disorder is a variant of bulimia nervosa with occasional, once a week, binge eating.

Pica. Pica is the eating of nonnutritional substances, for example, starch.

Rumination Disorder. The essential feature of rumination disorder is the repeated regurgitation of food, usually beginning in infancy or childhood.

Avoidant/Restrictive Food Intake Disorder. Previously called feeding disorder of infancy or childhood in DSM-IV, the main feature of this disorder is a lack of interest in food or eating resulting in failure to thrive.

Elimination Disorders

These are disorders of elimination caused by physiologic or psychological factors. There are two: *Encopresis,* which is the inability to maintain bowel control, and *Enuresis* which is the inability to maintain bladder control.

Sleep–Wake Disorders

Sleep–wake disorders involve disruptions in sleep quality, timing, and amount that result in daytime impairment and distress. They include the following disorders or disorder groups in DSM-5.

Insomnia Disorder. Difficulty falling asleep or staying asleep is characteristic of insomnia disorder. Insomnia can be an independent condition or it can be comorbid with another mental disorder, another sleep disorder, or another medical condition.

Hypersomnolence Disorder. Hypersomnolence disorder, or hypersomnia, occurs when a person sleeps too much and feels excessively tired in spite of normal or because of prolonged quantity of sleep.

Parasomnias. Parasomnias are marked by unusual behavior, experiences, or physiologic events during sleep. This category is divided into three subtypes: *non-REM sleep arousal disorders* involve incomplete awakening from sleep accompanied by either sleepwalking or sleep terror disorder; *Nightmare disorder* in which nightmares induce awakening repeatedly and cause distress and impairment; and *REM Sleep Behavior Disorder* which is characterized by vocal or motor behavior during sleep.

Narcolepsy. Narcolepsy is marked by sleep attacks, usually with loss of muscle tone (cataplexy).

Breathing-Related Sleep Disorders. There are three subtypes of breathing-related sleep disorders. The most common of the three is *Obstructive Sleep Apnea Hypopnea* in which apneas (absence of airflow) and hypopneas (reduction in airflow) occur repeatedly during sleep, causing snoring and daytime sleepiness. *Central Sleep Apnea* is the presence of Cheyne–Stokes breathing in addition to apneas and hypopneas. Finally, *Sleep-Related Hypoventilation* causes elevated CO_2 levels from decreased respiration.

Restless Legs Syndrome. Restless legs syndrome is the compulsive movement of legs during sleep.

Substance/Medication-Induced Sleep Disorder. This category includes sleep disorders that are caused by a drug or medication, for example, alcohol, caffeine.

Circadian Rhythm Sleep–Wake Disorders. Underlying these disorders is a pattern of sleep disruption that alters or misaligns a person's circadian system, resulting in insomnia or excessive sleepiness. There are six types: (1) *Delayed sleep phase type* is characterized by sleep–wake times that are several hours later than desired or conventional times, (2) *Advanced sleep phase type* is characterized by earlier than usual sleep-onset and wakeup times, (3) *Irregular sleep–wake type* is characterized by fragmented sleep throughout the 24-hour day with no major sleep period and no discernible sleep–wake circadian rhythm, (4) *Non–24-hour sleep–wake type* is a circadian period that is not aligned to the external 24-hour environment, most common among blind or visually impaired individuals, (5) *Shift work type* is from working on a nightly schedule on a regular basis, and (6) *Unspecified type* that does not meet any of the above criteria.

Sexual Dysfunctions

Sexual dysfunctions are divided into 10 disorders that are related to change in sexual desire or performance.

Delayed Ejaculation. Delayed ejaculation is the inability or marked delay in the ability to ejaculate during coitus or masturbation.

Erectile Disorder. Erectile disorder is the inability to achieve or maintain an erection sufficient for coital penetration.

Female Orgasmic Disorder. Female orgasmic disorder is the absence of the ability to achieve orgasm and/or a significant reduction in intensity of orgasmic sensations during masturbation or coitus.

Female Sexual Interest/Arousal Disorder. Female sexual interest/arousal disorder is absent or decreased interest in sexual fantasy or behavior which causes distress in the individual.

Genito-Pelvic Pain/Penetration Disorder. Genito-pelvic pain/penetration disorder replaces the terms vaginismus and dyspareunia (vaginal spasm and pain interfering with coitus). It is the anticipation of or actual pain during sex activities, particularly related to intromission.

Male Hypoactive Sexual Desire Disorder. Male hypoactive sexual desire disorder is absent or reduced sexual fantasy or desire in males.

Premature or Early Ejaculation. Premature ejaculation is manifested by ejaculation that occurs before or immediately after intromission during coitus.

Substance/Medication-Induced Sexual Dysfunction. Substance/medication-induced sexual dysfunction is impaired function due to substances, for example, fluoxetine.

Other unspecified sexual dysfunction would include sexual disorder due to a medical condition, for example, multiple sclerosis.

Gender Dysphoria

Gender dysphoria is characterized by a persistent discomfort with one's biologic sex and in some cases, the desire to have sex organs of the opposite sex. It is subdivided into *Gender Dysphoria in Children* and *Gender Dysphoria in Adolescents and Adults.*

Disruptive, Impulse-Control, and Conduct Disorders

Included in this category are conditions involving problems in the self-control of emotions and behaviors.

Oppositional Defiant Disorder. Oppositional defiant disorder is diagnosed in children and adolescents. Symptoms include anger, irritability, defiance, and refusal to comply with regulations.

Intermittent Explosive Disorder. Intermittent explosive disorder involves uncontrolled outbursts of aggression.

Conduct Disorder. Conduct disorder is diagnosed in children and adolescents and is characterized by fighting and bullying.

Pyromania. Repeated fire-setting is the distinguishing feature of pyromania.

Kleptomania. Repeated stealing is the distinguishing feature of kleptomania.

Substance-Related Disorders

Substance-Induced Disorders. Psychoactive and other substances may cause *intoxication* and *withdrawal syndrome* and induce psychiatric disorders including *bipolar and related disorders, obsessive-compulsive and related disorders, sleep disorders, sexual dysfunction, delirium,* and *neurocognitive disorders*.

Substance Use Disorders. Sometimes referred to as addiction, this is a group of disorders diagnosed by the substance abused—alcohol, cocaine, cannabis, hallucinogens, inhalants, opioids, sedative, stimulant, or tobacco.

Alcohol-Related Disorders. Alcohol-related disorders result in impairment caused by excessive use of alcohol. They include *alcohol use disorder* which is recurrent alcohol use with developing tolerance and withdrawal and *alcohol intoxication* which is simple drunkenness, and *alcohol withdrawal* which can involve delirium tremens (DTs).

Other Alcohol-Induced Disorders. This group of disorders includes psychotic, bipolar, depressive, anxiety, sleep, sexual, or neurocognitive disorders including amnestic disorder (also known as Korsakoff's syndrome). Wernicke's encephalopathy, a neurologic condition of ataxia, ophthalmoplegia, and confusion develops from chronic alcohol use. The two may coexist (Wernicke–Korsakoff syndrome). *Alcohol-induced persisting-dementia* is differentiated from Korsakoff's syndrome by multiple cognitive deficits.

Similar categories (intoxication, withdrawal, and induced disorders) exist for caffeine, cannabis, phencyclidine, other hallucinogens, inhalants, opioids, sedative, hypnotic, or anxiolytics, stimulants, and tobacco.

Gambling Disorder. Gambling disorder is classified as a *non–substance-related disorder*. It involves compulsive gambling with an inability to stop or cut down, leading to social and financial difficulties. Some clinicians believe sexual addiction should be classified in the same way; but it is not a DSM-5 diagnosis.

Neurocognitive Disorders (previously called Dementia, Delirium, Amnestic and Other Cognitive Disorders in DSM-IV)

These are disorders characterized by changes in brain structure and function that result in impaired learning, orientation judgment, memory, and intellectual functions. They are divided into three categories (Table 1-1).

Delirium. Delirium is marked by short-term confusion and cognition caused by substance intoxication or withdrawal (cocaine, opioids, phencyclidine), medication (cortisol), general medical condition (infection), or other causes (sleep deprivation).

Mild Neurocognitive Disorder. Mild neurocognitive disorder is a mild or modest decline in cognitive function. It must be distinguished from normal age-related cognitive change (normal age-related senescence).

Major Neurocognitive Disorder. Major neurocognitive disorder (a term that may be used synonymously with dementia which is still preferred by most psychiatrists) is marked by severe impairment in memory, judgment, orientation, and cognition. There are 13 subtypes (see Table 6-2): *Alzheimer's disease* which usually occurs in persons over age 65 and is manifested by progressive intellectual deterioration and dementia; *vascular dementia* which is a stepwise progression in cognitive deterioration caused by vessel thrombosis or hemorrhage; *frontotemporal lobar degeneration* which is marked by behavioral inhibition (also known as Picks disease); *Lewy body disease* which involves hallucinations with dementia; *Traumatic Brain Injury* from physical trauma; *HIV disease;* *Prion disease* which is caused by slow-growing transmissible prion protein; *Parkinson's*

Table 1-1
Major Subtypes of Neurocognitive Disorder (Dementia)

1. Alzheimer's Disease
2. Vascular dementia
3. Lewy body disease
4. Parkinson's disease
5. Frontotemporal dementia (Pick's disease)
6. Traumatic Brain Injury
7. HIV Infection
8. Substance/medication-induced dementia
9. Huntington's disease
10. Prion disease
11. Other medical condition (known as Amnestic Syndrome in DSM-IV-TR)
12. Multiple etiologies
13. Unspecified dementia

disease; Huntington's disease; caused by a medical condition; Substance/medication-induced, for example, alcohol causing Korsakoff's syndrome; *Multiple Etiologies* and *Unspecified dementia.*

Personality Disorders

Personality disorders are characterized by deeply engrained, generally lifelong maladaptive patterns of behavior that are usually recognizable at adolescence or earlier.

Paranoid Personality Disorder. Paranoid personality disorder is characterized by unwarranted suspicion, hypersensitivity, jealousy, envy, rigidity, excessive self-importance, and a tendency to blame and ascribe evil motives to others.

Schizoid Personality Disorder. Schizoid personality disorder is characterized by shyness, oversensitivity, seclusiveness, avoidance of close or competitive relationships, eccentricity, no loss of capacity to recognize reality, daydreaming, and an ability to express hostility and aggression.

Schizotypal Personality Disorder. Schizotypal personality disorder is similar to schizoid personality, but the person also exhibits slight losses of reality testing, has odd beliefs, and is aloof and withdrawn.

Obsessive-Compulsive Personality Disorder. OCPD is characterized by excessive concern with conformity and standards of conscience; patient may be rigid, overconscientious, over dutiful, over inhibited, and unable to relax (three *Ps*—punctual, parsimonious, precise).

Histrionic Personality Disorder. Histrionic personality disorder is characterized by emotional instability, excitability, over reactivity, vanity, immaturity, dependency, and self-dramatization that is attention seeking and seductive.

Avoidant Personality Disorder. Avoidant personality disorder is characterized by low levels of energy, easy fatigability, lack of enthusiasm, inability to enjoy life, and oversensitivity to stress.

Antisocial Personality Disorder. Antisocial personality disorder covers persons in conflict with society. They are incapable of loyalty, selfish, callous, irresponsible, impulsive, and unable to feel guilt or learn from experience; they have low level of frustration tolerance and a tendency to blame others.

Narcissistic Personality Disorder. Narcissistic personality disorder is characterized by grandiose feelings, sense of entitlement, lack of empathy, envy, manipulativeness, and need for attention and admiration.

Borderline Personality Disorder. Borderline personality disorder is characterized by instability, impulsiveness, chaotic sexuality, suicidal acts, self-mutilating behavior, identity problems, ambivalence, and feeling of emptiness and boredom.

Dependent Personality Disorder. This is characterized by passive and submissive behavior; person is unsure of him- or herself and becomes entirely dependent on others.

Personality Changes Due to Another Medical Condition. This category includes alterations to a person's personality due to a medical condition, for example, brain tumor.

Unspecified Personality Disorder. This category involves other personality traits that do not fit any of the patterns described above.

Paraphilic Disorders and Paraphilia

In *paraphilia*, a person's sexual interests are directed primarily toward objects rather than toward people, toward sexual acts not usually associated with coitus, or toward coitus performed under bizarre circumstances. A *paraphilic disorder* is acted out sexual behavior that can cause possible harm to another person. Included are: *exhibitionism* (genital exposure); *voyeurism* (watching sexual acts); *frotteurism* (rubbing against another person); *pedophilia* (sexual attraction toward children); *sexual masochism* (receiving pain); *sexual sadism* (inflicting pain); *fetishism* (arousal from an inanimate object); and *transvestism* (cross-dressing).

Other Mental Disorders

This is a residual category that includes four disorders that do not meet the full criteria for any of the previously described mental disorders: (1) *Other specified mental disorder due to another medical condition,* for example, dissociative symptoms secondary to temporal lobe epilepsy; (2) *Unspecified mental disorder due to another medical condition,* for example, temporal lobe epilepsy producing unspecified symptoms; (3) *Other specified mental disorder* in which symptoms are present but subthreshold for a specific mental illness; and (4) *Unspecified mental disorder* in which symptoms are present but subthreshold for any mental disorder.

Some clinicians use the term ***forme fruste*** (French, "unfinished form") to describe atypical or attenuated manifestation of a disease or syndrome, with the implication of incompleteness or partial presence of the condition or disorder. This term might apply to 3 and 4 above.

Medication-Induced Movement Disorders and Other Adverse Effects of Medication

Ten disorders are included: (1) *Neuroleptic or Other medication-induced parkinsonism* presents as rhythmic tremor, rigidity, akinesia, or bradykinesia that is reversible when the causative drug is withdrawn or its dosage reduced; (2) *Neuroleptic malignant syndrome* presents as muscle rigidity, dystonia, or hyperthermia; (3) *Medication-induced acute dystonia* consists of slow, sustained contracture of musculature causing postural deviations; (4) *Medication-induced acute akathisia* presents as motor restlessness with constant movement; (5) *Tardive dyskinesia* is characterized by involuntary movement of the lips, jaw, tongue, and by other involuntary dyskinetic movements; (6) *Tardive dystonia or akathisia* is a variant of tardive dyskinesia that involves extrapyramidal syndrome; (7) *Medication-induced postural tremor* is a fine tremor, usually at rest, that is caused by medication; (8) *Other medication-induced movement disorder* describes atypical extrapyramidal syndrome from a medication; (9) *Antidepressant discontinuation syndrome* is a withdrawal syndrome that arises after abrupt cessation of antidepressant drugs, for example, fluoxetine; and (10) *Other adverse effect of medication* includes changes in blood pressure, diarrhea etc. due to medication.

Other Conditions That May Be a Focus of Clinical Attention

These are conditions that may interfere with overall functioning but are not severe enough to warrant a psychiatric diagnosis. These conditions are not mental disorders but may aggravate an existing mental disorder.

A broad range of life problems and stressors are included in this section among which are: (1) *Relational Problem*s including *Problems Related to Family Upbringing,* such as problems with siblings or upbringing away from parents, and *Problems Related to Primary Support Group,* such as problems with a spouse or intimate partner, separation or divorce, family expressed emotion (EE), or uncomplicated bereavement; and (2) *Abuse and Neglect,* which includes *Child Maltreatment and Neglect Problems,* such as physical abuse, sexual abuse, neglect, or psychological abuse; and *Adult Maltreatment and Neglect*

Problems, which involves spouse or partner physical, sexual, and psychological violence and neglect, or adult abuse by a nonspouse or nonpartner. Borderline intellectual functioning is included here in DSM-5.

Conditions for Further Study

In addition to the diagnostic categories listed above, other categories of illness are listed in DSM-5 that requires further study before they become part of the official nomenclature. Some of these disorders are controversial.

There are eight disorders in this group: (1) *Attenuated Psychosis Syndrome* refers to subthreshold signs and symptoms of psychosis that develops in adolescence; (2) *Depressive Episodes With Short-duration Hypomania* are short episodes (2 to 3 days) of hypomania that occur with major depression; (3) *Persistent Complex Bereavement Disorder* is bereavement that persists over 1 year after loss; (4) *Caffeine Use Disorder* is dependence on caffeine with withdrawal syndrome; (5) *Internet Gaming Disorder* is the excessive use of internet that disrupts normal living; (6) *Neurobehavioral Disorder Associated With Prenatal Alcohol Exposure* covers all developmental disorders that occur in utero due to excessive alcohol use by mother, for example, fetal alcohol syndrome; (7) *Suicidal Behavior Disorder* is repeated suicide attempts that occur irrespective of diagnostic category of mental illness; and (8) *Nonsuicidal Self-Injury* is skin-cutting and other self-harm without suicidal intent.

For more detailed discussion of this topic, see Classification in Psychiatry, Section 9, p. 1151, in CTP/X.

2

Psychiatric History and Mental Status Examination

I. Introduction

A. Psychiatric history. The psychiatric history is the record of the patient's life; it allows the psychiatrist to understand who the patient is, where the patient has come from, and where the patient is likely to go in the future. The history is the patient's life story told in the patient's own words from his or her own point of view. It may include information about the patient from other sources, such as parents or spouse. A thorough psychiatric history is essential to making a correct diagnosis and formulating a specific and effective treatment plan.

B. Mental status. A patient's history remains stable, whereas the mental status can change daily or hourly. The mental status examination (MSE) is a description of the patient's appearance, speech, actions, and thoughts during the interview. It is a systematic format for recording findings about thinking, feeling, and behavior. A patient's history remains stable, whereas the mental status can change daily or hourly. Only phenomena observed at the time of the interview are recorded in the mental status. Other data are recorded in the history. A comprehensive psychiatric history and mental status are described below.

II. Psychiatric History

A. Identification

1. Name, age, marital status, sex, occupation, language if other than English; race, nationality, religion, if pertinent.
2. Previous admissions to a hospital for the same or a different condition.
3. Persons with whom the patient lives.

B. Chief complaint (CC)

1. Describe exactly why the patient came to the psychiatrist, preferably in the patient's own words.
2. If that information does not come from the patient, note who supplied it.

C. History of present illness (HPI)

1. Chronologic background and development of the symptoms or behavioral changes that culminated in the patient's seeking assistance.
2. Patient's life circumstances at the time of onset.
3. Personality when well; how illness has affected life activities and personal relations—changes in personality, interests, mood, attitudes toward others, dress, habits, level of tenseness, irritability, activity, attention, concentration, memory, speech.
4. Psychophysiological symptoms—nature and details of dysfunction; pain—location, intensity, fluctuation.

   5. Level of anxiety—generalized and nonspecific (free floating) or specifically related to particular situations, activities, or objects.
   6. How anxieties are handled—avoidance, repetition of feared situation.
   7. Use of drugs or other activities for alleviation.
D. Past psychiatric and medical history
   1. Emotional or mental disturbances—extent of incapacity, type of treatment, names of hospitals, length of illness, effect of treatment.
   2. Psychosomatic disorders: hay fever, arthritis, colitis, chronic fatigue, recurrent colds, skin conditions.
   3. Medical conditions—customary review of systems, sexually transmitted diseases, alcohol or other substance abuse, at risk for acquired immune deficiency syndrome (AIDS).
   4. Neurologic disorders—headache, craniocerebral trauma, loss of consciousness, seizures, or tumors.
E. Family history
   1. Elicited from patient and from someone else, because quite different descriptions may be given of the same people and events.
   2. Ethnic, national, and religious traditions.
   3. List other people in the home and descriptions of them—personality and intelligence—and their relationship to the patient.
   4. Role of illness in the family and family history of mental illness.
   5. Where does the patient live—neighborhood and particular residence of the patient; is the home crowded; privacy of family members from each other and from other families.
   6. Sources of family income, public assistance (if any) and attitudes about it; will the patient lose his or her job or apartment by remaining in the hospital.
   7. Child care arrangements.
F. Personal history (anamnesis)

 CLINICAL HINT:
It is seldom necessary to describe all of the following categories below for all patients. For example, early developmental history may not be as relevant for adults as for children and adolescents.

---

   1. *Early childhood (through 3 years of age)*
      a. Prenatal history and mother's pregnancy and delivery: length of pregnancy, spontaneity and normality of delivery, birth trauma, whether the patient was planned and wanted, birth defects.
      b. Feeding habits: breast fed or bottle fed, eating problems.
      c. Early development: maternal deprivation, language development, motor development, signs of unmet needs, sleep pattern, object constancy, stranger anxiety, separation anxiety.
      d. Toilet training: age, attitude of parents, feelings about it.
      e. Symptoms of behavior problems: thumb sucking, temper tantrums, tics, head bumping, rocking, night terrors, fears, bedwetting or bed soiling, nail biting, masturbation.

      f. Personality and temperament as a child: shy, restless, overactive, withdrawn, studious, outgoing, timid, athletic, friendly patterns of play, reactions to siblings.

      g. Early or recurrent dreams or fantasies.

2. *Middle childhood (3 to 11 years of age)*

      a. Early school history—feelings about going to school.

      b. Early adjustment, gender identification.

      c. Conscience development, punishment.

      d. Social relationships.

      e. Attitudes toward siblings and playmates.

3. *Later childhood (prepuberty through adolescence)*

      a. Peer relationships: number and closeness of friends, leader or follower, social popularity, participation in group or gang activities, idealized figures; patterns of aggression, passivity, anxiety, antisocial behavior.

      b. School history: how far the patient went in school; adjustment to school; relationships with teachers—teacher's pet or rebellious; favorite studies or interests; particular abilities or assets; extracurricular activities; sports; hobbies; relationships of problems or symptoms to any school period.

      c. Cognitive and motor development: learning to read and other intellectual and motor skills, minimal cerebral dysfunction, learning disabilities—their management and effects on the child.

      d. Particular adolescent emotional or physical problems: nightmares, phobias, bedwetting, running away, delinquency, smoking, drug or alcohol use, weight problems, feeling of inferiority.

      e. Psychosexual history.

         (1) Early curiosity, infantile masturbation, sex play.

         (2) Acquiring of sexual knowledge, attitude of parents toward sex, sexual abuse.

         (3) Onset of puberty, feelings about it, kind of preparation, feelings about menstruation, development of secondary sexual characteristics.

         (4) Adolescent sexual activity: crushes, parties, dating, petting, masturbation, wet dreams (nocturnal emissions), and attitudes toward them.

         (5) Attitudes toward same and opposite sex: timid, shy, aggressive, need to impress, seductive, sexual conquests, anxiety.

         (6) Sexual practices: sexual problems, homosexual and heterosexual experiences, paraphilias, promiscuity.

      f. Religious background: strict, liberal, mixed (possible conflicts), relationship of background to current religious practices.

4. *Adulthood*

      a. Occupational history: choice of occupation, training, ambitions, and conflicts; relations with authority, peers, and subordinates; number of jobs and duration; changes in job status; current job and feelings about it.

b. Social activity: whether patient has friends; whether he or she is withdrawn or socializing well; social, intellectual, and physical interests; relationships with same sex and opposite sex; depth, duration, and quality of human relations.

c. Adult sexuality.

    (1) Premarital sexual relationships, age of first coitus, sexual orientation.

    (2) Marital history: common-law marriages; legal marriages; description of courtship and role played by each partner; age at marriage; family planning and contraception; names and ages of children; attitudes toward raising children; problems of any family members; housing difficulties, if important to the marriage; sexual adjustment; extramarital affairs; areas of agreement and disagreement; management of money; role of in-laws.

    (3) Sexual symptoms: anorgasmia, impotence (erectile disorder), premature ejaculation, lack of desire.

    (4) Attitudes toward pregnancy and having children; contraceptive practices and feelings about them.

    (5) Sexual practices: paraphilias, such as sadism, fetishes, voyeurism; attitude toward fellatio, cunnilingus; coital techniques, frequency.

d. Military history: general adjustment, combat, injuries, referral to psychiatrists, type of discharge, veteran status.

e. Value systems: whether children are seen as a burden or a joy; whether work is seen as a necessary evil, an avoidable chore, or an opportunity; current attitude about religion; belief in heaven and hell.

III. Mental Status

A. Appearance

    1. Personal identification: may include a brief nontechnical description of the patient's appearance and behavior as a novelist might write it. Attitude toward examiner can be described here: cooperative, attentive, interested, frank, seductive, defensive, hostile, playful, ingratiating, evasive, or guarded.

    2. Behavior and psychomotor activity: gait, mannerisms, tics, gestures, twitches, stereotypes, picking, touching examiner, echopraxia, clumsy, agile, limp, rigid, retarded, hyperactive, agitated, combative, or waxy.

    3. General description: posture, bearing, clothes, grooming, hair, nails; healthy, sickly, angry, frightened, apathetic, perplexed, contemptuous, ill at ease, poised, old looking, young looking, effeminate, masculine; signs of anxiety—moist hands, perspiring forehead, restlessness, tense posture, strained voice, wide eyes; shifts in level of anxiety during interview or with particular topic; eye contact (50% is normal).

B. Speech: rapid, slow, pressured, hesitant, emotional, monotonous, loud, whispered, slurred, mumbled, stuttering, echolalia, intensity, pitch, ease, spontaneity, productivity, manner, reaction time, vocabulary, prosody.

C. Mood and affect

1. Mood (a pervasive and sustained emotion that colors the person's perception of the world): how does patient say he or she feels; depth, intensity, duration, and fluctuations of mood—depressed, despairing, irritable, anxious, terrified, angry, expansive, euphoric, empty, guilty, awed, futile, self-contemptuous, anhedonic, alexithymic.

2. Affect (the outward expression of the patient's inner experiences): how the examiner evaluates the patient's affects—broad, restricted, blunted or flat, shallow, amount and range of expression; difficulty in initiating, sustaining, or terminating an emotional response; whether the emotional expression is appropriate to the thought content, culture, and setting of the examination; examples should be given if emotional expression is not appropriate.

D. Thinking and perception

1. Form of thinking

   a. Productivity: overabundance of ideas, paucity of ideas, flight of ideas, rapid thinking, slow thinking, hesitant thinking; whether the patient speaks spontaneously or only when questions are asked; stream of thought, quotations from patient.

   b. Continuity of thought: whether the patient's replies really answer questions and are goal directed, relevant, or irrelevant; loose associations; lack of cause-and-effect relationships in the patient's explanations; illogical, tangential, circumstantial, rambling, evasive, persevering statements, blocking or distractibility.

   c. Language impairments: impairments that reflect disordered mentation, such as incoherent or incomprehensible speech (word salad), clang associations, neologisms.

2. Content of thinking

   a. Preoccupations about the illness, environmental problems.

   b. Obsessions, compulsions, phobias.

   c. Obsessions or plans about suicide, homicide.

   d. Hypochondriacal symptoms, specific antisocial urges or impulses.

3. Thought disturbances

   a. Delusions: content of any delusional system, its organization, the patient's convictions as to its validity, how it affects his or her life; persecutory delusions—isolated or associated with pervasive suspiciousness; mood-congruent or mood-incongruent.

   b. Ideas of reference and ideas of influence: how ideas began, their content, and the meaning that the patient attributes to them.

   c. Thought broadcasting—thoughts being heard by others.

   d. Thought insertion—thoughts being inserted into a person's mind by others.

4. Perceptual disturbances

   a. Hallucinations and illusions: whether the patient hears voices or sees visions; content, sensory system involvement, circumstances of the occurrence; hypnagogic or hypnopompic hallucinations; thought broadcasting.

    b. Depersonalization and derealization: extreme feelings of detachment from self or from the environment.

5. Dreams and fantasies

    a. Dreams: prominent ones, if the patient will tell them; nightmares.

    b. Fantasies: recurrent, favorite, or unshakable daydreams.

E. Sensorium

 CLINICAL HINT:

This section includes an assessment of several cognitive functions. Collectively, they help describe the overall intactness of the central nervous system, as different functions are served by different brain regions. Abnormalities of the sensorium are seen in delirium and dementia, and they raise the suspicion of an underlying medical or drug-related cause of symptoms. See Table 2-1 for a scored general intelligence test that can be used to increase the reliability and validity of the diagnosis of cognitive disorder.

---

    1. Alertness: awareness of environment, attention span, clouding of consciousness, fluctuations in levels of awareness, somnolence, stupor, lethargy, fugue state, coma.

    2. Orientation

        a. Time: whether the patient identifies the day or the approximate date and the time of day correctly; if in a hospital, whether the patient knows how long he or she has been there; whether the patient behaves as though oriented to the present.

        b. Place: whether patient knows where he or she is.

        c. Person: whether patient knows who the examiner is and the roles or names of the persons with whom the patient is in contact.

    3. Concentration and calculation: whether the patient can subtract 7 from 100 and keep subtracting 7s; if the patient cannot subtract 7s, whether easier tasks can be accomplished—4×9 and 5×4; whether the patient can calculate how many nickels are in $1.35; whether anxiety or some disturbance of mood or concentration seems to be responsible for difficulty.

    4. Memory: impairment, efforts made to cope with impairment—denial, confabulation, catastrophic reaction, circumstantiality used to conceal deficit; whether the process of registration, retention, or recollection of material is involved.

        a. Remote memory: childhood data, important events known to have occurred when the patient was younger or free of illness, personal matters, neutral material.

        b. Recent past memory: past few months.

        c. Recent memory: past few days, what did the patient do yesterday and the day before, what did the patient have for breakfast, lunch, and dinner.

Table 2-1
Scored General Intelligence Test[a]

Indications: When a cognitive disorder is suspected because of apparent intellectual defects, impairment in the ability to make generalizations, the ability to maintain a trend of thought, or to show good judgment, a scored test can be of value. It can confirm the diagnosis of impairment with greater reliability and validity.

Directions: Ask the following questions as part of the mental status examination. A conversational manner should be used and the questions may be adapted to cultural differences.

Scoring: If the patient obtains a score of 25 or under (out of a maximum of 40), it is indicative of a cognitive problem and further examination should follow.

Questions: There are 10 questions that follow:

1. What are houses made of? (Any material you can think of) **1–4**
   One point for each item, up to four.
2. What is sand used for? .... **1, 2, or 4**
   Four points for manufacture of glass. Two points for mixing with concrete, road building, or other constructive use. One point for play or sandboxes. Credit not cumulative.
3. If the flag floats to the south, from what direction is the wind? **3**
   Three points for north, no partial credits. It is permissible to say: "Which way is the wind coming from?"
4. Tell me the names of some fish **1–4**
   One point for each, up to four. If the subject stops with one, encourage him or her to go on.
5. At what time of day is your shadow shortest? **3**
   Noon, three points. If correct response is suspected of being a guess, inquire why.
6. Give the names of some large cities **1–4**
   One point for each, up to four. When any state is named as a city, no credit, i.e., New York unless specified as New York City. No credit for home town except when it is an outstanding city.
7. Why does the moon look larger than the stars? **2.3.4**
   Make it clear that the question refers to any particular star, and give assurance that the moon is actually smaller than any star. Encourage the subject to guess. Two points for "Moon is lower down." Three points for nearer or closer. Four points for generalized statement that nearer objects look larger than more distant objects.
8. What metal is attracted by a magnet? .... **2 or 4**
   Four points for iron, two for steel.
9. If your shadow points to the northeast, where is the sun? **4**
   Four points for southwest, no partial credits.
10. How many stripes are in the flag? **2**
    Thirteen, two points. A subject who responds 50 may be permitted to correct the mistake. Explain, if necessary, that the white stripes are included as well as the red ones.
11. What does ice become when it melts? **1**
    Water, one point.
12. How many minutes in an hour? **1**
    Sixty, one point.
13. Why is it colder at night than in the daytime? **1–3**
    Two points for "sun goes down," or any recognition of direct rays of sun as source of heat. Additional point for rotation of earth. Question may be reversed: "What makes it warmer in the daytime than at night?" Only one point for answer to reverse question.

[a]This test was developed by N.D.C. Lewis M.D. Adapted by B.J. Sadock. M.D.

    d. Immediate retention and recall: ability to repeat six figures after the examiner dictates them—first forward, then backward, then after a few minutes' interruption; other test questions; whether the same questions, if repeated, called forth different answers at different times.

    e. Effect of defect on patient: mechanisms the patient has developed to cope with the defect.

  5. Fund of knowledge

    a. Estimate of the patient's intellectual capability and whether the patient is capable of functioning at the level of his or her basic endowment.

b. General knowledge; questions should have relevance to the patient's educational and cultural background.

6. Abstract thinking: disturbances in concept formation; manner in which the patient conceptualizes or handles his or her ideas; similarities (e.g., between apples and pears), differences, absurdities; meanings of simple proverbs, such as "a rolling stone gathers no moss"; answers may be concrete (giving specific examples to illustrate the meaning) or overly abstract (giving generalized explanation); appropriateness of answers.

7. Insight: the recognition of having a mental disorder and degree of personal awareness and understanding of illness.

   a. Complete denial of illness.

   b. Slight awareness of being sick and needing help but denying it at the same time.

   c. Awareness of being sick but blaming it on others, external factors, or medical or unknown organic factors.

   d. Intellectual insight: admission of illness and recognition that symptoms or failures in social adjustment are due to irrational feelings or disturbances, without applying that knowledge to future experiences.

   e. True emotional insight: emotional awareness of the motives and feelings within and of the underlying meaning of symptoms; whether the awareness leads to changes in personality and future behavior; openness to new ideas and concepts about self and the important people in the patient's life.

 CLINICAL HINT:

Test for insight by asking: "Do you think you have a problem?" "Do you need treatment?" "What are your plans for the future?" Insight is severely impaired in cognitive disorders, psychosis, and borderline IQ.

---

8. Judgment

   a. Social judgment: subtle manifestations of behavior that are harmful to the patient and contrary to acceptable behavior in the culture; whether the patient understands the likely outcome of personal behavior and is influenced by that understanding; examples of impairment.

   b. Test judgment: the patient's prediction of what he or she would do in imaginary situations; for instance, what patient would do with a stamped, addressed letter found in the street or if medication was lost.

 CLINICAL HINT:

Judgment is severely impaired in manic episodes of bipolar disorders and in cognitive disorders (e.g., delirium and dementia).

A summary of questions to elicit psychiatric history and mental status data is provided in Table 2-2.

Table 2-2
Common Questions for the Psychiatric History and Mental Status

Topic	Questions	Comments and Helpful Hints
Identifying data: Name, age, sex, marital status, religion, education, address, phone number, occupation, source of referral	Be direct in obtaining identifying data. Request specific answers.	If patient cannot cooperate, get information from family member or friend; if referred by a physician, obtain medical record.
Chief complaint (CC): Brief statement in patient's own words of why patient is in the hospital or is being seen in consultation	Why are you going to see a psychiatrist? What brought you to the hospital? What seems to be the problem?	Record answers verbatim; a bizarre complaint points to psychotic process.
History of present illness (HPI): Development of symptoms from time of onset to present; relation of life events, conflicts, stressors: drugs; change from previous level of functioning	When did you first notice something happening to you? Were you upset about anything when symptoms began? Did they begin suddenly or gradually?	Record in patient's own words as much as possible. Get history of previous hospitalizations and treatment. Sudden onset of symptoms may indicate drug-induced disorder.
Previous psychiatric and medical disorders: Psychiatric disorders; psychosomatic, medical, neurologic illnesses (e.g., craniocerebral trauma, convulsions)	Did you ever lose consciousness? Have a seizure?	Ascertain extent of illness, treatment, medications, outcomes, hospitals, doctors. Determine whether illness serves some additional purpose (secondary gain).
Personal history: Birth and infancy: To the extent known by the patient, ascertain mother's pregnancy and delivery, planned or unwanted pregnancy, developmental landmarks—standing, walking, talking, temperament	Do you know anything about your birth? If so, from whom? How old was your mother when you were born? Your father?	Older mothers (>35) have high risk for Down syndrome baby; older father (>45) may contribute damaged sperm producing deficits including schizophrenia.
Childhood: Feeding habits, toilet training, personality (shy, outgoing), general conduct and behavior, relationship with parents or caregivers and peers, separations, nightmares, bedwetting, fears	Toilet training? Bedwetting? Sex play with peers? What is your first childhood memory?	Separation anxiety and school phobia associated with adult depression; enuresis associated with firesetting. Childhood memories before the age of 3 are usually imagined, not real.
Adolescence: Peer and authority relationship, school history, grades, emotional problems, drug use, age of puberty	Adolescents may refuse to answer questions, but they should be asked. Adults may distort memories of emotionally charged adolescent experience. Sexual molestation?	Poor school performance is a sensitive indicator of emotional disorder. Schizophrenia begins in late adolescence.
Adulthood: Work history, choice of career, marital history, children, education, finances, military history, religion	Open-ended questions are preferable. Tell me about your marriage. Be nonjudgmental: What role does religion play in your life, if any? What is your sexual preference in a partner?	Depending on chief complaint, some areas require more detailed inquiry. Manic patients frequently go into debt or are promiscuous. Overvalued religious ideas associated with paranoid personality disorder.

(continued)

Table 2-2
Common Questions for the Psychiatric History and Mental Status *(Continued)*

Topic	Questions	Comments and Helpful Hints
Sexual history: Sexual development, masturbation, anorgasmia, erectile disorder, premature ejaculation, paraphilia, sexual orientation, general attitudes and feelings	Are there or have there been any problems or concerns about your sex life? How did you learn about sex? Has there been any change in your sex drive?	Be nonjudgmental. Asking *when* masturbation began is a better approach than asking *do you* or *did you ever* masturbate.
Family history: Psychiatric, medical, and genetic illness in mother, father, siblings; age of parents and occupations; if deceased, date and cause; feelings about each family member, finances	Have any members in your family been depressed? Alcoholic? In a mental hospital? In jail? Describe your living conditions. Did you have your own room?	Genetic loading in anxiety, depression, suicide, schizophrenia. Get medication history of family (medications effective in family members for similar disorders may be effective in patient).
Mental status		
General appearance: Note appearance, gait, dress, grooming (neat or unkempt), posture, gestures, facial expressions. Does patient appear older or younger than stated age?	Introduce yourself and direct patient to take a seat. In the hospital, bring your chair to bedside; do not sit on the bed.	Unkempt and disheveled in cognitive disorder; pinpoint pupils in narcotic addiction; withdrawal and stooped posture in depression.
Motoric behavior: Level of activity: Psychomotor agitation or psychomotor retardation—tics, tremors, automatisms, mannerisms, grimacing, stereotypes, negativism, apraxia, echopraxia, waxy flexibility; emotional appearance—anxious, tense, panicky, bewildered, sad, unhappy: voice—faint, loud, hoarse; eye contact	Have you been more active than usual? Less active? You may ask about obvious mannerisms, e.g., "I notice that your hand still shakes, can you tell me about that?" Stay aware of smells, e.g., alcoholism/ketoacidosis.	Fixed posturing, odd behavior in schizophrenia. Hyperactive with stimulant (cocaine) abuse and in mania. Psychomotor retardation in depression; tremors with anxiety or medication side effect (lithium). Eye contact is normally made approximately half the time during the interview. Minimal eye contact in schizophrenia. Scanning of environment in paranoid states.
Attitude during interview: How patient relates to examiner—irritable, aggressive, seductive, guarded, defensive, indifferent, apathetic, cooperative, sarcastic	You may comment about attitude: You seem irritated about something; is that an accurate observation?	Suspiciousness in paranoia; seductive in hysteria; apathetic in conversion disorder (*la belle indifference*); punning (*witzelsucht*) in frontal lobe syndromes.
Mood: Steady or sustained emotional state—gloomy, tense, hopeless, ecstatic, resentful, happy, bashful, sad, exultant, elated, euphoric, depressed, apathetic, anhedonic, fearful, suicidal, grandiose, nihilistic	How do you feel? How are your spirits? Do you have thoughts that life is not worth living or that you want to harm yourself? Do you have plans to take your own life? Do you want to die? Has there been a change in your sleep habits?	Suicidal ideas in 25% of depressives; elation in mania. Early morning awakening in depression; decreased need for sleep in mania.

(continued)

Table 2-2
Common Questions for the Psychiatric History and Mental Status *(Continued)*

Topic	Questions	Comments and Helpful Hints
Affect: Feeling tone associated with idea—labile, blunt, appropriate to content, inappropriate, flat	Observe nonverbal signs of emotion, body movements, facies, rhythm of voice (prosody). Laughing when talking about sad subjects, e.g., death, is inappropriate.	Changes in affect usual with schizophrenia: loss of prosody in cognitive disorder, catatonia. Do not confuse medication adverse effect with flat affect.
Speech: Slow, fast, pressured, garrulous, spontaneous, taciturn, stammering, stuttering, slurring, staccato. Pitch, articulation, aphasia, coprolalia, echolalia, incoherent, logorrhea, mute, paucity, stilted	Ask patient to say "Methodist Episcopalian" to test for dysarthria.	Manic patients show pressured speech; paucity of speech in depression; uneven or slurred speech in cognitive disorders.
Perceptual disorders: Hallucinations—olfactory, auditory, haptic (tactile), gustatory, visual; illusions; hypnopompic or hypnagogic experiences; feeling of unreality, *déjà vu, éjà entendu,* macropsia	Do you ever see things or hear voices? Do you have strange experiences as you fall asleep or upon awakening? Has the world changed in any way? Do you have strange smells?	Hallucinations suggest schizophrenia. Tactile hallucinations suggest cocainism, delirium tremens (DTs). Olfactory hallucinations common in temporal lobe epilepsy. Visual hallucinations may be caused by toxins.
Thought content: Delusions— persecutory (paranoid), grandiose, infidelity, somatic, sensory, thought broadcasting, thought insertion, ideas of reference, ideas of unreality, phobias, obsessions, compul- sions, ambivalence, autism, dereism, blocking, suicidal or homicidal preoccupation, conflicts, nihilistic ideas, hypochondriasis, deperson- alization, derealization, flight of ideas, *idée* fixe, magical thinking, neologisms	Do you feel people want to harm you? Do you have special powers? Is anyone trying to influence you? Do you have strange body sensations? Are there thoughts that you can't get out of your mind? Do you think about the end of the world? Can people read your mind? Do you ever feel the TV is talking to you? Ask about fantasies and dreams.	Are delusions congruent with mood (grandiose delusions with elated mood) or incongruent? Mood-incongruent delusions point to schizophrenia. Illusions are common in delirium. Thought insertion is characteristic of schizophrenia.
Thought process: Goal-directed ideas, loosened associations, illogical, tangential, relevant, circumstantial, rambling, ability to abstract, flight of ideas, clang associations, perseveration	Ask meaning of proverbs to test abstraction, e.g., "People in glass houses should not throw stones." Concrete answer is, "Glass breaks." Abstract answers deal with univer- sal themes or moral issues. Ask similarity between bird and butterfly (both alive), bread and cake (both food).	Loose associations point to schizophrenia; flight of ideas, to mania; inability to abstract, to schizophrenia, brain damage.
Sensorium: Level of consciousness—alert, clear, confused, clouded, comatose, stuporous; orientation to time, place, person; cognition	What place is this? What is today's date? Do you know who I am? Do you know who you are?	Delirium or dementia shows clouded or wandering sensorium. Orientation to person remains intact longer than orientation to time or place.

(continued)

Table 2-2
Common Questions for the Psychiatric History and Mental Status (Continued)

Topic	Questions	Comments and Helpful Hints
Memory: Remote memory (long-term): Past several days, months, years	Where were you born? Where did you go to school? Date of marriage? Birthdays of children? What were last week's newspaper headlines?	Patients with dementia of the Alzheimer's type retain remote memory longer, than recent memory. Gaps in memory may be localized or filled in with confabulatory details. Hypermnesia is seen in paranoid personality.
Recent memory (short-term): Recall of events in past day or two	Where were you yesterday? What did you eat at your last meal?	In brain disease, recent memory loss (amnesia) usually occurs before remote memory loss.
Immediate memory (very short-term): Laying down of immediate information with ability to quickly recall data	Ask patient to repeat six digits forward, then backward (normal responses). Ask patient to try to remember three nonrelated items; test patient after 5 minutes.	Loss of memory occurs with cognitive, dissociative, or conversion disorder. Anxiety can impair immediate retention and recent memory. Anterograde memory loss (amnesia) occurs after taking certain drugs, e.g., benzodiazepines. Retrograde memory loss occurs after head trauma.
Concentration and calculation: Ability to pay attention; distractibility; ability to do simple math	Ask patient to count from 1 to 20 rapidly; do simple calculations (2×3, 4×9); do serial 7 test, i.e., subtract 7 from 100 and keep subtracting 7. How many nickels in $1.35?	Rule out medical cause for any defects versus anxiety or depression (pseudodementia). Make tests congruent with educational level of patient.
Information and intelligence: Use of vocabulary; level of education; fund of knowledge	Distance from New York City to Los Angeles. Name some vegetables. What is the largest river in the United States?	Check educational level to judge results. Rule out mental retardation, borderline intellectual functioning.
Judgment: Ability to understand relations between facts and to draw conclusions; responses in social situations	What is the thing to do if you find an envelope in the street that is sealed, stamped, and addressed?	Impaired in brain disease, schizophrenia, borderline intellectual functioning, intoxication.
Insight level: Realizing that there are physical or mental problems; denial of illness, ascribing blame to outside factors; recognizing need for treatment	Do you think you have a problem? Do you need treatment? What are your plans for the future?	Impaired in delirium, dementia, frontal lobe syndrome, psychosis, borderline intellectual functioning.

For more detailed discussion of this topic, see Chapter 7, Diagnosis and Psychiatry: Examination of the Psychiatric Patient, Section 7.1 p. 944, in CTP/X.

3

Medical Assessment and Laboratory Testing in Psychiatry

Recent developments in understanding the complexities and interplay of psychiatric and medical illnesses have led to new standards of medical assessment and laboratory testing in psychiatric patients. The widespread recognition of the pervasive problem of metabolic syndrome in clinical psychiatry and the shorter life expectancy of psychiatric patients compared to that of the general population have pushed medical assessment and laboratory testing in psychiatric patients to the forefront of attention for most clinicians. Factors that may contribute to medical comorbidity include abuse of tobacco, alcohol and drugs, poor dietary habits, and obesity. Further, many psychotropic medications are associated with health risks that include obesity, metabolic syndrome, and hyperprolactinemia. Consequently, monitoring the physical health of psychiatric patients has become a more prominent issue.

The following section describes the tests in detail with clinical relevance.

I. Neuroendocrine Tests

A. Thyroid function tests

1. Include tests for thyroxine (T_4) by competitive protein binding (T_4D); radioimmunoassay (T_4RIA) involving a specific antigen–antibody reaction; free T_4 index (FT_4I), triiodothyronine (T_3) uptake, and total serum T_3 measured by radioimmunoassay (T_3RIA).

2. Tests are used to rule out hypothyroidism, which can appear with symptoms of depression.

3. Up to 10% of patients complaining of depression and associated fatigue have incipient hypothyroid disease. Neonatal hypothyroidism results in mental retardation and is preventable if the diagnosis is made at birth.

4. Thyrotropin-releasing hormone (TRH) stimulation test indicated in patients with marginally abnormal thyroid test results suggest subclinical hypothyroidism, which may account for clinical depression.

5. **Procedure**

   a. At 8 AM after an overnight fast, have the patient lie down and warn of a possible urge to urinate after the injection.

   b. Measure baseline levels of thyroid-stimulating hormone, T_3, T_4, and T_3 resin uptake.

   c. Inject 500 μg of thyroid-releasing hormone intravenously.

   d. Measure thyroid-stimulating hormone levels at 15, 30, 60, and 90 minutes.

B. Dexamethasone suppression test (DST)
  1. Procedure
    a. Give 1 mg of dexamethasone orally at 11 PM.
    b. Measure plasma cortisol at 4 PM and 11 PM the next day (may also take 8 PM sample).
    c. Any plasma cortisol level above 5 µg/dL is abnormal (although the normal range should be adjusted according to the local assay so that 95% of normals are within the normal range).
    d. Baseline plasma cortisol level may be helpful.
  2. Indications
    a. To help confirm a diagnostic impression of major depressive disorder. Not routinely used because it is unreliable. Abnormal results may confirm need for somatic treatment.
    b. To follow a depressed nonsuppressor through treatment of depression.
    c. To differentiate major depression from minor dysphoria.
    d. Some evidence indicates that depressed nonsuppressors are more likely to respond positively to treatment with electroconvulsive therapy or tricyclic antidepressants.
    e. Proposed utility in predicting outcome of treatment, but DST results may normalize before depression resolves.
    f. Proposed utility in predicting relapse in patients who are persistent nonsuppressors or whose DST results revert to abnormal.
    g. Possible utility in differentiating delusional from nondelusional depression.
    h. Highly abnormal plasma cortisol levels (>10 µg/dL) are more significant than mildly elevated levels.
  3. Reliability. The problems associated with the DST include varying reports of sensitivity or specificity. False-positive and false-negative results are common. The sensitivity of the DST is considered to be 45% in major depressive disorders and 70% in major depressive episodes with psychotic features. The specificity is 90% compared with controls and 77% compared with other psychiatric diagnoses. Some evidence indicates that patients with a positive DST result (especially 10 µg/dL) will have a good response to somatic treatment, such as electroconvulsive therapy or cyclic antidepressant therapy.

C. Catecholamines
  1. Level of serotonin metabolite 5-hydroxyindoleacetic acid (5-HIAA) is elevated in the urine of patients with carcinoid tumors.
  2. Elevated levels are noted at times in patients who take phenothiazine medication and in those who eat foods high in serotonin (i.e., walnuts, bananas, and avocados).
  3. The amount of 5-HIAA in cerebrospinal fluid (CSF) is low in some people who are in a suicidal depression and in postmortem studies of those who have committed suicide in particularly violent ways.

4. Low CSF 5-HIAA levels are associated with violence in general.
5. Norepinephrine and its metabolic products—metanephrine, normetanephrine, and vanillylmandelic acid—can be measured in urine, blood, and plasma.
6. Plasma catecholamine levels are markedly elevated in pheochromocytoma, which is associated with anxiety, agitation, and hypertension.
7. High levels of urinary norepinephrine and epinephrine have been found in some patients with posttraumatic stress disorder (PTSD).
8. The norepinephrine metabolic 3-methoxy-4-hydroxyphenylglycol level is decreased in patients with severe depressive disorders, especially in those patients who attempt suicide.

D. **Other endocrine tests.** In addition to thyroid hormones, these hormones include the anterior pituitary hormone prolactin, growth hormone, somatostatin, gonadotropin-releasing hormone, and the sex steroids—luteinizing hormone, follicle-stimulating hormone, testosterone, and estrogen. Melatonin from the pineal gland has been implicated in seasonal affective disorder (called *seasonal pattern for recurrent major depressive disorder* in the fifth edition of the *Diagnostic and Statistical Manual of Mental Disorders* [DSM-5]).

II. Renal and Hepatic Tests

A. **Renal function tests.** Serum blood urea nitrogen (BUN) and creatinine are monitored in patients taking lithium (Eskalith). If the serum BUN or creatinine is abnormal, the patient's 2-hour creatinine clearance and, ultimately, the 24-hour creatinine clearance are tested. Table 3-1 summarizes other laboratory testing for patients taking lithium.

B. **Liver function tests (LFTs)**
1. Total bilirubin and direct bilirubin values are elevated in hepatocellular injury and intrahepatic bile stasis, which can occur with phenothiazine or tricyclic medication and with alcohol and other substance abuse.
2. Liver damage or disease, which is reflected by abnormal findings in LFTs, may manifest with signs and symptoms of a cognitive disorder, including disorientation and delirium.

Table 3-1
Other Laboratory Testing for Patients Taking Lithium

Test	Frequency
1. Complete blood count	Before treatment and yearly
2. Serum electrolytes	Before treatment and yearly
3. Fasting blood glucose	Before treatment and yearly
4. Electrocardiogram	Before treatment and yearly
5. Pregnancy testing for women of childbearing age[a]	Before treatment

[a]Test more frequently when compliance with treatment plan is uncertain.
Reprinted with permission from MacKinnon RA, Yudofsky SC. *Principles of the Psychiatric Evaluation.* Philadelphia, PA: JB Lippincott; 1991:106.

3. LFTs must be monitored routinely when using certain drugs, such as carbamazepine (Tegretol) and valproate (Depakene).

III. Blood Test for Sexually Transmitted Diseases (STDs)

A. Venereal Disease Research Laboratory (VDRL) test is used as a screening test for syphilis. If positive, the result is confirmed by using the specific fluorescent treponemal antibody-absorption test (FTA-ABS test), in which the spirochete *Treponema pallidum* is used as the antigen.

B. A positive HIV test result indicates that a person has been exposed to infection with the virus that causes AIDS.

IV. Tests Related to Psychotropic Drugs

A. Benzodiazepines

1. No special tests are needed. Among the benzodiazepines metabolized in the liver by oxidation, impaired hepatic function increases the half-life.

2. Baseline LFTs are indicated in patients with suspected liver damage. Urine testing for benzodiazepines is used routinely in cases of substance abuse.

B. Antipsychotics

1. As per FDA guidelines it is recommended that baseline values for HgA1c, lipid panel be established. In addition, it is a good clinical practice to obtain LFTs and a complete blood cell count as these may cause neutropenia. Antipsychotics are metabolized primarily in the liver, with metabolites excreted primarily in urine. Many metabolites are active. Peak plasma concentration usually is reached 2 to 3 hours after an oral dose. Elimination half-life is 12 to 30 hours but may be much longer. Steady state requires at least 1 week at a constant dose (months at a constant dose of depot antipsychotics).

2. Apart from clozapine (Clozaril), and some newer generation antipsychotics including quetiapine (Seroquel) and Aripiprazole (Abilify) most antipsychotics may cause an elevation in serum prolactin (secondary to tuberoinfundibular activity). A normal prolactin level may indicate either noncompliance or poor absorption. Side effects include leukocytosis, leucopenia, impaired platelet function, mild anemia (both aplastic and hemolytic), and agranulocytosis. Bone marrow and blood element side effects can occur abruptly, even when the dosage has remained constant. Low-potency antipsychotics are most likely to cause agranulocytosis, which is most common bone marrow side effect. These agents may cause hepatocellular injury and intrahepatic biliary stasis (indicated by elevated total and direct bilirubin and elevated transaminases). They also can cause electrocardiographic changes (not as frequently as with tricyclic antidepressants), including a prolonged QT interval; flattened, inverted, or bifid T waves; and U waves. Dose-plasma concentration relations differ widely among patients. Baseline EKG testing is recommended.

3. **Clozapine.** Because of the risk of agranulocytosis (1% to 2%), patients who are being treated with clozapine must have a baseline white blood cell (WBC) and differential count before the initiation of treatment, a WBC count every week for 6 months, biweekly thereafter for another 6 months and patients maintained after a year require monthly monitoring. Physicians and pharmacists who provide clozapine are required to be registered through Clozapine Risk Evaluation and Mitigation Strategy (REMS Program). These new guidelines replace the individual clozapine patient registries and the National Non-Rechallenge Master File (NNRMF).

Clinicians should be aware of the cardiac side effects and monitor creatine phosphokinase (CPK) and troponin as necessary based on signs and symptoms. Myocarditis and cardiomyopathy are well-known issues that can be fatal but preventable with appropriate monitoring and laboratory testing.

4. Newer generation antipsychotics with the exception of a few may increase appetite with subsequent weight gain and may cause hyperlipidemia and diabetes mellitus type II. Clinicians should take weight and waist measurements during each visit to guide patients with appropriate advice on nutrition and exercise as well as may dictate monitoring of blood sugar, and lipid testing.

C. **Tricyclic and tetracyclic drugs.** An electrocardiogram (EKG) should be given before starting a regimen or cyclic drugs to access for conduction delays, which may lead to heart blocks at therapeutic levels. Some clinicians believe that all patients receiving prolonged cyclic drug therapy should have an annual EKG. At therapeutic levels, the drugs suppress arrhythmias through a quinidinelike effect.

Blood levels should be tested routinely when using imipramine (Tofranil), desipramine (Norpramin), or nortriptyline (Pamelor) in the treatment of depressive disorders. Taking blood levels may also be of use in patients for whom there is an urgent need to know whether a therapeutic or toxic plasma level of the drug has been reached. Blood level tests should also include the measurement of active metabolites (e.g., imipramine is converted to desipramine, amitriptyline [Elavil] to nortriptyline). Some characteristics of tricyclic drug plasma levels are described as follows.

1. **Imipramine (Tofranil).** The percentage of favorable responses to imipramine correlates with plasma levels in a linear manner between 200 and 250 ng/mL, but some patients may respond at a lower level. At levels that exceed 250 ng/mL, there is no improved favorable response, and side effects increase.

2. **Nortriptyline (Pamelor).** The therapeutic window (the range within which a drug is most effective) of nortriptyline is between 50 and 150 ng/mL. There is a decreased response rate at levels greater than 150 ng/mL.

3. **Desipramine (Norpramin).** Levels of desipramine greater than 125 ng/mL correlate with a higher percentage of favorable responses.

4. **Amitriptyline (Elavil).** Different studies have produced conflicting results regarding blood levels of amitriptyline, but they range from 75 to 175 ng/mL.

5. **Procedure for determining blood concentrations.** The blood specimen should be drawn 10 to 14 hours after the last dose, usually in the morning after a bedtime dose. Patients must be receiving stable daily dosage for at least 5 days for the test to be valid. Some patients are unusually poor metabolizers of cyclic drugs and may have levels as high as 2,000 ng/mL while taking normal dosages and before showing a favorable clinical response. Such patients must be monitored closely for cardiac side effects. Patients with levels greater than 1,000 ng/mL are generally at risk for cardiotoxicity.

D. **Monoamine oxidase inhibitors (MAOIs).** Patients taking MAOIs are instructed to avoid tyramine-containing foods because of the danger of a potential hypertensive crisis. A baseline normal blood pressure (BP) must be recorded, and the BP must be monitored during treatment. MAOIs may also cause orthostatic hypotension as a direct drug side effect unrelated to diet. Other than their potential for causing elevated BP when taken with certain foods, MAOIs are relatively free of other side effects. A test used both in a research setting and in current clinical practice involves correlating the therapeutic response with the degree of platelet MAO inhibition.

E. **Lithium.** Patients receiving lithium should have baseline thyroid function tests, electrolyte monitoring, a WBC count, renal function tests (specific gravity, BUN, and creatinine), and a baseline EKG. The rationale for these tests is that lithium can cause renal concentrating defects, hypothyroidism, and leukocytosis; sodium depletion can cause toxic lithium levels; and approximately 95% of lithium is excreted in the urine. Lithium has also been shown to cause EKG changes, including various conduction defects.

Lithium is mostly clearly indicated in the prophylactic treatment of manic episodes (its direct antimanic effect may take up to 2 weeks) and is commonly coupled with antipsychotics for the treatment of acute manic episodes. Lithium itself may also have antipsychotic activity and has been shown to have antisuicidal properties. The maintenance level is 0.6 to 1.2 mEq/L, although acutely manic patients can tolerate up to 1.5 to 1.8 mEq/L. Some patients may respond at lower levels, whereas others may require higher levels. A response below 0.4 mEq/L is probably a placebo. Toxic reactions may occur with levels over 2.0 mEq/L. Regular lithium monitoring is essential; there is a narrow therapeutic range beyond which cardiac problems and central nervous system (CNS) effects can occur.

Lithium levels are drawn 8 to 12 hours after the last dose, usually in the morning after the bedtime dose. The level should be measured at least twice a week while stabilizing the patient and may be drawn monthly thereafter.

F. **Carbamazepine.** A pretreatment complete blood count, including platelet count, should be done. Reticulocyte count and serum iron tests are also desirable. These tests should be repeated weekly during the first 3 months of treatment and monthly thereafter. Carbamazepine can cause aplastic anemia, agranulocytosis, thrombocytopenia, and leucopenia. Because of the minor risk of hepatotoxicity, LFTs should be done every 3 to 6 months. The medication should be discontinued if the patient shows any signs of bone marrow suppression as measured with periodic complete blood counts. The therapeutic level of carbamazepine is 8 to 12 ng/mL, with toxicity most often reached at levels of 15 ng/mL. Most clinicians report that levels as high as 12 ng/mL are hard to achieve.

G. **Valproate.** Serum levels of valproic acid (Depakene) and divalproex (Depakote) are therapeutic in the range of 45 to 50 ng/mL. Above 125 ng/mL side effects occur, including thrombocytopenia. Serum levels should be obtained periodically, and LFTs should be obtained every 6 to 12 months. Valproate may cause hyperammonemic encephalopathy and clinicians should check ammonia levels if clinically indicated.

H. **Tacrine (Cognex).** Tacrine may cause liver damage. A baseline of liver function should be established, and follow-up serum transaminase levels should be obtained every other week for approximately 5 months. Patients who develop jaundice or who have bilirubin levels higher than 3 mg/dL must be withdrawn from the drug.

V. **Provocation of Panic Attacks with Sodium Lactate**

Up to 72% of patients with panic disorder have a panic attack when administered an intravenous (IV) injection of sodium lactate. Therefore, lactate provocation is used to confirm a diagnosis of panic disorder. Lactate provocation has also been used to trigger flashbacks in patients with PTSD. Hyperventilation, another known trigger of panic attacks in predisposed persons, is not as sensitive as lactate provocation in inducing panic attacks. Carbon dioxide inhalation also precipitates panic attacks in those so predisposed. Panic attacks triggered by sodium lactate are not inhibited by peripherally acting β-blockers but are inhibited by Alprazolam (Xanax) and tricyclic drugs.

VI. **Lumbar Puncture**

Lumbar puncture is of use in patients who have a sudden manifestation of new psychiatric symptoms, especially changes in cognition. The clinician should be especially vigilant if there is fever or neurologic symptoms such as seizure. Lumbar puncture is of use in diagnosing CNS infection (i.e., meningitis).

VII. **Urine Testing for Substance Abuse**

Several substances may be detected in a patient's urine if the urine is tested within a specific (and variable) period after ingestion. Knowledge of urine substance testing is becoming crucial for practicing physicians in view of the controversial issue of mandatory or random substance testing. Table 3-2 provides a summary of substances of abuse that can be tested in the urine.

Laboratory tests are also used in the detection of substances that may be contributing to cognitive disorders.

Table 3-2
Substances of Abuse That Can Be Tested in Urine

Substance	Length of Time Detected in Urine
Alcohol	7–12 hours
Amphetamine	48 hours
Barbiturate	24 hours (short acting)
	3 weeks (long acting)
Benzodiazepine	3 days
Cannabis	3 days to 4 weeks (depending on use)
Cocaine	6–8 hours (metabolites 2–4 days)
Codeine	48 hours
Heroin	36–72 hours
Methadone	3 days
Methaqualone	7 days
Morphine	48–72 hours
Phencyclidine (PCP)	8 days
Propoxyphene	6–48 hours

VIII. Screening Tests for Medical Illnesses

See Table 3-3. Rule out organic causes for the psychiatric disorder. A thorough screening battery of laboratory tests administered on admission may detect a significant degree of morbidity. The routine admission workup includes the following:

A. Complete blood cell count with differential.

B. Complete blood chemistries (including measurements of electrolytes, glucose, calcium, and magnesium and tests of hepatic and renal function).

C. Thyroid function tests.

D. Rapid plasma reagent (RPR) or VDRL test.

E. Urinalysis.

F. Urine toxicology screen.

G. EKG.

H. Vitamin B_{12} and folate levels.

I. Glycosylated hemoglobin (HgA1c) and lipid panel.

IX. Electrophysiology

A. Electroencephalogram (EEG)

1. First clinical application was by the psychiatrist Hans Berger in 1929.

2. Measures voltages between electrodes placed on the skin.

3. Provides gross description of electrical activity of CNS neurons.

4. Each person's EEG is unique, like a fingerprint.

5. For decades, researchers have attempted to correlate specific psychiatric conditions with characteristic EEG changes but have been unsuccessful.

6. EEG changes with age.

7. Normal EEG pattern does not rule out seizure disorder or medical disease; yield is higher in sleep-deprived subjects and with placement of nasopharyngeal leads.

Text continues on page 39.

Table 3-3
Psychiatric Indications for Diagnostic Tests

Test	Major Psychiatric Indications	Comments
Acid phosphatase	Cognitive/medical workup	Increased in prostate cancer, benign prostatic hypertrophy, excessive platelet destruction, bone disease
Adrenocorticotropic hormone (ACTH)	Cognitive/medical workup	Changed in steroid abuse; may be increased in seizures, psychoses, and Cushing's disease, and in response to stress Decreased in Addison's disease
Alanine aminotrans-ferase (ALT)	Cognitive/medical workup	Increased in hepatitis, cirrhosis, liver metastases Decreased in pyridoxine (vitamin B_6) deficiency
Albumin	Cognitive/medical workup	Increased in dehydration Decreased in malnutrition, hepatic failure, burns, multiple myeloma, carcinomas
Aldolase	Eating disorders Schizophrenia	Increased in patients who abuse ipecac (e.g., bulimic patients), some patients with schizophrenia
Alkaline phosphatase	Cognitive/medical workup Use of psychiatric medications	Increased in Paget's disease, hyperparathyroidism, hepatic disease, liver metastases, heart failure, phenothiazine use Decreased in pernicious anemia (vitamin B_{12} deficiency)
Ammonia, serum	Cognitive/medical workup	Increased in hepatic encephalopathy, liver failure, Reye's syndrome; increases with gastrointestinal hemorrhage and severe congestive heart failure
Amylase, serum	Eating disorders	May be increased in bulimia nervosa
Antinuclear antibodies	Cognitive/medical workup	Found in systemic lupus erythematosus (SLE) and drug-induced lupus (e.g., secondary to phenothi-azines, anticonvulsants); SLE can be associated with delirium, psychosis, mood disorder
Aspartate amino-transferase (AST)	Cognitive/medical workup	Increased in heart failure, hepatic disease, pancre-atitis, eclampsia, cerebral damage, alcoholism Decreased in pyridoxine (vitamin B_6) deficiency and terminal stages of liver disease
Bicarbonate, serum	Panic disorder	Decreased in hyperventilation syndrome, panic dis-order, anabolic steroid abuse
	Eating disorders	May be elevated in patients with bulimia nervosa, in laxative abuse, psychogenic vomiting
Bilirubin	Cognitive/medical workup	Increased in hepatic disease
Blood urea nitrogen (BUN)	Delirium Use of psychiatric medications	Elevated in renal disease, dehydration Elevations associated with lethargy, delirium If elevated, can increase toxic potential of psychi-atric medications, especially lithium and amanta-dine (Symmetrel)
Bromide, serum	Dementia	Bromide intoxication can cause psychosis, hallucina-tions, delirium
	Psychosis	Part of dementia workup, especially when serum chloride Is elevated
Caffeine level, serum	Anxiety/panic disorder	Evaluation of patients with suspected caffeinism
Calcium (Ca), serum	Cognitive/medical workup	Increased in hyperparathyroidism, bone metastases
	Mood disorders	Increase associated with delirium, depression, psychosis
	Psychosis	Decreased in hypoparathyroidism, renal failure
	Eating disorders	Decrease associated with depression, irritability, delir-ium, chronic laxative abuse

(continued)

Table 3-3
Psychiatric Indications for Diagnostic Tests (Continued)

Test	Major Psychiatric Indications	Comments
Carotid ultrasonography	Dementia	Occasionally included in dementia workup, especially to rule out multiinfarct dementia Primary value is in search for possible infarct causes
Catecholamines, urinary and plasma	Panic attacks Anxiety	Elevated in pheochromocytoma
Cerebrospinal fluid (CSF)	Cognitive/medical workup	Increased protein and cells in infection, positive VDRL in neurosyphilis, bloody CSF in hemorrhagic conditions
Ceruloplasmin, serum; copper, serum	Cognitive/medical workup	Low in Wilson's disease (hepatolenticular disease)
Chloride (Cl), serum	Eating disorders	Decreased in patients with bulimia and psychogenic vomiting
	Panic disorder	Mild elevation in hyperventilation syndrome, panic disorder
Cholecystokinin (CCK)	Eating disorders	Compared with controls, blunted in bulimic patients after eating meal (may normalize after treatment with antidepressants)
CO_2 inhalation; sodium bicarbonate infusion	Anxiety/panic attacks	Panic attacks produced in subgroup of patients
Coombs' test, direct and indirect	Hemolytic anemias secondary to psychiatric medications	Evaluation of drug-induced hemolytic anemias, such as those secondary to chlorpromazine, phenytoin, levodopa, and methyldopa
Copper, urine	Cognitive/medical workup	Elevated in Wilson's disease
Cortisol (hydrocortisone)	Cognitive/medical workup Mood disorders	Excessive level may indicate Cushing's disease associated with anxiety, depression, and a variety of other conditions
Creatine phosphokinase (CPK)	Use of antipsychotic agents Use of restraints Substance abuse	Increased in neuroleptic malignant syndrome, intramuscular injection rhabdomyolysis (secondary to substance abuse), patients in restraint, patients experiencing dystonic reactions; asymptomatic elevation with use of antipsychotic drugs. Increased in myocarditis and cardiomyopathy.
Creatinine, serum	Cognitive/medical workup	Elevated in renal disease (see BUN)
Dopamine (DA) (levodopa stimulation of dopamine)	Depression	Inhibits prolactin Test used to assess functional integrity of dopaminergic system, which is impaired in Parkinson's disease, depression
Doppler ultrasonography	Erectile disorder (ED) Cognitive/medical workup	Carotid occlusion, transient ischemic attack (TIA), reduced penile blood flow in ED
Electrocardiogram (EKG)	Panic disorder	Among patients with panic disorder, 10–40% show mitral valve prolapse
Electroencephalogram (EEG)	Cognitive/medical workup	Seizures, brain death, lesions; shortened rapid eye movement (REM) latency in depression High-voltage activity in stupor, low-voltage fast activity in excitement, functional nonorganic cases (e.g., dissociative states); alpha activity present in the background, which responds to auditory and visual stimuli Biphasic or triphasic slow bursts seen in dementia of Creutzfeldt–Jakob disease

(continued)

Table 3-3
Psychiatric Indications for Diagnostic Tests *(Continued)*

Test	Major Psychiatric Indications	Comments
Epstein-Barr virus (EBV); cytomegalovirus (CMV)	Cognitive/medical workup	Part of herpesvirus group EBV is causative agent for infectious mononucleosis, which can present with depression, fatigue, and personality change
	Anxiety	CMV can produce anxiety, confusion, mood disorders
	Mood disorders	EBV may be associated with chronic mononucleosis-like syndrome associated with chronic depression and fatigue
Erythrocyte sedimentation rate (ESR)	Cognitive/medical workup	An increase in ESR represents a nonspecific test of infectious, inflammatory, autoimmune, or malignant disease; sometimes recommended in the evaluation of anorexia nervosa
Estrogen	Mood disorder	Decreased in menopausal depression and premenstrual syndrome; variable changes in anxiety
Ferritin, serum	Cognitive/medical workup	Most sensitive test for iron deficiency
Folate (folic acid), serum	Alcohol abuse	Usually measured with vitamin B_{12} deficiencies associated with psychosis, paranoia, fatigue, agitation, dementia, delirium
	Use of specific medications	Associated with alcoholism, use of phenytoin, oral contraceptives, estrogen
Follicle-stimulating hormone (FSH)	Depression	High normal in anorexia nervosa, higher values in postmenopausal women; low levels in patients with panhypopituitarism
Glucose, fasting blood (FBS)	Panic attacks Anxiety Delirium	Very high FBS associated with delirium
	Depression	Very low FBS associated with delirium, agitation, panic attacks, anxiety, depression
Glutamyl transaminase, serum	Alcohol abuse	Increased in alcohol abuse, cirrhosis, liver disease
Gonadotropin-releasing hormone (GnRH)	Cognitive/medical workup	Decreased in schizophrenia; increase in anorexia; variable in depression, anxiety
Growth hormone (GH)	Depression Anxiety Schizophrenia	Blunted GH responses to insulin-induced hypoglycemia in depressed patients; increased GH responses to dopamine agonist challenge in schizophrenic patients; increased in some cases of anorexia
Hematocrit (Hct); hemoglobin (Hb)	Cognitive/medical workup	Assessment of anemia (anemia may be associated with depression and psychosis)
Hepatitis A viral antigen (HAAg)	Mood disorders Cognitive/medical workup	Less severe, better prognosis than hepatitis B; may present with anorexia, depression
Hepatitis B surface antigen (HBsAg); hepatitis B core antigen (HBcAg)	Mood disorders Cognitive/medical workup	Active hepatitis B infection indicates greater degree of infectivity and progression to chronic liver disease May present with depression
Holter monitor	Panic disorder	Evaluation of panic-disordered patients with palpitations and other cardiac symptoms
HIV	Cognitive/medical workup	CNS Involvement; AIDS dementia organic personality disorder, organic mood disorder, acute psychosis
17-Hydroxycorticosteroid	Depression	Deviations detect hyperadrenocorticalism, which can be associated with major depression Increased in steroid abuse

(continued)

Table 3-3
Psychiatric Indications for Diagnostic Tests (Continued)

Test	Major Psychiatric Indications	Comments
5-Hydroxyin-doleacetic acid (5-HIAA)	Depression Suicide Violence	Decreased in CSF in aggressive or violent patients with suicidal or homicidal impulses May be indicator of decreased impulse control and predictor of suicide
Iron, serum	Cognitive/medical workup	Iron-deficiency anemia
Lactate dehydroge-nase (LDH)	Cognitive/medical workup	Increased in myocardial infarction, pulmonary infarc-tion, hepatic disease, renal infarction, seizures, cerebral damage, megaloblastic (pernicious) anemia, factitious elevations secondary to rough handling of blood specimen tube
Lupus anticoagulant (LA)	Use of phenothiazines	An antiphospholipid antibody, which has been described in some patients using phenothiazines, especially chlorpromazine; often associated with elevated PTT; associated with anticardiolipin antibodies
Lupus erythematosus (LE) test	Depression Psychosis Delirium Dementia	Positive test associated with systemic LE, which may present with various psychiatric disturbances, such as psychosis, depression, delirium, dementia; also tested with antinuclear antibody (ANA) and anti-DNA antibody tests
Luteinizing hormone (LH)	Depression	Low in patients with panhypopituitarism; decrease associated with depression
Magnesium, serum	Alcohol abuse Cognitive/medical workup	Decreased in alcoholism; low levels associated with agitation, delirium, seizures
Monoamine oxidase (MAO), platelet	Depression	Low in depression; has been used to monitor MAO inhibitor therapy
MCV (mean cor-puscular volume) (average volume of a red blood cell)	Alcohol abuse	Elevated in alcoholism and vitamin B_{12} and folate deficiency
Melatonin	Seasonal affective disorder	Produced by light and pineal gland and decreased in seasonal affective disorder
Metal (heavy) intox-ication (serum or urinary)	Cognitive/medical workup	Lead—apathy, irritability, anorexia, confusion Mercury—psychosis, fatigue, apathy, decreased memory, emotional lability, "mad hatter" Manganese—manganese madness, Parkinson-like syndrome Aluminum—dementia Arsenic—fatigue, blackouts, hair loss
3-Methoxy-4-hydroxy-phenylglycol (MHPG)	Depression Anxiety	Most useful in research; decreases in urine may indicate decreases centrally; may predict response to certain antidepressants
Myoglobin, urine	Phenothiazine use Substance abuse Use of restraints	Increased in neuroleptic malignant syndrome; in phencyclidine (PCP), cocaine, or lysergic acid diethylamide (LSD) intoxication; and in patients in restraints
Nicotine	Anxiety Nicotine addiction	Anxiety, smoking
Nocturnal penile tumescence	Erectile disorder (ED)	Quantification of penile circumference changes, penile rigidity, frequency of penile tumescence Evaluation of erectile function during sleep Erections associated with REM sleep Helpful in differentiation between organic and functional causes of ED

Table 3-3
Psychiatric Indications for Diagnostic Tests *(Continued)*

Test	Major Psychiatric Indications	Comments
Parathyroid hormone (parathormone)	Anxiety	Low level causes hypocalcemia and anxiety
	Cognitive/medical workup	Dysregulation associated with wide variety of organic mental disorders
Partial thromboplastin time (PTT)	Treatment with antipsychotics, heparin	Monitor anticoagulant therapy; increased in presence of lupus anticoagulant and anticardiolipin antibodies
Phosphorus, serum	Cognitive/medical workup	Increased in renal failure, diabetic acidosis hypoparathyroidism, hypervitaminosis D; decreased in cirrhosis, hypokalemia, hyperparathyroidism, panic attacks, hyperventilation syndrome
	Panic disorder	
Platelet count	Use of psychotropic medications	Decreased by certain psychotropic medications (carbamazepine, clozapine, phenothiazines)
Porphobilinogen (PBG)	Cognitive/medical workup	Increased in acute porphyria
Porphyria-synthesizing enzyme	Psychosis	Acute neuropsychiatric disorder can occur in acute porphyria attack, which may be precipitated by barbiturates, imipramine
	Cognitive/medical workup	
Potassium (K), serum	Cognitive/medical workup	Increased in hyperkalemic acidosis; increase associated with anxiety in cardiac arrhythmia
	Eating disorders	Decreased in cirrhosis, metabolic alkalosis, laxative abuse, diuretic abuse; decrease is common in bulimic patients and in psychogenic vomiting, anabolic steroid abuse
Prolactin, serum	Use of antipsychotic medications	Antipsychotics, by decreasing dopamine, increased prolactin synthesis and release, especially in women
	Cocaine use	Elevated prolactin levels may be seen secondary to cocaine withdrawal
	Pseudoseizures	Lack of prolactin rise after seizure suggests pseudoseizure
Protein, total serum	Cognitive/medical workup	Increased in multiple myeloma, myxedema, lupus Decreased in cirrhosis, malnutrition, overhydration
	Use of psychotropic medications	Low serum protein can result in greater sensitivity to conventional doses of protein-bound medications (lithium is not protein-bound)
Prothrombin time (PT)	Cognitive/medical workup	Elevated in significant liver damage (cirrhosis)
Reticulocyte count (estimate of red blood cell production in bone marrow)	Cognitive/medical workup	Low in megaloblastic or iron-deficiency anemia and anemia of chronic disease
	Use of carbamazepine	Must be monitored in patient taking carbamazepine
Salicylate, serum	Organic hallucinosis Suicide attempts	Toxic levels may be seen in suicide attempts; may also cause organic hallucinosis with high levels
Sodium (Na), serum	Cognitive/medical workup	Decreased with water intoxication, syndrome of inappropriate secretion of antidiuretic hormone (SIADH) Decrease in hypoadrenalism, myxedema, congestive heart failure, diarrhea, polydipsia, use of carbamazepine, anabolic steroids
	Use of lithium	Low levels associated with greater sensitivity to conventional dose of lithium

(continued)

Table 3-3
Psychiatric Indications for Diagnostic Tests *(Continued)*

Test	Major Psychiatric Indications	Comments
Testosterone, serum	Erectile disorder (ED)	Increased in anabolic steroid abuse
		May be decreased in organic workup of ED
	Inhibited sexual desire	Decrease may be seen with inhibited sexual desire
		Follow-up of sex offenders treated with medroxyprogesterone
		Decreased with medroxyprogesterone treatment
Thyroid function tests	Cognitive/medical workup	Detection of hypothyroidism or hyperthyroidism
	Depression	Abnormalities can be associated with depression, anxiety, psychosis, dementia, delirium, lithium treatment
Urinalysis	Cognitive/medical workup	Provides clues to cause of various cognitive disorders (assessing general appearance, pH, specific gravity, bilirubin, glucose, blood, ketones, protein); specific gravity may be affected by lithium
	Pretreatment workup of lithium	
	Drug screening	
Urinary creatinine	Cognitive/medical workup	Increased in renal failure, dehydration
	Substance abuse	Part of pretreatment workup for lithium; sometimes used in follow-up evaluations of patients treated with lithium
	Lithium use	
Venereal Disease Research Laboratory (VDRL)	Syphilis	Positive (high titers) in secondary syphilis (may be positive or negative in primary syphilis); rapid plasma reagent (RPR) test also used
		Low titers (or negative) in tertiary syphilis
Vitamin A, serum	Depression	Hypervitaminosis A is associated with a variety of mental status changes, headache
	Delirium	
Vitamin B_{12}, serum	Cognitive/medical workup	Part of workup of megaloblastic anemia and dementia
	Dementia	B_{12} deficiency associated with psychosis, paranoia, fatigue, agitation, dementia, delirium
	Mood disorder	Often associated with chronic alcohol abuse
White blood cell (WBC) count	Use of psychiatric medications	Leukopenia and agranulocytosis associated with certain psychotropic medications, such as phenothiazines, carbamazepine, clozapine
		Leukocytosis associated with lithium and neuroleptic malignant syndrome

Table by Richard B. Rosse, M.D., Lynn H. Deutsch, D.O., and Stephen J. Deutsch, M.D., Ph.D.

8. Indications

    a. General cognitive and medical workup; evaluation of delirium and dementia.

    b. Part of routine workup for any first-break psychosis.

    c. Can help diagnose some seizure disorders (e.g., epilepsy).

        (1) Grand mal seizures—onset characterized by epileptic recruiting rhythm of rhythmic, synchronous high-amplitude spikes between 8 and 12 Hz (cycles per second). After 15 to 30 seconds, spikes may become grouped and separated by slow waves (correlation with clonic phase). Finally, a quiescent phase of low-amplitude delta (slow) waves occurs.

(2) Petit mal seizures—sudden onset of bilaterally synchronous generalized spike-and-wave pattern with high-amplitude and characteristic 3-Hz frequency.

d. Helpful in diagnosing space-occupying lesions and vascular lesions of the CNS and encephalopathies, among others.

e. Can detect characteristic changes caused by specific drugs.

f. EEG exquisitely sensitive to drug changes.

g. Diagnosis of brain death.

9. **EEG waves**

   a. Beta, 14 to 30 Hz.

   b. Alpha, 8 to 13 Hz.

   c. Theta, 4 to 7 Hz.

   d. Delta, 0.5 to 3 Hz.

B. **Polysomnography**

1. Records EEG during sleep; often used with EKG, electrooculography (EOG), electromyography (EMG), chest expansion, and recording of penile tumescence, blood oxygen saturation, body movement, body temperature, galvanic skin response (GSR), and gastric acid levels.

2. **Indications**—to assist in the diagnosis of the following:

   a. Sleep disorders—insomnias, hypersomnias, parasomnias, sleep apnea, nocturnal myoclonus, and sleep-related bruxism.

   b. Childhood sleep-related disorders—enuresis, somnambulism (sleepwalking), and sleep terror disorder (pavor nocturnus).

   c. Other conditions—erectile disorder, seizure disorders, migraine and other vascular headaches, substance abuse, gastroesophageal reflux, and major depressive disorder.

   d. Comments

      (1) Rapid eye movement (REM) latency correlates with major depressive disorder; degree of decreased REM latency correlates with degree of depression.

      (2) Shortened REM latency as a diagnostic test for major depressive disorder seems to be slightly more sensitive than DST.

      (3) Use with DST or TRH stimulation test can improve sensitivity. Preliminary data indicate that depressed DST nonsuppressors are extremely likely to have shortened REM latency.

3. **Polysomnographic findings in major depressive disorder**

   a. Most depressed patients (80% to 85%) exhibit hyposomnia.

   b. In depressed patients, slow-wave (delta-wave) sleep is decreased and sleep stages III and IV are shorter.

   c. In depressed patients, the time between onset of sleep and onset of first REM period (REM latency) is shorter.

   d. In depressed patients, a greater proportion of REM sleep take place early in the night (opposite true for nondepressed controls).

   e. More REMs during the entire night (REM density) have been observed in depressed patients than in nondepressed controls.

C. **Evoked potentials**
   1. Evoked potentials are brain electrical activity elicited by stimuli.
   2. Visual, auditory, and somatosensory evoked potentials can detect abnormalities of peripheral and central neural conduction.
   3. Can differentiate some functional complaints from organic complaints (e.g., studies with visual evoked potentials can be used to evaluate hysterical blindness).
   4. Can be useful for detecting underlying neurologic illness (e.g., demyelinating disorder).

X. **Drug-Assisted Interview**
   Although rarely used the drug-assisted interview may be helpful in some circumstances. Common use of amobarbital (Amytal)—a barbiturate with a medium half-life of 8 to 42 hours—led to popular name, *Amytal interview*. Other drugs used include benzodiazepines such as diazepam and lorazepam.
   A. **Diagnostic indications.** Catatonia; supposed conversion disorder; unexplained muteness; differentiating functional from organic stupors (organic conditions should worsen, and functional conditions should improve because of decreased anxiety).
   B. **Therapeutic indications.** As an interview aid for patients with disorders of repression and dissociation.
      1. Abreaction of PTSD.
      2. Recovery of memory in dissociative amnesia and fugue.
      3. Recovery of function in conversion disorder.
   C. **Procedure**
      1. Have patient recline in an environment in which cardiopulmonary resuscitation is readily available should hypotension or respiratory depression develop.
      2. Explain to the patient that medication should help him or her to relax and feel like talking.
      3. Insert a narrow-bore needle into a peripheral vein.
      4. Inject 5% solution of sodium amobarbital (500 mg dissolved in 10 mL of sterile water) at a rate no faster than 1 mL/min (50 mg/min).
      5. Begin interview by discussing neutral topics. Often, it is helpful to prompt the patient with known facts about his or her life.
      6. Continue infusion until either sustained lateral nystagmus or drowsiness is noted.
      7. To maintain level of narcosis, continue infusion at a rate of 0.5 to 1.0 mL/5 min (25 to 50 mg/5 min).
      8. Have the patient recline for at least 15 minutes after the interview is terminated and until the patient can walk without supervision.
      9. Use the same method every time to avoid dosage errors.
   D. **Contraindications**
      1. Upper respiratory infection or inflammation.
      2. Severe hepatic or renal impairment.

3. Hypotension.
4. History of porphyria.
5. Barbiturate addiction.

XI. Biochemical Markers and Pharmacogenomic Testing

Many potential biochemical markers, including neurotransmitters and their metabolites, may help in the diagnosis and treatment of psychiatric disorders. Research in this area is still evolving.

A. Monoamines

1. Plasma homovanillic as (pHVA), a major dopamine metabolite, may have value in identifying schizophrenic patients who respond to antipsychotics.

2. 3-Methoxy-4-hydroxyphenylglycol (MHPG) is a norepinephrine metabolite.

3. 5-Hydroxyindoleacetic acid is associated with suicidal behavior, aggression, poor impulse control, and depression. Elevated levels may be associated with anxious, obsessional, and inhibited behaviors.

4. Pharmacogenomics is defined as an individual's genetic variability to drug response. It has some utility for psychotropic drugs and some examples are:

   a. Pharmacodynamic gene testing includes serotonin transporter (SLC6A4), which predicts response and adverse effects of SSRI and SNRI antidepressants.

   b. Another serotonin receptor 2C (5-HT2c) mutation may predict weight gain with atypical antipsychotics.

   c. The pharmacokinetic genes for P450 enzyme system are relevant for predicting rate of metabolism as well as dose adjustment.

B. Alzheimer's disease

1. Apolipoprotein E allele—associated with increased risk for Alzheimer's disease. Reduced glucose metabolism noted on PET in some asymptomatic middle-aged persons, similar to findings in Alzheimer's patients.

2. Neural thread protein—reported to be increased in patients with Alzheimer's disease. CSF neural thread protein is marketed as a diagnostic test.

3. Other potentials CSF tests include CSF tau (increased), CSF amyloid (decreased), ratio of CSF albumin to serum albumin (normal in Alzheimer's disease, elevated in vascular dementia), and inflammatory markers (e.g., CSF acute-phase reactive proteins). The gene for the amyloid precursor protein is considered to be possible etiologic significance, but further research is needed.

For more detailed discussion of this topic, see Chapter 7, Diagnosis and Psychiatry: Examination of the Psychiatric Patient, Section 7.6, Medical Assessment and Laboratory Testing in Psychiatry, p. 1008, in CTP/X.

Brain Imaging

I. Introduction

Imaging of the central nervous system (CNS) can be broadly divided into two domains: structural and functional. Structural imaging provides detailed, non-invasive visualization of the morphology of the brain. Functional imaging provides a visualization of the spatial distribution of specific biochemical processes. Structural imaging includes x-ray CT and magnetic resonance imaging (MRI). Functional imaging includes positron emission tomography (PET), single-photon emission computed tomography (SPECT), functional MRI (fMRI), and magnetic resonance spectroscopy (MRS). With the limited exception of PET scanning, functional imaging techniques are still research tools that are not yet ready for routine clinical use. This chapter describes the indications, usage, and descriptions of the current imagining methods in use today.

II. Uses of Neuroimaging

A. Indications for neuroimaging in clinical practice

1. **Neurologic deficits.** In a neurologic examination, any change that can be localized to the brain or spinal cord requires neuroimaging. Consider neuroimaging for patients with new-onset psychosis and acute changes in mental status.

 CLINICAL HINT:

The clinical examination always assumes priority, and neuroimaging is ordered on the basis of clinical suspicion of a central nervous system (CNS) disorder.

---

2. **Dementia.** The most common cause of dementia is Alzheimer's disease, which does not have a characteristic appearance on routine neuroimaging but, rather, is associated with diffuse loss of brain volume. One treatable cause of dementia that requires neuroimaging for diagnosis is *normal pressure hydrocephalus*, a disorder of the drainage of cerebrospinal fluid (CSF).

3. **Strokes.** Strokes are easily seen on MRI scans. In addition to major strokes, extensive atherosclerosis in brain capillaries can cause countless tiny infarctions of brain tissue; patients with this phenomenon may develop dementia as fewer and fewer neural pathways participate in cognition. This state, called *vascular dementia*, is characterized on MRI scans by patches of increased signal in the white matter.

4. **Degenerative disorders.** Certain degenerative disorders of basal ganglia structures, associated with dementia, may have a characteristic appearance

on MRI scans. Huntington's disease typically produces atrophy on the caudate nucleus; thalamic degeneration can interrupt the neural links to the cortex. Space-occupying lesions can cause dementia and are apparent with neuroimaging techniques (e.g., chronic subdural hematomas, cerebral contusions, brain tumors).

5. Chronic infections. Chronic infections, including neurosyphilis, cryptococcosis, tuberculosis, and Lyme disease, may produce a characteristic enhancement of the meninges, especially at the base of the brain. Serologic studies are needed to complete the diagnosis. Human immunodeficiency virus (HIV) infection can cause dementia directly, in which case is seen a diffuse loss of brain volume, or it can allow proliferation to the Creutzfeldt–Jakob virus to yield progressive multifocal leukoencephalopathy, which affects white matter tracts and appears as increased white matter signal on MRI scans. Multiple sclerosis (MS) plaques easily seen on MRI scans are periventricular patches of increased signal intensity.

III. Brain Imaging Methods
A. Computed tomography (CT)
1. Clinical indications—dementia or depression, general cognitive and medical workup, and routine workup for any first-break psychosis.
2. Research
   a. Differentiating subtypes of Alzheimer's disease.
   b. Cerebral atrophy in alcohol abusers.
   c. Cerebral atrophy in benzodiazepine abusers.
   d. Cortical and cerebellar atrophy in schizophrenia.
   e. Increased ventricle size in schizophrenia.
   f. Type—CT scans may be performed with or without contrast. The contrast CT enhances the visualization of diseases such as tumors, strokes, abscesses, and other infections.
B. Magnetic resonance imaging (MRI). Used to distinguish structural brain abnormalities that may be associated with a patient's behavioral changes.
1. Measures radiofrequencies emitted by different elements in the brain following the application of an external magnetic field and produces slice images.
2. Measures structure, not function.
3. Provides much higher resolution than CT, particularly in gray matter.
4. No radiation involved; minimal or no risk to patients from strong magnetic fields.
5. Can image deep midline structures well.
6. Does not actually measure tissue density; measures density of particular nucleus being studied.
7. A major problem is the time needed to make a scan (5 to 40 minutes).
8. May offer information about cell function in the future, but stronger magnetic fields are needed.
9. The ideal technique for evaluating MS and other demyelinating diseases.

   10. MRI scans are contraindicated when the patient has a pacemaker, aneurysm clips, or ferromagnetic foreign bodies.
C. Positron emission tomography (PET)
   1. Positron emitters (e.g., carbon-11 or fluorine-18) are used to label glucose, amino acids, neurotransmitter precursors, and many other molecules (particularly high-affinity ligands), which are used to measure receptor densities.
   2. Can follow the distribution and fate of these molecules.
   3. Produces slice images, as CT does.
   4. Labeled antipsychotics can map out location and density of dopamine receptors.
   5. Dopamine receptors have been shown to decrease with age (through PET).
   6. Can assess regional brain function and blood flow.
   7. 2-Deoxyglucose (a glucose analogue) is absorbed into cells as easily as glucose but is not metabolized. Can be used to measure regional glucose uptake.
   8. Measure brain function and physiology.
   9. Potential for increasing our understanding of brain function and sites of action of drugs.
   10. Research.
      a. Usually compares laterality, anteroposterior gradients, and cortical-to-subcortical gradients.
      b. Findings reported in schizophrenia.
         (1) Cortical hypofrontality (also found in depressed patients).
         (2) Steeper subcortical-to-cortical gradient.
         (3) Uptake decreased in left compared with right cortex.
         (4) Higher rate of activity in left temporal lobe.
         (5) Lower rate of metabolism in left basal ganglia.
         (6) Higher density of dopamine receptors (replicated studies needed).
         (7) Greater increase in metabolism in anterior brain regions in response to unpleasant stimuli, but this finding is not specific to patients with schizophrenia.
         (8) Ability to differentiate between normal aging, mild cognitive impairment, and Alzheimer's disease by determining regional cerebral patterns of plaques and tangles associated with Alzheimer's disease.
D. Brain electrical activity mapping (BEAM)
   1. Topographic imaging of EEG and evoked potentials.
   2. Shows areas of varying electrical activity in the brain through scalp electrodes.
   3. New data-processing techniques produce new ways of visualizing massive quantities of data produced by EEG and evoked potentials.
   4. Each point on the map is given a numeric value representing its electrical activity.

    5. Each value is computed by linear interpolation among the three nearest electrodes.

    6. Some preliminary results show differences in schizophrenic patients. Evoked potentials differ spatially and temporally; asymmetric beta-wave activity is increased in certain regions; delta-wave activity is increased, most prominently in the frontal lobes.

E. Regional cerebral blood flow (rCBF)

    1. Yields a two-dimensional cortical image representing blood flow to different brain areas.

    2. Blood flow is believed to correlate directly with neuronal activity.

    3. Xenon-133 (radioisotope that emits low-energy gamma rays) is inhaled. Cross blood–brain barrier freely but is inert.

    4. Detectors measure rate at which xenon-133 is cleared from specific brain areas and compare with calculated control to obtain a mean transit time for the tracer.

    5. Gray matter—clears quickly.

    6. White matter—clears slowly.

    7. rCBF may have great potential in studying diseases that involve a decrease in the amount of brain tissue (e.g., dementia, ischemia, atrophy).

    8. Highly susceptible to transient artifacts (e.g., anxiety, hyperventilation, low carbon dioxide pressure, high rate of CBF).

    9. Test is fast, equipment relatively inexpensive.

    10. Low levels of radiation.

    11. Compared with PET, spatial resolution less but temporal resolution better.

    12. Preliminary data show that in schizophrenia patients, CBF in the dorsolateral frontal lobe may be decreased and CBF in the left hemisphere may be increased during activation (e.g., when subjected to the Wisconsin Card Sorting Test).

    13. No differences have been found in resting schizophrenic patients.

    14. Still under development.

F. Single-photon emission computed tomography (SPECT)

    1. Adaptation of rCBF techniques to obtain slice tomograms rather than two-dimensional surface images.

    2. Presently can obtain tomograms 2, 6, and 10 cm above and parallel to the canthomeatal line.

    3. Aids in diagnosis of Alzheimer's disease. Typically shows decreased in bilateral temporoparietal perfusion in Alzheimer's disease and single-perfusion defects or multiple areas of hypoperfusion in vascular dementia.

G. Functional MRI (fMRI)

    1. May provide functional brain images with clarity of MRI.

    2. fMRI can be correlated with high-resolution, three-dimensional MRI.

    3. Schizophrenic patients show less frontal activation and more left temporal activation during a word fluency task in comparison with controls.

    4. Used in research clinical settings in other disorders (e.g., panic disorder, phobias, and substance-related disorders).

H. Magnetic resonance spectroscopy (MRS)

1. Uses powerful magnetic fields to evaluate brain function and metabolism.
2. Provides information regarding brain intracellular pH and phospholipids, carbohydrate, protein, and high-energy phosphate metabolism.
3. Can provide information about lithium and fluorinated psychopharmacologic agents.
4. Has detected decreased adenosine triphosphate and inorganic orthophosphate levels, suggestive of dorsal prefrontal hypoactivity, in schizophrenic patients in comparison with controls.
5. Further use in research is expected with refinements in technique.

I. Magnetoencephalography

1. Research tool.
2. Uses conventional and computerized EEG data.
3. Detects magnetic fields associated with neuronal electrical activity in cortical and deep brain structures.
4. Noninvasive with no radiation exposure.

For more detailed discussion of this topic, see Chapter 1, Nuclear Magnetic Resonance Imaging, Section 1.16, p. 259, in CTP/X.

5
Major Neurocognitive Disorders

The major neurocognitive disorders consist of three conditions: (1) delirium, (2) dementia, and (3) other cognitive disorders such as Lewy body disease among others. These three categories are discussed in this chapter. Another category called major and minor neurocognitive disorder due to another medical condition is described in Chapter 6.

Cognition includes memory, language, orientation, judgment, conducting inter-personal relationships, performing actions (praxis), and problem solving. Cognitive disorders reflect disruption in one or more of these domains and are frequently complicated by behavioral symptoms.

I. Delirium

Delirium is marked by short-term confusion, acute onset of fluctuating cognitive impairment, and a disturbance of consciousness with reduced ability to attend. Delirium is a syndrome, not a disease, and it has many causes, all of which result in a similar pattern of signs and symptoms relating to the patient's level of consciousness and cognitive impairment.

A. Epidemiology

Delirium is a common disorder. About 1% of elderly persons age 55 years or older have delirium (13% in the age 85 years and older group in the community). Among elderly emergency department patients, 5% to 10% have delirium while 15% to 21% of those on admission to medical wards meet criteria for delirium. Approximately 10% to 15% of surgical patients, 30% of open-heart surgery patients, and more than 50% of patients treated for hip fractures have delirium. The highest rate of delirium is found in postcardiotomy patients—more than 90% in some studies. An estimated 20% of patients with severe burns and 30% to 40% of patients with acquired immune deficiency syndrome (AIDS) have episodes of delirium while they are hospitalized. The incidence and prevalence rates for delirium across settings are shown in Table 5-1.

B. Risk factors

1. **Advanced age.** A major risk factor for the development of delirium. Approximately 30% to 40% of hospitalized patients older than age 65 years have an episode of delirium, and another 10% to 15% of elderly persons exhibit delirium on admission to the hospital.

2. **Nursing home residents.** Of residents older than age 75 years, 60% have repeated episodes of delirium.

3. **Preexisting brain damage.** Such as dementia, cerebrovascular disease, and tumor.

4. **Other risk factors.** A history of delirium, alcohol dependence, and malnutrition.

Table 5-1
Delirium Prevalence and Incidence in Multiple Settings

Population	Prevalence Range (%)	Incidence Range (%)
General medical inpatients	10–30	3–16
Medical and surgical inpatients	10–15	10–55
General surgical inpatients	N/A	9–15 postoperatively
Critical care unit patients	16	16–83
Cardiac surgery inpatients	16–34	7–34
Orthopedic surgery patients	50	18–50
Emergency department	5–10	N/A
Terminally ill cancer patients	23–28	83
Institutionalized elderly	44	33
In the community	1–13	

N/A, not available.

5. Male gender. An independent risk factor for delirium according to DSM-5.

There are numerous predisposing risk factors for delirium. See Table 5-2.

C. Etiology. The major causes of delirium are central nervous system (CNS) disease (e.g., epilepsy), systemic disease (e.g., cardiac failure), and either intoxication or withdrawal from pharmacologic or toxic agents. When evaluating patients with delirium, clinicians should assume that any drug that a patient has taken may be etiologically relevant to the delirium. See Table 5-3. Delirium is also identified by other names, see Table 5-4.

Table 5-2
Predisposing Factors for Delirium

Demographic characteristics
Age 65 years and older
Male sex

Cognitive status
Dementia
Cognitive impairment
History of delirium
Depression

Functional status
Functional dependence
Immobility
History of falls
Low level of activity

Sensory impairment
Hearing
Visual

Decreased oral intake
Dehydration
Malnutrition

Drugs
Treatment with psychoactive drugs
Treatment with drugs with anticholinergic
   properties
Alcohol abuse

Coexisting medical conditions
Severe medical diseases
Chronic renal or hepatic disease
Stroke
Neurologic disease
Metabolic derangements
Infection with human immunodeficiency virus
Fractures or trauma
Terminal diseases

Adapted from Inouye SK. Delirium in older persons. *N Engl J Med.* 2106;354(11):1157.

Table 5-3
Precipitating Factors for Delirium

Drugs	**Surgery**
Sedative–hypnotics	Orthopedic surgery
Narcotics	Cardiac surgery
Anticholinergic drugs	Prolonged cardiopulmonary bypass
Treatment with multiple drugs	Noncardiac surgery
Alcohol or drug withdrawal	**Environmental**
Primary neurologic diseases	Admission to intensive care unit
Stroke, nondominant hemispheric	Use of physical restraints
Intracranial bleeding	Use of bladder catheter
Meningitis or encephalitis	Use of multiple procedures
	Pain
Intercurrent illnesses	Emotional stress
Infections	Prolonged sleep depravation
Iatrogenic complications	
Severe acute illness	
Hypoxia	
Shock	
Anemia	
Fever or hypothermia	
Dehydration	
Poor nutritional status	
Low serum albumin levels	
Metabolic derangements	

Adapted from Inouye SK. Delirium in older persons. *N Engl J Med.* 2106;354(11):1157.

D. Diagnosis and clinical features

The syndrome of delirium is almost always caused by one or more systemic or cerebral derangements that affect brain function. There are four subcategories based on several causes: (1) general medical condition (e.g., infection), (2) substance induced (e.g., cocaine, opioids, phencyclidine [PCP]), (3) multiple causes (e.g., head trauma and kidney disease), and (4) other or multiple etiologies (e.g., sleep deprivation, mediation). See Table 5-5.

The core features of delirium include:

1. **Altered consciousness.** Such as decreased level of consciousness.
2. **Altered attention.** Can include diminished ability to focus, sustain, or shift attention.

Table 5-4
Delirium by Other Names

Intensive care unit psychosis
Acute confusional state
Acute brain failure
Encephalitis
Encephalopathy
Toxic metabolic state
Central nervous system toxicity
Paraneoplastic limbic encephalitis
Sundowning
Cerebral insufficiency
Organic brain syndrome

Table 5-5
Common Causes of Delirium

Central nervous system disorder	Seizure (postictal, nonconvulsive status, status)
	Migraine
	Head trauma, brain tumor, subarachnoid hemorrhage, subdural, epidural hematoma, abscess, intracerebral hemorrhage, cerebellar hemorrhage, nonhemorrhagic stroke, transient ischemia
Metabolic disorder	Electrolyte abnormalities
	Diabetes, hypoglycemia, hyperglycemia, or insulin resistance
Systemic illness	Infection (e.g., sepsis, malaria, erysipelas, viral, plague, Lyme disease, syphilis, or abscess)
	Trauma
	Change in fluid status (dehydration or volume overload)
	Nutritional deficiency
	Burns
	Uncontrolled pain
	Heat stroke
	High altitude (usually >5000 m)
Medications	Pain medications (e.g., postoperative meperidine (Demerol) or morphine (Duramorph))
	Antibiotics, antivirals, and antifungals
	Steroids
	Anesthesia
	Cardiac medications
	Antihypertensives
	Antineoplastic agents
	Anticholinergic agents
	Neuroleptic malignant syndrome
Serotonin syndrome	
Over-the-counter preparations	Herbals, teas, and nutritional supplements
Botanicals	Jimsonweed, oleander, foxglove, hemlock, dieffenbachia, and *Amanita phalloides*
Cardiac	Cardiac failure, arrhythmia, myocardial infarction, cardiac assist device, cardiac surgery
Pulmonary	Chronic obstructive pulmonary disease, hypoxia, SIADH, acid–base disturbance
Endocrine	Adrenal crisis or adrenal failure, thyroid abnormality, parathyroid abnormality
Hematological	Anemia, leukemia, blood dyscrasia, stem cell transplant
Renal	Renal failure, uremia, SIADH
Hepatic	Hepatitis, cirrhosis, hepatic failure
Neoplasm	Neoplasm (primary brain, metastases, paraneoplastic syndrome)
Drugs of abuse	Intoxication and withdrawal
Toxins	Intoxication and withdrawal
	Heavy metals and aluminum

SIADH, syndrome of inappropriate secretion of antidiuretic hormone.

3. **Disorientation.** Especially to time and space.
4. **Decreased memory.**
5. **Rapid onset.** Usually hours to days.
6. **Brief duration.** Usually days to weeks.
7. **Fluctuation in sensorium.**
8. **Sometimes worse at night (sundowning)**. May range from periods of lucidity to quite severe cognitive impairment and disorganization.
9. **Disorganization of thought.** Ranging from mild tangentiality to frank incoherence.

10. **Perceptual disturbances.** Such as illusions and hallucinations.
11. **Disruption of the sleep-wake cycle.** Often manifested as fragmented sleep at night, with or without daytime drowsiness.
12. **Mood alterations.** From subtle irritability to obvious dysphoria, anxiety, or even euphoria.
13. **Altered neurological function.** E.g., autonomic hyperactivity or instability, myoclonic jerking, and dysarthria.

E. **Physical and laboratory examinations**

Delirium is usually diagnosed at the bedside and is characterized by the sudden onset of symptoms. The physical examination often reveals clues to the cause of the delirium. The presence of a known physical illness or a history of head trauma or alcohol or other substance dependence increases the likelihood of the diagnosis.

The laboratory workup of a patient with delirium should include standard tests and additional studies indicated by the clinical situation. In delirium, the EEG characteristically shows a generalized slowing of activity and may be useful in differentiating delirium from depression or psychosis. The EEG of a delirious patient sometimes shows focal areas of hyperactivity. See Tables 5-6 to 5-8.

F. **Differential diagnosis**

1. **Delirium versus dementia.** The time to development of symptoms is usually short in delirium, and, except for vascular dementia caused by stroke, it is usually gradual and insidious in dementia. A patient with dementia is usually alert; a patient with delirium has episodes of decreased consciousness. Occasionally, delirium occurs in a patient with dementia, a condition known as *beclouded dementia*. A dual diagnosis of delirium can be made when there is a definite history of pre-existing dementia. See Table 5-9.

2. **Delirium versus schizophrenia or depression.** The hallucinations and delusions of patients with schizophrenia are more constant and better organized than those of patients with delirium. Patients with hypoactive symptoms of delirium may appear somewhat similar to severely depressed patients, but they can be distinguished on the basis of an EEG.

3. **Dissociative disorders.** May show spotty amnesia but lack the global cognitive impairment and abnormal psychomotor and sleep patterns of delirium.

   For a complete list of differentiation from dementia, see Table 5-10.

G. **Course and prognosis.** The symptoms of delirium usually persist as long as the causally relevant factors are present, although delirium generally lasts less than a week. After identification and removal of the causative factors, the symptoms of delirium usually recede over a 3- to 7-day period, although some symptoms may take up to 2 weeks to resolve completely. Recall of what occurred during a delirium, once it is over, is characteristically spotty. The occurrence of delirium is associated with a high mortality rate in the ensuing year, primarily because of the serious nature of the associated medical conditions that lead to delirium. Periods of delirium

Table 5-6
Physical Examination of the Delirious Patient

Parameter	Finding	Clinical Implication
1. Pulse	Bradycardia	Hypothyroidism
		Stokes–Adams syndrome
		Increased intracranial pressure
	Tachycardia	Hyperthyroidism
		Infection
		Heart failure
2. Temperature	Fever	Sepsis
		Thyroid storm
		Vasculitis
3. Blood pressure	Hypotension	Shock
		Hypothyroidism
		Addison's disease
	Hypertension	Encephalopathy
		Intracranial mass
4. Respiration	Tachypnea	Diabetes
		Pneumonia
		Cardiac failure
		Fever
		Acidosis (metabolic)
	Shallow	Alcohol or other substance intoxication
5. Carotid vessels	Bruits or decreased pulse	Transient cerebral ischemia
6. Scalp and face	Evidence of trauma	
7. Neck	Evidence of nuchal rigidity	Meningitis
		Subarachnoid hemorrhage
8. Eyes	Papilledema	Tumor
		Hypertensive encephalopathy
	Pupillary dilatation	Anxiety
		Autonomic overactivity (e.g., delirium tremens)
9. Mouth	Tongue or cheek lacerations	Evidence of generalized tonic–clonic seizures
10. Thyroid	Enlarged	Hyperthyroidism
11. Heart	Arrhythmia	Inadequate cardiac output, possibility of emboli
	Cardiomegaly	Heart failure
		Hypertensive disease
12. Lungs	Congestion	Primary pulmonary failure
		Pulmonary edema
		Pneumonia
13. Breath	Alcohol	
	Ketones	Diabetes
14. Liver	Enlargement	Cirrhosis
		Liver failure
15. Nervous system		
a. Reflexes—muscle stretch	Asymmetry with Babinski's signs	Mass lesion
		Cerebrovascular disease
		Preexisting dementia
	Snout	Frontal mass
		Bilateral posterior cerebral artery occlusion
b. Abducent nerve (sixth cranial nerve)	Weakness in lateral gaze	Increased intracranial pressure
c. Limb strength	Asymmetrical	Mass lesion
		Cerebrovascular disease
d. Autonomic	Hyperactivity	Anxiety
		Delirium

From Strub RL, Black FW. *Neurobehavioral Disorders: A Clinical Approach.* Philadelphia, PA: FA Davis; 1981:121, with permission.

Table 5-7
Screening Laboratory Tests

General tests
Complete blood cell count
Erythrocyte sedimentation rate
Electrolytes
Glucose
Blood urea nitrogen and serum creatinine
Liver function tests
Serum calcium and phosphorus
Thyroid function tests
Serum protein
Levels of all drugs
Urinalysis
Pregnancy test for women of childbearing age
Electrocardiography

Ancillary laboratory tests
Blood
Blood cultures
Rapid plasma reagin test
Human immunodeficiency virus (HIV) testing (enzyme-linked immunosorbent assay (ELISA)
   and Western blot)
Serum heavy metals
Serum copper
Ceruloplasmin
Serum B_{12}, red blood cell (RBC) folate levels

Urine
Culture
Toxicology
Heavy metal screen

Electrography
Electroencephalography
Evoked potentials
Polysomnography
Nocturnal penile tumescence

Cerebrospinal fluid
Glucose, protein
Cell count
Cultures (bacterial, viral, fungal)
Cryptococcal antigen
Venereal Disease Research Laboratory test

Radiography
Computed tomography
Magnetic resonance imaging
Positron emission tomography
Single photon emission computed tomography

Courtesy of Eric D. Caine, M.D., and Jeffrey M. Lyness, M.D.

are sometimes followed by depression or posttraumatic stress disorder (PTSD).

1. **Treatment.** The primary goal is to treat the underlying cause. When the underlying condition is anticholinergic toxicity, the use of physostig-mine salicylate (Antilirium), 1 to 2 mg intravenously or intramuscularly, with repeated doses in 15 to 30 minutes may be indicated. Physical support is necessary so that delirious patients do not get into situations in which they may have accidents. Patients with delirium should be neither

Table 5-8
Laboratory Workup of the Patient with Delirium

Standard studies
Blood chemistries (including electrolytes, renal and hepatic indexes, and glucose)
Complete blood count with white cell differential
Thyroid function tests
Serologic tests for syphilis
Human immunodeficiency virus (HIV) antibody test
Urinalysis
Electrocardiogram
Electroencephalogram
Chest radiograph
Blood and urine drug screens
Additional tests when indicated
Blood, urine, and cerebrospinal fluid cultures
B_{12}, folic acid concentrations
Computed tomography or magnetic resonance imaging brain scan
Lumbar puncture and CSF examination

> sensory deprived nor overly stimulated by the environment. Delirium can sometimes occur in older patients wearing eye patches after cataract surgery ("black-patch delirium"). Such patients can be helped by placing pinholes in the patches to let in some stimuli or by occasionally removing one patch at a time during recovery.
>
> **2. Pharmacotherapy.** The two major symptoms of delirium that may require pharmacologic treatment are psychosis and insomnia. A commonly used drug for psychosis is haloperidol (Haldol), a butyrophenone antipsychotic drug. The initial dose may range from 2 to 6 mg intramuscularly, repeated in an hour if the patient remains agitated. The effective total daily dose of haloperidol may range from 5 to 40 mg for most patients with delirium. As soon as the patient is calm, oral medication

Table 5-9
Clinical Differentiation of Delirium and Dementia[a]

	Delirium	**Dementia**
History	Acute disease	Chronic disease
Onset	Rapid	Insidious (usually)
Duration	Days to weeks	Months to years
Course	Fluctuating	Chronically progressive
Level of consciousness	Fluctuating	Normal
Orientation	Impaired, at least periodically	Intact initially
Affect	Anxious, irritable	Labile but not usually anxious
Thinking	Often disordered	Decreased amount
Memory	Recent memory markedly impaired	Both recent and remote impaired
Perception	Hallucinations common (especially visual)	Hallucinations less common (except sundowning)
Psychomotor function	Retarded, agitated, or mixed	Normal
Sleep	Disrupted sleep–wake cycle	Less disruption of sleep–wake cycle
Attention and awareness	Prominently impaired	Less impaired
Reversibility	Often reversible	Majority not reversible

[a]Demented patients are more susceptible to delirium, and delirium superimposed on dementia is common.

Table 5-10
Frequency of Clinical Features of Delirium Contrasted with Dementia

Feature	Dementia	Delirium
Onset	Slow	Rapid
Duration	Months to years	Hours to weeks
Attention	Preserved	Fluctuates
Memory	Impaired remote memory	Impaired recent and immediate memory
Speech	Word-finding difficulty	Incoherent (slow or rapid)
Sleep–wake cycle	Fragmented sleep	Frequent disruption (e.g., day–night reversal)
Thoughts	Impoverished	Disorganized
Awareness	Unchanged	Reduced
Alertness	Usually normal	Hypervigilant or reduced vigilance

Adapted from Lipowski ZJ. *Delirium: Acute Confusional States.* Oxford: Oxford University Press; 1990.

in liquid concentrate or tablet form should begin. Droperidol (Inapsine) is a butyrophenone available as an alternative intravenous formulation, although careful monitoring of the electrocardiogram (ECG) may be prudent with this treatment. It prolongs the QTc interval and carries a black-box warning. Phenothiazines should be avoided in delirious patients because these drugs are associated with significant anticholinergic activity that may add to confusion.

Use of second-generation antipsychotics, such as risperidone (Risperdal), clozapine (Clozaril), olanzapine (Zyprexa), quetiapine (Seroquel), ziprasidone (Geodon), aripiprazole (Abilify), and asenapine (saphris) may be considered for delirium management, but clinical trial experience with these agents for delirium is limited. Insomnia is best treated with benzodiazepines with short or intermediate half-lives (e.g., lorazepam [Ativan] 1 to 2 mg at bedtime). Benzodiazepines with long half-lives and barbiturates should be avoided unless they are being used as part of the treatment for the underlying disorder (e.g., alcohol withdrawal).

Current trials are ongoing to see if dexmedetomidine (Precedex) is a more effective medication than haloperidol in the treatment of agitation and delirium in patients receiving mechanical ventilation in an intensive care unit. See Table 5-11.

II. Dementia

Dementia, also referred to as major neurocognitive disorder in DSM-5, is marked by severe impairment in memory, judgment, orientation, and cognition. The subcategories are (1) dementia of the Alzheimer's type, which usually occurs in persons older than 65 years of age and is manifested by progressive intellectual disorientation and dementia, delusions, or depression; (2) vascular dementia, caused by vessel thrombosis or hemorrhage; (3) human immunodeficiency virus (HIV) disease; (4) head trauma; (5) Pick's disease or frontotemporal lobar degeneration; (6) Prion disease such as Creutzfeldt–Jakob disease, which is caused by a slow-growing transmittable virus; (7) substance induced, caused by toxin or medication (e.g., gasoline

Table 5-11
Pharmacologic Treatment

Pharmacologic Agent	Dosage	Side Effects	Comments
Typical antipsychotics			
Haloperidol (Haldol)	0.5–1 mg p.o. 2×/day (may be given every 4–6 hours as needed, too)	Extrapyramidal side (EPS) effects Prolonged QTc	Most commonly used Can be given intramuscularly
Atypical antipsychotics		All can prolong QTc duration	
Risperidone (Risperdal)	0.5–1 mg/day	EPS concerns	Limited data in delirium
Olanzapine (Zyprexa)	5–10 mg/day	Metabolic syndrome	Higher mortality in dementia patients
Quetiapine (Seroquel)	25–150 mg/day	More sedating	
Benzodiazepine			
Lorazepam (Ativan)	0.5–3 mg/day and as needed every 4 hours	Respiratory depression, paradoxical agitation	Best use in delirium secondary to alcohol or benzodiazepine withdrawal Can worsen delirium

fumes, atropine); (8) multiple etiologies; and (9) not specified (if cause is unknown).

A. **Epidemiology.** The prevalence of dementia is rising. The prevalence of moderate to severe dementia in different population groups is approximately 5% in the general population older than 65 years of age, 20% to 40% in the general population older than 85 years of age, 15% to 20% in outpatient general medical practices, and 50% in chronic care facilities. Of all patients with dementia, 50% to 60% have the most common type of dementia, dementia of the Alzheimer's type (Alzheimer's disease). The second most common type of dementia is vascular dementia, which is causally related to cerebrovascular diseases. Other common causes of dementia, each representing 1% to 5% of all cases, include head trauma, alcohol-related dementias, and various movement disorder–related dementias, such as Huntington's disease and Parkinson's disease. See Table 5-12.

B. **Etiology.** The most common causes of dementia in individuals older than 65 years of age are (1) Alzheimer's disease, (2) vascular dementia, and (3) mixed vascular and Alzheimer's dementia. Other illnesses that account for approximately 10% include Lewy body dementia; Pick's disease; frontotemporal dementias; normal-pressure hydrocephalus (NPH); alcoholic dementia; infectious dementia, such as that due to infection with HIV or syphilis; and Parkinson's disease.

C. **Diagnosis, signs, and symptoms.** The major defects in dementia involve orientation, memory, perception, intellectual functioning, and reasoning. Marked changes in personality, affect, and behavior can occur. Dementias are commonly accompanied by hallucinations (20% to 30% of patients) and delusions (30% to 40%). Symptoms of depression and anxiety are

Table 5-12
Causes of Dementia

Tumor Primary cerebral[a]	**Physiologic** Epilepsy[a] Normal-pressure hydrocephalus[a]
Trauma Hematomas[a] Posttraumatic dementia[a]	**Metabolic** Vitamin deficiencies[a] Chronic metabolic disturbances[a]
Infection (chronic) Metastatic[a] Syphilis Creutzfeldt–Jakob disease[b] AIDS dementio complex[c]	Chronic anoxic states[a] Chronic endocrinopathies[a] **Degenerative dementias** Alzheimer's disease[b] Pick's disease (dementias of frontal lobe type)[b] Parkinson's disease[a]
Cardiac/vascular Single infarction[a] Multiple infarctions[b] Large infarction Locunar infarction Binswanger's disease (subcortical arteriosclerotic encephalopathies) Hemodynamic type[a]	Progressive supranuclear palsy[c] Idiopathic cerebral ferrocalcinosis (Fahr's disease)[c] Wilson's disease[a] **Demyellinating disease** Multiple sclerosis[c] **Drugs and toxins** Alcohol[a]
Congenital/hereditary Huntington's disease[c] Metachromatic leukodystrophy[c]	Heavy metals[a] Carbon monoxide poisoning[a] Medications[a] Irradiation[a]
Primary psychiatric Pseudodementia[a]	

[a]Variable or mixed pattern.
[b]Predominantly cortical pattern.
[c]Predominantly subcortical pattern.
Table by Eric D. Caine, M.D., Hillel Grossman, M.D., and Jeffrey M. Lyness, M.D.

present in 40% to 50% of patients with dementia. Dementia is diagnosed according to etiology (Table 5-13).

D. Laboratory tests. First, identify a potentially reversible cause for the dementia, and then identify other treatable medical conditions that may otherwise worsen the dementia (cognitive decline is often precipitated by other medical illness). The workup should include vital signs, complete blood cell count with differential sedimentation rate (ESR), complete blood chemistries, serum B_{12} and folate levels, liver and renal function tests, thyroid function tests, urinalysis, urine toxicology, ECG, chest roentgenography, computed tomography (CT) or magnetic resonance imaging (MRI) of the head, and lumbar puncture. Single-photon emission computed tomography (SPECT) can be used to detect patterns of brain metabolism in certain types of dementia. See Table 5-14.

E. Differential diagnosis

1. Age-associated memory impairment (normal aging). There is a decreased ability to learn new material and a slowing of thought processes as a consequence of normal aging. In addition, there is a syndrome of benign senescent forgetfulness, which does not show a progressively deteriorating course.

Table 5-13
Possible Etiologies of Dementia

Degenerative dementias
Alzheimer's disease
Frontotemporal dementias (e.g., Pick's disease)
Parkinson's disease
Lewy body dementia
Idiopathic cerebral ferrocalcinosis (Fahr's disease)
Progressive supranuclear palsy

Miscellaneous
Huntington's disease
Wilson's disease
Metachromatic leukodystrophy
Neuroacanthocytosis

Psychiatric
Pseudodementia of depression
Cognitive decline in late-life schizophrenia

Physiologic
Normal-pressure hydrocephalus

Metabolic
Vitamin deficiencies (e.g., vitamin B_{12}, folate)
Endocrinopathies (e.g., hypothyroidism)
Chronic metabolic disturbances (e.g., uremia)

Tumor
Primary or metastatic (e.g., meningioma or metastatic breast or lung cancer)

Traumatic
Dementia pugilistica, posttraumatic dementia
Subdural hematoma

Infection
Prion diseases (e.g., Creutzfeldt–Jakob disease, bovine spongiform encephalitis,
    Gerstmann–Sträussler syndrome)
Acquired immune deficiency syndrome (AIDS)
Syphilis

Cardiac, vascular, and anoxia
Infarction (single or multiple or strategic lacunar)
Binswanger's disease (subcortical arteriosclerotic encephalopathy)
Hemodynamic insufficiency (e.g., hypoperfusion or hypoxia)

Demyelinating diseases
Multiple sclerosis

Drugs and toxins
Alcohol
Heavy metals
Irradiation
Pseudodementia due to medications (e.g., anticholinergics)
Carbon monoxide

2. **Depression.** Depression in the elderly may present as symptoms of cognitive impairment, which has led to the term *pseudodementia* (Table 5-15).

The apparently demented patient is really depressed and responds well to antidepressant drugs or electroconvulsive therapy (ECT). Many demented patients also become depressed as they begin to comprehend their progressive cognitive impairment. In patients with both dementia

Table 5-14
Comprehensive Workup of Dementia

Physical examination, including thorough neurologic examination
Vital signs
Mental status examination
Review of medications and drug levels
Blood and urine screens for alcohol, drugs, and heavy metals[a]
Physiologic workup
   Serum electrolytes/glucose/Ca^{++}, Mg^{++}
   Liver, renal function tests
   SMA-12 or equivalent serum chemistry profile
   Urinalysis
   Complete blood cell count with differential cell type count
   Thyroid function tests (including TSH level)
   RPR (serum screen)
   FTA-ABS (if CNS disease suspected)
   Serum B_{12}
   Folate levels
   Urine corticosteroids[a]
   Erythrocyte sedimentation rate (Westergren)
   Antinuclear antibody[a] (ANA), C_3C_4, Anti-DS DNA[a]
   Arterial blood gases[a]
   HIV screen[a,b]
   Urine porphobilinogens[a]
Chest radiograph
Electrocardiogram
Neurologic workup
   CT or MRI of head[a]
   SPECT[b]
   Lumbar puncture[a]
   EEG[a]
   Neuropsychological testing[c]

[a]All indicated by history and physical examination.
[b]Requires special consent and counseling.
[c]May be useful in differentiating dementia from other neuropsychiatric syndromes if it cannot be done clinically.
Adapted from Stoudemire A, Thompson TL. Recognizing and treating dementia. *Geriatrics* 1981;36:112.

and depression, a treatment trial with antidepressants is often warranted. ECT may be of help in refractory cases. Table 5-16 differentiates dementia from depression.

3. **Delirium.** Also characterized by global cognitive impairment. Demented patients often have a superimposed delirium. Dementia tends to be chronic and lacks the prominent features of rapid fluctuations, sudden onset, impaired attention, changing level of consciousness, psychomotor disturbance, acutely disturbed sleep–wake cycle, and prominent hallucinations or delusions that characterize delirium.

F. **Course and prognosis.** Dementia may be progressive, remitting, or stable. Because about 15% of dementias are reversible (e.g., hypothyroidism, CNS syphilis, subdural hematoma, vitamin B_{12} deficiency, uremia, hypoxia), the course in these cases depends on how quickly the cause is reversed. If the cause is reversed too late, the patient may have residual deficits with a subsequently stable course if extensive brain damage has not occurred. For

Table 5-15
Major Clinical Features Differentiating Pseudodementia from Dementia

Pseudodementia	Dementia
Clinical course and history	
Family always aware of dysfunction and its severity	Family often unaware of dysfunction and its severity
Onset can be dated with some precision	Onset can be dated only within broad limits
Symptoms of short duration before medical help is sought	Symptoms usually of long duration before medical help is sought
Rapid progression of symptoms after onset	Slow progression of symptoms throughout course
History of previous psychiatric dysfunction common	History of previous psychiatric dysfunction unusual
Complaints and clinical behavior	
Patients usually complain much of cognitive loss	Patients usually complain little of cognitive loss
Patients' complaints of cognitive dysfunction usually detailed	Patients' complaints of cognitive dysfunction usually vague
Patients emphasize disability	Patients conceal disability
Patients highlight failures	Patients delight in accomplishments, however trivial
Patients make little effort to perform even simple tasks	Patients struggle to perform tasks
	Patients rely on notes, calendars, and so on to keep up
Patients usually communicate strong sense of distress	Patients often appear unconcerned
Affective change often pervasive	Affect labile and shallow
Loss of social skills often early and prominent	Social skills often retained
Behavior often incongruent with severity of cognitive dysfunction	Behavior usually compatible with severity of cognitive dysfunction
Nocturnal accentuation of dysfunction uncommon	Nocturnal accentuation of dysfunction common
Clinical features related to memory, cognitive, and intellectual dysfunctions	
Attention and concentration often well preserved	Attention and concentration usually faulty
"Don't know" answers typical	Near-miss answers frequent
On tests of orientation, patients often give "don't know" answers	On tests of orientation, patients often mistake unusual for usual
Memory loss for recent and remote events usually severe	Memory loss for recent events usually more severe than for remote events
Memory gaps for specific periods or events common	Memory gaps for specific periods unusual[a]
Marked variability in performance on tasks of similar difficulty	Consistently poor performance on tasks of similar difficulty

[a]Except when caused by delirium, trauma, seizures, and so on.
Reprinted with permission from Wells CE. Pseudodementia. *Am J Psychiatry*. 1979;136:898.

dementia with no identifiable cause (e.g., dementia of the Alzheimer's type), the course is likely to be one of slow deterioration. The patient may become lost in familiar places, lose the ability to handle money, later fail to recognize family members, and eventually become incontinent of stool and urine.

G. Treatment. Treatment is generally supportive. Ensure proper treatment of any concurrent medical problems. Maintain proper nutrition, exercise, and activities. Provide an environment with frequent cues for orientation to day, date, place, and time. As functioning decreases, nursing home placement may be necessary. Often, cognitive impairment may become

Table 5-16
Dementia Versus Depression

Feature	Dementia	Pseudodementia
Age	Usually elderly	Nonspecific
Onset	Vague	Days to weeks
Course	Slow, worse at night	Rapid, even through day
History	Systemic illness or drugs	Mood disorder
Awareness	Unaware, unconcerned	Aware, distressed
Organic signs	Often present	Absent
Cognition[a]	Prominent impairment	Personality changes
Mental status examination	Consistent, spotty deficits	Variable deficits in different modalities
	Approximates, confabulates, perseverates	Apathetic, "I don't know"
	Emphasizes trivial accomplishments	Emphasizes failures
	Shallow or stable mood	Depressed
Behavior	Appropriate to degree of cognitive impairment	Incongruent with degree of cognitive impairment
Cooperation	Cooperative but frustrated	Uncooperative with little effort
CT and EEG	Abnormal	Normal

[a]Benzodiazepines and barbiturates worsen cognitive impairments in the demented patient, whereas they help the depressed patient to relax.

worse at night (sundowning). Some nursing homes have successfully developed a schedule of nighttime activities to help manage this problem.

1. **Psychological.** Supportive therapy, group therapy, and referral to organizations for families of demented patients can help them to cope and feel less frustrated and helpless.

2. **Pharmacologic.** In general, barbiturates and benzodiazepines should be avoided because they can worsen cognition. For agitation, low doses of an antipsychotic may be effective (e.g., 2 mg of haloperidol orally or intramuscularly or 0.25 to 1.0 mg of risperidone per day orally). However, black-box warnings have been issued for conventional and atypical antipsychotics alerting clinicians to reports of elevated mortality in demented, agitated elderly patients treated with these agents. Some studies also question their efficacy. Practice is evolving in this area as few alternatives are available. When using antipsychotics, use the lowest effective dose and review progress frequently. Some clinicians suggest a short-acting benzodiazepine for sleep (e.g., 0.25 mg of triazolam [Halcion] orally), but this may cause further memory deficits the next day.

III. Dementia of the Alzheimer's Type (DAT)

  A. Definition. A progressive dementia in which all known reversible causes have been ruled out. Two types—with late onset (onset after age 65) and with early onset (onset before or at age 65).

  B. Diagnosis, signs, and symptoms. Multiple cognitive deficits with behavioral disturbances. See Table 5-17.

  C. Epidemiology. Most common cause of dementia. DAT accounts for 50% to 60% of all dementias. May affect as many as 5% of persons over age 65 and 15% to 20% of persons age 85 or older. Risk factors include female sex, history of head injury, and having a first-degree relative with the disorder.

Table 5-17
Clinical Criteria for Dementia of the Alzheimer's Type (DAT)

Memory loss
Inability to learn nee material
Steady decline in cognition
Long-term memory affected
Abstract thinking impaired
Language impairment
Insidious onset
Judgment impaired
Agnosia
Apraxia
Behavioral changes, e.g.,
  Paranoia
  Agitation
  Anxiety
  Depression
Visuospatial skills impaired
Progressive course

Incidence increases with age. Patients with DAT occupy more than 50% of nursing home beds.

D. Etiology. Genetic factors play a role; up to 40% of patients have a family history of DAT. Concordance rate for monozygotic twins is 43%, versus 8% for dizygotic twins. Several cases have documented autosomal dominant transmission. Down syndrome is associated with DAT. The gene for amyloid precursor protein on chromosome 21 may be involved. The neurotransmitters most often implicated are acetylcholine and norepinephrine. Both are believed to be hypoactive. Degeneration of cholinergic neurons in the nucleus basalis of Meynert in addition to decreased brain concentrations of acetylcholine and its key synthetic enzyme choline acetyltransferase have been noted. Further evidence for a cholinergic hypothesis includes the beneficial effects of cholinesterase inhibitors and the further impairment of cognition associated with anticholinergics. Some evidence has been found of a decrease in norepinephrine-containing neurons in the locus ceruleus. Decreased levels of corticotropin and somatostatin may also be involved. Other proposed causes include abnormal regulation of cell membrane phospholipid metabolism, aluminum toxicity, and abnormal brain glutamate metabolism.

E. Neuropathology. The characteristic neuropathologic changes, first described by Alois Alzheimer, are neurofibrillary tangles, senile plaques, and granulovacuolar degenerations. These changes can also appear with normal aging, but they are always present in the brains of DAT patients. They are most prominent in the amygdala, hippocampus, cortex, and basal forebrain. A definitive diagnosis of Alzheimer's disease can be made only by histopathology. The aluminum toxicity etiologic theory is based on the fact that these pathologic structures in the brain contain high amounts of aluminum. The clinical diagnosis of DAT should be considered only either possible or probable in Alzheimer's disease. Other abnormalities that have been found in DAT patients include diffuse cortical atrophy on CT or MRI, enlarged ventricles, and decreased brain acetylcholine metabolism.

Table 5-18
Approved Medications for Alzheimer's Disease

Medication	Preparations	Initial Dosage	Maintenance Dosage	Comment
Tacrine (Cognex)	10-, 20-, 30-, and 40-mg capsules	10 mg 4×/day	30 or 40 mg 4×/day	Reversible direct hepatotoxicity in approximately one-third of patients, requiring initial biweekly transaminase monitoring. Not commonly used.
Donepezil (Aricept)	5- and 10-mg tablets	5 mg/day	5–10 mg/day	10 mg may be somewhat more efficacious, but with more adverse effects.
Rivastigmine (Exelon)	1.5-, 3.0-, 4.5-, and 6.0-mg capsules	1.5 mg 2×/day	3.0, 4.5, or 6.0 mg 2×/day	Doses of 4.5 mg 2×/day may be most optimal. May be taken with food.
Galatamine (Reminyl)	4-, 8-, and 12-mg capsules; solution, 4 mg per mL	4 mg 2×/day	8 or 12 mg 2×/day	8 mg 2×/day has fewer adverse events.
Memantine (Namenda)	5- and 10-mg tablets	5 mg per day	10 mg 2×/day	10 mg per day was effective in a trial in nursing home patients.
Rivastigmine (Exelon)	4.6 mg/24 h, 9.5 mg/24 h and 13.3 mg/24 h transdermal patch	4.6 mg/24 h	Increase after 4 weeks to 9.5 mg/24 h	In severe Alzheimer's disease can be increased to 13.3 mg/24 h

The finding of low levels of acetylcholine explains why these patients are highly susceptible to the effects of anticholinergic medication and has led to development of choline-replacement strategies for treatment.

F. Course and prognosis

1. Onset usually insidious in a person's 50s or 60s; slowly progressive.
2. Aphasia, apraxia, and agnosia often present after several years.
3. Motor and gait disturbances may develop later; patient may become bedridden.
4. Mean survival is 8 years; ranges from 1 to 20 years.

G. Treatment. Donepezil (Aricept), rivastigmine (Exelon), galatamine (Remynal), and tacrine (Cognex) are cholinesterase inhibitors. These drugs can enhance cognition and slow the cognitive decline in some patients with mild to moderate Alzheimer's disease. The most recently introduced drug, mementine (Namenda), acts on glutamate receptors. None of these alters the underlying disease process. Tacrine is rarely used because of liver toxicity. See Table 5-18.

IV. Vascular Dementia

A. Definition. The second most common type of dementia is that resulting from cerebrovascular disease. Vascular dementia usually progresses in a stepwise fashion with each recurrent infarct. Some patients notice one specific moment when their functioning became worse and improved slightly over subsequent days until their next infarct. Other patients have a progressively downhill course.

   1. Binswanger's disease

      Binswanger's disease, also known as *subcortical arteriosclerotic encephalopathy,* is characterized by the presence of many small infarctions of the white matter that spare the cortical regions Although Binswanger's disease was previously considered a rare condition, the advent of sophisticated and powerful imaging techniques, such as MRI, has revealed that the condition is more common than previously thought.

B. Diagnosis, signs, and symptoms. Multiple cognitive impairments and behavioral changes are present. Neurologic signs are common; small- and medium-sized cerebral vessels are usually affected. Infarcts may be caused by occlusive plaque or thromboembolism. Physical findings may include carotid bruit, funduscopic abnormalities, and enlarged cerebral chambers. Cognitive impairment may be patchy, with some areas intact. See Table 5-13.

C. Epidemiology. This accounts for 15% to 30% of all dementias, most common in persons 60 to 70 years of age and is less common than DAT. It is more common in men than in women and onset is at an earlier age than onset of DAT. Risk factors include hypertension, heart disease, and other risk factors for stroke.

D. Laboratory tests. CT or MRI will show infarcts.

E. Differential diagnosis

   1. DAT. Vascular dementia may be difficult to differentiate from DAT. Obtain a good history of the course of the disease, noting whether the onset was abrupt, whether the course was insidious or stepwise, and whether neurologic impairment was present. Identify vascular disease risk factors and obtain brain image. If a patient has features of both vascular dementia and DAT, then the diagnosis should be dementia with multiple causes.

   2. Depression. Patients with vascular dementia may become depressed, like patients with pseudodementia, as previously described. Depression is unlikely to produce focal neurologic findings. If present, depression should be diagnosed and treated.

   3. Strokes and transient ischemic attacks (TIAs). Generally do not lead to a progressively demented patient. TIAs are brief episodes of focal neurologic dysfunction lasting less than 24 hours (usually 5 to 15 minutes). A patient with a completed stroke may have some cognitive deficits, but unless the loss of brain tissue is massive, a single stroke generally will not cause dementia.

F. Treatment. The treatment is to identify and reverse the cause of the strokes. Hypertension, diabetes, and cardiac disease must be treated. Nursing home placement may be necessary if impairment is severe. Treatment is supportive and symptomatic. Antidepressants, psychostimulants, antipsychotic medication, and benzodiazepines can be used, but any psychoactive drug may cause adverse effects in a brain-damaged patient.

V. Frontotemporal Dementia (Pick's Disease)
This relatively rare primary degenerative dementia is clinically similar to DAT. Pick's disease accounts for approximately 5% of all irreversible dementias. The frontal lobe is prominently involved, and frontal signs of disinhibited behavior may present early. With a relative preservation of cognitive functions, Klüver–Bucy syndrome (hypersexuality, hyperorality, and placidity) is more common in Pick's disease than in DAT. The frontal and temporal lobes show atrophy, neuronal loss, gliosis, and intraneural deposits called *Pick's bodies*. The diagnosis often is made at autopsy, although CT or MRI can reveal prominent frontal lobe involvement.

VI. Huntington's Disease
  A. Definition. A genetic autosomal dominant disease with complete penetrance (chromosome 4) characterized by choreoathetoid movement and dementia. The chance for the development of the disease in a person who has one parent with Huntington's disease is 50%.
  B. Diagnosis. Onset usually is in a patient's 30s to 40s (the patient frequently already has children). Choreiform movements usually present first and become progressively more severe. Dementia presents later, often with psychotic features. Dementia may first be described by the patient's family as a personality change. Look for a family history.
  C. Associated psychiatric symptoms and complications
    1. Personality changes (25%).
    2. Schizophreniform (25%).
    3. Mood disorder (50%).
    4. Presentation with sudden-onset dementia (25%).
    5. Development of dementia in 90% of patients.
  D. Epidemiology. Incidence is two to six cases a year per 100,000 persons. More than 1,000 cases have been traced to two brothers who immigrated to Long Island from England. Incidence is equal in men and women.
  E. Pathophysiology. Atrophy of brain with extensive involvement of the basal ganglia and the caudate nucleus in particular.
  F. Differential diagnosis. When choreiform movements are first noted, they are often misinterpreted as inconsequential habit spasms or tics. Up to 75% of patients with Huntington's disease are initially misdiagnosed with a primary psychiatric disorder. Features distinguishing it from DAT are the high incidence of depression and psychosis and the classic choreoathetoid movement disorder.
  G. Course and prognosis. The course is progressive and usually leads to death 15 to 20 years after diagnosis. Suicide is common.
  H. Treatment. Institutionalization may be needed as chorea progresses. Symptoms of insomnia, anxiety, and depression can be relieved with benzodiazepines and antidepressants. Psychotic symptoms can be treated

with antipsychotic medication, usually of the atypical or second-generation group. Genetic counseling is the most important intervention.

VII. Parkinson's Disease

A. Definition. An idiopathic movement disorder with onset usually late in life, characterized by bradykinesia, resting tremor, pill-rolling tremor, masklike face, cogwheel rigidity, and shuffling gait. Intellectual impairment is common, and 40% to 80% of patients become demented. Depression is extremely common.

B. Epidemiology. Annual prevalence in the Western Hemisphere is 200 cases per 100,000 persons.

C. Etiology. Unknown for most patients. Characteristic findings are decreased cells in the substantia nigra, decreased dopamine, and degeneration of dopaminergic tracts. Parkinsonism can be caused by repeated head trauma and a contaminant of an illicitly made synthetic heroin, *N*-methyl-4-phenyl-1,2,3,6-tetrahydropyridine (MPTP).

D. Treatment. Levodopa (Larodopa) is a dopamine precursor and is often prepared with carbidopa (Sinemet), a dopa decarboxylase inhibitor, to increase brain dopamine levels. Amantadine (Symadine) has also been used synergistically with levodopa. Some surgeons have tried implanting adrenal medulla tissue into the brain to produce dopamine, with equivocal results. Depression is treatable with antidepressants or ECT.

VIII. Lewy Body Disease

Lewy body disease is a dementia clinically similar to Alzheimer's disease and often characterized by hallucinations, parkinsonian features, and extrapyramidal signs (Table 5-19). Lewy inclusion bodies are found in the cerebral cortex (Table 5-20). The exact incidence is unknown. These patients

Table 5-19
Clinical Criteria for Dementia with Lewy Bodies (DLB)

The patient must have sufficient cognitive decline to interfere with social or occupational functioning. Of note early in the illness, memory symptoms may not be as prominent as attention, frontosubcortical skills, and visuospatial ability. Probable DLB requires two or more core symptoms, whereas possible DLB only requires one core symptom.

Core features
Fluctuating levels of attention and alertness
Recurrent visual hallucinations
Parkinsonian features (cogwheeling, bradykinesia, and resting tremor)

Supporting features
Repeated falls
Syncope
Sensitivity to neuroleptics
Systematized delusions
Hallucinations in other modalities (e.g., auditory, tactile)

Adapted from McKeith LG, Galasko D, Kosaka K. Consensus guidelines for the clinical and pathologic diagnosis of dementia with Lewy bodies (DLB): Report of the consortium on DLB international workshop. *Neurology.* 1996;47:1113–1124.

Table 5-20
Distinguishing Features of Subcortical and Cortical Dementias

Characteristic	Subcortical Dementia	Cortical Dementia	Recommended Tests
Language	No aphasia (anomia, if severe)	Aphasia early	Fast Scale Administration (FAS) test Boston Naming test WAIS-R vocabulary test
Memory	Impaired recall (retrieval) > recognition (encoding)	Recall and recognition impaired	Wechsler memory scale; Symbol Digit Paired Associate Learning (Brandt)
Attention and immediate recall	Impaired	Impaired	WAIS-R digit span
Visuospatial skills	Impaired	Impaired	Picture arrangement, object assembly and block design; WAIS subtests
Calculation	Preserved until late	Involved early	Mini-Mental State
Frontal system abilities (executive function)	Disproportionately affected	Degree of impairment consistent with other involvement	Wisconsin Card Sorting Test; Odd Man Out test; Picture Absurdities
Speed of cognitive processing	Slowed early	Normal until late in disease	Trail making A and B: Paced Auditory Serial Addition Test (PASAT)
Personality	Apathetic, inert	Unconcerned	MMPI
Mood	Depressed	Euthymic	Beck and Hamilton depression scales
Speech	Dysarthric	Articulate until late	Verbal fluency (Rosen, 1980)
Posture	Bowed or extended	Upright	
Coordination	Impaired	Normal until late	
Motor speed and control	Slowed	Normal	Finger-tap; grooved pegboard
Adventitious movements	Chorea, tremor tics, dystonia	Absent (Alzheimer's dementia—some myoclonus)	
Abstraction	Impaired	Impaired	Category test (Halstead Battery)

From Pajeau AK, Román GC. HIV encephalopathy and dementia. In: J Biller, RG Kathol, eds. *The Psychiatric Clinics of North America: The Interface of Psychiatry and Neurology.* Vol. 15. Philadelphia, PA: WB Saunders; 1992:457.

often have Capgras syndrome (reduplicative paramnesia) as party of the clinical picture.

IX. HIV-Related Dementia

HIV encephalopathy is associated with dementia and is termed *acquired immune deficiency syndrome* (AIDS) *dementia complex,* or *HIV dementia.* The annual rate of HIV dementia is approximately 14%. An estimated 75% of patients with AIDS have involvement of the CNS at the time of autopsy. This finding is often paralleled by the appearance of parenchymal abnormalities on MRI scans. Other infectious dementias are caused by *Cryptococcus* or *Treponema pallidum.*

Table 5-21
Criteria for Clinical Diagnosis of HIV Type 1–Associated Dementia Complex

Laboratory evidence for systemic human immunodeficiency virus (HIV) type 1 infection with confirmation by Western blot, polymerase chain reaction, or culture.

Acquired abnormality in at least *two* cognitive abilities for a period of at least 1 month: attention and concentration, speed of processing information, abstraction and reasoning, visuospatial skills, memory and learning, and speech and language. The decline should be verified by reliable history and mental status examination. History should be obtained from an informant, and examination should be supplemented by neuropsychological testing.

Cognitive dysfunction causes impairment in social or occupational functioning. Impairment should not be attributable solely to severe systemic illness.

At least *one* of the following:

Acquired abnormality in motor function verified by clinical examination (e.g., slowed rapid movements, abnormal gait, incoordination, hyperreflexia, hypertonia, or weakness), neuropsychological tests (e.g., fine motor speed, manual dexterity, or perceptual motor skills), or both.

Decline in motivation or emotional control or a change in social behavior. This may be characterized by a change in personality with apathy, inertia, irritability, emotional lability, or a new onset of impaired judgment or disinhibition.

This does not exclusively occur in the context of a delirium.

Evidence of another etiology, including active central nervous system opportunistic infection, malignancy, psychiatric disorders (e.g., major depression), or substance abuse, if present, is *not* the cause of the previously mentioned symptoms and signs.

Adapted from Working Group of the American Academy of Neurology AIDS Task Force. Nomenclature and research case definitions for neurologic manifestations of human immunodeficiency virus–type 1 (HIV-1) infection. *Neurology.* 1991;41:778–785.

The diagnosis of AIDS dementia complex is made by confirmation of HIV infection and exclusion of alternative pathology to explain cognitive impairment. The American Academy of Neurology AIDS Task Force research criteria in adults and adolescents are listed in Table 5-21. The criteria for AIDS dementia complex require laboratory evidence for systemic HIV, at least two cognitive deficits, and the presence of motor abnormalities or personality changes. Cognitive, motor, and behavioral changes are assessed using physical, neurologic, and psychiatric examinations, in addition to neuropsychological testing.

X. Head Trauma-Related Dementia

Dementia can be a sequela of head trauma. The so-called punch-drunk syndrome (dementia pugilistica) occurs in boxers after repeated head trauma over many years. It is characterized by emotional lability, dysarthria, and impulsivity. It has also been observed in professional football players who developed dementia after repeated concussions over many years.

XI. Substance-Induced Persisting Dementia

To make the diagnosis of alcohol-induced persisting dementia, the criteria for dementia must be met. Because amnesia can also occur in the context of Korsakoff's psychosis, it is important to distinguish between memory impairment accompanied by other cognitive deficits (i.e., dementia) and amnesia caused by thiamine deficiency. Other cognitive functions, such as attention and concentration, may also be impaired in Wernicke–Korsakoff syndrome. In addition, alcohol abuse is frequently associated with mood changes, so poor concentration and other cognitive symptoms often observed in the context of a major depression must also be ruled out. Alcohol-related dementia has been estimated to account for approximately 4% of dementias.

XII. Other Dementias

Other dementias include those associated with Wilson's disease, supranuclear palsy, NPH (dementia, ataxia, incontinence), and brain tumors.

Systemic causes of dementia include thyroid disease, pituitary diseases (Addison's disease and Cushing's disease), liver failure, dialysis, nicotinic acid deficiency (pellagra causes the three Ds: dementia, dermatitis, diarrhea), vitamin B_{12} deficiency, folate deficiency, infections, heavy-metal intoxication, and chronic alcohol abuse.

For more detailed discussion of this topic, see Delirium, Section 10.2, p. 1178, and Section 57.3g, p. 4008, for Dementia, Section 10.3, p. 1191 and for Alzheimer Disease and Other Neurocognitive Disorders, Section 57.3f, p. 4078 in CTP/X.

6

Major or Minor Neurocognitive Disorder Due to Another Medical Condition (Amnestic Disorder)

This chapter *Major or Minor Neurocognitive Disorder Due to Another Medical Condition* was previously classified as amnestic disorder in the last edition of the *Diagnostic and Statistical Manual of Mental Disorders* (DSM-IV-TR) because each of the disorders described below is associated with amnesia.

I. Introduction
These disorders are a broad category that includes a variety of diseases and conditions that present with amnesia or loss of memory.

II. Epidemiology
A. No adequate studies have reported on incidence or prevalence.
B. Most commonly found in alcohol-use disorders and in head injury.
C. Frequency of amnesia related to chronic alcohol abuse has decreased, and the frequency of amnesia related to head trauma has increased.

III. Etiology
The most common form is caused by thiamine deficiency associated with alcohol dependence. It may also result from head trauma, surgery, hypoxia, infarction, and herpes simplex encephalitis. Typically, any process that damages certain diencephalic and medial temporal structures (e.g., mammillary bodies, fornix, and hippocampus) can cause the disorder. See Table 6-1.

IV. Diagnosis, Signs, and Symptoms
The essential feature is the acquired impaired ability to learn and recall new information coupled with the inability to recall past events. Impaired recent, short-term memory and long-term memory are caused by systemic medical or primary cerebral disease. Patient is normal in other areas of cognition.

These disorders are diagnosed according to their etiology: disorder resulting from a general medical condition, those caused by substances, and NOS.

V. Clinical Features and Subtypes
A. Impairment in the ability to learn new information (anterograde amnesia).
B. The inability to recall previously remembered knowledge (retrograde amnesia).
C. Short-term and recent memory are usually impaired and patients cannot remember what they had for breakfast or lunch or the name of the doctors.

Table 6-1
Major Causes of Neurocognitive Disorders due to Another Medical Condition

Thiamine deficiency (Korsakoff's syndrome)
Hypoglycemia
Primary brain conditions
Seizures
Head trauma (closed and penetrating)
Cerebral tumors (especially thalamic and temporal lobe)
Cerebrovascular diseases (especially thalamic and temporal lobe)
Surgical procedures on the brain
Encephalitis due to herpes simplex
Hypoxia (including nonfatal hanging attempts and carbon monoxide poisoning)
Transient global amnesia
Electroconvulsive therapy
Multiple sclerosis
Substance-related causes
Alcohol use disorders
Neurotoxins
Benzodiazepines (and other sedative-hypnotics)
Many over-the-counter preparations

D. Memory for over-learned information or events from the remote past, such as childhood experiences, is preserved, but memory for events from the less remote past (the past decade) is impaired.

E. The onset of symptoms can be sudden, as in trauma, cerebrovascular events, and neurotoxic chemical assaults, or gradual, as in nutritional deficiency and cerebral tumors. The amnesia can be of short duration specified by DSM-5 as transient if less than 1 month, or chronic if lasting more than 1 month.

F. Subtle and gross changes in personality can occur and patients maybe apathetic, lack initiative, have unprovoked episodes of agitation, or appear to be overly friendly or agreeable. Patients with these disorders can also appear bewildered and confused, and may attempt to cover their confusion with confabulatory answers to questions.

G. Patients with these disorders do not have good insight into their neuropsychiatric conditions.

VI. Pathophysiology

A. Structures involved in memory loss include diencephalic structures, such as dorsomedial and midline nuclei of the thalamus and mid-temporal lobe structures such as the hippocampus, the mammillary bodies, and the amygdala.

B. Amnesia is usually the result of bilateral damage to these structures, and left hemisphere may be more critical than the right hemisphere in the development of memory disorders. Many studies of memory and amnesia in animals have suggested that other brain areas may also be involved in the symptoms accompanying amnesia.

C. Frontal lobe involvement can result in such symptoms as confabulation and apathy, which can be seen in patients with amnestic disorders.

VII. Treatment

Identify the cause and intervene to reverse if possible. If an illness or trauma is present, institute supportive medical procedures such as fluids, and blood pressure maintenance measures.

VIII. Types of Disorders

Three types exist: (1) Disorders due to a general medical condition (such as head trauma or hypoxia), (2) those caused by toxins or medications (such as due to carbon monoxide poisoning or chronic alcohol consumption), and (3) those classified as a category not otherwise specified (NOS) for cases in which the etiology is unclear. There are three modifiers for this condition: mild, moderate and severe.

A. Cerebrovascular diseases

Cerebrovascular diseases affecting the bilateral medial thalamus, particularly the anterior portions, are often associated with symptoms of disorder that cause amnesia. A few case studies report these disorders resulting from the rupture of an aneurysm of the anterior communicating artery, resulting in infarction of the basal forebrain region.

B. Multiple sclerosis

The most common cognitive complaints in patients with multiple sclerosis involve impaired memory, which occurs in 40% to 60% of patients. Characteristically, digit span memory is normal, but immediate recall and delayed recall of information are impaired. The memory impairment can affect both verbal and nonverbal materials.

C. Korsakoff's syndrome

1. Korsakoff's syndrome is a syndrome caused by thiamine deficiency, most commonly associated with the poor nutritional habits of people with chronic alcohol abuse. Other causes of poor nutrition (e.g., starvation), gastric carcinoma, hemodialysis, hyperemesis gravidarum, prolonged intravenous hyperalimentation, and gastric plication can also result in thiamine deficiency.

2. Korsakoff's syndrome is often associated with Wernicke's encephalopathy, which is the associated syndrome of confusion, ataxia, and ophthalmoplegia. Although the confusion clears up within a month or so, the amnesia either accompanies or follows untreated Wernicke's encephalopathy in approximately 85% of all cases.

3. Patients with Korsakoff's syndrome typically demonstrate a change in personality as well, such that they display a lack of initiative, diminished spontaneity, and a lack of interest or concern. Confabulation, apathy, and passivity are often prominent symptoms in the syndrome.

4. **Treatment.** Administration of thiamine may prevent the development of additional amnestic symptoms, but the treatment seldom reverses severe amnestic symptoms once they are present. Approximately one-third to one-fourth of all patients recover completely, and approximately one-fourth of all patients have no improvement of their symptoms.

D. **Alcoholic blackouts**

Occurs with severe alcohol abuse. Characteristically, these persons awake in the morning with a conscious awareness of being unable to remember a period the night before during which they were intoxicated. Sometimes, specific behaviors (hiding money in a secret place and provoking fights) are associated with the blackouts.

E. **Electroconvulsive therapy (ECT)**

ECT treatments are usually associated with retrograde amnesia for a period of several minutes before the treatment and anterograde amnesia after the treatment. The anterograde amnesia usually resolves within 5 hours. Mild memory deficits may remain for 1 to 2 months after a course of ECT treatments, but the symptoms are completely resolved 6 to 9 months after the treatment.

F. **Head injury**

Head injuries (both closed and penetrating) can result in a wide range of neuropsychiatric symptoms, including dementia, depression, personality changes, and neurocognitive disorder secondary to another medical condition. These disorders caused by head injuries are commonly associated with a period of retrograde amnesia leading up to the traumatic incident and amnesia for the traumatic incident itself. The severity of the brain injury correlates somewhat with the duration and severity of the syndrome causing amnesia, but the best correlate of eventual improvement is the degree of clinical improvement in the amnesia during the first week after the patient regains consciousness.

G. **Transient global amnesia**

This disorder is associated with abrupt episodes of profound amnesia in all modalities. The patient is fully alert, and distant memory is intact. The attack occurs suddenly and usually lasts several hours. The patient is bewildered and confused after an episode and may repeatedly ask others about what happened. It is usually associated with cerebrovascular disease, but also with episodic medical conditions (e.g., seizures). It is most common in old age (over 65).

1. **Pathology and laboratory examination.** Laboratory findings, diagnostic of these disorders, may be obtained using quantitative neuropsychological testing. Standardized tests also are available to assess recall of well-known historical events or public figures to characterize an individual's inability to remember previously learned information. Performance on such tests varies among individuals with these disorders. Subtle deficits in other cognitive functions may be noted in individuals with these disorders. Memory deficits, however, constitute the predominant feature of the mental status examination and account largely for any functional deficits. No specific or diagnostic features are detectable on imaging studies such as magnetic resonance imaging (MRI) or computed tomography (CT). Damage of mid-temporal lobe structures is common, however, and may be reflected in enlargement of third ventricle or temporal horns or in structural atrophy detected by MRI.

Table 6-2
Comparison of Syndrome Characteristics in Alzheimer's Disease and Amnestic Disorder

Characteristic	Alzheimer's Dementia	Amnestic Disorder
Onset	Insidious	Can be abrupt
Course	Progressive deterioration	Static or improvement
Anterograde memory	Impaired	Impaired
Retrograde memory	Impaired	Temporal gradient
Episodic memory	Impaired	Impaired
Semantic memory	Impaired	Intact
Language	Impaired	Intact
Praxis or function	Impaired	Intact

2. **Differential diagnosis**

   a. Delirium and dementia, but these disorders involve impairments in many other areas of cognition, e.g., confusion, and disorientation.

   b. Factitious disorders may simulate amnesia, but the amnestic deficits will be inconsistent. There is often secondary gain to forgetting.

   c. Patients with dissociative disorders are more likely to have lost their orientation to self and may have more selective memory deficits than do patients with the above-described disorders. They can also lay down new memories. Dissociative disorders also often associated with emotionally stressful life events involving money, the legal system, or troubled relationships.

   d. The deficits in Alzheimer's disease extend beyond memory to general knowledge (semantic memory), language, praxis, and general function. These are spared in neurocognitive disorders due to another medical condition (Table 6-2).

   e. The dementias associated with Parkinson's disease, acquired immune deficiency syndrome (AIDS), and other subcortical disorders demonstrate disproportionate impairment of retrieval but relatively intact encoding and consolidation and, thus, can be distinguished from the above-mentioned disorders.

   f. Subcortical pattern dementias are also likely to display motor symptoms, such as bradykinesia, chorea, or tremor, that are not components of the disorders described above.

H. **Normal Aging**

   Some minor impairment in memory may accompany normal aging, but the DSM-5 requirement that the memory impairment causes significant impairment in social or occupational functioning should exclude normal aging from the diagnosis.

   1. **Course and prognosis**

      a. Generally neurocognitive disorder due to a medical condition has a static course. Little improvement is seen over time, but also no progression of the disorder occurs.

      b. Acute amnesias, such as transient global amnesia, resolve entirely over hours to days.

    c. These disorders associated with head trauma improve steadily in the months subsequent to the trauma.

    d. Amnesia secondary to processes that destroy brain tissue, such as stroke, tumor, and infection, are irreversible, although, again, static, once the acute infection or ischemia has been staunched.

2. Treatment

    a. Treat the underlying cause of the disorder, for example, infection and trauma.

    b. Supportive prompts about the date, the time, and the patient's location can be helpful and can reduce the patient's anxiety.

    c. After the resolution of the episode, psychotherapy of some type (cognitive, psychodynamic, or supportive) may help patients incorporate the amnestic experience into their lives.

For more detailed discussion of this topic, see Chapter 10, Neurocognitive Disorders, Section 10.4, Amnestic Disorders and Mild Cognitive Impairment, p. 1222, in CTP/X.

7

Mental Disorders Due to a General Medical Condition

I. Introduction

General medical conditions may cause and be associated with a variety of mental disorders. The psychiatrist should always be aware of (1) any general medical condition that a patient may have and (2) any prescription, nonprescription, or illegal substances that a patient may be taking. The psychiatric conditions discussed below may be caused or associated with a general medical condition.

II. Mood Disorder Due to a General Medical Condition

A. Epidemiology

1. Appears to affect men and women equally.
2. As much as 50% of all poststroke patients experience depressive illness. A similar prevalence pertains to individuals with pancreatic cancer.
3. Forty percent of patients with Parkinson's disease are depressed.
4. Major and minor depressive episodes are common after certain illnesses such as Huntington's disease, human immunodeficiency virus (HIV) infection, and multiple sclerosis (MS).
5. Depressive disorders associated with terminal or painful conditions carry the greatest risk of suicide.

 CLINICAL HINT:
Depressive disorders associated with terminal or painful conditions carry the greatest risk of suicide.

B. Diagnosis and clinical features

1. Patients with depression may experience psychological symptoms (e.g., sad mood, lack of pleasure or interest in usual activities, tearfulness, concentration disturbance, and suicidal ideation) or somatic symptoms (e.g., fatigue, sleep disturbance, and appetite disturbance), or both psychological and somatic symptoms.
2. Diagnosis in the medically ill can be confounded by the presence of somatic symptoms related purely to medical illness, not to depression. In an effort to overcome the underdiagnosis of depression in the medically ill, most practitioners favor including somatic symptoms in identifying mood syndromes.

C. Differential diagnosis

1. **Substance-induced mood disorder.** Mood disorder due to a general medical condition can be distinguished from substance-induced

mood disorder by examination of time course of symptoms, response to correction of suspect medical conditions or discontinuation of substances, and, occasionally, urine or blood toxicology results.

2. Delirium. Mood changes occurring during the course of delirium are acute and fluctuating and should be attributed to that disorder.

3. Pain syndromes. Pain syndromes can depress mood, but do so through psychological, not physiologic means, and may appropriately lead to a diagnosis of primary mood disorder.

4. Sleep disorders, anorexia, and fatigue. In the medically ill, somatic complaints, such as sleep disturbance, anorexia, and fatigue, may be counted toward a diagnosis of major depressive episode or mood disorder due to a general medical condition, unless those complaints are purely attributable to the medical illness.

D. Course and prognosis. Prognosis for mood symptoms is best when etiologic medical illnesses or medications are most susceptible to correction (e.g., treatment of hypothyroidism and cessation of alcohol use).

E. Treatment

1. Pharmacotherapy. The underlying medical cause should be treated as effectively as possible. Standard treatment approaches for the corresponding primary mood disorder should be used, although the risk of toxic effects from psychotropic drugs may require more gradual dose increases. Standard antidepressant medications, including tricyclic drugs, monoamine oxidase inhibitors (MAOIs), selective serotonin reuptake inhibitors (SSRIs), and psychostimulants, are effective in many patients. Electroconvulsive therapy (ECT) may be useful in patients who do not respond to medication.

2. Psychotherapy. At a minimum, psychotherapy should focus on psychoeducational issues. The concept of a behavioral disturbance secondary to medical illness may be new or difficult for many patients and families to understand. Specific intrapsychic, interpersonal, and family issues are addressed as indicated in psychotherapy.

III. Psychotic Disorder Due to a General Medical Condition

To establish the diagnosis of psychotic disorder due to a general medical condition, the clinician first must exclude syndromes in which psychotic symptoms may be present in association with cognitive impairment (e.g., delirium and dementia of the Alzheimer's type). Disorders in this category are not associated usually with changes in the sensorium.

A. Epidemiology

1. The incidence and prevalence in the general population are unknown.

2. As much as 40% of individuals with temporal lobe epilepsy (TLE) experience psychosis.

3. The prevalence of psychotic symptoms is increased in selected clinical populations, such as nursing home residents, but it is unclear how to extrapolate these findings to other patient groups.

B. Etiology. Virtually any cerebral or systemic disease that affects brain function can produce psychotic symptoms. Degenerative disorders, such as Alzheimer's disease or Huntington's disease, can present initially with new-onset psychosis, with minimal evidence of cognitive impairment at the earliest stages.

C. Diagnosis and clinical features. Two subtypes exist for psychotic disorder due to a general medical condition: *with delusions*, to be used if the predominant psychotic symptoms are delusional, and *with hallucinations*, to be used if hallucinations of any form comprise the primary psychotic symptoms. To establish the diagnosis of a secondary psychotic syndrome, determine that the patient is not delirious, as evidenced by a stable level of consciousness. Conduct a careful mental status assessment to exclude significant cognitive impairments, such as those encountered in dementia or amnestic disorder.

D. Differential diagnosis

1. Psychotic disorders and mood disorders. Features may present with symptoms identical or similar to psychotic disorder due to a general medical condition; however, in primary disorders, no medical or substance cause is identifiable, despite laboratory workup.

2. Delirium. May be present with psychotic symptoms, however delirium-related psychosis is acute and fluctuating, commonly associated with disturbance in consciousness and cognitive defects.

3. Dementia. Psychosis resulting from dementia may be diagnosed as psychotic disorder due to a general medical condition, except in the case of vascular dementia, which should be diagnosed as vascular dementia with delusions.

4. Substance-induced psychosis. Most cases of nonauditory hallucinations are due to medical conditions, substances, or both. Auditory hallucinations can occur in primary and induced psychoses. Stimulant (e.g., amphetamine and cocaine) intoxication psychosis may involve a perception of bugs crawling under the skin (formication). Diagnosis may be assisted by chronology of symptoms, response to removal of suspect substances or alleviation of medical illnesses, and toxicology results.

E. Course and prognosis. Psychosis caused by certain medications (e.g., immunosuppressants) may gradually subside even when use of those medications is continued. Minimizing doses of such medications consistent with therapeutic efficacy often facilitates resolution of psychosis. Certain degenerative brain disorders (e.g., Parkinson's disease) can be characterized by episodic lapses into psychosis, even as the underlying medical condition advances. If abuse of substances persists over a lengthy period, psychosis (e.g., hallucinations from alcohol) may fail to remit even during extended intervals of abstinence.

F. Treatment. The principles of treatment for a secondary psychotic disorder are similar to those for any secondary neuropsychiatric disorder, namely, rapid identification of the etiologic agent and treatment of the underlying cause. Antipsychotic medication may provide symptomatic relief.

IV. Anxiety Disorder Due to a General Medical Condition
The individual experiences anxiety that represents a direct physiologic, not emotional, consequence of a general medical condition. In *substance-induced anxiety disorder*, the anxiety symptoms are the product of a prescribed medication or stem from intoxication or withdrawal from a nonprescribed substance, typically a drug of abuse.

A. Epidemiology
1. Medically ill individuals in general have higher rates of anxiety disorder than do the general population.
2. Rates of panic and generalized anxiety are especially high in neurologic, endocrine, and cardiology patients, although this finding does not necessarily prove a physiologic link.
3. Approximately one-third of patients with hypothyroidism and two-thirds of patients with hyperthyroidism may experience anxiety symptoms.
4. As much as 40% of patients with Parkinson's disease have anxiety disorders. Prevalence of most anxiety disorders is higher in women than in men.

B. Etiology. Causes most commonly described in anxiety syndromes include substance-related states (intoxication with caffeine, cocaine, amphetamines, and other sympathomimetic agents; withdrawal from nicotine, sedative–hypnotics, and alcohol), endocrinopathies (especially pheochromocytoma, hyperthyroidism, hypercortisolemic states, and hyperparathyroidism), metabolic derangements (e.g., hypoxemia, hypercalcemia, and hypoglycemia), and neurologic disorders (including vascular, trauma, and degenerative types). Many of these conditions are either inherently transient or easily remediable.

C. Diagnosis and clinical features. Anxiety stemming from a general medical condition or substance may present with physical complaints (e.g., chest pain, palpitation, abdominal distress, diaphoresis, dizziness, tremulousness, and urinary frequency), generalized symptoms of fear and excessive worry, outright panic attacks associated with fear of dying or losing control, recurrent obsessive thoughts or ritualistic compulsive behaviors, or phobia with associated avoidant behavior.

D. Differential diagnosis
1. **Primary anxiety disorders.** Anxiety disorder due to a general medical condition symptomatically can resemble corresponding primary anxiety disorders. Acute onset, lack of family history, and occurrence within the context of acute medical illness or introduction of new medications or substances suggest a nonprimary cause.
2. **Delirium.** Individuals with delirium commonly experience anxiety and panic symptoms, but these fluctuate and are accompanied by other delirium symptoms such as cognitive loss and inattentiveness; furthermore, anxiety symptoms diminish as delirium subsides.
3. **Dementia.** Dementia often is associated with agitation or anxiety, especially at night (called *sundowning*), but an independent anxiety

diagnosis is warranted only if it becomes a source of prominent clinical attention.

4. **Psychosis.** Patients with psychosis of any origin can experience anxiety commonly related to delusions or hallucinations.

5. **Mood disorders.** Depressive disorders often present with anxiety symptoms, mandating that the clinician inquire broadly about depressive symptoms in any patient whose primary complaint is anxiety.

6. **Adjustment disorders.** Adjustment disorders with anxiety arising within the context of reaction to medical or other life stressors should not be diagnosed as anxiety disorder due to a general medical condition.

E. **Course and prognosis**

1. Medical conditions responsive to treatment or cure (e.g., correction of hypothyroidism and reduction in caffeine consumption) often provide concomitant relief of anxiety symptoms, although such relief may lag the rate or extent of improvement in the underlying medical condition.

2. Chronic, incurable medical conditions associated with persistent physiologic insult (e.g., chronic obstructive pulmonary disease) or recurrent relapse to substance use can contribute to seeming refractoriness of associated anxiety symptoms.

3. In medication-induced anxiety, if complete cessation of the offending factor (e.g., immunosuppressant therapy) is not possible, dose reduction, when clinically feasible, often brings substantial relief.

F. **Treatment.** Aside from treating the underlying causes, clinicians have found benzodiazepines helpful in decreasing anxiety symptoms; supportive psychotherapy (including psychoeducational issues focusing on the diagnosis and prognosis) may also be useful. The efficacy of other, more specific therapies in secondary syndromes (e.g., antidepressant medications for panic attacks, SSRIs for obsessive-compulsive symptoms, behavior therapy for simple phobias) is unknown, but they may be of use.

V. Sleep Disorder Due to a General Medical Condition

A. **Diagnosis.** Sleep disorders can manifest in four ways: by an excess of sleep (hypersomnia), by a deficiency of sleep (insomnia), by abnormal behavior or activity during sleep (parasomnia), and by a disturbance in the timing of sleep (circadian rhythm sleep disorders). Primary sleep disorders occur unrelated to any other medical or psychiatric illness.

B. **Treatment.** The diagnosis of a secondary sleep disorder hinges on the identification of an active disease process known to exert the observed effect on sleep. Treatment first addresses the underlying neurologic or medical disease. Symptomatic treatments focus on behavior modification, such as improvement of sleep hygiene. Pharmacologic options can also be used, such as benzodiazepines for restless legs syndrome or nocturnal myoclonus, stimulants for hypersomnia, and tricyclic antidepressant medications for manipulation of rapid eye movement (REM) sleep.

VI. Sexual Dysfunction Due to a General Medical Condition

Sexual dysfunction often has psychological and physical underpinnings. *Sexual dysfunction due to a general medical condition* subsumes multiple forms of medically induced sexual disturbance, including erectile dysfunction, pain during sexual intercourse, low sexual desire, and orgasmic disorders.

A. Epidemiology

1. Little is known regarding the prevalence of sexual dysfunction due to general medical illness.
2. Prevalence rates for sexual complaints are highest for female hypoactive sexual desire and orgasm problems and for premature ejaculation in men.
3. High rates of sexual dysfunction are described in patients with cardiac conditions, cancer, diabetes, and HIV.
4. Forty to 50% of individuals with MS describe sexual dysfunction.
5. Cerebrovascular accident impairs sexual functioning, with the possibility that, in men, greater impairment follows right hemispheric cerebrovascular injury than left hemispheric injury.
6. Delayed orgasm can affect as much as 50% of individuals taking SSRIs.

B. Etiology.
The type of sexual dysfunction is affected by the cause, but specificity is rare; that is, a given cause can manifest as one (or more than one) of several syndromes. General categories include medications and drugs of abuse, local disease processes that affect the primary or secondary sexual organs, and systemic illnesses that affect sexual organs via neurologic, vascular, or endocrinologic routes.

C. Course and prognosis.
Varies widely, depending on the cause. Drug-induced syndromes generally remit with discontinuation (or dose reduction) of the offending agent. Endocrine-based dysfunctions also generally improve with restoration of normal physiology. By contrast, dysfunctions caused by neurologic disease can run protracted, even progressive, courses.

D. Treatment.
When reversal of the underlying cause is not possible, supportive and behaviorally oriented psychotherapy with the patient (and perhaps the partner) may minimize distress and increase sexual satisfaction (e.g., by developing sexual interactions that are not limited by the specific dysfunction). Support groups for people with specific types of dysfunctions are available. Other symptom-based treatments can be used in certain conditions; for example, sildenafil (Viagra) administration or surgical implantation of a penile prosthesis may be used in the treatment of male erectile dysfunction.

VII. Mental Disorders Due to a General Medical Condition Not Elsewhere Classified

There are three additional diagnostic categories for clinical presentations of mental disorders due to a general medical condition that do not meet the diagnostic criteria for specific diagnoses. The first of the diagnoses is catatonic disorder due to a general medical condition. The second is personality change due to a general medical condition. The third diagnosis is mental disorder not otherwise specified due to a general medical condition.

A. Catatonia due to a medical condition. Catatonia can be caused by a variety of medical or surgical conditions. It is characterized usually by fixed posture and waxy flexibility. Mutism, negativism, and echolalia may be associated features.

1. **Epidemiology.** Catatonia is an uncommon condition. Among inpatients with catatonia, 25% to 50% are related to mood disorders (e.g., major depressive episode, recurrent, with catatonic features), and approximately 10% are associated with schizophrenia. Data are scant on catatonia's rate of occurrence due to medical conditions or substances.

2. **Diagnosis and clinical features.** Peculiarities of movement are the most characteristic feature, usually rigidity. Hyperactivity and psychomotor agitation can also occur. A thorough medical workup is necessary to confirm the diagnosis.

3. **Course and prognosis.** The course and prognosis are intimately related to the cause. Neoplasms, encephalitis, head trauma, diabetes, and other metabolic disorders can manifest with catatonic features. If the underlying disorder is treatable, the catatonic syndrome will resolve.

4. **Treatment.** Treatment must be directed to the underlying cause. Antipsychotic medications may improve postural abnormalities even though they have no effect on the underlying disorder. Schizophrenia must always be ruled out in patients who present with catatonic symptoms. ECT has been shown to be a useful first-choice method of treatment.

B. Personality change due to a general medical condition. Personality change means that the person's fundamental means of interacting and behaving have been altered. When a true personality change occurs in adulthood, the clinician should always suspect brain injury. Almost every medical disorder can be accompanied by personality change, however.

1. **Epidemiology.** No reliable epidemiologic data exist on personality trait changes in medical conditions. Specific personality trait changes for particular brain diseases—for example, passive and self-centered behaviors in patients with dementia of the Alzheimer's type—have been reported. Similarly, apathy has been described in patients with frontal lobe lesions.

2. **Etiology**
   a. Diseases that preferentially affect the frontal lobes or subcortical structures are more likely to manifest with prominent personality change.
   b. Head trauma is a common cause. Frontal lobe tumors, such as meningiomas and gliomas, can grow to considerable size before coming to medical attention because they can be neurologically silent (i.e., without focal signs).
   c. Progressive dementia syndromes, especially those with a subcortical pattern of degeneration, such as acquired immune deficiency

syndrome (AIDS) dementia complex, Huntington's disease, or progressive supranuclear palsy, often cause significant personality disturbance.

d. MS can impinge on the personality, reflecting subcortical white matter degeneration.

e. Exposure to toxins with a predilection for white matter, such as irradiation, can also produce significant personality change disproportionate to the cognitive or motor impairment.

3. Diagnosis and clinical features. The diagnostic criteria for personality change due to a general medical condition include: Impaired control of emotions, impulses, labile and shallow emotions with euphoria or apathy. Facile jocularity when frontal lobes are involved with indifference, apathy, lack of concern, temper outbursts, and can result in violent behavior. Patients make inappropriate jokes, sexual advances, show antisocial conduct, and assaultive behavior. They are unable to anticipate legal consequences of actions. The diagnosis should be suspected in patients who have no history of mental disorder, and whose personality changes occur abruptly or over a relatively brief time.

4. Course and prognosis. Course depends on the nature of the medical or neurologic insult. Personality changes resulting from medical conditions likely to yield to intervention (e.g., correction of hypothyroidism) are more amenable to improvement than are personality changes due to medical conditions that are static (e.g., brain injury after head trauma) or progressive in nature (e.g., Huntington's disease).

5. Treatment

a. Pharmacotherapy. Lithium carbonate (Eskalith), carbamazepine (Tegretol), and valproic acid (Depakote) have been used for the control of affective lability and impulsivity. Aggression or explosiveness can be treated with lithium, anticonvulsant medications, or a combination of lithium and an anticonvulsant agent. Centrally active β-adrenergic receptor antagonists, such as propranolol (Inderal), have some efficacy as well. Apathy and inertia have occasionally improved with psychostimulant agents.

b. Psychotherapy. Families should be involved in the therapy process, with a focus on education and understanding the origins of the patient's inappropriate behaviors. Issues such as competency, disability, and advocacy are frequently of clinical concern with these patients in light of the unpredictable and pervasive behavior change.

VIII. Mental Disorders Due to a General Medical Condition
   A. Epilepsy
      1. Ictal and postictal confusional syndromes.
      2. Prevalence of psychosis in epilepsy is 7%.
      3. Epilepsy is three to seven times more common in psychotic patients.
      4. Lifetime prevalence of psychosis in patients with epilepsy is 10%.
      5. Seizures versus pseudoseizures (Table 7-1).

Table 7-1
Clinical Features Distinguishing Seizures and Pseudoseizures[a]

Features	Seizure	Pseudoseizure
Aura	Common stereotyped	Rare
Timing	Nocturnal common	Only when awake
Incontinence	Common	Rare
Cyanosis	Common	Rare
Postictal confusion	Yes	No
Body movement	Tonic or clonic	Nonstereotyped and asynchronous
Self-injury	Common	Rare
EEG	May be abnormal	Normal
Affected by suggestion	No	Yes
Secondary gain	No	Yes

[a]Some patients with organic seizure disorders may also have pseudoseizures.

6. TLE
   a. TLE is the most likely type to produce psychiatric symptoms.
   b. Often involves schizophrenia like psychosis.
   c. Often difficult to distinguish from schizophrenia with aggressiveness.
   d. Varied and complex auras that may masquerade as functional illness (e.g., hallucinations, depersonalization, derealization).
   e. Automatisms, autonomic effects, and visceral sensations (e.g., epigastric aura, stomach churning, salivation, flushing, tachycardia, dizziness).
   f. Altered perceptual experiences (e.g., distortions, hallucinations, depersonalization, feeling remote, feeling something has a peculiar significance [*déjà vu, jamais vu*]).
   g. Hallucinations of taste and smell are common and may be accompanied by lip smacking or pursing, chewing, or tasting and swallowing movements.
   h. Subjective disorders of thinking and memory.
   i. Strong affective experiences, most commonly fear and anxiety.

CLINICAL HINT:
If patient complains of only smelling bad odors (burning hair, feces), then TLE is the most likely diagnosis.

B. **Brain tumors**
   1. Neurologic signs, headache, nausea, vomiting, seizures, visual loss, papilledema, virtually any psychiatric symptoms are possible.
   2. Symptoms often are caused by raised intracranial pressure or mass effects rather than by direct effects of tumor.
   3. Suicidal ideation is present in 10% of patients, usually during headache paroxysms.
   4. Although rarely seen in a psychiatric practice, most patients with brain tumors have psychiatric symptoms.

        a. Slow tumors produce personality change.

        b. Rapid tumors produce cognitive change.

    5. Frontal lobe tumors—depression, inappropriate affect, disinhibition, dementia, impaired coordination, psychotic symptoms. Often misdiagnosed as primary degenerative dementia; neurologic signs often are absent. May have bowel or bladder incontinence.

    6. Temporal lobe tumors—anxiety, depression, hallucinations (especially gustatory and olfactory), TLE symptoms, schizophrenia like psychosis. May have impaired memory and speech.

    7. Parietal lobe tumors—fewer psychiatric symptoms (anosognosia, apraxia, aphasia); may be mistaken for hysteria.

    8. Colloid cysts—not a tumor. Located in third ventricle and can place pressure on diencephalon. Can produce depression, psychosis, mood lability, and personality change. Classically produces position-dependent intermittent headaches.

C. Head trauma. Head trauma can result in an array of mental symptoms.

    1. Pathophysiology

        a. An estimated 2 million incidents involve head trauma each year.

        b. Most commonly occurs in people 15 to 25 years of age and has a male-to-female predominance of approximately 3 to 1.

        c. Virtually all patients with serious head trauma, more than half of patients with moderate head trauma, and about 10% of patients with mild head trauma have ongoing neuropsychiatric sequelae resulting from the head trauma.

    2. Symptoms. The most common cognitive problems are decreased speed in information processing, decreased attention, increased distractibility, deficits in problem solving and in the ability to sustain effort, and problems with memory and learning new information. A variety of language disabilities can also occur. Behaviorally, the major symptoms involve depression, increased impulsivity, increased aggression, and changes in personality.

    3. Treatment. Standard antidepressants can be used to treat depression, and either anticonvulsants or antipsychotics can be used to treat aggression and impulsivity. Other approaches to the symptoms include lithium, calcium channel blockers, and β-adrenergic receptor antagonists. Clinicians must support patients through individual or group psychotherapy and should support the major caretakers through couples and family therapy. All involved parties need help to adjust to any changes in the patient's personality and mental abilities.

D. Demyelinating disorders

    1. Multiple sclerosis

        a. More common in Northern Hemisphere.

        b. Psychiatric changes are common (75%).

        c. Depression is seen early in course.

        d. With frontal lobe involvement, disinhibition and manic-like symptoms occur, including euphoria.

    e. Intellectual deterioration is common (60%), ranging from mild memory loss to dementia.

    f. Psychosis is reported, but rates are unclear.

    g. Hysteria is common, especially late in disease.

    h. Symptoms are exacerbated by physical or emotional trauma.

    i. MRI is needed for workup.

  2. Amyotrophic lateral sclerosis (ALS)

    a. Rare progressive noninherited disease causing asymmetric muscle atrophy.

    b. Atrophy of all muscle except cardiac and ocular.

    c. Deterioration of anterior horn cells.

    d. Rapidly progressive, usually fatal within 4 years.

    e. Concomitant dementia rare. Patients with pseudobulbar palsy may show emotional lability.

E. Infectious diseases

  1. Herpes simplex encephalitis

    a. Most commonly affects the frontal and temporal lobes.

    b. Symptoms often include anosmia, olfactory and gustatory hallucinations, and personality changes and can also involve bizarre or psychotic behaviors.

    c. Complex partial epilepsy may also develop in patients with herpes simplex encephalitis.

    d. Although the mortality rate for the infection has decreased, many patients exhibit personality changes, symptoms of memory loss, and psychotic symptoms.

  2. Rabies encephalitis

    a. The incubation period ranges from 10 days to 1 year, after which symptoms of restlessness, overactivity, and agitation can develop.

    b. Hydrophobia, present in up to 50% of patients.

    c. Is fatal within days or weeks.

  3. Neurosyphilis (general paresis)

    a. Appears 10 to 15 years after the primary *Treponema* infection.

    b. Penicillin has made it a rare disorder, although AIDS is associated with reintroducing neurosyphilis into medical practice in some urban settings.

    c. Generally affects the frontal lobes and results in personality changes, development of poor judgment, irritability, and decreased care for self.

    d. Delusions of grandeur develop in 10% to 20% of affected patients.

    e. Progresses with the development of dementia and tremor, until patients are paretic.

  4. Chronic meningitis. Now seen more often than in the recent past because of the immunocompromised condition of people with AIDS. The usual causative agents are *Mycobacterium tuberculosis*, *Cryptococcus*, and *Coccidioides*. The usual symptoms are headache, memory impairment, confusion, and fever.

5. Lyme disease

   a. Caused by infection with the spirochete *Borrelia burgdorferi* transmitted through the bite of the deer tick (*Ixodes scapularis*).

   b. About 16,000 cases are reported annually in the United States.

   c. Associated with impaired cognitive functioning and mood changes (i.e., memory lapses, difficulty concentrating, irritability, depression).

   d. No clear-cut diagnostic test is available.

   e. About 50% of patients become seropositive to *B. burgdorferi*.

   f. Treatment consists of a 14- to 21-day course of doxycycline (Vibramycin).

   g. Specific psychotropic drugs can be targeted to treat the psychiatric sign or symptom (e.g., diazepam [Valium] for anxiety).

   h. Approximately 60% of persons develop a chronic condition if left untreated.

   i. Support groups provide emotional support that help improve quality of life.

6. Prion disease.

Prion disease is a group of related disorders caused by a transmissible infectious protein known as a *prion*. Included in this group are Creutzfeldt–Jakob disease (CJD), Gerstmann–Sträussler syndrome (GSS), fatal familial insomnia (FFI), and kuru. Collectively, these disorders are also known as *subacute spongiform encephalopathy* because of shared neuropathologic changes that consist of (1) spongiform vacuolization, (2) neuronal loss, and (3) astrocyte proliferation in the cerebral cortex. Amyloid plaques may or may not be present.

   a. Etiology. Prions are mutated proteins generated from the human prion protein gene (PrP), which is located on the short arm of chromosome 20. The PrP mutates into a disease-related isoform PrP-Super-C (PrP^{Sc}) that can replicate and is infectious. The neuropathologic changes that occur in prion disease are presumed to be caused by direct neurotoxic effects of PrP^{Sc}.

   b. Creutzfeldt–Jakob disease. Is an invariably fatal, rapidly progressive disorder that occurs mainly in middle-aged or older adults. It manifests initially with fatigue, flu-like symptoms, and cognitive impairment. Psychiatric manifestations are protean and include emotional lability, anxiety, euphoria, depression, delusions, hallucinations, or marked personality changes. The disease progresses over months, leading to dementia, akinetic mutism, coma, and death. The rates of CJD range from 1 to 2 cases per 1 million persons a year, worldwide. No known treatment exists and death usually occurs within 6 months after diagnosis.

   c. Variant CJD. The mean age of onset is 29 years. Clinicians must be alert to the diagnosis in young people with behavioral and psychiatric abnormalities in association with cerebellar signs such as ataxia or myoclonus. The psychiatric presentation of CJD is not specific. Most patients reported depression, withdrawal, anxiety, and sleep disturbance. Paranoid delusions have occurred. No cure exists, and death usually occurs within 2 to 3 years after diagnosis. Prevention is dependent on careful monitoring of cattle for disease and feeding them grain instead of meat by-products.

d. **Kuru.** Found in New Guinea and is caused by cannibalistic funeral rituals in which the brains of the deceased are eaten. Women are more affected by the disorder than men, presumably because they participate in the ceremony to a greater extent. Death usually occurs within 2 years after symptoms develop. Neuropsychiatric signs and symptoms consist of ataxia, chorea, strabismus, delirium, and dementia. The cerebellum is most affected. Since the cessation of cannibalism in New Guinea, the incidence of the disease has decreased drastically.

e. **Gerstmann–Sträussler–Scheinker disease.** Is characterized by ataxia, chorea, and cognitive decline leading to dementia. The disease is inherited and affected families have been identified over several generations. Genetic testing can confirm the presence of the abnormal genes before onset. Pathologic changes characteristic of prion disease are present: spongiform lesions, neuronal loss, and astrocyte proliferation. Amyloid plaques have been found in the cerebellum. Onset of the disease occurs between 30 and 40 years of age. The disease is fatal within 5 years of onset.

f. **Fatal familial insomnia.** Primarily affects the thalamus. A syndrome of insomnia and autonomic nervous system dysfunction consisting of fever, sweating, labile blood pressure, and tachycardia occurs that is debilitating. Onset is in middle adulthood, and death usually occurs in 1 year. No treatment currently exists.

F. Immune disorders

1. **Systemic lupus erythematosus.** An autoimmune disease that involves inflammation of multiple organ systems. Between 5% and 50% of patients have mental symptoms at the initial presentation, and approximately 50% eventually show neuropsychiatric manifestations. The major symptoms are depression, insomnia, emotional lability, nervousness, and confusion. Treatment with steroids commonly induces further psychiatric complications, including mania and psychosis.

2. **Autoimmune disorders affecting brain neurotransmitters.** A group of autoimmune receptor-seeking disorders have been identified that cause an encephalitis that mimics schizophrenia. Among those is anti-NMDA (*N*-methyl D-aspartate)-receptor encephalitis that causes dissociative symptoms, amnesia, and vivid hallucinations. The disorder occurs mostly in women. There is no treatment although intravenous immunoglobulins have proved useful. Recovery does occur but some patients might require prolonged intensive care. There is increasing interest in the role of the immune system not only in schizophrenia-like illnesses but also in mood and bipolar disorders.

G. Endocrine disorders

1. **Thyroid disorders.** Hyperthyroidism is characterized by confusion, anxiety, and an agitated, depressive syndrome. Patients may also complain

of being easily fatigued and of feeling generally weak. Insomnia, weight loss despite increased appetite, tremulousness, palpitations, and increased perspiration are also common symptoms. Serious psychiatric symptoms include impairments in memory, orientation, and judgment; manic excitement; delusions; and hallucinations.

2. **Parathyroid disorders**
   a. Dysfunction of the parathyroid gland results in the abnormal regulation of calcium metabolism.
   b. Excessive secretion of parathyroid hormone causes hypercalcemia, which can result in delirium, personality changes, and apathy in 50% to 60% of patients and cognitive impairments in approximately 25% of patients.
   c. Neuromuscular excitability, which depends on proper calcium ion concentration, is reduced, and muscle weakness may appear.
   d. Hypocalcemia can occur with hypoparathyroid disorders and can result in neuropsychiatric symptoms of delirium and personality changes.
   e. Other symptoms of hypocalcemia are cataract formation, seizures, extrapyramidal symptoms, and increased intracranial pressure.

3. **Adrenal disorders**
   a. **Addison's disease: adrenal insufficiency.**
      (1) Most common causes are adrenocortical atrophy or tubercular or fungal infection.
      (2) Patients may have apathy, irritability, fatigue, and depression.
      (3) Rarely have confusion or psychosis.
      (4) Treatment with cortisone or the equivalent is usually effective.
   b. **Cushing's syndrome**
      (1) Excessive cortisol produced by an adrenocortical tumor or hyperplasia.
      (2) Causes secondary mood disorder of agitated depression and often suicide.
      (3) Patient may have memory deficits, decreased concentration, and psychosis.
      (4) Physical findings include truncal obesity, moon facies, buffalo hump, purple striae, hirsutism, and excessive bruising.
      (5) Severe depression can follow the termination of steroid therapy.

4. **Pituitary disorders.** Patients with total pituitary failure can exhibit psychiatric symptoms, particularly postpartum women who have hemorrhaged into the pituitary, a condition known as *Sheehan's syndrome*. Patients have a combination of symptoms, especially of thyroid and adrenal disorders, and can show virtually any psychiatric symptom.

H. Metabolic disorders

1. **Hepatic encephalopathy**
   a. Can result in hepatic encephalopathy, characterized by asterixis, hyperventilation, EEG abnormalities, and alterations in consciousness.

    b. The alterations in consciousness can range from apathy to drowsiness to coma.

    c. Associated psychiatric symptoms are changes in memory, general intellectual skills, and personality.

2. Uremic encephalopathy

    a. Renal failure is associated with alterations in memory, orientation, and consciousness. Restlessness, crawling sensations on the limbs, muscle twitching, and persistent hiccups are associated symptoms.

    b. In young people with brief episodes of uremia, the neuropsychiatric symptoms tend to be reversible; in elderly people with long episodes of uremia, the neuropsychiatric symptoms can be irreversible.

3. Hypoglycemic encephalopathy

    a. Can be caused either by excessive endogenous production of insulin or by excessive exogenous insulin administration.

    b. Premonitory symptoms include nausea, sweating, tachycardia, and feelings of hunger, apprehension, and restlessness.

    c. As the disorder progresses, disorientation, confusion, and hallucinations, as well as other neurologic and medical symptoms, can develop. Stupor and coma can occur, and a residual and persistent dementia can sometimes be a serious neuropsychiatric sequela of the disorder.

4. Diabetic ketoacidosis

    a. Begins with feelings of weakness, easy fatigability, and listlessness and increasing polyuria and polydipsia.

    b. Headache and sometimes nausea and vomiting appear.

    c. Patients with diabetes mellitus have an increased likelihood of chronic dementia with general arteriosclerosis.

5. Acute intermittent porphyria

    a. An autosomal dominant disorder that affects more women than men and has its onset between ages 20 and 50.

    b. Psychiatric symptoms include anxiety, insomnia, lability of mood, depression, and psychosis.

    c. Some studies have found that between 0.2% and 0.5% of chronic psychiatric patients may have undiagnosed porphyrias.

 CLINICAL HINT:
Barbiturates can precipitate and aggravate the disorder and thus are contraindicated in patients with porphyria.

I. Nutritional disorders

  1. Niacin deficiency

    a. Seen in association with alcohol abuse, vegetarian diets, and extreme poverty and starvation.

    b. Neuropsychiatric symptoms include apathy, irritability, insomnia, depression, and delirium; the medical symptoms include dermatitis, peripheral neuropathies, and diarrhea.

c. Course has traditionally been described as "five Ds": dermatitis, diarrhea, delirium, dementia, and death.

d. The response to treatment with nicotinic acid is rapid, but dementia from prolonged illness may improve only slowly and incompletely.

2. Thiamine (vitamin B₁) deficiency.

a. Leads to beriberi, characterized chiefly by cardiovascular and neurologic changes, and to Wernicke–Korsakoff syndrome, which is most often associated with chronic alcohol abuse.

b. Psychiatric symptoms include apathy, depression, irritability, nervousness, and poor concentration; severe memory disorders can develop with prolonged deficiencies.

3. Cobalamin (vitamin B₁₂) deficiency.

a. Mental changes such as apathy, depression, irritability, and moodiness are common. In a few patients, encephalopathy and its associated delirium, delusions, hallucinations, dementia, and, sometimes, paranoid features are prominent and are sometimes called megaloblastic madness.

b. The neurologic manifestations of vitamin B₁₂ deficiency can be rapidly and completely arrested by early and continued administration of parenteral vitamin therapy.

J. Toxins

1. Mercury. Mercury poisoning can be caused by either inorganic or organic mercury. Inorganic mercury poisoning results in the "mad hatter" syndrome with depression, irritability, and psychosis. Associated neurologic symptoms are headache, tremor, and weakness. Organic mercury poisoning can be caused by contaminated fish or grain and can result in depression, irritability, and cognitive impairment. Associated symptoms are sensory neuropathies, cerebellar ataxia, dysarthria, paresthesias, and visual field defects. Mercury poisoning in pregnant women causes abnormal fetal development. No specific therapy is available, although chelation therapy with dimercaprol has been used in acute poisoning.

2. Lead. It takes several months for toxic symptoms to appear. When lead reaches levels above 200 mg/mL, symptoms of severe lead encephalopathy occur, with dizziness, clumsiness, ataxia, irritability, restlessness, headache, and insomnia. Later, an excited delirium occurs, with associated vomiting and visual disturbances, and progresses to convulsions, lethargy, and coma. The treatment of choice to facilitate lead excretion is intravenous administration of calcium disodium edetate (calcium disodium versenate) daily for 5 days.

3. Manganese. Sometimes called *manganese madness* and causes symptoms of headache, irritability, joint pains, and somnolence. An eventual picture appears of emotional lability, pathologic laughter, nightmares, hallucinations, and compulsive and impulsive acts associated with periods of confusion and aggressiveness. Lesions involving the basal ganglia and pyramidal system result in gait impairment, rigidity, monotonous or whispering speech, tremors of the extremities and tongue, masked facies (manganese mask), micrographia, dystonia, dysarthria, and loss of equilibrium. The psychological effects tend to clear 3 or 4 months after the patient's removal from the site of exposure, but neurologic symptoms tend to remain stationary or to progress. No specific treatment exists for manganese poisoning, other than removal from the source of poisoning.

4. **Arsenic.** Most commonly results from prolonged exposure to herbicides containing arsenic or from drinking water contaminated with arsenic. Early signs of toxicity are skin pigmentation, gastrointestinal complaints, renal and hepatic dysfunction, hair loss, and a characteristic garlic odor to the breath. Encephalopathy eventually occurs, with generalized sensory and motor loss. Chelation therapy with dimercaprol has been used successfully to treat arsenic poisoning.

For more detailed discussion of this topic, see Other Cognitive and Mental Disorders due to Another Medical Condition, Chapter 10, Section 10.5, p. 1233 and Psychosomatic Medicine, Chapter 27, p. 2177 in CTP/X.

8

Substance-Related and Addictive Disorders

I. Introduction

This chapter covers substance dependence and substance abuse with descriptions of the clinical phenomena associated with the use of 11 designated classes of pharmacologic agents: alcohol; amphetamines or similarly acting agents; caffeine; cannabis; cocaine; hallucinogens; inhalants; nicotine; opioids; phencyclidine (PCP) or similar agents; and a group that includes sedatives, hypnotics, and anxiolytics. A residual 12th category includes a variety of agents not in the 11 designated classes, such as anabolic steroids and nitrous oxide.

Substance abuse problems cause significant disabilities for a relatively high percentage of the population. Illicit substance abuse affects multiple areas of functioning, and comorbid diagnosis occurs in about 60% to 75% of patients with substance-related disorders. About 40% of the U.S. population has used an illicit substance at one time, and about 15% of persons over the age of 18 are estimated to have one of these disorders in their lifetime. Substance-induced syndromes can mimic the full range of psychiatric illnesses, including mood, psychotic, and anxiety disorders. In clinical practice, substance use disorders must always be considered in the differential diagnosis. Additionally, patients who are diagnosed with primary substance use disorders must be evaluated for another psychiatric disorder (dual diagnosis) that may be contributing to the substance abuse or dependence.

Classification

Brain-altering compounds are referred to as *substances* in *DSM-5* and the related disorders as *substance-related disorders*. Diagnostic criteria for these generally capture patterns of toxicity, that is changes in mood, behavior, and cognition, as well as impairment in social or occupational functioning, tolerance, or dependence that results from continued and prolonged use of the offending drug or toxin. There are many classes of substances that are associated with these disorders.

The signs and symptoms of substance use disorder according to DSM-5 are listed below:

1. A maladaptive pattern of substance use leading to clinically significant impairment or distress
2. Recurrent substance use in situations in which it is physically hazardous (e.g., driving an automobile or operating a machine when impaired by substance use)

3. Continued use leading to impairment in school or work
4. Development of tolerance
5. Characteristic withdrawal syndrome depending on substance
6. Persistent desire to cut down or decrease substance use
7. Drug-seeking behavior

II. Terminology

A. Dependence. The term *dependence* is used in one of two ways. In behavioral dependence, substance-seeking activities and related evidence of pathologic use patterns are emphasized with or without physical dependence. Physical dependence indicates an altered physiologic state due to repeated administration of a drug, the cessation of which results in a specific syndrome. (See withdrawal syndrome below.) See Table 8-1.

Table 8-1
Diagnosis of Substance Dependence

1. A need for markedly increased amounts of the substance
2. Diminished effect
3. Characteristic withdrawal syndrome
4. Taken in larger amounts or over a longer period
5. Unable to cut down or control substance use
6. Significant amount of time is spent in activities necessary to obtain the substance
7. Important activities are sacrificed because of substance abuse

B. Abuse. Use of any drug, usually by self-administration, in a manner that deviates from approved social or medical patterns. See Table 8-2.

Table 8-2
Diagnosis of Substance Abuse

1. Recurrent drug use and inability to fulfill obligations
2. Engaging in physically hazardous activities
3. Legal problems
4. Interpersonal problems

C. Misuse. Similar to abuse but usually applies to drugs prescribed by physicians that are not used properly.

D. Addiction. The repeated and increased use of a substance, the deprivation of which gives rise to symptoms of distress and an irresistible urge to use the agent again and which leads also to physical and mental deterioration. The term is no longer included in the official nomenclature, having been replaced by the term dependence, but it is a useful term in common usage.

E. Intoxication. A reversible syndrome caused by a specific substance (e.g., alcohol) that effects one or more of the following mental functions: memory, orientation, mood, judgment, and behavioral, social, or occupational functioning. See Table 8-3.

Table 8-3
Diagnosis of Substance Intoxication

1. Slurred speech
2. Dizziness
3. Incoordination
4. Unsteady gait
5. Nystagmus
6. Impairment in attention or memory
7. Stupor or coma
8. Double vision

F. Withdrawal. A substance-specific syndrome that occurs after stopping or reducing the amount of the drug or substance that has been used regularly over a prolonged period of time. The syndrome is characterized by physiologic signs and symptoms in addition to psychological changes such as disturbances in thinking, feeling, and behavior. Also called *abstinence syndrome* or *discontinuation syndrome.* See Table 8-4.

Table 8-4
Diagnosis of Substance Withdrawal

1. Substance-specific syndrome develops after stopping or decreasing prolonged use
2. Syndrome leads to impaired functioning.
3. Not caused by a known general medical condition

G. Tolerance. Phenomenon in which, after repeated administration, a given dose of a drug produces a decreased effect or increasingly larger doses must be administered to obtain the effect observed with the original dose. *Behavioral tolerance* reflects the ability of the person to perform tasks despite the effects of the drug.

H. Cross-tolerance. Refers to the ability of one drug to be substituted for another, each usually producing the same physiologic and psychological effect (e.g., diazepam and barbiturates). Also known as *cross-dependence.*

I. Co-dependence. Term used to refer to family members affected by or influencing the behavior of the substance abuser. Related to the term *enabler,* which is a person who facilitates the abuser's addictive behavior (e.g., providing drugs directly or money to buy drugs). Enabling also includes the unwillingness of a family member to accept addiction as a medical–psychiatric disorder or to deny that the person is abusing a substance.

J. Neuroadaptation. Neurochemical or neurophysiologic changes in the body that result from the repeated administration of a drug. Neuroadaptation accounts for the phenomenon of the metabolizing system in the body. *Cellular or pharmacodynamics* adaptation refers to the ability of the nervous system to function despite high blood levels of the offending substance.

III. Evaluation

Substance-abusing patients are often difficult to detect and evaluate. Not easily categorized, they almost always underestimate the amount of substance used, are prone to use denial, are often manipulative, and often fear the consequences of acknowledging the problem. Because these patients may be unreliable, it is necessary to obtain information from other sources, such as family members. Perhaps more than other disorders, understanding the interpersonal, social, and genetic contexts of those behaviors is central to evaluation and treatment.

When dealing with these patients, clinicians must present clear, firm, and consistent limits, which will be tested frequently. Such patients usually require a confrontational approach. Although clinicians may feel angered by being manipulated, they should not act on these feelings.

Psychiatric conditions are difficult to evaluate properly in the presence of ongoing substance abuse, which itself causes or complicates symptoms seen in other disorders. Substance abuse is frequently associated with personality disorders (e.g., antisocial, borderline, and narcissistic). Depressed, anxious, or psychotic patients may self-medicate with either prescribed or nonprescribed substances.

 CLINICAL HINT:
Substance-induced disorders should always be considered in the evaluation of depression, anxiety, or psychosis. Underlying substance use is often present when psychiatric disorders do not respond to usual treatments.

A. **Toxicology.** Urine or blood tests are useful in confirming suspected substance use. The two types of tests are screening and confirmatory. Screening tests tend to be sensitive but not specific (many false-positives). Confirm positive screening results with a specific confirmatory test for an identified drug. Although most drugs are well detected in urine, some are best detected in blood (e.g., barbiturates and alcohol). Absolute blood concentrations can sometimes be useful (e.g., a high concentration in the absence of clinical signs of intoxication would imply tolerance). Urine toxicology is usually positive for up to 2 days after the ingestion of most drugs. See Table 8-5.

B. **Physical examination**
   1. Carefully consider whether concomitant medical conditions are substance-related. Look specifically for the following:
      a. **Subcutaneous or intravenous abusers:** AIDS, scars from intravenous or subcutaneous injections, abscesses, infections from contaminated injections, bacterial endocarditis, drug-induced or infectious hepatitis, thrombophlebitis, tetanus.
      b. **Snorters of cocaine, heroin, or other drugs:** deviated or perforated nasal septum, nasal bleeding, and rhinitis.
      c. **Cocaine freebasers; smokers of crack, marijuana, or other drugs; inhalant abusers:** bronchitis, asthma, chronic respiratory conditions.

C. **History.** Determine the pattern of abuse. Is it continuous or episodic? When, where, and with whom is the substance taken? Is the abuse recreational or

Table 8-5
Drugs of Abuse that Can Be Tested in Urine

Drug	Length of Time Detected in Urine
Alcohol	7–12 hours
Amphetamine	48 hours
Barbiturate	24 hours (short-acting)
	3 weeks (long-acting)
Benzodiazepine	3 days
Cocaine	6–8 hours (metabolites 2–4 days)
Codeine	48 hours
Heroin	36–72 hours
Marijuana (tetrahydrocannabinol)	3 days–4 weeks (depending on use)
Methadone	3 days
Methaqualone	7 days
Morphine	48–72 hours
Phencyclidine	8 days
Propoxyphene	6–48 hours

confined to certain social contexts? Find out how much of the patient's life is associated with obtaining, taking, withdrawing from, and recovering from substances. How much do the substances affect the patient's social and work functioning? How does he or she get and pay for the substances? Always specifically describe the substance and route of administration rather than the category (i.e., use "intravenous heroin withdrawal" rather than "opioid withdrawal"). If describing polysubstance abuse, list all substances. Substance abusers typically abuse multiple substances.

   D. Diagnoses. Abuse is the chronic use of a substance that leads to impairment or distress and eventually produces dependence on the drug with tolerance and withdrawal symptoms. See Table 8-1.

   E. Treatment. In general, the management of dependence involves observation for possible overdose, evaluation for polysubstance intoxication and concomitant medical conditions, and supportive treatment, such as protecting the patient from injury. The management of abuse or dependence involves abstinence and long-term treatment often relies on creating adaptive social supports and problem solving, with psychopharmacologic strategies generally managing withdrawal, substituting for dependence antagonizing substance effects or mediating craving and reward mechanisms.

IV. Specific Substance-Related Disorders
   A. Alcohol-related disorders
      The high prevalence of alcohol abuse and dependence makes the assessment of alcohol use a key part of any psychiatric or medical evaluation. Almost any presenting clinical problem can be related to the effects of alcohol abuse. Although alcoholism does not describe a specific mental disorder, the disorders associated with alcoholism generally can be divided into three groups: (1) disorders related to the direct effects of alcohol on the brain (including alcohol intoxication, withdrawal, withdrawal delirium, and hallucinosis); (2) disorders related to behavior associated with alcohol (alcohol abuse and

dependence); and (3) disorders with persisting effects (including alcohol-induced persisting amnestic disorder, dementia, Wernicke's encephalopathy, and Korsakoff's syndrome).

B. Alcohol dependence and abuse

1. **Definitions.** Alcohol dependence is a pattern of compulsive alcohol use, defined by the presence of three or more major areas of impairment related to alcohol occurring within the same 12 months. These areas may include tolerance or withdrawal, spending a great deal of time using the substance, returning to use despite adverse physical or psychological consequences, and repeated unsuccessful attempts to control alcohol intake. Alcohol abuse is diagnosed when alcohol is used in physically hazardous situations (e.g., driving). Alcohol abuse differs from alcohol dependence in that it does not include tolerance and withdrawal or a compulsive use pattern; rather, it is defined by negative consequences of repeated use. Alcohol abuse can develop into alcohol dependence, and maladaptive patterns of alcohol consumption may include continuous heavy use, weekend intoxication, or binges interspersed with periods of sobriety.

2. **Pharmacology**

   a. **Pharmacokinetics.** About 90% of alcohol is absorbed through the stomach, the remainder from the small intestine. It is rapidly absorbed, highly water-soluble, and distributed throughout the body. Peak blood concentration is reached in 30 to 90 minutes. Rapid consumption of alcohol and consumption of alcohol on an empty stomach enhance absorption and decrease the time to peak blood concentration. Rapidly rising blood alcohol concentrations correlate with degree of intoxication. Intoxication is more pronounced when blood concentrations are rising rather than falling. Ninety percent of alcohol is metabolized by hepatic oxidation; the rest is excreted unchanged by the kidneys and lungs. Alcohol is converted by alcohol dehydrogenase into acetaldehyde, which is converted to acetic acid by aldehyde dehydrogenase. The body metabolizes about 15 dL of alcohol per hour, which is equivalent to one moderately sized drink (12 g of ethanol—the content of 12 oz of beer, 4 oz of wine, or 1 to 1.5 oz of an 80-proof liquor). Patients who use alcohol excessively have upregulated enzymes that metabolize alcohol quickly.

   b. **Neuropharmacology.** Alcohol is a depressant that produces somnolence and decreased neuronal activity. It can be categorized with the other sedative–anxiolytics, such as benzodiazepines, barbiturates, and carbamates. These agents are cross-tolerant with alcohol, produce similar profiles of intoxication and withdrawal, and are potentially lethal in overdose, especially when taken with other depressant drugs. According to the various theories regarding the mechanism of action of alcohol on the brain, alcohol may affect cell membrane fluidity, dopamine-mediated pleasure centers, benzodiazepine receptor complexes, glutamate-gated ionophore receptors that bind N-methyl-D-aspartate (NMDA), and the production of opioidlike alkaloids.

Table 8-6
Alcohol Epidemiology

Condition	Population (%)
Ever had a drink	90
Current drinker	60–70
Temporary problems	40+
Abuse[a]	Male: 10+
	Female: 5+
Dependence[a]	Male: 10
	Female: 3–5

[a]20–30% of psychiatric patients.

3. **Epidemiology.** Approximately 10% of women and 20% of men have met the diagnostic criteria for alcohol abuse during their lifetimes, and 3% to 5% of women and 10% of men have met the diagnostic criteria for the more serious diagnosis of alcohol dependence. See Table 8-6. The lifetime risk for alcohol dependence is about 10% to 15% for men and 3% to 5% for women. Whites have the highest rate of alcohol use—56%. Sixty percent of alcohol abusers are men. The higher the educational level, the more likely is the current use of alcohol, in contrast to the pattern for illicit drugs. Among religious groups, alcohol dependence is highest among liberal Protestants and Catholics. The orthodox religions appear to be protective against alcohol dependence in all religious groups. About 200,000 deaths each year are directly related to alcohol abuse, and about 50% of all automotive fatalities involve drunken drivers. Compared with other groups, whites have the highest rate of alcohol use, about 60%. See Table 8-7.

4. **Etiology.** Data supporting genetic influences in alcoholism include the following: (1) close family members have a fourfold increased risk; (2) the identical twin of an alcoholic person is at higher risk than a fraternal twin; and (3) adopted-away children of alcoholic persons have a fourfold increased risk. The familial association is strongest for the son of an alcohol-dependent father. Ethnic and cultural differences are found in susceptibility to alcohol and its effects. For example, many Asians show acute toxic effects (e.g., intoxication, flushing, dizziness, headache) after consuming only minimal amounts of alcohol. Some ethnic groups, such as Jews and Asians, have lower rates of alcohol dependence, whereas others, such as Native Americans, Inuits, and some groups of Hispanic men, show high rates. These findings have led to a genetic theory about the cause of alcoholism, but a definitive cause remains unknown.

5. **Comorbidity.** The sedative effect and its ready availability make alcohol the most commonly used substance for the relief of anxiety, depression, and insomnia. However, long-term use may cause depression, and withdrawal in a dependent person may cause anxiety. Proper evaluation of depressed or anxious patients who drink heavily may

Table 8-7
Epidemiologic Data for Alcohol-Related Disorders

Whites have a higher rate of alcohol use
Men are more likely to be binge and heavy drinkers
Alcohol use is highest in western states and lowest in southern states
70% of adults with college degrees are current drinkers compared with 40% among those with high
  school education
Alcohol-related disorders appear among all socioeconomic classes

require observation and reevaluation after a period of sobriety lasting up to several weeks. Many psychotic patients medicate themselves with alcohol when prescribed medications do not sufficiently reduce psychotic symptoms or when prescription medications are not available. In bipolar patients, heavy alcohol use often leads to a manic episode. Among patients with personality disorders, those with antisocial personalities are particularly likely to exhibit long-standing patterns of alcohol dependence. Alcohol abuse is prevalent in persons with other substance use disorders, and the correlation between alcohol dependence and nicotine dependence is particularly high.

6. **Diagnosis, signs, and symptoms**
    a. **Alcohol dependence.** Tolerance is a phenomenon in the drinker, who with time requires greater amounts of alcohol to obtain the same effect. The development of tolerance, especially marked tolerance, usually indicates dependence. Mild tolerance for alcohol is common, but severe tolerance, such as that possible with opioids and barbiturates, is uncommon. Tolerance varies widely among persons. Dependence may become apparent in the tolerant patient only when he or she is forced to stop drinking and withdrawal symptoms develop. The clinical course of alcohol dependence is given in Table 8-8.
    b. **Alcohol abuse.** Chronic use of alcohol that leads to dependence, tolerance, or withdrawal. See Tables 8-1 and 8-4.
7. **Evaluation.** The proper evaluation of the alcohol user requires some suspicion on the part of the evaluator. In general, most people, when questioned, minimize the amount of alcohol they consume.

Table 8-8
Clinical Course of Alcohol Dependence

Age at first drink[a]	13–15 years
Age at first intoxication[a]	15–17 years
Age at first problem[a]	16–22 years
Age at onset of dependence	25–40 years
Age at death	60 years
Fluctuating course of abstention, temporary control, alcohol problems	
Spontaneous remission in 20%	

[a]Same as general population.
Table from Marc A. Schuckitt, M.D.

CLINICAL HINT:
When obtaining a history of the degree of alcohol use, it can be helpful to phrase questions in a manner likely to elicit positive responses. For example, ask "How much alcohol do you drink?" rather than "Do you drink alcohol?"

Other questions that may provide important clues include how often and when the patient drinks, how often he or she has blackouts (amnesia while intoxicated), and how often friends or relatives have told the patient to cut down on drinking. Always look for subtle signs of alcohol abuse, and always inquire about the use of other substances. Physical findings may include palmar erythema, Dupuytren's contractures, and telangiectasia. Does the patient seem to be accident-prone (head injury, rib fracture, motor vehicle accidents)? Is he or she often in fights? Often absent from work? Are there social or family problems? Laboratory assessment can be helpful. Patients may have macrocytic anemia secondary to nutritional deficiencies. Serum liver enzymes and γ-glutamyltransferase (GGT) may be elevated. An elevation of liver enzymes can also be used as a marker of a return to drinking in a previously abstinent patient (Table 8-9). The following subtypes of alcohol dependence have been described:

a. **Type A:** late onset, mild dependence, few alcohol-related problems, and little psychopathology (sometimes called *Type I*).
b. **Type B:** severe dependence, early onset of alcohol-related problems, strong history of family alcohol use, high number of life stressors, severe psychopathology, polysubstance use, and high psychopathology (sometimes called *Type II*).
c. **Affiliative drinkers:** tend to drink daily in moderate amounts in social settings.
d. **Schizoid-isolated drinkers:** tend to drink alone and subject to binge drinking.

 Table 8-9
State Markers of Heavy Drinking Useful in Screening for Alcoholism

Test	Relevant Range of Results
γ-Glutamyltransferase (GGT)	>30 U/L
Carbohydrate-deficient transferrin (CDT)	>20 mg/L
Mean corpuscular volume (MCV)	>91 μm³
Uric acid	>6.4 mg/dL for men
	>5.0 mg/dL for women
Aspartate aminotransferase (AST)	>45 IU/L
Alanine aminotransferase (ALT)	>45 IU/L
Triglycerides	>160 mg/dL
Adapted from Marc A. Schuckitt, M.D.	

  e. **Gamma alcohol dependence:** persons unable to stop drinking once they start.
8. **Treatment.** The goal is the prolonged maintenance of total sobriety. Relapses are common. Initial treatment requires detoxification, on an inpatient basis if necessary, and treatment of any withdrawal symptoms. Coexisting mental disorders should be treated when the patient is sober.

 CLINICAL HINT:
When doing individual therapy, if the patient comes to a session under the influence of alcohol, the session should not be held. If suicidal ideation is expressed, hospitalization should be obtained.

---

  a. **Insight.** Critically necessary but is often difficult to achieve. The patient must acknowledge that he or she has a drinking problem. Severe denial may have to be overcome before the patient will cooperate in seeking treatment. Often, this requires the collaboration of family, friends, employers, and others. The patient may need to be confronted with the potential loss of career, family, and health if he or she continues to drink. Individual psychotherapy has been used, but group therapy may be more effective. Group therapy may also be more acceptable to many patients who perceive alcohol dependence as a social problem rather than a personal psychiatric problem.
  b. **Alcoholics Anonymous (AA) and Al-Anon.** Supportive organizations, such as AA (for patients) and Al-Anon (for families of patients), can be effective in maintaining sobriety and helping the family to cope. AA emphasizes the inability of the member to cope alone with addiction to alcohol and encourages dependence on the group for support; AA also utilizes many techniques of group therapy. Most experts recommend that a recovered alcohol-dependent patient maintain lifelong sobriety and discourage attempts by recovered patients to learn to drink normally. (A dogma of AA is, "It's the first drink that gets you drunk.")
  c. **Psychosocial interventions.** These are often necessary and very effective. Family therapy should focus on describing the effects of alcohol use on other family members. Patients must be forced to relinquish the perception of their right to be able to drink and recognize the detrimental effects on the family.
  d. **Psychopharmacotherapy**
    (1) **Disulfiram (Antabuse).** A daily dosage of 250 to 500 mg of disulfiram may be used if the patient desire's enforced sobriety. The usual dosage is 250 mg/day. Patients taking disulfiram have an extremely unpleasant reaction when they ingest even small amounts of alcohol. The reaction, caused by an accumulation of acetaldehyde resulting from the inhibition of aldehyde dehydrogenase,

includes flushing, headache, throbbing in the head and neck, dyspnea, hyperventilation, tachycardia, hypotension, sweating, anxiety, weakness, and confusion. Life-threatening complications, although uncommon, can occur. Patients with pre-existing heart disease, cerebral thrombosis, diabetes, and several other conditions cannot take disulfiram because of the risk of a fatal reaction. Disulfiram is useful only temporarily to help establish a long-term pattern of sobriety and to change long-standing alcohol-related coping mechanisms.

 CLINICAL HINT:
Advise patients using Antabuse not to use any after-shave lotions or colognes that contain alcohol. Inhalation of the alcohol can produce a reaction.

---

(2) Naltrexone
- **(A) (ReVia).** This agent decreases the craving for alcohol, probably by blocking the release of endogenous opioids, thereby aiding the patient to achieve the goal of abstinence by preventing the "high" associated with alcohol consumption. A dosage of 50 mg once daily is recommended for most patients.
- **(B) (Vivitrol).** This formulation of naltrexone is an extended-release injectable suspension administered by intramuscular injection every 4 weeks or once a month. The recommended dose is 380 mg once a month and pretreatment with oral naltrexone is not required before using Vivitrol. The side effects and other cautions are similar to oral naltrexone.

(3) Acamprosate (Campral). This drug is used with patients who have already achieved abstinence. It helps patients remain abstinent by a yet unexplained mechanism involving neuronal excitation and inhibition. It is taken in a delayed-release tablet in dosages 666 mg (2 tabs 333 mg) three times daily.

(4) Topiramate (Topamax). This drug is an anticonvulsant approved for the treatment of epilepsy and migraine. It is used as an off-label agent for maintaining alcohol abstinence. Numerous studies suggest that at a mean dose of 200 mg/day it showed less cravings and subsequent intake of alcohol compared to naltrexone. Slow titration at 25 mg/wk is recommended to prevent cognitive side effects. The exact mechanism of action is unclear but is considered an alternative treatment to FDA-approved medications. See Table 8-10.

9. Medical complications. Alcohol is toxic to numerous organ systems. Complications of chronic alcohol abuse and dependence (or associated

Table 8-10
Medications for Treating Alcohol Dependence

Disulfiram (Antabuse)
Action: Inhibits intermediate metabolism of alcohol, causing a build-up of acetaldehyde and a reaction of flushing, sweating, nausea, and tachycardia if a patient drinks alcohol.
Contraindications: Concomitant use of alcohol or alcohol-containing preparations or metronidazole; coronary artery disease; severe myocardial disease.
Precautions: High impulsivity—likely to drink while using it; psychoses (current or history); diabetes mellitus; epilepsy, hepatic dysfunction, hypothyroidism; renal impairment; rubber contact dermatitis.
Serious adverse reactions: Hepatitis; optic neuritis; peripheral neuropathy, psychotic reactions, Pregnancy Category C.
Common side effects: Metallic after-taste; dermatitis.
Examples of drug interactions: Amitryptyline; anticoagulants such as warfarin; diazepam; isoniazid; metronidazole; phenytoin; theophylline; any non–prescription drug containing alcohol.
Usual adult dosage: *Oral dose:* 250 mg daily (range 125–500 mg).
Before prescribing: (1) warn that the patient should not take disulfiram for at least 12 hours after drinking and that a disulfiram alcohol reaction can occur up to 2 weeks after the last dose; and (2) warn about alcohol in the diet (e.g., sauces and vinegar) and in medications and toiletries.
Follow-up: Monitor liver function tests periodically.

Naltrexone (ReVia) and Vivitrol (Extended-Release Injectable Formulation)
Action: Blocks opioid receptors, resulting in reduced craving and reduced reward in response to drinking.
Contraindications: Currently using opioids or in acute opioid withdrawal; anticipated need for opi-oid analgesics; acute hepatitis or liver failure.
Precautions: Other hepatic disease; renal impairment; history of suicide attempts. If opioid analgesia is required larger doses may be required and respiratory depression may be deeper and more prolonged.
Serious adverse reactions: Will precipitate severe withdrawal if patient dependent on opioids; hepatotoxicity (uncommon at usual doses). Pregnancy Category C.
Common side effects: Nausea; abdominal pain; constipation; dizziness; headache; anxiety; fatigue.
Examples of drug interactions: Opioid analgesics (blocks action); yohimbine (use with naltrexone increases negative drug effects).
Usual adult dosage: *Intramuscular dose:* Administered every 4 weeks or once a month. The recommended dose is 380 mg once a month and pretreatment with oral naltrexone is not required before using Vivitrol.
Before prescribing: Evaluate for possible current opioid use; consider a urine toxicology screen for opioids, including synthetic opioids. Obtain liver function tests.
Follow-up: Monitor liver function tests periodically.

Acamprosate (Campral)
Action: Affects glutamate and GABA neurotransmitter systems, but its alcohol-related action is unclear.
Contraindications: Severe renal impairment (CrCl <30 mL/min).
Precautions: Moderate renal impairment (dose adjustment for CrCl between 30 and 50 mL/min); depression or suicidality.
Serious adverse reactions: Anxiety; depression. Rare events include the following: suicide attempt, acute kidney failure, heart failure, mesenteric arterial occlusion, cardiomyopathy, deep thrombo-phlebitis, and shock. Pregnancy Category C.
Common side effects: Diarrhea; flatulence; nausea; abdominal pain; infection; flu syndrome; chills; somnolence; decreased libido, amnesia; confusion.
Examples of drug interactions: No clinically relevant interactions known.
Usual adult dosage: *Oral dose:* 666 mg (two 333-mg tablets) three times daily or, for patients with moderate renal impairment (CrCl 30–50 mL/min), reduce to 333 mg (one tablet) three times daily.
Before prescribing: Establish abstinence.

(continued)

Table 8-10
Medications for Treating Alcohol Dependence *(Continued)*

Topiramate (Topamax)
Action: Affects multiple neurotransmitter systems including glutamate and GABA as well as blocks voltage-dependent sodium channels. Its action in alcohol-related conditions is unknown.
Contraindications: Increased intraocular pressure; liver problems, kidney stones; hyperammonemia; secondary angle-closure glaucoma.

Precautions: Acute myopia and secondary angle-closure glaucoma; oligohidrosis and hyperthermia; metabolic acidosis; suicidal behavior and ideation; cognitive dysfunction.
Serious adverse reactions: Double vision or rapidly decreasing vision; renal stones; cognitive dysfunctions; Pregnancy Category D.
Common side effects: Tiredness; drowsiness; dizziness; nervousness; numbness or tingly feeling; coordination problems; diarrhea; weight loss.
Examples of drug interactions: Co-administration with other antiepileptic drugs may lower topiramate's plasma concentration; concomitant use with oral contraceptives may decrease the efficacy of oral contraceptives and administration with carbonic anhydrase inhibitors may increase the severity of metabolic acidosis.
Usual adult dosage: *Oral dose:* 200 mg daily dose for alcohol-related disorders. The dose should be gradually increased by 25 mg/wk to prevent cognitive effects.
Before prescribing: Evaluate for renal stones, suicidality and any vision-related problems.

---

nutritional deficiencies) are listed in Table 8-11. Alcohol use during pregnancy is toxic to the developing fetus and can cause congenital defects in addition to fetal alcohol syndrome.

C. Alcohol intoxication

1. **Definition.** Alcohol intoxication, also called simple drunkenness, is the recent ingestion of a sufficient amount of alcohol to produce acute maladaptive behavioral changes.

2. **Diagnosis, signs, and symptoms.** Whereas mild intoxication may produce a relaxed, talkative, euphoric, or disinhibited person, severe intoxication often leads to more maladaptive changes, such as aggressiveness, irritability, labile mood, impaired judgment, and impaired social or work functioning, among others.

    Persons exhibit at least one of the following: slurred speech, incoordination, unsteady gait, nystagmus, memory impairment, stupor. Severe intoxication can lead to withdrawn behavior, psychomotor retardation, blackouts, and eventually obtundation, coma, and death. Common complications of alcohol intoxication include motor vehicle accidents, head injury, rib fracture, criminal acts, homicide, and suicide. Stages of alcohol intoxication and effects on behavior at different blood alcohol levels are presented in Table 8-12.

3. **Evaluation.** A thorough medical evaluation should be conducted including a physical examination and blood chemistry screen and standard liver function tests; consider a possible subdural hematoma or a concurrent infection. Always evaluate for possible intoxication with other substances. Alcohol is frequently used in combination with other central nervous system (CNS) depressants, such as benzodiazepines and barbiturates. The CNS depressant effects of such combinations can be synergistic and potentially fatal. Blood alcohol levels are seldom important in the clinical evaluation (except to determine legal intoxication) because tolerance varies.

Table 8-11
Neurologic and Medical Complications of Alcohol Use

Alcohol intoxication
Acute intoxication
Pathologic intoxication (atypical, complicated, unusual)
Blackouts

Alcohol withdrawal syndromes
Tremulousness (shakes or jitters)
Alcoholic hallucinosis (horrors)
Withdrawal seizures (rum fits)
Delirium tremens (shakes)

Nutritional diseases of the nervous system secondary to alcohol abuse
Wernicke–Korsakoff syndrome
Cerebellar degeneration
Peripheral neuropathy
Optic neuropathy (tobacco-alcohol amblyopia)
Pellagra

Alcoholic diseases of uncertain pathogenesis
Central pontine myelinolysis
Marchiafava–Bignami disease
Fetal alcohol syndrome
Myopathy
Alcoholic dementia (?)
Alcoholic cerebral atrophy

Systemic diseases due to alcohol with secondary neurologic complications
Liver disease
  Hepatic encephalopathy
  Acquired (nonwilsonian) chronic hepatocerebral degeneration
Gastrointestinal diseases
  Malabsorption syndromes
  Postgastrectomy syndromes
  Possible pancreatic encephalopathy
Cardiovascular diseases
  Cardiomyopathy with potential cardiogenic emboli and cerebrovascular disease
  Arrhythmias and abnormal blood pressure leading to cerebrovascular disease
Hematologic disorders
  Anemia, leukopenia, thrombocytopenia (could possibly lead to hemorrhagic cerebrovascular
    disease)
Infectious disease, especially meningitis (especially pneumococcal and meningococcal)
Hypothermia and hyperthermia
Hypotension and hypertension
Respiratory depression and associated hypoxia
Toxic encephalopathies (alcohol and other substances)
Electrolyte imbalances leading to acute confusional states and rarely focal neurologic signs and
  symptoms
  Hypoglycemia
  Hyperglycemia
  Hyponatremia
  Hypercalcemia
  Hypomagnesemia
  Hypophosphatemia

Increased incidence of trauma
Epidural, subdural, and intracerebral hematoma
Spinal cord injury
Posttraumatic seizure disorders
Compressive neuropathies and brachial plexus injuries (Saturday night palsies)
Posttraumatic symptomatic hydrocephalus (normal-pressure hydrocephalus)
Muscle crush injuries and compartmental syndromes

Reprinted from Rubino FA. Neurologic complications of alcoholism. *Psychiatr Clin North Am* 1992;15:361, with permission.

Table 8-12
Impairment Likely to Be Seen at Different Blood Alcohol Concentrations

Level (mg/dL)	Likely Impairment
20–30	Slowed motor performance and decreased thinking ability
30–80	Increases in motor and cognitive problems
80–200	Increases in incoordination and judgment errors
	Mood lability
	Deterioration in cognition
200–300	Nystagmus, marked slurring of speech, and alcoholic blackouts
>300	Impaired vital signs and possible death

Table from Marc A. Schuckitt, M.D.

a. A variant of alcohol intoxication is called *alcohol idiosyncratic intoxication.* It is characterized by maladaptive behavior (often aggressive or assaultive) after the ingestion of a small amount of alcohol that would not cause intoxication in most people (i.e., pathologic intoxication). The behavior must be atypical for the person when he or she is not drinking. Brain-damaged persons may also be more susceptible to alcohol idiosyncratic intoxication.

b. Blackouts consist of episodes of intoxication during which the patient exhibits complete anterograde amnesia and appears awake and alert. They occasionally can last for days, during which the intoxicated person performs complex tasks, such as long-distance travel, with no subsequent recollection. Brain-damaged persons may be more susceptible to blackouts.

4. Treatment

a. Usually only supportive.

b. May give nutrients (especially thiamine, vitamin B_{12}, folate).

c. Observation for complications (e.g., combativeness, coma, head injury, falling) may be required.

d. Alcoholic idiosyncratic intoxication is a medical emergency that requires steps to prevent the patient from harming others or self. Lorazepam (Ativan) 1 to 2 mg by mouth or intramuscularly or haloperidol (2 to 5 mg by mouth or intramuscularly) can be used for agitation. Physical restraints may be necessary.

D. Alcohol-induced psychotic disorder, with hallucinations (previously known as alcohol hallucinosis). Vivid, persistent hallucinations (often visual and auditory), without delirium, following (usually within 2 days) a decrease in alcohol consumption in an alcohol-dependent person. May persist and progress to a more chronic form that is clinically similar to schizophrenia. Rare. The male-to-female ratio is 4:1. The condition usually requires at least 10 years of alcohol dependence. If the patient is agitated, possible treatments include benzodiazepines (e.g., 1 to 2 mg of lorazepam [Ativan] orally or intramuscularly, 5 to 10 mg of diazepam [Valium]) or low doses of a high-potency antipsychotic (e.g., 2 to 5 mg of haloperidol [Haldol] orally or intramuscularly as needed every 4 to 6 hours).

E. Alcohol withdrawal. Begins within several hours after cessation of, or reduction in, prolonged (at least days) heavy alcohol consumption. At least two of the following must be present: autonomic hyperactivity, hand tremor, insomnia, nausea or vomiting, transient illusions or hallucinations, anxiety, grand mal seizures, and psychomotor agitation. May occur with perceptual disturbances (e.g., hallucinations) and intact reality testing.

F. Alcohol withdrawal delirium (delirium tremens [DTs]). Usually occurs only after recent cessation of or reduction in severe, heavy alcohol use in medically compromised patients with a long history of dependence. Less common than uncomplicated alcohol withdrawal. Occurs in 1% to 3% of alcohol-dependent patients.

1. **Diagnosis, signs, and symptoms**
   a. Delirium.
   b. Marked autonomic hyperactivity—tachycardia, sweating, fever, anxiety, or insomnia.
   c. Associated features—vivid hallucinations that may be visual, tactile, or olfactory; delusions; agitation; tremor; fever; and seizures or the so-called rum fits (if seizures develop, they always occur before delirium).
   d. Typical features—paranoid delusions, visual hallucinations of insects or small animals, and tactile hallucinations.

2. **Medical workup**
   a. Complete history and physical.
   b. Laboratory tests—complete blood cell count with differential; measurement of electrolytes, including calcium and magnesium; blood chemistry panel; liver function tests; measurement of bilirubin, blood urea nitrogen, creatinine, fasting glucose, prothrombin time, albumin, total protein, hepatitis type B surface antigen, vitamin B, folate, serum amylase; stool guaiac; urinalysis and urine drug screen; electrocardiogram (ECG); and chest roentgenography. Other possible tests include electroencephalogram (EEG), lumbar puncture, computed tomography of the head, and gastrointestinal series.

3. **Treatment**
   a. Take vital signs every 6 hours.
   b. Observe the patient constantly.
   c. Decrease stimulation.
   d. Correct electrolyte imbalances and treat coexisting medical problems (e.g., infection, head trauma).
   e. If the patient is dehydrated, hydrate.
   f. Chlordiazepoxide (Librium): 25 to 100 mg orally every 6 hours (other sedative–hypnotics can be substituted, but this is the convention). Use as needed for agitation, tremor, or increased vital signs (temperature, pulse, blood pressure). In the treatment of alcohol withdrawal delirium in the geriatric patient, lorazepam (Ativan) 1 to 2 mg by mouth, intravenously, or intramuscularly every 4 hours may be used with a 50% decrease in dose on day 2 and day 3 (see Table 8-13).

Table 8-13
Drug Therapy for Alcohol Intoxication, and Withdrawal and Maintenance

Clinical Problem	Drug	Route	Dosage[a]	Comment
Tremulousness and mild to moderate agitation	Chlordiazepoxide	Oral	25–100 mg every 4–6 hours	Initial dose can be repeated every 2 hours until patient is calm; subsequent doses must be individualized and titrated.
	Diazepam	Oral	5–20 mg every 4–6 hours	
Hallucinosis	Lorazepam	Oral	2–10 mg every 4–6 hours	
Extreme agitation	Chlordiazepoxide	Intravenous	0.5 mg/kg at 12.5 mg/min	Give until patient is calm; subsequent doses must be individualized and titrated.
Withdrawal seizures	Diazepam	Intravenous	0.15 mg/kg at 2.5 mg/min	
Delirium tremens	Lorazepam	Intravenous	0.1 mg/kg at 2.0 mg/min	
Maintenance	Acamprosate	Oral	2 g/day	Only used after patient has achieved abstinence.

[a]Scheduled doses should be held for somnolence.
Adapted from Koch-Weser J, Sellers EM, Kalant J. Alcohol Intoxication and withdrawal. *N Engl J Med* 1976;294:757.

g. Thiamine: 100 mg orally one to three times a day.

h. Folic acid: 1 mg orally daily.

i. One multivitamin daily.

j. Magnesium sulfate: 1 g intramuscularly every 6 hours for 2 days (in patients who have had postwithdrawal seizures).

k. After the patient is stabilized, taper chlordiazepoxide by 20% every 5 to 7 days.

l. Provide medication for adequate sleep.

m. Treat malnutrition if present.

n. This regimen allows for a very flexible dosage of chlordiazepoxide. If prescribing a sedative on a standing regimen, be sure that the medication will be held if the patient is asleep or not easily aroused. The necessary total dose of benzodiazepine varies greatly among patients owing to inherent individual differences, differing levels of alcohol intake, and concomitant use of other substances. Because many of these patients have impaired liver function, it also may be difficult to estimate the elimination half-life of the sedative accurately.

o. In general, antipsychotics should be used cautiously because they can precipitate seizures. If the patient is agitated and psychotic and shows signs of benzodiazepine toxicity (ataxia, slurred speech) despite being agitated, then consider using an antipsychotic such as haloperidol or fluphenazine (Prolixin, Permitil), which is less likely to precipitate seizures.

G. Alcohol-induced persisting amnestic disorder. Disturbance in short-term memory resulting from prolonged heavy use of alcohol; rare in persons under the age of 35. The classic names for the disorder are *Wernicke's encephalopathy* (an acute set of neurologic symptoms) and *Korsakoff's syndrome* (a chronic condition).

    1. Wernicke's encephalopathy (also known as *alcoholic encephalopathy*). An acute syndrome caused by thiamine deficiency. Characterized by nystagmus, abducens and conjugate gaze palsies, ataxia, and global confusion. Other symptoms may include confabulation, lethargy, indifference, mild delirium, anxious insomnia, and fear of the dark. Thiamine deficiency usually is secondary to chronic alcohol dependence. Treat with 100 to 300 mg of thiamine per day until ophthalmoplegia resolves. The patient may also require magnesium (a cofactor for thiamine metabolism). With treatment, most symptoms resolve except ataxia, nystagmus, and sometimes peripheral neuropathy. The syndrome may clear in a few days or weeks or progress to Korsakoff's syndrome.

    2. Korsakoff's syndrome (also known as *Korsakoff's psychosis*). A chronic condition, usually related to alcohol dependence, wherein alcohol represents a large portion of the caloric intake for years. Caused by thiamine deficiency. Rare. Characterized by retrograde and anterograde amnesia. The patient also often exhibits confabulation, disorientation, and polyneuritis. In addition to thiamine replacement, clonidine (Catapres) and propranolol (Inderal) may be of some limited use. Often coexists with alcohol-related dementia. Twenty-five percent of patients recover fully, and 50% recover partially with long-term oral administration of 50 to 100 mg of thiamine per day.

H. Substance-induced persisting dementia. This diagnosis should be made when other causes of dementia have been excluded and a history of chronic heavy alcohol abuse is evident. The symptoms persist past intoxication or withdrawal states. The dementia is usually mild. Management is similar to that for dementia of other causes.

I. Opioid-related disorders

    1. Introduction. Opioids have been used for analgesic and other medicinal purposes for thousands of years, but they also have a long history of misuse for their psychoactive effects. Prescription opioids, which are widely available, have significant abuse liability, and continued opioid misuse can result in syndromes of abuse and dependence and cause disturbances in mood, behavior, and cognition that can mimic other psychiatric disorders.

        Opioids include the natural drug opium and its derivatives, in addition to synthetic drugs with similar actions. The natural drugs derived from opium include morphine and codeine; the synthetic opioids include methadone, oxycodone, hydromorphone (Dilaudid), levorphanol (Levo-Dromoran), pentazocine (Talwin), meperidine (Demerol), and propoxyphene (Darvon). Heroin is considered a semisynthetic drug and has the strongest euphoriant property, thus producing the most craving.

Opioids affect opioid receptors. μ-opioid receptors mediate analgesia, respiratory depression, constipation, and dependence; δ-opioid receptors mediate analgesia, diuresis, and sedation. Opioids also affect dopaminergic and noradrenergic systems. Dopaminergic reward pathways mediate addiction. Heroin is more lipid-soluble than morphine and more potent. It crosses the blood–brain barrier more rapidly, has a faster onset of action, and is more addictive.

2. **Epidemiology.** In developed countries, the opioid drug most associated with abuse is heroin, with an estimated 1,000,000 heroin users reported in the United States. The lifetime rate of heroin use in the United States is about 2%. Dependence on opioids other than heroin is seen most often in persons who have become dependent in the course of medical treatment. The male-to-female ratio of persons with heroin dependence is about 3:1. Most users are in their 30s and 40s. Heroin is exclusively a drug of abuse and is most commonly used by patients of lower socioeconomic status, who often engage in criminal activities to pay for drugs. Of note, prescription opiate abuse is fast becoming a major public health problem.

3. **Route of administration.** Depends on the drug. Opium is smoked. Heroin is typically injected (intravenously or subcutaneously) or inhaled (snorted) nasally, and it may be combined with stimulants for intravenous injection (speedball). Heroin snorting and smoking are increasingly popular owing to increased drug purity and concerns about HIV risk. Pharmaceutically available opioids are typically taken orally, but some are also injectable.

 CLINICAL HINT:
Look for "track marks" on extremities (including hands and feet), indicating chronic injection of substances.

---

4. **Dose.** Often difficult to determine by history for two reasons. First, the abuser has no way of knowing the concentration of the heroin he or she has bought and may underestimate the amount taken (which can lead to accidental overdose if the person suddenly obtains one bag containing 15% heroin when the typical amount is 5%). Second, the abuser may overstate the dosage in an attempt to get more methadone.

5. **Diagnosis.** Opioid use disorder is a pattern of maladaptive use of an opioid drug, leading to clinically significant impairment or distress and occurring within a 12-month period.

   a. **Intoxication**

      (1) **Objective signs and symptoms.** CNS depression, decreased gastrointestinal motility, respiratory depression, analgesia, nausea and vomiting, slurred speech, hypotension, bradycardia, pupillary constriction, seizures (in overdose). Tolerant patients still have pupillary constriction and constipation.

- **(2) Subjective signs and symptoms.** Euphoria (heroin intoxication, described as a total-body orgasm), at times anxious dysphoria, tranquility, decreased attention and memory, drowsiness, and psychomotor retardation.
- **(3) Overdose.** Can be a medical emergency and is usually accidental and often results from combined use with other CNS depressants (e.g., alcohol or sedative–hypnotics). Clinical signs include pinpoint pupils, respiratory depression, and CNS depression.
- **(4) Treatment**
  - **(A)** ICU admission and support of vital functions (e.g., intravenous fluids).
  - **(B)** Immediately administer 0.8 mg of naloxone (Narcan) (0.01 mg/kg for neonates), an opioid antagonist, intravenously and wait 15 minutes.
  - **(C)** If no response, give 1.6 mg intravenously and wait 15 minutes.
  - **(D)** If still no response, give 3.2 mg intravenously and suspect another diagnosis.
  - **(E)** If successful, continue at 0.4 mg/hr intravenously.
  - **(F)** Always consider possible polysubstance overdose. A patient successfully treated with naloxone may wake up briefly only to succumb to subsequent overdose symptoms from another, slower-acting drug (e.g., sedative–hypnotic) taken simultaneously. Remember that naloxone will precipitate rapid withdrawal symptoms. It has a short half-life and must be administered continuously until the opioid has been cleared (up to 3 days for methadone). Babies born to opioid-abusing mothers may experience intoxication, overdose, or withdrawal.

 CLINICAL HINT:
Consider opiate addiction irrespective of socioeconomic status. Prescription opiate addiction far exceeds heroin use.

- **b. Tolerance, dependence, and withdrawal.** Develop rapidly with long-term opioid use, which changes the number and sensitivity of opioid receptors and increases the sensitivity of dopaminergic, cholinergic, and serotonergic receptors. Produce profound effects on noradrenergic systems. Occur after cessation of long-term use or after abrupt cessation, as with administration of an opioid antagonist. Symptoms are primarily related to rebound hyperactivity of noradrenergic neurons of the locus ceruleus. Withdrawal is seldom a medical emergency. Clinical signs are flulike and include drug craving, anxiety, lacrimation, rhinorrhea, yawning, sweating, insomnia, hot and cold flashes, muscle aches, abdominal cramping, dilated pupils, piloerection, tremor, restlessness, nausea and vomiting, diarrhea, and increased vital signs. Intensity depends on previous dose and on rate of decrease. Less intense with drugs that have long half-lives, such as methadone; more intense with drugs that have short half-lives, such as meperidine. Patients have severe craving for opioid drugs and will demand and manipulate for opioids. Beware of malingerers and look for piloerection, dilated pupils, tachycardia, and hypertension. If objective signs are absent, do not give opioids for withdrawal.

(1) Detoxification. If objective withdrawal signs are present, give 10 mg of methadone. If withdrawal persists after 4 to 6 hours, give an additional 5 to 10 mg, which may be repeated every 4 to 6 hours. Total dose in 24 hours equals the dose for the second day (seldom >40 mg). Give twice a day or every day and decrease dosage by 5 mg/day for heroin withdrawal; methadone withdrawal may require slower detoxification. Pentazocine-dependent patients should be detoxified on pentazocine because of its mixed opioid receptor agonist and antagonist properties. Many nonopioid drugs have been tried for opioid detoxification, but the only promising one is clonidine (Catapres), which is a centrally acting agent that effectively relieves the nausea, vomiting, and diarrhea associated with opioid withdrawal (it is not effective for most other symptoms). Give 0.1 to 0.2 mg every 3 hours as needed, not to exceed 0.8 mg/day. Titrate dose according to symptoms. When dosage is stabilized, taper over 2 weeks. Hypotension is a side effect. Clonidine is short-acting and not a narcotic.

The general approach in withdrawal is one of support, detoxification, and progression to methadone maintenance or abstinence. Patients dependent on multiple drugs (e.g., an opioid and a sedative–hypnotic) should be maintained on a stable dosage of one drug while being detoxified from the other. Naltrexone (a long-acting oral opioid antagonist) can be used with clonidine to expedite detoxification. It is orally effective, and when given three times a week (100 mg on weekdays and 150 mg on weekends), it blocks the effects of heroin. After detoxification, oral naltrexone has been effective in helping to maintain abstinence for up to 2 months.

Ultrarapid detoxification is the procedure of precipitating withdrawal with opioid antagonists under general anesthesia. Further research is needed to determine whether the use of this expensive and intensive method, which adds anesthetic risk to the detoxification process, is of any benefit.

c. Opioid intoxication delirium

Opioid intoxication delirium is most likely to happen when opioids are used in high doses, are mixed with other psychoactive compounds, or are used by a person with pre-existing brain damage or a CNS disorder (e.g., epilepsy).

d. Opioid-induced psychotic disorder

Opioid-induced psychotic disorder can begin during opioid intoxication. Clinicians can specify whether hallucinations or delusions are the predominant symptoms.

e. Opioid-induced mood disorder

Opioid-induced mood disorder can begin during opioid intoxication. Opioid-induced mood disorder symptoms can have a manic, depressed, or mixed nature, depending on a person's response to opioids. A person coming to psychiatric attention with opioid-induced mood disorder usually has mixed symptoms, combining irritability, expansiveness, and depression.

f. Opioid-induced sleep disorder and opioid-induced sexual dysfunction

Hypersomnia is likely to be more common with opioids than insomnia. The most common sexual dysfunction is likely to be impotence.

g. Unspecified opioid-related disorder

The DSM-5 includes diagnoses for other opioid-related disorders with symptoms of delirium, abnormal mood, psychosis, abnormal sleep, and sexual dysfunction. Clinical situations that do not fit into these categories exemplify appropriate cases for the use of the DSM-5 diagnosis of unspecified opioid-related disorder.

6. **Opioid substitutes.** The main long-term treatment for opiate dependence, methadone maintenance, is a slow, extended detoxification. Most patients can be maintained on daily doses of 60 mg or less. Although often criticized, methadone maintenance programs do decrease rates of heroin use. A sufficient methadone dosage is necessary; the use of plasma methadone concentrations may help to determine the appropriate dosage.

Levomethadyl (ORLAAM, also known as LAAM) is a longer-acting opioid than methadone. Due to its potential for serious and possibly life-threatening, proarrhythmic effects, LAAM was taken off the market.

Buprenorphine (Buprenex) is a partial μ-opioid receptor agonist that is of use for both detoxification and maintenance treatment. Treatment is given three days a week because it is long-acting. A dosage of 8 to 16 mg a day appears to reduce heroin use.

7. **Therapeutic communities.** Residential programs that emphasize abstinence and group therapy in a structured environment (e.g., Phoenix House).

8. **Other interventions.** Education about HIV transmission, free needle-exchange programs, individual and group psychotherapies, self-help groups (e.g., Narcotics Anonymous), and outpatient drug-free programs are also of benefit.

J. **Sedative–hypnotic, and anxiolytic-related disorders**

1. **Introduction.** The drugs associated with this group have a sedative or calming effect and are also used as antiepileptics, muscle relaxants, and anesthetics. These include the benzodiazepines, for example, diazepam (Valium) and flunitrazepam (Rohypnol); barbiturates, for example, secobarbital (seconal); and the barbituratelike substances, which include methaqualone (formerly known as quaalude) and meprobamate (Miltown).

Drugs of this class are used to treat insomnia and anxiety. Alcohol and all drugs of this class are cross-tolerant and their effects are additive. They all have agonist effects on the γ-aminobutyric acid type A (GABA$_A$) receptor complex. Sedatives, hypnotics, and anxiolytics are the most commonly prescribed psychoactive drugs and are taken orally. Dependence develops only after at least several months of daily use, but persons vary widely in this respect. Many middle-aged patients begin taking benzodiazepines for insomnia or anxiety, become dependent, and then seek multiple physicians to prescribe them. Sedative–hypnotics are used illicitly for their euphoric effects, to augment the effects of other CNS depressant drugs (e.g., opioids and alcohol), and to temper the excitatory and anxiety-producing effects of stimulants (e.g., cocaine).

The major complication of sedative, hypnotic, or anxiolytic intoxication is overdose, with associated CNS and respiratory depression. Although mild intoxication is not in itself dangerous (unless the patient is driving or operating machinery), the possibility of a covert overdose must always be considered. The lethality of benzodiazepines is low and overdose has been reduced by the use of the specific benzodiazepine antagonist flumazenil (Romazicon) in emergency department settings.

Sedative, hypnotic, or anxiolytic intoxication is similar to alcohol intoxication, but idiosyncratic aggressive reactions are uncommon. These drugs are often taken with other CNS depressants (e.g., alcohol), which can produce additive effects. Withdrawal is dangerous and can lead to delirium or seizures. See Table 8-14.

2. Epidemiology. About 6% of persons have used these drugs illicitly, usually by under age 40. The highest prevalence of illicit use is between the ages of 26 to 35, with a female-to-male ratio of 3:1 and a white-to-black ratio of 2:1. Barbiturate abuse is more common in those over age 40.

3. Diagnosis

 a. Intoxication. See Table 8-15. Intoxication also can cause disinhibition and amnesia.

Table 8-14
Signs and Symptoms of the Benzodiazepine Discontinuation Syndrome

The following signs and symptoms may be seen when benzodiazepine therapy is discontinued; they reflect the return of the original anxiety symptoms (recurrence), worsening of the original anxiety symptoms (rebound), or emergence of new symptoms (true withdrawal):
Disturbances of mood and cognition
 Anxiety, apprehension, dysphoria, pessimism, irritability, obsessive rumination, and paranoid ideation
Disturbances of sleep
 Insomnia, altered sleep–wake cycle, and daytime drowsiness
Physical signs and symptoms
 Tachycardia, elevated blood pressure, hyperreflexia, muscle tension, agitation/motor restlessness, tremor, myoclonus, muscle and joint pain, nausea, coryza, diaphoresis, ataxia, tinnitus, and grand mal seizures
Perceptual disturbances
 Hyperacusis, depersonalization, blurred vision, illusions, and hallucinations

Table 8-15
Signs and Symptoms of Substance Intoxication and Withdrawal

Substance	Intoxication	Withdrawal
Opioid	Drowsiness Slurred speech Impaired attention or memory Analgesia Anorexia Decreased sex drive Hypoactivity	Craving for drug Nausea, vomiting Muscle aches Lacrimation, rhinorrhea Pupillary dilation Piloerection Sweating Diarrhea Fever Insomnia Yawning
Amphetamine or cocaine	Perspiration, chills Tachycardia Pupillary dilation Elevated blood pressure Nausea, vomiting Tremor Arrhythmia Fever Convulsions Anorexia, weight loss Dry mouth Impotence Hallucinations Hyperactivity Irritability Aggressiveness Paranoid ideation	Dysphoria Fatigue Sleep disorder Agitation Craving
Sedative, hypnotic, or anxiolytic	Slurred speech Incoordination Unsteady gait Impaired attention or memory	Nausea, vomiting Malaise, weakness Autonomic hyperactivity Anxiety, irritability Increased sensitivity to light and sound Coarse tremor Marked insomnia Seizures

b. Withdrawal. See Table 8-15. Can range from a minor to a potentially life-threatening condition requiring hospitalization. Individual differences in tolerance are large. All sedatives, hypnotics, and anxiolytics are cross-tolerant with each other and with alcohol. Drugs with a short half-life (e.g., alprazolam) may induce a more rapid onset of withdrawal and a more severe withdrawal than drugs with a long half-life (e.g., diazepam). The degree of tolerance can be measured with the pentobarbital challenge test (see Table 8-16), which identifies the dose of pentobarbital needed to prevent withdrawal. True withdrawal, a return of original anxiety symptoms (recurrence) or worsening of original anxiety symptoms (rebound), can be precipitated by drug discontinuation. Guidelines for treatment of benzodiazepine withdrawal are presented in Table 8-17. Dose equivalents are presented in Table 8-18.

Table 8-16
Pentobarbital^a Challenge Test

1. Give 200 mg of pentobarbital orally.
2. Observe patient for intoxication after 1 hour (e.g., sleepiness, slurred speech, or nystagmus).
3. If patient is not intoxicated, give another 100 mg of pentobarbital every 2 hours (maximum 500 mg over 6 hours).
4. Total dose given to produce mild intoxication is equivalent to daily abuse level of barbiturates.
5. Substitute 30 mg of phenobarbital (longer half-life) for each 100 mg of pentobarbital.
6. Decrease dose by about 10% a day.
7. Adjust rate if signs of intoxication or withdrawal are present.

^{a}Other drugs can also be used.

c. Other sedative-, hypnotic-, or anxiolytic-induced disorders

(1) Delirium. Delirium that is indistinguishable from DTs associated with alcohol withdrawal is seen more commonly with barbiturate withdrawal

(2) Persisting dementia. This diagnosis is controversial, because uncertainty exists whether a persisting dementia is caused by the substance use itself or by associated features of the substance use.

(3) Persisting amnestic disorder. This condition may be underdiagnosed. One exception is the increased number of reports of amnestic episodes associated with short-term use of benzodiazepines with short half-lives (e.g., triazolam [Halcion]).

Table 8-17
Guidelines for Treatment of Benzodiazepine Withdrawal

1. Evaluate and treat concomitant medical and psychiatric conditions.
2. Obtain drug history and urine and blood samples for drug and ethanol assay.
3. Determine required dose of benzodiazepine or barbiturate for stabilization, guided by history, clinical presentation, drug-ethanol assay, and (in some cases) challenge dose.
4. Detoxification from supratherapeutic dosages:
    a. Hospitalize if there are medical or psychiatric indications, poor social supports, or polysubstance dependence or the patient is unreliable.
    b. Some clinicians recommend switching to longer-acting benzodiazepine for withdrawal (e.g., diazepam, clonazepam); others recommend stabilizing on the drug that the patient was taking or on phenobarbital.
    c. After stabilization, reduce dosage by 30% on the second or third day and evaluate the response, keeping in mind that symptoms occur sooner after decreases in benzodiazepines with short elimination half-lives (e.g., lorazepam) than after decreases in those with longer elimination half-lives (e.g., diazepam).
    d. Reduce dosage further by 10–25% every few days if tolerated.
    e. Use adjunctive medications if necessary; carbamazepine, β-adrenergic receptor antagonists, valproate, clonidine, and sedative antidepressants have been used, but their efficacy in the treatment of the benzodiazepine abstinence syndrome has not been established.
5. Detoxification from therapeutic dosages:
    a. Initiate 10–25% dose reduction and evaluate response.
    b. Dose, duration of therapy, and severity of anxiety influence the rate of taper and need for adjunctive medications.
    c. Most patients taking therapeutic doses have uncomplicated discontinuation.
6. Psychological interventions may assist patients in detoxification from benzodiazepines and in the long-term management of anxiety.

Adapted from Domenic A. Ciraulo M.D., and Ofra Sarid-Segal, M.D.

Table 8-18
Approximate Therapeutic Equivalent Doses of Benzodiazepines

Generic Name	Trade Name	Dose (mg)
Alprazolam	Xanax	1
Chlordiazepoxide	Librium	25
Clonazepam	Klonopin	0.5–1
Clorazepate	Tranxene	15
Diazepam	Valium	10
Estazolam	ProSom	1
Flurazepam	Dalmane	30
Lorazepam	Ativan	2
Oxazepam	Serax	30
Prazepam	Paxipam	80
Temazepam	Restoril	20
Triazolam	Halcion	0.25
Quazepam	Doral	15
Zolpidem[a]	Ambien	10

[a]An imidazopyridine benzodiazepine agonist.
Adapted from Domenic A. Ciraulo, M.D., and Ofra Sarid-Segal, M.D.

(4) Psychotic disorders. Agitation, delusions, and hallucinations are usually visual, but sometimes tactile or auditory features develop after about 1 week of abstinence. Psychotic symptoms associated with intoxication or withdrawal are more common with barbiturates than with benzodiazepines.

(5) Other disorders. Sedative and hypnotic use has also been associated with mood disorders, anxiety disorders, sleep disorders, and sexual dysfunctions.

(6) Unspecified sedative-, hypnotic-, or anxiolytic-related disorders. When none of the previously discussed diagnostic categories is appropriate the likely diagnosis is unspecified sedative-, hypnotic-, or anxiolytic-related disorder.

K. Stimulant-related disorders. Amphetamines and amphetamine-like substances are among the most widely used substance in the Western Hemisphere and exert their major effect by releasing catecholamines, primarily dopamine, from presynaptic stores, particularly in the "reward pathway" of dopaminergic neurons projecting from the ventral tegmentum to the cortex and the limbic areas. Legitimate indications include attention-deficit disorders, and narcolepsy, but are also used in the treatment of obesity, dementia, fibromyalgia, and depression. Methylphenidate (Ritalin) appears less addictive than other amphetamines, possibly because it has a different mechanism of action (inhibits dopamine reuptake). Effects are euphoric and anorectic. Amphetamines are usually taken orally but also can be injected, nasally inhaled, or smoked. The clinical syndromes associated with amphetamines are similar to those associated with cocaine, although the oral route of amphetamine administration produces a less rapid euphoria and consequently is less addictive. Intravenous amphetamine abuse is highly addictive.

CLINICAL HINT:
Amphetamines are commonly abused by students, long-distance truck drivers, and other persons who desire prolonged wakefulness and attentiveness.

Amphetamines can induce a paranoid psychosis similar to paranoid schizophrenia. Intoxication usually resolves in 24 to 48 hours. Amphetamine abuse can cause severe hypertension, cerebrovascular disease, and myocardial infarction and ischemia. Neurologic symptoms range from twitching to tetany to seizures, coma, and death as doses escalate. Tremor, ataxia, bruxism, shortness of breath, headache, fever, and flushing are common but less severe physical effects.

1. **Epidemiology.** In the United States, about 7% of the population used psychostimulants, with the highest use in the 18- to 25-year-old age group, followed by the 12- to 17-year-old age group. The lifetime prevalence of amphetamine dependence and abuse is 1.5%, with about equal use in men and women.

2. **Drugs**
   a. **Major amphetamines.** Amphetamine, dextroamphetamine (Dexedrine), methamphetamine (Desoxyn, "speed"), and methylphenidate (Ritalin).
   b. **Related substances.** Ephedrine, phenylpropanolamine (PPA), khat, and methcathinone ("crank").
   c. **Substituted (designer) amphetamines** (also classified as hallucinogens). These have neurochemical effects on both serotonergic and dopaminergic systems resulting in amphetamine-like and hallucinogen-like behavioral effects (e.g., 3,4-methylenedioxymethamphetamine [MDMA, "ecstasy"]; 2.5-dimethoxy-4-methylamphetamine (DOM), also referred to as "STP" *N*-ethyl-3,4-methylenedioxyamphetamine [MDEA]; 5-methoxy-3,4-methylenedioxyamphetamine [MMDA]). MDMA use is associated with increased self-confidence and sensory sensitivity; and peaceful feelings with insight, empathy, and a sense of personal closeness with other people. Effects are activating and energizing with a hallucinogenic character but less disorientation and perceptual disturbance than are seen with classic hallucinogens. MDMA is associated with hyperthermia, particularly when used in close quarters in combination with increased physical activity, as is common at "raves." Heavy or long-term use may be associated with serotonergic nerve damage.
   d. **"Ice."** Pure form of methamphetamine (inhaled, smoked, or injected). It is particularly powerful and psychological effects can last for hours. It is a synthetic drug, and manufactured domestically.

3. **Diagnosis and clinical features**
   a. **Intoxication and withdrawal.** Autonomic nervous system hyperactivity and behavioral changes. See Tables 8-19 and 8-20.

Table 8-19
Diagnostic Criteria for Stimulant Intoxication

A. Behavioral and physical signs and symptoms of stimulant use.
B. Characteristic effects of elation and euphoria.
C. Perceived improvement in mental and physical tasks.
D. Agitation and irritability.
E. Dangerous sexual behavior and aggression.
F. Tachycardia, hypertension, and mydriasis.

 CLINICAL HINT:

Amphetamine can also produce psychotic symptoms similar to paranoid schizophrenia (amphetamine-induced psychosis); unlike schizophrenia, it clears in a few days and a positive finding in a urine drug screen reveals the correct diagnosis.

---

b. **Stimulant intoxication delirium.** In general, result from high doses and sustained use. Combination with other substances in persons with brain damage may lead to delirium.

c. **Stimulant-induced psychotic disorder.** Presence of paranoid delusions and hallucinations. Formication (sensation of bugs crawling under the skin) is also associated with cocaine use. More common in intravenous and crack users. The treatment of choice is antipsychotic medication like haloperidol (Haldol).

d. **Stimulant-induced mood disorder.** This includes the stimulant-induced bipolar and depressive disorders. These can be present in intoxication or withdrawal but generally intoxication is associated with mania and withdrawal with depressive episodes.

e. **Stimulant-induced anxiety disorder.** This can occur during intoxication or withdrawal and symptoms may mimic panic and phobic disorders.

f. **Stimulant-induced obsessive-compulsive disorder.** The symptoms may occur during intoxication or withdrawal and high doses may lead to time-limited stereotyped behaviors or rituals (picking and arranging) as seen in obsessive-compulsive disorder.

Table 8-20
Diagnostic Criteria for Stimulant Withdrawal

A. Anxiety, dysphoric mood, and lethargy.
B. Tremulousness, fatigue, and headache.
C. Nightmares, profuse sweating, and muscle cramps.
D. Insatiable hunger and stomach cramps.
E. Depression and suicidal ideation.
F. Symptoms last 2–4 days and resolve in 1 week.

g. Stimulant-induced sexual dysfunction. Amphetamines can be used to reverse sexual side effects of serotonergic agents like fluoxetine (Prozac). They are often misused to enhance sexual experience and high and long-term use may lead to erectile and sexual dysfunction.

h. Stimulant-induced sleep disorder. May begin during intoxication or withdrawal. Intoxication may lead to insomnia and sleep deprivation while withdrawal may cause hypersomnolence and nightmares.

4. Treatment. Symptomatic. Benzodiazepines for agitation. Fluoxetine (Prozac) or bupropion (Wellbutrin) has been used for maintenance therapy after detoxification.

5. Cocaine. One of the most addictive of the commonly abused substances, referred to as *coke, blow, cane,* or *freebase.* The effects of cocaine are pharmacologically similar to those of other stimulants, but its widespread use warrants a separate discussion. Before it was well known that cocaine was highly addictive, it was widely used as a stimulant and euphoriant. Cocaine is usually inhaled but can be smoked or injected. Crack is smoked, has a rapid onset of action, and is highly addictive. The onset of action of smoked cocaine is comparable with that of intravenously injected cocaine, and the drug is equally addictive in this circumstance. The euphoria is intense, and a risk for dependence develops after only one dose. Like amphetamines, cocaine can be taken in binges lasting up to several days. This phenomenon is partly the result of greater euphoric effects derived from subsequent doses (sensitization). During binges, the abuser takes the cocaine repeatedly until exhausted or out of the drug. There follows a crash of lethargy, hunger, and prolonged sleep, followed by another binge. With repeated use, tolerance develops to the euphoriant, anorectic, hyperthermic, and cardiovascular effects.

Intravenous cocaine use is associated with risks for the same conditions as other forms of intravenous drug abuse, including AIDS, septicemia, and venous thrombus.

 CLINICAL HINT:
Long-term snorting can lead to a rebound rhinitis, which is often self-treated with nasal decongestants; it also causes nosebleeds and eventually may lead to a perforated nasal septum.

Other physical sequelae include cerebral infarctions, seizures, myocardial infarctions, cardiac arrhythmias, and cardiomyopathies.

a. Epidemiology. About 10% of the U.S. population has tried cocaine, and the lifetime rate of cocaine abuse or dependence is about 2%. It is most common in persons in the 18- to 25-year-old age group, with a male-to-female ration of 2:1. All races and socioeconomic groups are equally affected.

b. Cocaine intoxication. Can cause restlessness, agitation, anxiety, talkativeness, pressured speech, paranoid ideation, aggressiveness, increased sexual interest, heightened sense of awareness, grandiosity, hyperactivity, and other manic symptoms. Physical signs include tachycardia, hypertension, pupillary dilation, chills, anorexia, insomnia, and stereotyped movements. Cocaine use has also been associated with sudden death from cardiac complications and delirium. Delusional disorders are typically paranoid. Delirium may involve tactile or olfactory hallucinations. Delusions and hallucinations may occur in up to 50% of all persons who use cocaine. Delirium may lead to seizures and death.

  c. **Withdrawal.** The most prominent sign of cocaine withdrawal is the craving for cocaine. The tendency to develop dependence is related to the route of administration (lower with snorting, higher with intravenous injection or smoking freebase cocaine). Withdrawal symptoms include fatigue, lethargy, guilt, anxiety, and feelings of helplessness, hopelessness, and worthlessness. Long-term use can lead to depression, which may require antidepressant treatment. Observe for possible suicidal ideation. Withdrawal symptoms usually peak in several days, but the syndrome (especially depressive symptoms) may last for weeks.

  d. **Treatment.** Treatment is largely symptomatic. Agitation can be treated with restraints, benzodiazepines, or, if severe (delirium or psychosis), low doses of high-potency antipsychotics (only as a last resort because the medications lower the seizure threshold). Somatic symptoms (e.g., tachycardia, hypertension) can be treated with β-adrenergic receptor antagonists (β blockers). Evaluate for possible medical complications.

L. **Cannabis-related disorders.** Cannabis is the most widely used illegal drug in the world, with an estimated 19 million users in 2012. *Cannabis sativa* is a plant from which cannabis or marijuana is derived. All parts of the plant contain psychoactive cannabinoids of which Δ-9-tetrahydrocannabinol (THC) is the main active euphoriant (many other active cannabinoids are probably responsible for the other varied effects). Sometimes, purified THC also is abused. Cannabinoids usually are smoked but also can be eaten (onset of effect is delayed, but one can eat very large doses).

  1. **Epidemiology.** There is a 5% lifetime rate of cannabis abuse or dependence with those aged 18 to 21 being the highest users, but all age groups are affected. Use is highest among whites compared to other ethnic groups. Approximately 1% of eighth graders, 4% of tenth graders, and 7% of twelfth graders reported daily use of marijuana.

  2. **Diagnosis and clinical features**

  Many reports indicate that long-term cannabis use is associated with cerebral atrophy, seizure susceptibility, chromosomal damage, birth defects, impaired immune reactivity, alterations in testosterone concentrations, and dysregulation of menstrual cycles; however, these reports have been inconclusive.

  a. **Cannabis use disorder.** People who use cannabis daily over weeks to months are most likely to become dependent.

  b. **Cannabis intoxication.** When cannabis is smoked, euphoric effects appear within minutes, peak in 30 minutes, and last 2 to 4 hours.

Motor and cognitive effects can last 5 to 12 hours. Symptoms include euphoria or dysphoria, anxiety, suspiciousness, inappropriate laughter, time distortion, social withdrawal, impaired judgment, and the following objective signs: conjunctival injection, increased appetite, dry mouth, and tachycardia. It also causes a dose-dependent hypothermia and mild sedation. Often used with alcohol, cocaine, and other drugs. Can cause depersonalization and, rarely, hallucinations. More commonly causes mild persecutory delusions, which seldom require medication. In very high doses, can cause mild delirium with panic symptoms or a prolonged cannabis psychosis (may last up to 6 weeks). Long-term use can lead to anxiety or depression and an apathetic amotivational syndrome. Chronic respiratory disease and lung cancer are long-term risks secondary to inhalation of carcinogenic hydrocarbons. Results of urinary testing for THC are positive for up to 4 weeks after intoxication.

c. **Cannabis intoxication delirium.** It is characterized by marked impairment on cognition and performance tasks.

d. **Cannabis withdrawal.** Cessation of daily cannabis use results in withdrawal symptoms within 1 to 2 weeks of cessation. These include irritability, nervousness, anxiety, insomnia, disturbed or vivid dreaming, decreased appetite, weight loss, depressed mood, restlessness, headache, chills, stomach pain, sweating, and tremors.

e. **Cannabis-induced psychotic disorder.** Cannabis-induced psychotic disorder is diagnosed in the presence of a cannabis-induced psychosis. Cannabis-induced psychotic disorder is rare; transient paranoid ideation is more common.

f. **Cannabis-induced anxiety disorder.** This disorder is a common diagnosis for acute cannabis intoxication, which in many persons induces short-lived anxiety states often provoked by paranoid thoughts.

g. **Unspecified cannabis-related disorders.** This includes cannabis disorders that cannot be classified as those specified above.

   (1) **Flashbacks.** Sensations related to cannabis intoxication after the short-term effects of the substance have disappeared.

   (2) **Cognitive impairment.** The long-term use of cannabis may produce subtle forms of cognitive impairment in the higher cognitive functions of memory, attention, and organization and in the integration of complex information.

   (3) **Amotivational syndrome.** It is associated with long-term heavy cannabis use and described as becoming apathetic and anergic, usually gaining weight, and appearing slothful.

3. **Therapeutic uses.** Cannabis and its primary active components (Δ-9-THC) have been used successfully to treat nausea secondary to cancer chemotherapy, to stimulate appetite in patients with AIDS, and in the treatment of glaucoma.

Medical use of marijuana. Marijuana has been used as a medicinal herb for centuries. Currently, cannabis is a controlled substance with a high potential for abuse and no medical use recognized by the Drug Enforcement Agency (DEA). The U.S. Supreme Court ruled that the manufacture and distribution of marijuana are illegal under any circumstances. Despite this ruling numerous states (20) have passed laws exempting patients who use cannabis under a physician's supervision from state criminal penalties.

4. Treatment. Treatment of cannabis use rests on the same principles as treatment of other substances of abuse—abstinence and support. Treatment of intoxication usually is not required. Anxiolytics may be useful for anxiety and antipsychotics for hallucinations or delusions.

M. Hallucinogen-related disorders. Hallucinogens have been used for thousands of years, and drug-induced hallucinogenic states have been part of social and religious rituals. Hallucinogens are natural and synthetic substances, also known as psychedelics or psychotomimetics because they produce hallucinations, a loss of contact with reality, and an experience of expanded or heightened consciousness. The classic, naturally occurring hallucinogens are psilocybin (from some mushrooms) and mescaline (from peyote cactus); others are harmine, harmaline, ibogaine, and dimethyltryptamine. The classic substituted amphetamines include MDMA, MDEA, 2,5-dimethoxy-4-methylamphetamine (DOM, STP), dimethyltryptamine (DMT), MMDA, and trimethoxyamphetamine (TMA), which are also commonly classified with amphetamines. See Table 8-21.

1. General considerations. Hallucinogens usually are eaten, sucked out of paper (buccally ingested), or smoked. This category includes many different drugs with different effects. Hallucinogens act as sympathomimetics and cause hypertension, tachycardia, hyperthermia, and dilated pupils. Psychological effects range from mild perceptual changes to frank hallucinations; most users experience only mild effects. Usually used sporadically because of tolerance, which develop rapidly and remit within several days of abstinence. Physical dependence or withdrawal does not occur, but psychological dependence can develop. Hallucinogens often are contaminated with anticholinergic drugs. Hallucinogen potency is associated with binding affinity at the serotonin-5-HT2 receptor, where these drugs act as partial agonists.

2. Epidemiology. Hallucinogen use is most common among young men (ages 15 to 35), with white men having the highest use compared to women and other ethnic groups. The lifetime use of hallucinogen in the United States is about 12%.

3. Hallucinogen intoxication (hallucinosis)
   a. Diagnosis, signs, and symptoms. In a state of full wakefulness and alertness, maladaptive behavioral changes (anxiety, depression, ideas of reference, paranoid ideation); changes in perception (hallucinations, illusions, depersonalization); pupillary dilation, tachycardia or palpitations, sweating, blurring of vision, tremors, and incoordination. Panic reactions ("bad trips") can occur even in experienced users. The user typically becomes convinced that the disturbed perceptions

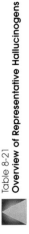

Table 8-21
Overview of Representative Hallucinogens

Agent	Locale	Chemical Classification	Biologic Sources	Common Route	Typical Dose	Duration of Effects
Lysergic acid diethylamine	Global	Indolealkylamine	Lysergic acid, semisynthetic	Oral	75 mcg	6–12 hours
Mescaline	Southwestern United States	Phenethylamine	Peyote cactus, *Lophophora williamsii, Lophophora diffusa*	Oral	200–400 mg or 4–6 cactus buttons	10–12 hours
Methylenedioxy-methamphetamine	Global	Phenethylamine	Synthetic	Oral	50–150 mg	4–6 hours
Psilocybin	Southern United States, Mexico, South America	Phosphorylated hydroxylated DMT	Psilocybin mushrooms	Oral	5 mg or 8 g of dried mushroom	4–6 hours
DMT[a]	South America, synthetic	Substituted tryptamine	Leaves of *Virola calophylla*	As a snuff, IV, smoked	0.2 mg/kg IV	30 minutes
Ibogaine	West Central Africa	Indolealkylamine	*Tabernanthe iboga* powdered root	Oral	200–400 mg	8–48 hours
Ayahuasca	South America East Amazon	Harmine, other β carbolines	Bark or leaves of liana vine	Orally as a tea	300–400 mg	4–8 hours
Morning glory seeds	American temperate zones	D-Lysergic acid alkaloids	Seeds of *Ipomoea violacea, Turbina corymbosa*	Orally as a tea	7–13 seeds	3 hours

[a]DMT, dimethyltryptamine.

126

Table 8-22
Diagnosis of Hallucinogen Intoxication

Behavioral and perceptual changes
Amnesia for the entire period of psychoses
Physiologic changes
1. Pupillary dilatation
2. Tachycardia
3. Sweating
4. Palpitations
5. Blurred vision
6. Tremors
7. Incoordination

are real. In the typical bad trip, the user feels as if he or she is going mad, has damaged his or her brain, and will never recover. See Table 8-22.

b. Treatment. Involves reassurance and keeping the patient in contact with trusted, supportive people (friends, nurses). Diazepam (20 mg orally) can rapidly curtail hallucinogen intoxication and is considered superior to "talking down" the patient, which may take hours. If the patient is psychotic and agitated, high-potency antipsychotics, such as haloperidol (Haldol), fluphenazine (Prolixin), or thiothixene (Navane), may be used (avoid low-potency antipsychotics because of anticholinergic effects). A controlled environment is necessary to prevent possible dangerous actions resulting from grossly impaired judgment. Physical restraints may be required. Prolonged psychosis resembling schizophreniform disorder occasionally develops in vulnerable patients. Delusional syndromes and mood (usually depressive) disorders may also develop.

4. Hallucinogen persisting perception disorder. A distressing repeated experience of impaired perception after cessation of hallucinogen use (i.e., a **flashback**). The patient may require low doses of a benzodiazepine (for an acute episode) or antipsychotic drug (if persistent). Anticonvulsants such as valproic acid (Depakene) and carbamazepine (Tegretol) have also been of use. See Table 8-23.

Phencyclidine (PCP; 1-1-phenylcyclohexyl-piperidine), also known as *angel dust*, is a dissociative anesthetic with hallucinogenic effects.

Table 8-23
Diagnosis of Hallucinogen Persisting Perception Disorder (Flashbacks)

Spontaneous and transitory recurrences of the substance-induced experience
Visual distortion and geometric hallucinations
Auditory hallucinations
Flashes of color
Trail of images from moving objects
Macropsia and micropsia
Time expansion and relived intense emotion
Episodes lasts a few seconds to a few minutes

Similarly acting drugs include ketamine (Ketalar), also referred to as *special K*. PCP commonly causes paranoia and unpredictable violence, which often brings abusers to medical attention. The primary pharmacodynamic effect is antagonism of the NMDA subtype of glutamate receptors.

a. **Epidemiology.** About 14% of 18- to 25-year-old men and women have used PCP in their lifetime; however, its use is declining. PCP is associated with 3% of substance abuse deaths and 32% of substance-related disorders.

b. **PCP intoxication**

(1) **Diagnosis, signs, and symptoms.** Belligerence, assaultiveness, agitation, impulsiveness, unpredictability, and the following signs: nystagmus, increased blood pressure or heart rate, numbness or diminished response to pain, ataxia, dysarthria, muscle rigidity, seizures, and hyperacusis.

Typically, PCP is smoked with marijuana (a laced joint) or tobacco, but it can be eaten, injected, or inhaled nasally. PCP should be considered in patients who describe unusual experiences with marijuana or LSD. PCP may remain detectable in blood and urine for more than 1 week.

Effects are dose-related. At low doses, PCP acts as a CNS depressant, producing nystagmus, blurred vision, numbness, and incoordination. At moderate doses, PCP produces hypertension, dysarthria, ataxia, increased muscle tone (especially in the face and neck), hyperactive reflexes, and sweating. At higher doses, PCP produces agitation, fever, abnormal movements, rhabdomyolysis, myoglobinuria, and renal failure. Overdose can cause seizures, severe hypertension, diaphoresis, hypersalivation, respiratory depression, stupor (with eyes open), coma, and death. Violent actions are common with intoxication. Because of the analgesic effects of PCP, patients may have no regard for their own bodies and may severely injure themselves while agitated and combative. Psychosis, sometimes persistent (may resemble schizophreniform disorder), may develop. This is especially likely in patients with underlying schizophrenia. Other possible complications include delirium, mood disorder, and delusional disorder. Ketamine, derived from PCP, produces a similar clinical picture.

(2) **Treatment.** Isolate the patient in a nonstimulating environment. Do not try to talk down the intoxicated patient, as you might with a patient with anxiety disorder; wait for the PCP to clear first. Urine acidification may increase drug clearance (ascorbic acid or ammonium chloride), but it may be ineffective and increase the risk for renal failure. Screen for other drugs. If the patient is acutely agitated, use benzodiazepines. If agitated and psychotic, an antipsychotic may be used. Avoid antipsychotics with potent intensive anticholinergic properties, because high-dose PCP has anti-

cholinergic actions. If physical restraint is required, immobilize the patient completely to prevent self-injury. Recovery is usually rapid. Protect the patient and staff. Always evaluate for concomitant medical conditions. Treatment for ketamine intoxication is similar.

5. **Hallucinogen intoxication delirium.** It is a relatively rare disorder and an estimated 25% of all PCP-related emergency room patients may meet the criteria for hallucinogen intoxication delirium. Hallucinogens are often mixed with other substances, and these interactions can produce clinical delirium.

6. **Hallucinogen-induced psychotic disorders.** If psychotic symptoms are present in the absence of retained reality testing, a diagnosis of hallucinogen-induced psychotic disorder may be warranted. A protracted psychotic episode may be difficult to distinguish from a nonorganic psychotic disorder.

7. **Hallucinogen-induced mood disorder.** Mood disorder symptoms accompanying hallucinogen abuse can vary and abusers may experience manic-like symptoms with grandiose delusions or depression-like feelings and ideas or mixed symptoms.

8. **Hallucinogen-induced anxiety disorder.** Hallucinogen-induced anxiety disorder also varies in its symptom pattern, but patients frequently report panic disorder with agoraphobia.

   a. **Clinical features of hallucinogens**

   Lysergic acid diethylamide (LSD). Common physiologic symptoms include dilated pupils, increased deep tendon motor reflexes, muscle tension, mild motor incoordination and ataxia. Increased heart rate, respiration, and blood pressure are modest in degree and variable, as are nausea, decreased appetite, and salivation.

   (1) Phenethylamines. Their chemical structure is similar to those of the neurotransmitters dopamine and norepinephrine. It was the first hallucinogen isolated from the peyote cactus.

   (2) Mescaline. It is consumed as peyote "buttons," picked from the small blue-green cacti *Lophophora williamsii* and *Lophophora diffusa*. The buttons are the dried, round, fleshy cacti tops and Mescaline is the active hallucinogenic alkaloid in the buttons. Use of peyote is legal for the Native American Church members in some states.

   (3) Psilocybin analogs. Psilocybin is usually ingested as mushrooms. Many species of psilocybin-containing mushrooms are found worldwide. Various studies indicate that psilocybin is helpful in reducing morbid anxiety about death and dying. It may play an important role in palliative care medicine in the future.

   (4) Phencyclidine (PCP). PCP ingestion may lead to experiencing speedy feelings, euphoria, bodily warmth, tingling, peaceful floating sensations, and, occasionally, feelings of depersonalization, isolation, and estrangement. Nystagmus, hypertension, and hyperthermia are common effects of PCP.

(5) Ketamine. Ketamine is a dissociative anesthetic agent, and has become a drug of abuse. It causes hallucinations and a dissociated state in which the patient has an altered sense of the body and reality and little concern for the environment. It is being used in an infusion form as a rapidly acting antidepressant agent with resolution of suicidal ideation.

(6) Additional hallucinogens. Canthinones, Ibogaine, Ayahuasca, and Salvia Divinorum.

N. **Inhalant-related disorders.** Inhalant drugs (also called inhalants or volatile substances) are volatile hydrocarbons that are inhaled for psychotropic effects. They include gasoline, kerosene, plastic and rubber cements, airplane and household glues, paints, lacquers, enamels, paint thinners, aerosols, polishes, fingernail polish remover, and cleaning fluids. Inhalants typically are abused by adolescents in lower socioeconomic groups.

 CLINICAL HINT:
Some persons use "poppers" (amyl nitrate, butyl nitrate) during sex to intensify orgasm through vasodilation, which produces light-headedness, giddiness, and euphoria. With the introduction of sildenafil (Viagra) used to produce penile erections, a special warning must be given to those who use nitrate-containing drugs, because the combination can cause cardiovascular collapse and death.

1. **Clinical features.** Symptoms of mild intoxication are similar to intoxication with alcohol or sedative–hypnotics. Psychological effects include mild euphoria, belligerence, assaultiveness, impaired judgment, and impulsiveness. Physical effects include ataxia, confusion, disorientation, slurred speech, dizziness, depressed reflexes, and nystagmus. These can progress to delirium and seizures. Possible toxic effects include brain damage, liver damage, bone marrow depression, peripheral neuropathies, and immunosuppression. See Table 8-24. Rarely a withdrawal syndrome can develop. It is characterized by irritability, sleep disturbances, jitters, sweats, nausea, vomiting, tachycardia, and sometimes hallucinations and delusions. Short-term treatment is

 Table 8-24
Diagnosis of Inhalant Intoxication

Maladaptive behavioral changes
Diminished social and occupational functioning
Impaired judgment
Impulsive behavior
Presence of at least two physical symptoms
1. Nausea
2. Anorexia
3. Nystagmus
4. Depressed reflexes
5. Diplopia

supportive medical care (e.g., fluids and monitoring of blood pressure). Inhalant-related disorders also encompass other diagnosis including, inhalant intoxication delirium, inhalant-induced persisting dementia, inhalant-induced psychotic disorder, and Inhalant-induced mood and anxiety disorders. The clinical symptoms are similar to those induced by other substances.

O. Caffeine-related disorders. Caffeine is the most widely consumed psychoactive substance in the world. Caffeine is present in coffee, tea, chocolate, cola and other carbonated beverages, cocoa, cold medications, and over-the-counter stimulants. (See Table 8-25 for the typical caffeine content of foods and medications.) Caffeine use is associated with five disorders: Caffeine use disorder, caffeine intoxication and withdrawal, as well as caffeine-induced anxiety and sleep disorder. Intoxication is characterized by restlessness, nervousness, excitement, insomnia, flushed face, diuresis, gastrointestinal disturbance, muscle twitching, rambling flow of thought and speech, tachycardia or cardiac arrhythmia, periods of inexhaustibility, and psychomotor agitation. Habitual use can result in psychiatric symptoms. High doses can increase symptoms of psychiatric disorders (e.g., anxiety, psychosis). Tolerance develops. Withdrawal is usually characterized by headache and lasts 4 to 5 days. Treatment is symptomatic. A short course of a benzodiazepine (diazepam, 15 mg per day for 2 to 5 days) may help alleviate withdrawal agitation and insomnia.

P. Tobacco-related disorders. Tobacco use disorder is among the most prevalent, deadly, and costly of substance dependencies. Nicotine is taken through tobacco smoking and chewing. Nicotine dependence is the most prevalent and deadly substance use disorder. Nicotine activates nicotine acetylcholine receptors in addition to the dopamine reward system and increases multiple stimulatory neurohormones. It is rapidly absorbed when inhaled and reaches the CNS within 15 seconds.

Table 8-25
Typical Caffeine Content of Foods and Medications

Substance	Caffeine Content
Brewed coffee	100 mg/6 oz
Instant coffee	70 mg/6 oz
Decaffeinated coffee	4 mg/6 oz
Leaf or bag tea	40 mg/6 oz
Instant tea	25 mg/6 oz
Caffeinated soda	45 mg/12 oz
Cocoa beverage	5 mg/6 oz
Chocolate milk	4 mg/6 oz
Dark chocolate	20 mg/1 oz
Milk chocolate	6 mg/1 oz
Caffeine-containing cold remedies	25–50 mg/tablet
Caffeine-containing analgesics	25–65 mg/tablet
Stimulants	100–350 mg/tablet
Weight-loss aids	75–200 mg/tablet

Adapted from *DSM-IV-TR* and Barone JJ, Roberts HR. Caffeine consumption. *Food Chem Toxicol* 1996;34:119.

1. **Epidemiology.** About 25% of Americans smoke, 25% are former smokers, and 50% have never smoked. The mean age of onset of smoking is 16 years of age, and few persons start after 20 years of age. Worldwide, about 1 billion people smoke 6 trillion cigarettes a year.
2. **Diagnosis.** Tobacco-related disorder is characterized by craving, persistent and recurrent use, tolerance, and withdrawal upon stopping.
   a. **Nicotine dependence.** Develops rapidly and is strongly affected by environmental conditioning. Often coexists with dependence on other substances (e.g., alcohol, marijuana). Treatments for dependence include hypnosis, aversive therapy, acupuncture, nicotine nasal sprays and gums, transdermal nicotine (nicotine patches), clonidine, and a variety of other non-nicotine psychopharmacologic agents. Bupropion (Zyban) at doses of 300 mg/day may increase the quit rate in smokers with and without depression. The combined use of systemic nicotine administration and behavioral counseling has resulted in sustained abstinence rates of 60%. High relapse rates. Chantix (varenicline) is a partial nicotine agonist for $\alpha_4\beta_2$ nicotinic acetylcholine receptor subtypes. It is usually dosed at 1 mg b.i.d. following 1 week titration beginning at 0.5 mg/day for several days. Psychiatrists should be aware of the effects of abstinence from smoking on blood concentrations of psychotropic drugs (Table 8-26). Smoking is more habit-forming than chewing. Smoking is associated with chronic obstructive pulmonary disease, cancers, coronary heart disease, and peripheral vascular disease. Tobacco chewing is associated with peripheral vascular disease.
   b. **Nicotine withdrawal.** Characterized by nicotine craving, irritability, frustration, anger, anxiety, difficulty concentrating, restlessness, bradycardia, and increased appetite. The withdrawal syndrome may last for up to several weeks and is often superimposed on withdrawal from other substances.
3. **Treatment.** A summary of treatment techniques is given in Table 8-27.

Q. **Other (or unknown substance-related disorders)**
   1. **γ-Hydroxybutyrate (GHB).** GHB is a neurotransmitter in the brain related to sleep regulation. It is a CNS depressant and induces anesthesia

Table 8-26
Effect of Abstinence from Smoking on Blood Concentrations of Psychiatric Medicines

Abstinence increases blood concentrations			
Clomipramine	Desmethyldiazepam	Haloperidol	Nortriptyline
Clozapine	Doxepin	Imipramine	Propranolol
Desipramine	Fluvoxamine	Oxazepam	
Abstinence does not increase blood concentrations			
Amitriptyline	Ethanol	Midazolam	
Chlordiazepoxide	Lorazepam	Triazolam	
Effects of abstinence unclear			
Alprazolam	Chlorpromazine	Diazepam	

Adapted from John R. Hughes, M.D.

Table 8-27
Scientifically Proven Treatments for Smoking

Psychosocial therapy
Behavior therapy
Hypnosis
Pharmacologic therapies
Nicotine gum
Nicotine patch
Nicotine gum + patch
Nicotine nasal spray
Nicotine inhaler
Nicotine lozenges
Bupropion
Bupropion + nicotine patch
Clonidine[a]
Varenicline (Chantix)
Nortriptyline[a]

[a]Not an FDA-approved use.
Adapted from John R. Hughes, M.D.

and long-term sedation. A form of GHB (Xyrem) is FDA approved for the treatment of narcolepsy though it is a controlled substance (CIII) requiring extra paper work. GHB is abused for intoxication and referred to as liquid ecstasy. It may cause nausea, respiratory problems, seizures, coma, and death.

2. **Nitrate inhalants.** These include amyl, butyl nitrate and are called poppers in popular culture. These induce mild euphoria, altered sense of time, and increased sexual feelings. It may cause toxic syndrome characterized by nausea, vomiting, hypotension, and drowsiness.

3. **Nitrous oxide.** Also called as laughing gas is an anesthetic agent and can be abused for inducing light-headedness and floating, experienced as pleasurable and sexual.

4. **Anabolic steroids.** Anabolic steroids are a family of drugs comprising the natural male hormone testosterone and a group of more than 50 synthetic analogs of testosterone. They are Drug Enforcement Agency Schedule III controlled substances that are illegally used to enhance physical performance and appearance and to increase muscle bulk. Examples of commonly used anabolic steroids are listed in Table 8-28. An estimated 1 million Americans have used illegal steroids at least once. Use has been increasing among male adolescents and young adults. People drawn to these drugs are usually involved in athletics. Reinforcement occurs when the drugs produce desired results, such as enhanced performance and appearance. Anabolic steroid users typically use a variety of ergogenic (performance-enhancing) drugs to gain muscle, lose fat, or lose water for body-building competitions. These drugs include thyroid hormones and stimulants. Dehydroepiandrosterone (DHEA) and androstenedione are adrenal androgens marketed as food supplements and sold over the counter. Steroids initially produce euphoria and hyperactivity, which can

Table 8-28
Examples of Commonly Used Anabolic Steroids^a

Compounds usually administered orally
Fluoxymesterone (Halotestin, Android-F, Ultandren)
Methandienone (formerly called *methandrostenolone*) (Dianabol)
Methyltestosterone (Android, Testred, Virilon)
Mibolerone (Cheque Drops)^b
Oxandrolone (Anavar)
Oxymetholone (Anadrol, Hemogenin)
Mesterolone (Mestoranum, Proviron)
Stanozolol (Winstrol)

Compounds usually administered intramuscularly
Nandrolone decanoate (Deca-Durabolin)
Nandrolone phenpropionate (Durabolin)
Methenolone enanthate (Primobolan depot)
Boldenone undecylenate (Equipoise)^b
Stanozolol (Winstrol-V)^b
Testosterone esters blends (Sustanon, Sten)
Testosterone cypionate
Testosterone enanthate (Delatestryl)
Testosterone propionate (Testoviron, Androlan)
Testosterone undecanoate (Andriol, Restandol)
Trenbolone acetate (Finajet, Finaplix)^b
Trenbolone hexahydrobencylcarbonate (Parabolan)

^{a}Many of the brand names listed are foreign but are included because of the widespread illicit use of foreign steroid preparations in the United States.
^{b}Veterinary compound.
Adapted from Harrison G. Pope, Jr., M.D., and Kirk J. Brower, M.D.

give way to hostility, irritability, anxiety, somatization, depression, manic symptoms, and violent outbursts ("roid rage"). Steroids are addictive. Abstinence can produce depression, anxiety, and worry about physical appearance. Physical complications of abuse include acne, premature balding, gynecomastia, testicular atrophy, yellowing of the skin and eyes, clitoral enlargement, menstrual abnormalities, and hirsutism.

Treatment includes psychotherapy to cope with body image distortions and the profound physical side effects of prolonged steroid use. As with other substances of abuse, abstinence is the goal. Frequent urine testing is indicated.

5. **Other substances**
Other substances commonly abused include:
a. Nutmeg - produces hallucinations
b. Catnip - causes disorganized thinking
c. Betel Nuts - causes euphoria and alertness
d. Kava - may cause panic states
e. Ephedra - may cause anxiety
f. Chocolate - contains anandamide which is a psychostimulant

For more detailed discussion of this topic, see Chapter 11, Substance-Related Disorders, Section, 11.1-11.11, p. 1282 in CTP/X.

Schizophrenia Spectrum and Other Psychotic Disorders

I. Introduction

Schizophrenia is usually discussed as a single disease but it probably comprises a group of disorders along a spectrum with heterogeneous etiologies and is characterized by disturbances in cognition, emotion, perception, thinking, and behavior. Schizophrenia is well established as a brain disorder, with structural and functional abnormalities visible in neuroimaging studies and a genetic component as seen in twin studies. The disorder is usually chronic, with a course encompassing a prodromal phase, an active phase, and a residual phase. The active phase has symptoms such as hallucinations, delusions, and disorganized thinking. The prodromal and residual phases are characterized by attenuated forms of active symptoms, such as odd beliefs and magical thinking, as well as deficits in self-care and interpersonal relatedness. Since the 1970s, the number of schizophrenic patients in hospitals has decreased by over 50% (deinstitutionalization). Of those being treated, over 80% are managed as out-patients. A brief history of the disorder is to be found in Table 9-1.

II. Epidemiology

A. Incidence and prevalence. In the United States, the lifetime prevalence of the disease is about 1%, which means that 1 in 100 persons will develop the disorder during his or her lifetime. It is found in all societies and in all geographic areas. Worldwide, 2 million new cases appear each year. In the United States, only about 0.05% of the total population is treated for schizophrenia in any single year and only about half of all patients obtain treatment of any kind. There are over 2 million persons suffering from schizophrenia in the United States.

B. Gender and age. Equally prevalent between men and women; usually onset is earlier in men. Peak age of onset between 15 and 35 (50% of cases occur before age 25). Onset before age 10 (called early-onset schizophrenia) or after age 45 (called late-onset) is uncommon.

C. Infection and birth season. Persons born in winter are more likely to develop the disease than those born in spring or summer (applies to both Northern and Southern Hemispheres). Increased in babies born to mothers who have influenza during pregnancy.

D. Race and religion. Jews are affected less often than Protestants and Catholics, and prevalence is higher in non-white populations.

E. Medical and mental illness. Higher mortality rate from accidents and natural causes than in general population. Leading cause of death in

Table 9-1
History of Schizophrenia

1852—Schizophrenia was first formally described by Belgian psychiatrist Benedict Morel, who called it *démence précoce*.
1896—Emil Kraepelin, a German psychiatrist, applied the term *dementia praecox* to a group of illnesses beginning in adolescence that ended in dementia.
1911—Swiss psychiatrist Eugen Bleuler introduced the term *schizophrenia*. No signs or symptoms are pathognomonic; instead, a cluster of characteristic findings indicates the diagnosis. He introduced the concept of the fundamental symptoms, called the *four A's*: (1) associational disturbances, (2) affective disturbances, (3) autism, and (4) ambivalence.

schizophrenic patients is suicide (10% kill themselves). Over 40% of schizophrenic patients abuse drugs and alcohol. The prevalence of diabetes mellitus type II and metabolic abnormalities is higher and treatment with atypical antipsychotics agents may increase the risk of developing diabetes and the metabolic syndrome.

F. Socioeconomics. More common among lower rather than higher socioeconomic groups; high prevalence among recent immigrants; most common in cities with over 1 million population. Direct and indirect costs resulting from schizophrenic illness in the United States are over $100 billion per year.

III. Etiology

Owing to the heterogeneity of the symptomatic and prognostic presentations of schizophrenia, no single factor is considered causative. The stress diathesis model is most often used, which states that the person in whom schizophrenia develops has a specific biologic vulnerability, or diathesis, that is triggered by stress and leads to schizophrenic symptoms. Stresses may be genetic, biologic, and psychosocial or environmental.

A. Genetic. Both single-gene and polygenic theories have been proposed (Table 9-2). Although neither theory has been definitively substantiated, the polygenic theory appears to be more consistent with the presentation of schizophrenia. Some data indicate that the age of the father has a correlation with the development of schizophrenia and that those born from fathers older than the age of 60 years were vulnerable to developing the disorder.

1. Consanguinity. Incidence in families is higher than in the general population, and monozygotic (MZ) twin concordance is greater than dizygotic (DZ) (Table 9-3).

Table 9-2
Features Consistent with Polygenic Inheritance[a]

Disorder can be transmitted with two normal parents.
Presentation of disorder ranges from very severe to less severe.
More severely affected persons have a greater number of ill relatives than mildly affected persons do.
Risk decreases as the number of shared genes decreases.
Disorder present in both mother's and father's side of family.

[a]The number of affected genes determines a person's risk and symptomatic picture.

Table 9-3
Prevalence of Schizophrenia in Specific Populations

Population	Prevalence (%)
General population	1–1.5
First-degree relative[a]	10–12
Second-degree relative	5–6
Child of two schizophrenic parents	40
Dizygotic twin	12–15
Monozygotic twin	45–50

[a]Schizophrenia is not a sex-linked disorder; it does not matter which parent has the disorder in terms of risk.

2. Adoption studies

　　a. The prevalence of schizophrenia is greater in the biologic parents of schizophrenic adoptees than in adoptive parents.

　　b. MZ twins reared apart have the same concordance rate as twins reared together.

　　c. Rates of schizophrenia are not increased in children born to unaffected parents but raised by a schizophrenic parent.

B. Biologic

　　1. Dopamine hypothesis. Schizophrenic symptoms may result from increased limbic dopamine activity (positive symptoms) and decreased frontal dopamine activity (negative symptoms). Dopaminergic pathology may be secondary to abnormal receptor number or sensitivity, or abnormal dopamine release (too much or too little). The theory is based on psychotogenic effects of drugs that increase dopamine levels (e.g., amphetamines, cocaine) and the antipsychotic effects of dopamine receptor antagonists (e.g., haloperidol [Haldol]). Dopamine receptors D1 through D5 have been identified. The D1 receptor may play a role in negative symptoms. Specific D3 and D4 receptor agonist and antagonist drugs are under development. Levels of the dopamine metabolite homovanillic acid may correlate with the severity and potential treatment responsiveness of psychotic symptoms. Limitations of the theory include the responsiveness of all types of psychoses to dopamine-blocking agents, which implicates dopaminergic abnormalities in psychoses of multiple causes. The complex interplay of different neurotransmitter systems, including serotonin–dopamine interactions, in addition to the effects of amino acid neurotransmitters on monoamine render single-neurotransmitter theories incomplete.

　　2. Norepinephrine hypothesis. Increased norepinephrine levels in schizophrenia lead to increased sensitization to sensory input.

　　3. γ-Aminobutyric acid (GABA) hypothesis. Decreased GABA activity results in increased dopamine activity.

　　4. Serotonin hypothesis. Serotonin metabolism apparently is abnormal in some chronically schizophrenic patients, with both hyperserotoninemia and hyposerotoninemia being reported. Specifically, antagonism at the serotonin 5-HT2 receptor has been emphasized as important in reducing psychotic symptoms and the development of movement disorders related to D2 antagonism. Research on mood disorders has been implicated serotonin activity in suicidal and impulsive behavior, which schizophrenic patients can also exhibit.

5. **Glutamate hypothesis.** Hypofunction of the glutamate *N*-methyl-D-aspartate (NMDA)-type receptor is theorized to cause both positive and negative symptoms of schizophrenia based on the observed psychotogenic effects of the NMDA antagonists phencyclidine and ketamine (Ketalar), in addition to the observed therapeutic effects (in research settings) of the NMDA agonists glycine and D-cycloserine.

6. **Neurodevelopmental theories.** This is evidence for abnormal neuronal migration during the second trimester of fetal development. Abnormal neuronal functioning may lead to the emergence of symptoms during adolescence.

C. **Psychosocial and environmental**

1. **Family factors.** Patients whose families have high levels of expressed emotion (EE) have higher relapse rate than those whose families have low EE levels. EE has been defined as any overly involved, intrusive behavior, be it hostile and critical or controlling and infantilizing. Relapse rates are better when family behavior is modified to lower EE. Most observers believe that family dysfunction is a consequence, rather than a cause, of schizophrenia.

2. **Other psychodynamic issues.** Knowing what psychological and environmental stresses are most likely to trigger psychotic decompensation in a patient helps the clinician to address these issues supportively and, in the process, helps the patient to feel and remain more in control.

D. **Infectious theory.** Evidence for a slow virus etiology includes neuropathologic changes consistent with past infections: gliosis, glial scarring, and antiviral antibodies in the serum and cerebrospinal fluid (CSF) of some schizophrenia patients. Increased frequency of perinatal complications and seasonality of birth data also support an infectious theory.

IV. **Diagnosis, Signs, and Symptoms**

Schizophrenia is a disorder whose diagnosis is based on observation and description of the patient. Abnormalities are often present on most components of the mental status examination. There are no pathognomonic signs or symptoms. According to the fifth edition of the *Diagnostic Statistical Manual of Mental Disorders* (DSM-5) at least two of the following five signs or symptoms must be present for at least 1 month. See Table 9-4. (1) Hallucinations; (2) delusions; (3) disorganized speech; (4) disorganized behavior; or (5) negative symptoms (e.g., flat affect, abulia). See Table 9-5. The signs and symptoms should be present for at least 6 months for the disorder to be confirmed. Other diagnostic features of schizophrenia are listed below.

Table 9-4
Signs and Symptoms of Schizophrenia

Positive symptoms
Hallucinations
Delusions
Disorganized speech
Disorganized behavior
Loose associations

Negative symptoms
Affective flattening
Alogia
Avolition
Anhedonia
Attention

Signs and symptoms must be present for at least 6 months before a diagnosis can be made.

A. **Overall functioning.** Level of functioning declines or fails to achieve the expected level.

B. **Thought content.** Abnormal (e.g., delusions, ideas of reference, poverty of content). Delusion and hallucinations are not necessary to make the diagnosis if other signs and symptoms are present.

C. **Form of thought.** Illogical (e.g., derailment, loosening of associations, incoherence, circumstantially, tangentiality, overinclusiveness, neologisms, blocking, echolalia—all incorporated as a thought disorder).

D. **Perception.** Distorted (e.g., hallucinations: visual, olfactory, tactile, and, most frequently, auditory).

Table 9-5
Negative Symptoms in Schizophrenia

I. Affective flattening or blunting
    a. Unchanged facial expressions
    b. Decreased spontaneous movements
    c. Paucity of expressive gesture
    d. Poor eye contact
    e. Affective nonresponsivity
    f. Inappropriate affect
    g. Lack of vocal inflections
II. Alogia
    a. Poverty of speech
    b. Poverty of content of speech
    c. Blocking
    d. Increased latency of response
III. Avolition-apathy
    a. Grooming and hygiene
    b. Impersistence at work or school
    c. Physical anergia
IV. Anhedonia-asociality
    a. Recreational interests and activities
    b. Sexual interest and activities
    c. Intimacy and closeness
    d. Relationship and friends
V. Attention
    a. Social inattentiveness
    b. Inattentiveness during testing

E. **Affect.** Abnormal (e.g., flat, blunted, silly, labile, inappropriate).

F. **Sense of self.** Impaired (e.g., loss of ego boundaries, gender confusion, inability to distinguish internal from external reality).

G. **Volition.** Altered (e.g., inadequate drive or motivation and marked ambivalence).

H. **Interpersonal functioning.** Impaired (e.g., social withdrawal and emotional detachment, aggressiveness, sexual inappropriateness).

I. **Psychomotor behavior.** Abnormal or changed (e.g., agitation vs. withdrawal, grimacing, posturing, rituals, catatonia).

J. **Cognition.** Impaired (e.g., concreteness, inattention, impaired information processing).

V. **Types**

DSM-5 no longer classifies schizophrenia based on subtypes. They are included in this text because the authors believe them to be of clinical significance and they are still used by most clinicians in the United States and around the world.

A. **Paranoid**
1. Characterized mainly by the presence of delusions of persecution or grandeur.
2. Frequent auditory hallucinations related to a single theme, usually persecutory.
3. Patients typically are tense, suspicious, guarded, reserved, and sometimes hostile or aggressive.
4. None of the following: incoherence, loosening of associations, flat or grossly inappropriate affect, catatonic behavior, grossly disorganized behavior. Intelligence remains intact.
5. Age of onset later than catatonic or disorganized type, and the later the onset, the better the prognosis.

B. **Disorganized (formerly called hebephrenia)**
1. Characterized by marked regression to primitive, disinhibited, and chaotic behavior.
2. Incoherence, marked loosening of associations, flat or grossly inappropriate affect, pronounced thought disorder.
3. Dilapidated appearance, incongruous grinning and grimacing.
4. Early onset, usually before age 25.
5. Does not meet criteria for catatonic type.

C. **Catatonic**
1. Classic feature is a marked disturbance in motor function called waxy flexibility.
2. May involve rigidity, stupor, posturing, echopraxia; patients may hold awkward positions for long periods of time.
3. Purposeless excitement with risk of injury to self or others may occur.
4. Speech disturbances such as echolalia or mutism may occur.
5. May need medical care for associated malnutrition, exhaustion, or hyperpyrexia.

CLINICAL HINT:
Patient may emerge from catatonic state suddenly and, without warning, be quite violent.

D. Undifferentiated type
   1. Prominent delusions, hallucinations, incoherence, or grossly disturbed behavior.
   2. Does not meet the criteria for paranoid, catatonic, or disorganized type.
E. Residual type
   1. Absence of prominent delusions, hallucinations, incoherence, or grossly disorganized behavior.
   2. Continuing evidence of the disturbance through two or more residual symptoms (e.g., emotional blunting, social withdrawal).
F. Other subtypes
   1. **Negative and positive symptoms.** Another system classifies schizophrenia into one that is based on the presence of positive or negative symptoms. The negative symptoms include affective flattening or blunting, poverty of speech or speech content, blocking, poor grooming, lack of motivation, anhedonia, social withdrawal, cognitive defects, and attentional deficits. Positive symptoms include loose associations, hallucinations, bizarre behavior, and increased speech (Table 9-5). Patients with positive symptoms have a better prognosis than those with negative symptoms.
   2. **Paraphrenia.** Sometimes used as a synonym for *paranoid schizophrenia*. The term also is used for either a progressively deteriorating course of illness or the presence of a well-systematized delusional system. These multiple meanings have reduced the usefulness of the term.
   3. **Simple deteriorative schizophrenia (simple schizophrenia).** Characterized by a gradual, insidious loss of drive and ambition. Patients with the disorder are usually not overtly psychotic and do not experience persistent hallucinations or delusions. The primary symptom is the withdrawal of the patient from social and work-related situations.
   4. **Early-onset schizophrenia.** Schizophrenia that develops in childhood. Very rare.
   5. **Late-onset schizophrenia.** Onset after age 45. More common in women, most often of the paranoid type, with good response to medication.
   6. *Bouffée Délirante* (Acute Delusional Psychosis). The diagnosis is similar to the DSM-5 diagnosis of schizophreniform disorder on the basis of a symptom duration of less than 3 months. About 40% of patients with progress to being classified as having schizophrenia.
   7. **Oneiroid.** Refers to a dream-like state in which patients may be deeply perplexed and not fully oriented in time and place. When an oneiroid state is present, clinicians should be particularly careful to examine patients for medical or neurologic causes of the symptoms.

VI. Laboratory and Psychological Tests

A. EEG. Most schizophrenic patients have normal EEG findings, but some have decreased alpha and increased theta and delta activity, paroxysmal abnormalities, and increased sensitivity to activation procedures (e.g., sleep deprivation).

B. Evoked potential studies. Initial hypersensitivity to sensory stimulation, with later compensatory blunting of information processing at higher cortical levels.

C. Immunologic studies. In some patients, atypical lymphocytes and decreased numbers of natural killer cells.

D. Endocrinologic studies. In some patients, decreased levels of luteinizing hormone and follicle-stimulating hormone; diminished release of prolactin and growth hormone following stimulation by gonadotropin-releasing hormone or thyrotropin-releasing hormone.

E. Neuropsychological testing. Thematic apperception test and Rorschach test usually reveal bizarre responses. When compared with the parents of normal controls, the parents of schizophrenic patients show more deviation from normal values in projective tests (may be a consequence of living with schizophrenic family member). Halstead–Reitan battery reveals impaired attention and intelligence, decreased retention time, and disturbed problem-solving ability in approximately 20% to 35% of patients. Schizophrenic patients have lower IQs when compared with nonschizophrenic patients, although the range of IQ scores is wide. Decline in IQ occurs with progression of the illness.

VII. Pathophysiology

A. Neuropathology. No consistent structural defects; changes noted include decreased number of neurons, increased gliosis, and disorganization of neuronal architecture. There is degeneration in the limbic system, especially the amygdala, hippocampus, and the cingulate cortex. The basal ganglia, including the substantia nigra and dorsolateral prefrontal cortex are also involved. Abnormal functioning in basal ganglia and cerebellum may account for movement disorders in schizophrenic patients.

B. Brain imaging

1. **Computed tomography (CT).** Cortical atrophy in 10% to 35% of patients; enlargement of the lateral and third ventricle in 10% to 50% of patients; atrophy of the cerebellar vermis and decreased radiodensity of brain parenchyma. Abnormal CT findings may correlate with the presence of negative symptoms (e.g., flattened affect, social withdrawal, psychomotor retardation, lack of motivation, neuropsychiatric impairment, increased frequency of extrapyramidal symptoms resulting from antipsychotic medications, and poor premorbid history).

2. **Magnetic resonance imaging (MRI).** Ventricles in MZ twins with schizophrenia are larger than those of unaffected siblings. Reduced volume of hippocampus, amygdala, and parahippocampal gyrus. Reduced limbic volume correlating with disease severity.

3. **Magnetic resonance spectroscopy.** Decreased metabolism of the dorsolateral prefrontal cortex.
4. **Positron emission tomography (PET).** In some patients, decreased frontal and parietal lobe metabolism, relatively high rate of posterior metabolism, and abnormal laterality.
5. **Cerebral blood flow (CBF).** In some patients, decreased resting levels of frontal blood flow, increased parietal blood flow, and decreased whole-brain blood flow. When PET and CBF studies are considered together with CT findings, dysfunction of the frontal lobe is most clearly implicated. Frontal lobe dysfunction may be secondary, however, to disease elsewhere in the brain.

C. **Physical findings.** Minor (soft) neurologic findings occur in 50% to 100% of patients: increased prevalence of primitive reflexes (e.g., grasp reflex), abnormal stereognosis and two-point discrimination, and dysdiadochokinesia (impairment in ability to perform rapidly alternating movements). Paroxysmal saccadic eye movements (inability to follow object through space with smooth eye movements) occur in 50% to 80% of schizophrenic patients and in 40% to 45% of first-degree relatives of schizophrenic patients (compared with an 8% to 10% prevalence in nonschizophrenic persons). This may be a neurophysiologic marker of a vulnerability to schizophrenia. Resting heart rates have been found to be higher in schizophrenic patients than in controls and may reflect a hyperaroused state.

VIII. Psychodynamic Factors

Understanding a patient's dynamics (or psychological conflicts and issues) is critical for complete understanding of the symbolic meaning of symptoms. A patient's internal experience is usually one of confusion and overwhelming sensory input, and defense mechanisms are the ego's attempt to deal with powerful affects. Three major primitive defenses interfere with reality testing: (1) psychotic projection—attributing inner sensations of aggression, sexuality, chaos, and confusion to the outside world, as opposed to recognizing them as emanating from within; boundaries between inner and outer experience are confused; projection is the major defense underlying paranoid delusions; (2) reaction formation—turning a disturbing idea or impulse into its opposite; and (3) psychotic denial—transforming confusing stimuli into delusions and hallucinations.

IX. Differential Diagnosis

A. **Medical and neurologic disorders.** Present with impaired memory, orientation, and cognition; visual hallucinations; signs of CNS damage. Many neurologic and medical disorders can present with symptoms identical to those of schizophrenia, including substance intoxication (e.g., cocaine, phencyclidine) and substance-induced psychotic disorder, CNS infections (e.g., herpes encephalitis), vascular disorders (e.g., systemic lupus erythematosus), complex partial seizures (e.g., temporal lobe epilepsy), and degenerative disease (e.g., Huntington's disease).

B. **Schizophreniform disorder.** Symptoms may be identical to those of schizophrenia but last for less than 6 months. Also, deterioration is less pronounced and the prognosis is better.

C. **Brief psychotic disorder.** Symptoms last less than 1 month and proceed from a clearly identifiable psychosocial stress.

D. **Mood disorders.** Both manic episodes and major depressive episodes of bipolar I disorder and major depressive disorder may present with psychotic symptoms. The differential diagnosis is particularly important because of the availability of specific and effective treatments for the mood disorders. DSM-5 states that mood symptoms in schizophrenia must be brief relative to the essential criteria. Also, if hallucinations and delusions are present in a mood disorder, they develop in the context of the mood disturbance and do not persist. Other factors that help differentiate mood disorders from schizophrenia include family history, premorbid history, course (e.g., age at onset), prognosis (e.g., absence of residual deterioration following the psychotic episode), and response to treatment. Patients may experience postpsychotic depressive disorder of schizophrenia (i.e., a major depressive episode occurring during the residual phase of schizophrenia). True depression in these patients must be differentiated from medication-induced adverse effects, such as sedation, akinesia, and flattening of affect.

E. **Schizoaffective disorder.** Mood symptoms develop concurrently with symptoms of schizophrenia, but delusions or hallucinations must be present for 2 weeks in the absence of prominent mood symptoms during some phase of the illness. The prognosis of this disorder is better than that expected for schizophrenia and worse than that for mood disorders.

F. **Other specified or unspecified related disorder.** An atypical psychosis with a confusing clinical picture (e.g., persistent auditory hallucinations as the only symptom, and many culture-bound syndromes).

G. **Delusional disorders.** Nonbizarre, systematized delusions that last at least 6 months in the context of an intact, relatively well-functioning personality in the absence of prominent hallucinations or other schizophrenic symptoms. Onset is in middle to late adult life.

H. **Personality disorders.** In general, no psychotic symptoms, but, if present, they tend to be transient and not prominent. The most important personality disorders in this differential diagnosis are schizotypal, schizoid, borderline, and paranoid.

I. **Factitious disorder and malingering.** No laboratory test or biologic marker can objectively confirm the diagnosis of schizophrenia. Schizophrenic symptoms are therefore possible to feign for either clear secondary gain (malingering) or deep psychological motivations (factitious disorder).

J. **Pervasive developmental disorders.** Pervasive developmental disorders (e.g., autistic disorder) are usually recognized before 3 years of age. Although behavior may be bizarre and deteriorated, no delusions, hallucinations, or clear formal thought disorder is present (e.g., loosening of associations).

K. **Intellectual disability.** Intellectual, behavioral, and mood disturbances that suggest schizophrenia. However, intellectual disability involves no

Table 9-6
Differential Diagnosis of Schizophrenia-Like Symptoms

Medical and Neurologic
Substance induced—amphetamine, hallucinogens, belladonna alkaloids, alcohol hallucinosis, barbiturate withdrawal, cocaine, phencyclidine
Epilepsy—especially temporal lobe epilepsy
Neoplasm, cerebrovascular disease, or trauma—especially frontal or limbic
Other conditions
Acute intermittent porphyria
AIDS
Vitamin B_{12} deficiency
Carbon monoxide poisoning
Cerebral lipoidosis
Creutzfeldt-Jakob disease
Fabry's disease
Fahr's disease
Hallervorden-Spatz disease
Heavy metal poisoning
Herpes encephalitis
Homocystinuria
Huntington's disease
Metachromatic leukodystrophy
Neurosyphilis
Normal pressure hydrocephalus
Pellagra
Systemic lupus erythematosus
Wernicke-Korsakoff syndrome
Wilson's disease

Psychiatric
Atypical psychosis
Autistic disorder
Brief psychotic disorder
Delusional disorder
Factitious disorder with predominantly psychological signs and symptoms
Malingering
Mood disorders
Normal adolescence
Obsessive-compulsive disorder
Personality disorders—schizotypal, schizoid, borderline, paranoid
Schizoaffective disorder
Schizophrenia
Schizophreniform disorder

overt psychotic symptoms and involves a constant low level of functioning rather than a deterioration. If psychotic symptoms are present, a diagnosis of schizophrenia may be made concurrently.

L. Shared cultural beliefs. Seemingly odd beliefs shared and accepted by a cultural group are not considered psychotic. See Table 9-6.

X. Course and Prognosis

A. Course. Prodromal symptoms of anxiety, perplexity, terror, or depression generally precede the onset of schizophrenia, which may be acute or insidious. Prodromal symptoms may be present for months before a definitive diagnosis is made. Onset is generally in the late teens and early 20s; women generally are older at onset than men. Precipitating events (e.g., emotional trauma, use of drugs, a separation) may trigger episodes of illness in predisposed persons. Classically, the course of schizophrenia is one of deterioration over time, with acute exacerbations superimposed on a chronic picture. Vulnerability to stress is lifelong. Postpsychotic depressive episodes may occur in the residual phase. Other comorbidities include substance use disorders, obsessive-compulsive disorder, hyponatremia secondary to polydipsia, smoking, and HIV infection.

CLINICAL HINT:
During the course of the illness, the more florid positive psychotic symptoms, such as bizarre delusions and hallucinations, tend to diminish in intensity, whereas the more residual negative symptoms, such as poor hygiene, flattened emotional response, and various oddities of behavior, tend to increase.

Relapse rates are approximately 40% in 2 years on medication and 80% in 2 years off medication. Suicide is attempted by 50% of patients; 10% are successful. Violence is a risk, particularly in untreated patients. Risk factors include persecutory delusions, a history of violence, and neurologic deficits. The risk for sudden death and medical illness is increased, and life expectancy is shortened.

B. **Prognosis.** See Table 9-7. In terms of overall prognosis, some investigators have described a loose rule of thirds: approximately one-third of patients lead somewhat normal lives, one-third continue to experience significant symptoms but can function within society, and the remaining one-third are markedly impaired and require frequent hospitalization. Approximately 10% of this final third of patients require long-term institutionalization. In general, women have a better prognosis than do men.

Table 9-7
Features Weighting Toward Good or Poor Prognosis in Schizophrenia

Good Prognosis	Poor Prognosis
Late onset	Early onset
Obvious precipitating factors	No precipitating factors
Acute onset	Insidious onset
Good premorbid social, sexual, and work histories	Poor premorbid social, sexual, and work histories
Mood disorder symptoms (especially depressive disorders)	Withdrawn, autistic behavior
Married	Single, divorced, or widowed
Family history of mood disorders and family history of schizophrenia	
Good support systems	Poor support systems
Positive symptoms	Negative symptoms
Female sex	Neurologic signs and symptoms
	History of perinatal trauma
	No remissions in 3 years
	Many relapses
	History of assaultiveness

XI. Treatment

Clinical management of the schizophrenic patient may include hospitalization and antipsychotic medication in addition to psychosocial treatments, such as behavioral, family, group, individual, and social skills and rehabilitation therapies. Any of these treatment modalities can be given on an inpatient or outpatient basis. Indications for hospitalization include posing a danger to others, suicidality, severe symptomatology leading to poor self-care or risk for injury secondary to disorganization, diagnostic evaluation, failure to respond to treatment in less restrictive settings, complicating comorbidities, and the need to alter complex drug treatment regimens.

A. Pharmacologic. The antipsychotics include the first-generation dopamine receptor antagonists and the second-generation agents such as serotonin–dopamine antagonists (SDAs), such as risperidone (Risperdal) and clozapine (Clozaril). See Table 9-8.

   1. Choice of drug.

   a. First-generation antipsychotics (also known as typical antipsychotics, or dopamine receptor antagonists)—the classic antipsychotic

Table 9-8
Commonly Used Antipsychotic Medications

Antipsychotic Medication	Recommended Dose Range (mg/day)	Chlorpromazine Equivalents (mg/day)	Half-Life (hours)
First-generation agents (typical)			
Phenothiazine			
Chlorpromazine (Thorazine)	300–1000	100	5–7
Fluphenazine (Prolixin Decanoate)	5–20	2	32–34
Mesoridazine (Serentil)	150–400	50	35–37
Perphenazine (Trilafon)	16–64	10	9–11
Thioridazine (Mellaril)	300–800	100	23–25
Trifluoperazine (Stelazine)	15–50	5	23–25
Butyrophenone			
Haloperidol (Haldol)	5–20	2	20–22
Others			
Loxapine (Loxitane)	30–100	10	3–5
Molindone (Moban)	30–100	10	23–25
Thiothixene (Navane)	15–50	5	33–35
Second-generation agents (atypical or novel)			
Aripiprazole (Abilify)	10–30	N/A	74–76
Clozapine (Clozaril)	150–600	N/A	11–13
Olanzapine (Zyprexa)	10–30	N/A	32–34
Paliperidone (Invega)	3–6	N/A	24
Quetiapine (Seroquel)	300–800	N/A	5–7
Risperidone (Risperdal)	2–8	N/A	23–25
Ziprasidone (Geodon)	120–200	N/A	6–8
Asenapine (Saphris)	10–20	N/A	24
Cariprazine (Vraylar)	1.5-6	N/A	48–96
Iloperidone (Fanapt)	6–24	N/A	18–31
Aripiprazole Long Acting (Maintena)	300–400	N/A	4 weeks
Aripiprazole Long Acting (Aristada)	441–882	N/A	4 weeks
Paliperidone Lond Acting (Sustenna)	39–234	N/A	4 weeks
Lurasidone (Latuda)	40–160	N/A	18
Quetiapine XR (Seroquel XR)	400–800	N/A	7
Brexpiprazole (Rexulti)	2–4	N/A	91

drugs, which are often effective in the treatment of positive symptoms of schizophrenia. High-potency agents (e.g., haloperidol) are more likely to cause extrapyramidal side effects such as akathisia, acute dystonia, and pseudoparkinsonism. Low-potency agents (e.g., chlorpromazine [Thorazine]) are more sedating, hypotensive, and anticholinergic. These agents can cause tardive dyskinesia at a rate of roughly 5% per year of exposure. A significant portion of patients are either unresponsive to or intolerant of these drugs. The newer, second-generation antipsychotic drugs—described below—are usually preferred and used more frequently than the first-generation antipsychotics. They are equally if not more effective and have fewer side effects.

b. **Second-generation antipsychotics** (also known as atypical, novel, or SDAs)—the newer-generation antipsychotic drugs that provide potent 5-HT2 receptor blockade and varying degrees of D2 receptor blockade, in addition to other receptor effects. In comparison with the dopamine receptor antagonists, these drugs improve two classes of disabilities typical of schizophrenia: (1) positive symptoms such as hallucinations, delusions, disordered thought, and agitation, and (2) negative symptoms such as withdrawal, flat affect, anhedonia, poverty of speech, and cognitive impairment. They cause fewer extrapyramidal side effects, do not elevate prolactin levels (with the exception of risperidone), and are less likely to cause tardive dyskinesia. Clozapine is the most atypical in that it causes minimal or no extrapyramidal side effects, regardless of dosage; seldom causes tardive dyskinesia; and is extremely effective in treating refractory patients despite weak D2 receptor blockade. As a group, these agents can be highly sedating and some agents (Olanzapine, Quetiapine, and Clozapine) may cause weight gain in excess of that associated with the dopamine receptor antagonists. The second-generation drugs are widely prescribed as first-line treatment for patients with schizophrenia. They include aripiprazole (Abilify), asenapine (Saphris), brexpiprazole (Rexulti), cariprazine (Vraylar), iloperidone (Fanapt), paliperidone (Invega) and long acting (Sustenna), lurasidone (Latuda), risperidone (Risperdal), olanzapine (Zyprexa), clozapine (Clozaril), and ziprasidone (Geodon).

2. **Dosage.** A moderate fixed dose that is maintained for 4 to 6 weeks (or longer in more chronic cases) is recommended for acute psychotic episodes. High dosages of antipsychotics (>1 g of chlorpromazine equivalents) and rapid neuroleptization are no longer recommended, as they increase side effects without enhancing efficacy. Typical therapeutic dosages are 4 to 6 mg of risperidone a day, 10 to 20 mg of olanzapine (Zyprexa) a day, and 6 to 20 mg of haloperidol a day. First-episode patients may respond well to lower dosages, whereas selected chronic or refractory patients may rarely require higher dosages. An antipsychotic response develops gradually. Agitation can be managed with benzodiazepines (e.g., 1 to 2 mg of lorazepam [Ativan] three or four

times daily) on a standing or as-needed basis while an antipsychotic response is awaited. Patients who are noncompliant because of lack of insight may benefit from long-acting injectable antipsychotics (e.g., 25 mg of fluphenazine decanoate [Prolixin] intramuscularly every 2 weeks or 100 to 200 mg of haloperidol decanoate intramuscularly every 4 weeks). Second-generation long-acting antipsychotics include risperidone (Consta) 25 to 50 mg intramuscular every 2 weeks. Other agents include long-acting paliperidone (Invega Sustenna) and aripiprazole (Maintena). Patients should first be treated with oral preparations of these drugs to establish efficacy and tolerability. Patients who are treated with long-acting haloperidol must be converted to the depot drug via a loading-dose strategy or with oral supplementation until the depot preparation reaches steady-state levels (4 months).

3. **Maintenance.** Schizophrenia is usually a chronic illness, and long-term treatment with antipsychotic medication is usually required to decrease the risk for relapse. If a patient has been stable for approximately 1 year, then the medication can be gradually decreased to the minimum effective dosage, possibly at the rate of 10% to 20% per month. During dosage reduction, patients and their families must be educated to recognize and report warning signs of relapse, including insomnia, anxiety, withdrawal, and odd behavior. Strategies for dose reduction must be individualized based on the severity of past episodes, stability of symptoms, and tolerability of medication.

4. **Other drugs.** If standard antipsychotic medication alone is ineffective, several other drugs have been reported to cause varying degrees of improvement. The addition of lithium may be helpful in a significant percentage of patients; propranolol (Inderal), benzodiazepines, valproic acid (Depakene) or divalproex (Depakote), and carbamazepine (Tegretol) have been reported to lead to improvement in some cases.

B. **Electroconvulsive therapy (ECT).** Can be effective for acute psychosis and catatonic subtype. Patients in whom the illness has lasted less than 1 year are most responsive. ECT is a promising treatment for refractory positive symptoms. It has been shown to have synergistic efficacy with antipsychotic drugs.

C. **Psychosocial.** Antipsychotic medication alone is not as effective in treating schizophrenic patients as are drugs coupled with psychosocial interventions.

1. **Behavior therapy.** Desired behaviors are positively reinforced by rewarding them with specific tokens, such as trips or privileges. The intent is to generalize reinforced behavior to the world outside the hospital ward.

2. **Group therapy.** Focus is on support and social skills development (activities of daily living). Groups are especially helpful in decreasing social isolation and increasing reality testing.

3. **Family therapy.** Family therapy techniques can significantly decrease relapse rates for the schizophrenic family member. High-EE family

interaction can be diminished through family therapy. Multiple family groups, in which family members of schizophrenic patients discuss and share issues, have been particularly helpful.

4. **Supportive psychotherapy.** Traditional insight-oriented psychotherapy is not usually recommended in treating schizophrenic patients because their egos are too fragile. Supportive therapy, which may include advice, reassurance, education, modeling, limit setting, and reality testing, is generally the therapy of choice. The rule is that as much insight as a patient desires and can tolerate is an acceptable goal. A type of supportive therapy called personal therapy involves a heavy reliance on the therapeutic relationship, with instillation of hope and imparting of information.

 CLINICAL HINT:
Even though a patient is in a catatonic or withdrawn state, they are often very aware of the environment and cognizant of what is being said around them.

5. **Social skills training.** Attempts to improve social skills deficits, such as poor eye contact, lack of relatedness, inaccurate perceptions of others, and social inappropriateness, by means of supportive structurally based and sometimes manually based therapies (often in group settings), which utilize homework, videotapes, and role playing.

6. **Case management.** Responsible for the schizophrenic patient's concrete needs and coordination of care. Case managers participate in coordinating treatment planning and communication between various providers. They help patients to make appointments, obtain housing and financial benefits, and navigate the health care system (advocacy), and also provide outreach and crisis management to keep patients in treatment.

7. **Support groups.** The National Alliance for the Mentally Ill (NAMI), the National Mental Health Association (NMHA), and similar groups provide support, information, and education for patients and their families. NAMI-sponsored support groups are available in most states.

XII. Interviewing Techniques

A. **Understanding.** The most important task is to understand as well as possible what schizophrenic patients may be feeling and thinking. Schizophrenic patients are described as having extremely fragile ego structures, which leave them open to an unstable sense of self and others; primitive defenses; and a severely impaired ability to modulate external stress.

B. **Other critical tasks.** The other critical task for the interviewer is to establish contact with the patient in a manner that allows for a tolerable balance of autonomy and interaction.

1. The patient has both a deep wish for and a terrible fear of interpersonal contact, called the need–fear dilemma.
2. The fear of contact may represent the fear of a fundamental intrusion, resulting in delusional fears of personal and world annihilation in addition to loss of control, identity, and self.
3. The wish for contact may represent fears that, without human interaction, the person is dead, nonhuman, mechanical, or permanently trapped.
4. Schizophrenic patients may project their own negative, bizarre, and frightening self-images onto others, leading the interviewer to feel as uncomfortable, scared, or angry as the patient. Aggressive or hostile impulses are particularly frightening to these patients and may lead them to disorganization in thought and behavior.
5. Offers of help may be experienced as coercion, attempts to force the person into helplessness, or a sense of being devoured.
6. There is no one right thing to say to a schizophrenic patient. The most important task of the interviewer is to help to diminish the inner chaos, loneliness, and terror that the schizophrenic patient is feeling. The challenge is to convey empathy without being regarded as dangerously intrusive.

   CLINICAL HINTS:

- *Efforts to convince the patient that a delusion is not real generally lead to more tenacious assertions of delusional ideas.*
- *How patients experience the world (e.g., dangerous, bizarre, overwhelming, invasive) is conveyed through their thought content and process. Listen for the feelings behind the delusional ideas—are they afraid, sad, angry, hopeless? Do they feel as though they have no privacy, no control? What is their image of themselves?*
- *Acknowledge the patient's feelings simply and clearly. For example, when the patient says, "When I walk into a room, people can see inside my head and read my thoughts," the clinician might respond with, "What is that like for you?"*
- *Careful listening can convey that the clinician believes the person is human with something important to say.*

For more detailed discussion of this topic, see Chapter 12, Schizophrenia and Other Psychotic Disorders, Section 12.1–12.16, p. 1405–1573, in CTP/X.

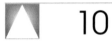

10

Schizophreniform, Schizoaffective, Delusional, and Other Psychotic Disorders

I. Schizophreniform Disorder

A. Definition. Symptoms similar to those of schizophrenia except that they last at least 1 month and resolve within 6 months, and then return to baseline level of functioning.

B. Epidemiology. Little is known about the incidence, prevalence, and sex ratio of schizophreniform disorder. The disorder is most common in adolescents, males, and young adults and is less than half as common as schizophrenia. A lifetime prevalence rate of 0.2% and a 1-year prevalence rate of 0.1% have been reported.

C. Etiology. In general, schizophreniform patients have more mood symptoms and a better prognosis than do schizophrenic patients. Schizophrenia occurs more often in families of patients with mood disorders than in families of patients with schizophreniform disorder. Cause remains unknown.

D. Diagnosis, signs, and symptoms. A rapid-onset psychotic disorder with hallucinations, delusions, or both. Although many patients with schizophreniform disorder may experience functional impairment at the time of an episode, they are unlikely to report a progressive decline in social and occupational functioning. See Table 10-1.

E. Differential diagnosis.

1. Schizophrenia. Schizophrenia is diagnosed if the duration of the prodromal, active, and residual phases lasts for more than 6 months.

2. Brief psychotic disorder. Symptoms occur for less than 1 month and a major stressor need not be present.

3. Mood and anxiety disorders. Can be highly comorbid with schizophrenia and schizophreniform. A thorough longitudinal history is important in elucidating the diagnosis because the presence of psychotic symptoms exclusively during periods of mood disturbance is an indication of a primary mood disorder.

4. Substance-induced psychosis. A detailed history of medication use and toxicologic screen.

5. Psychosis due to a medical condition. A detailed history and physical examination and, when indicated, performing laboratory tests or imaging studies.

F. Course and prognosis. Good prognostic features include absence of blunted or flat affect, good premorbid functioning, confusion and disorientation at the height of the psychotic episode, shorter duration, acute

Table 10-1
Signs and Symptoms of Schizophreniform Disorder

Symptoms last at least 1 mo but less than 6 mo.
  Symptom profile similar to schizophrenia with two or more psychotic symptoms
  Psychotic symptoms develop early in the episode with unusual behavior
  Emotional turmoil and confusion during the episode
  Overall good premorbid functioning
  Lack of blunted affect

onset, and onset of prominent psychotic symptoms within 4 weeks of any first noticeable change in behavior. Most estimates of progression to schizophrenia range between 60% and 80%. Some will have a second or third episode during which they will deteriorate into a more chronic condition of schizophrenia. Others remit and then have periodic recurrences.

G. Treatment. Hospitalization is often necessary and antipsychotic medications should be used to treat psychotic symptoms. Consideration can be given to withdrawing or tapering the medication if the psychosis has been completely resolved for 6 months. The decision to discontinue medication must be individualized based on treatment response, side effects, and other factors. A trial of lithium (Eskalith), carbamazepine (Tegretol), or valproate (Depakene) may be warranted for treatment and prophylaxis if a patient has a recurrent episode. Psychotherapy is critical in helping patients to understand and deal with their psychotic experiences. Electroconvulsive therapy may be indicated for some patients, especially those with marked catatonic or depressed features.

II. Schizoaffective Disorder

A. Definition. A disorder with concurrent features of both schizophrenia and mood disorder that cannot be diagnosed as either one separately. In current diagnostic systems, the diagnosis of schizoaffective disorder may fall into one of the six categories. See Table 10-2.

B. Epidemiology. Lifetime prevalence is less than 1%. The depressive type of schizoaffective disorder may be more common in older persons than in younger persons, and the bipolar type may be more common in young adults than in older adults. The prevalence of the disorder has been reported to be lower in men than in women, particularly married women; the age of onset for women is later than that for men, as in schizophrenia. Men with schizoaffective disorder are likely to exhibit antisocial behavior and to have a markedly flat or inappropriate affect.

Table 10-2
Categories of Schizoaffective Disorder

1. Patients with schizophrenia who have mood symptoms
2. Patients with mood disorder who have symptoms of schizophrenia
3. Patients with both mood disorder and schizophrenia
4. Patients with a third psychosis unrelated to schizophrenia and mood disorder
5. Patients whose disorder is on a continuum between schizophrenia and mood disorder
6. Patients with some combination of the above

Table 10-3
Signs and Symptoms of Schizoaffective Disorder

A. Mood symptoms including depressive, manic, or a mixed episode in combination with symptoms of schizophrenia.
B. Delusions or hallucinations are present with mood symptoms for 2 wks.
C. The mood component is present for the majority (>50%) of the total illness.
D. Schizoaffective disorder should not be used if the symptoms are caused by substance abuse or a secondary medical condition.

    C. Etiology. Some patients may be misdiagnosed; they are actually schizo-phrenic with prominent mood symptoms or have a mood disorder with prominent psychotic symptoms. The prevalence of schizophrenia is not increased in schizoaffective families, but the prevalence of mood dis-orders is. Patients with schizoaffective disorder have a better prognosis than patients with schizophrenia and a worse prognosis than patients with mood disorders.

    D. Diagnosis, signs, and symptoms. There will be signs and symptoms of schizophrenia coupled with manic or depressive episodes. The disorder is divided into two subtypes: (1) bipolar, if there is both a manic and depres-sive cycling, and (2) depressive, if the disturbance only includes major depressive episodes. See Table 10-3.

    E. Differential diagnosis. Any medical, psychiatric, or drug-related condi-tion that causes psychotic or mood symptoms must be considered.

    F. Course and prognosis. Poor prognosis is associated with positive family history of schizophrenia, early and insidious onset without precipitating factors, predominance of psychotic symptoms, and poor premorbid his-tory. Schizoaffective patients have a better prognosis than schizophrenic patients and a worse prognosis than mood disorder patients. Schizoaffec-tive patients respond more often to lithium and are less likely to have a deteriorating course than are schizophrenic patients.

    G. Treatment. Antidepressant or antimanic treatments should be used com-bined with antipsychotic medications to control psychotic signs and symptoms. Selective serotonin reuptake inhibitors (SSRIs; e.g., fluoxetine [Prozac] and sertraline [Zoloft]) are often used as first-line agents but treatment with antidepressants mirrors treatment of bipolar depression. Care should be taken not to precipitate a cycle of rapid switches from depression to mania with the antidepressant. In manic cases, the use of electroconvulsive therapy should be considered. Patients benefit from a combination of family therapy, social skills training, and cognitive reha-bilitation.

III. Delusional Disorder

    A. Definition. Disorder in which the primary or sole manifestation is a nonbi-zarre delusion that is fixed and unshakable. The delusions are usually about situations that can occur and are possible in real life, such as being followed, infected, or loved at a distance. Bizarre delusions are considered impossible, such as being impregnated by an alien being from another planet.

Table 10-4
Epidemiologic Features of Delusional Disorder

Incidence[a]	0.7–3.0
Prevalence[a]	24–30
Age at onset (range)	18–80 (mean, 34–45 yrs)
Type of onset	Acute or gradual
Sex ratio	Somewhat more frequently female
Prognosis	Best with early, acute onset
Associated features	Widowhood, celibacy often present, history of substance abuse, head injury not infrequent

[a]Incidence and prevalence figures represent cases per 100,000 population.
Adapted from Kendler KS. Demography of paranoid psychosis (delusional disorder). *Arch Gen Psychiatry* 1982;39:890, with permission.

B. Epidemiology. Delusional disorders account for only 1% to 2% of all admissions to inpatient mental health facilities. The mean age of onset is about 40 years, but the range for age of onset runs from 18 years of age to the 90s. A slight preponderance of female patients exists. Men are more likely to develop paranoid delusions than women, who are more likely to develop delusions of erotomania. Many patients are married and employed, but some association is seen with recent immigration and low socioeconomic status. See Table 10-4.

C. Etiology

1. **Genetic.** Genetic studies indicate that delusional disorder is neither a subtype nor an early or prodromal stage of schizophrenia or mood disorder. The risk for schizophrenia or mood disorder is not increased in first-degree relatives; however, there is a slight increase of delusional thinking, particularly suspiciousness, in families of patients with delusional disorder.

2. **Biologic.** The neurologic conditions most commonly associated with delusions affect the limbic system and the basal ganglia. Delusional disorder can also arise as a response to stimuli in the peripheral nervous system (e.g., paresthesias perceived as rays coming from outer space).

3. **Psychosocial.** Delusional disorder is primarily psychosocial in origin. Common background characteristics include a history of physical or emotional abuse; cruel, erratic, and unreliable parenting; and an overly demanding or perfectionistic upbringing. Basic trust (Erik Erikson) does not develop, with the child believing that the environment is consistently hostile and potentially dangerous. Other psychosocial factors include a history of deafness, blindness, social isolation and loneliness, recent immigration or other abrupt environmental changes, and advanced age. See Table 10-5.

D. Laboratory and psychological tests. No laboratory test can confirm the diagnosis. Projective psychological tests reveal a preoccupation with paranoid or grandiose themes and issues of inferiority, inadequacy, and anxiety.

Table 10-5
Risk Factors Associated With Delusional Disorder

Advanced age
Sensory impairment or isolation
Family history
Social isolation
Personality features (e.g., unusual interpersonal sensitivity)
Recent immigration

E. **Pathophysiology.** No known pathophysiology except when patients have discrete anatomic defects of the limbic system or basal ganglia.

F. **Psychodynamic factors.** Defenses used: (1) denial, (2) reaction formation, and (3) projection. Major defense is projection—symptoms are a defense against unacceptable ideas and feelings. Patients deny feelings of shame, humiliation, and inferiority; turn any unacceptable feelings into their opposites through reaction formation (inferiority into grandiosity); and project any unacceptable feelings outward onto others.

G. **Diagnosis, signs, and symptoms.** Delusions last at least 1 month and are well systematized and nonbizarre as opposed to fragmented and bizarre. The patient's emotional response to the delusional system is congruent with and appropriate to the content of the delusion. The personality remains intact or deteriorates minimally. The fact that patients often are hypersensitive and hypervigilant may lead to social isolation despite their high-level functioning capacities. Under nonstressful circumstances, patients may be judged to be without evidence of mental illness. See Table 10-6.

1. **Persecutory.** Patients with this subtype are convinced that they are being persecuted or harmed. The persecutory beliefs are often associated with querulousness, irritability, and anger. Most common type.

2. **Jealous** (also called conjugal paranoia, pathologic jealousy). Delusional disorder with delusions of infidelity has been called *conjugal paranoia* when it is limited to the delusion that a spouse has been unfaithful. The eponym *Othello syndrome* has been used to describe morbid jealousy that can arise from multiple concerns. The delusion usually afflicts men, often those with no prior psychiatric illness. May be associated with violence, including homicide.

Table 10-6
Signs and Symptoms of Delusional Disorder

A. Presence of one or more delusions which are present for at least 1 mo.
B. Criterion for schizophrenia has never been met.
C. No marked impairment in functioning and no odd behavior.
D. Short duration of mood episodes compared to the length of delusional thinking.
E. Delusions are not secondary to medical condition or drug use.

Types of Delusions

Jealous type	Mixed type
Grandiose type	Erotomanic type
Persecutory type	Unspecified type
Somatic type	

3. **Erotomanic.** Patient believes that someone, usually of higher socioeconomic status, is in love with him or her. Criteria can include (1) a delusional conviction of amorous communication; (2) object of much higher rank; (3) object being the first to fall in love; (4) object being the first to make advances; (5) sudden onset (within a 7-day period); (6) object remains unchanged; (7) patient rationalizes paradoxical behavior of the object; (8) chronic course; and (9) absence of hallucinations. More common in women. Accounts for stalking behavior.

4. **Somatic.** Belief that patient is suffering from an illness; common delusions are of parasites, foul odors coming from the body, misshapen body parts (dysmorphophobia), or of fatal illness.

5. **Grandiose.** Persons think they have special powers or are deities.

6. **Shared delusional disorder** (also known as *folie à deux*). Two people have the same delusional belief. Most common in mother–daughter relationships. Discussed further below.

H. **Differential diagnosis**

1. **Psychotic disorder resulting from a general medical condition with delusions.** Conditions that may mimic delusional disorder include hypothyroidism and hyperthyroidism, Parkinson's disease, multiple sclerosis, Alzheimer's disease, tumors, and trauma to the basal ganglia. Many medical and neurologic illnesses can be present with delusions (Table 10-7). The most common sites for lesions are the basal ganglia and the limbic system.

Table 10-7
Potential Medical Etiologies of Delusional Syndromes

Disease or Disorder Class	Examples
Neurodegenerative disorders	Alzheimer's disease, Pick's disease, Huntington's disease, basal ganglia calcification, multiple sclerosis, metachromatic leukodystrophy
Other central nervous system disorders	Brain tumors, especially temporal lobe and deep hemispheric tumors; epilepsy, especially complex partial seizure disorder; head trauma (subdural hematoma); anoxic brain injury; fat embolism
Vascular disease	Atherosclerotic vascular disease, especially when associated with diffuse, temporoparietal, or subcortical lesions; hypertensive encephalopathy; subarachnoid hemorrhage, temporal arteritis
Infectious disease	Human immunodeficiency virus or acquired immune deficiency syndrome, encephalitis lethargica, Creutzfeldt–Jakob disease, syphilis, malaria, acute viral encephalitis
Metabolic disorder	Hypercalcemia, hyponatremia, hypoglycemia, uremia, hepatic encephalopathy, porphyria
Endocrinopathies	Addison's disease, Cushing's syndrome, hyper- or hypothyroidism, panhypopituitarism
Vitamin deficiencies	Vitamin B_{12} deficiency, folate deficiency, thiamine deficiency, niacin deficiency
Medications	Adrenocorticotropic hormones, anabolic steroids, corticosteroids, cimetidine, antibiotics (cephalosporins, penicillin), disulfiram, anticholinergic agents
Substances	Amphetamines, cocaine, alcohol, cannabis, hallucinogens
Toxins	Mercury, arsenic, manganese, thallium

2. **Substance-induced psychotic disorder with delusions.** Intoxication with sympathomimetics (e.g., amphetamines, marijuana, or levodopa [Larodopa]) is likely to result in delusional symptoms.

3. **Paranoid personality disorder.** No true delusions are present, although overvalued ideas that verge on being delusional may be present. Patients are predisposed to delusional disorders.

4. **Paranoid schizophrenia.** More likely to present with prominent auditory hallucinations, personality deterioration, and more marked disturbance in role functioning. Age at onset tends to be younger in schizophrenia than in delusional disorder. Delusions are more bizarre.

5. **Major depressive disorder.** Depressed patients may have paranoid delusions secondary to major depressive disorder, but the mood symptoms and associated characteristics (e.g., vegetative symptoms, positive family history, response to antidepressants) are prominent.

6. **Bipolar I disorder.** Manic patients may have grandiose or paranoid delusions that are clearly secondary to the primary and prominent mood disorder; associated with such characteristics as euphoric and labile mood, positive family history, and response to lithium.

I. **Course and prognosis.** Delusional disorder is considered a fairly stable diagnosis. About 50% of patients have recovered at long-term follow-up, 20% show decreased symptoms, and 30% exhibit no change. A good prognosis is associated with high levels of occupational, social, and functional adjustments; female sex; onset before age 30 years; sudden onset; short duration of illness; and the presence of precipitating factors. Although reliable data are limited, patients with persecutory, somatic, and erotic delusions are thought to have a better prognosis than patients with grandiose and jealous delusions.

J. **Treatment.** Patients rarely enter therapy voluntarily; rather, they are brought by concerned friends and relatives. Establishing rapport is difficult; patient's hostility is fear-motivated.

1. **Hospitalization.** Hospitalization is necessary if the patient is unable to control suicidal or homicidal impulses; if impairment is extreme (e.g., refusal to eat because of a delusion about food poisoning); or if a thorough medical workup is indicated.

2. **Psychopharmacotherapy.** Patients tend to refuse medications because of suspicion. Severely agitated patients may require intramuscular antipsychotic medication. Otherwise, oral antipsychotics may be tried. Delusional disorder may preferentially respond to pimozide (Orap). Delusional patients are more likely to react to drug side effects with delusional ideas; thus, a very gradual increase in dose is recommended to diminish the likelihood of disturbing adverse effects. Antidepressants may be of use with severe depression. SSRIs may be helpful in somatic type.

3. **Psychotherapy.** Individual therapy seems to be more effective than group therapy; insight-oriented, supportive, cognitive, and behavioral therapies are often effective. A good therapeutic outcome depends

Table 10-8
Diagnosis and Management of Delusional Disorder

Rule out other causes of paranoid features
Confirm the absence of other psychopathology
Assess consequences of delusion-related behavior
   Demoralization
   Despondency
   Anger, fear
   Depression
Impact of search for "medical diagnosis," "legal solution," "proof of infidelity," and so on
   (e.g., financial, legal, personal, occupational)
Assess anxiety and agitation
Assess potential for violence, suicide
Assess need for hospitalization
Institute pharmacologic and psychological therapies
Maintain connection through recovery

on a psychiatrist's ability to respond to the patient's mistrust of others and the resulting interpersonal conflicts, frustrations, and failures. The mark of successful treatment may be a satisfactory social adjustment rather than abatement of the patient's delusions. See Table 10-8.

CLINICAL HINTS: PSYCHOTHERAPY

- *Do not argue with or challenge the patient's delusions. A delusion may become even more entrenched if the patient feels that it must be defended.*
- *Do not pretend that the delusion is true. However, do listen to the patient's concerns about the delusion and try to understand what the delusion may mean, specifically in terms of the patient's self-esteem.*
- *Respond sympathetically to the fact that the delusion is disturbing and intrusive in the patient's life.*
- *Understand that the delusional system may be a means of grappling with profound feelings of shame and inadequacy, and that the patient may be hypersensitive to any imagined slights or condescension.*
- *Be straightforward and honest in all dealings with the patient, as these patients are hypervigilant about being tricked or deceived. Explain side effects of medications and reasons for prescribing (e.g., to help with anxiety, irritability, insomnia, anorexia); be reliable and on time for appointments; schedule regular appointments.*
- *Examine what triggered the first appearance of the delusion. Similar stresses or experiences in the patient's life may exacerbate delusional symptoms. Help the patient develop alternative means of responding to stressful situations.*

IV. Brief Psychotic Disorder

    A. Definition. An acute and transient psychotic condition that involves the sudden onset of psychotic symptoms, that last for less than 1 month and follow a severe and obvious stress in the patient's life. Remission is full with return to premorbid level of functioning.

Table 10-9
Signs and Symptoms of Brief Psychotic Disorder

1. Psychotic symptoms with an abrupt inset that last at least 1 day but less than 1 mo
2. Not associated with a mood disorder, a substance-related disorder, or a psychotic disorder caused by a general medical condition
3. Presence of at least one major symptom of psychosis, such as hallucinations, delusions, and disorganized thoughts
4. Labile mood, confusion, and impaired attention
5. Emotional volatility, strange or bizarre behavior, screaming or muteness, and impaired memory of recent events
6. Symptom patterns include acute paranoid reactions and reactive confusion, excitation, and depression

B. Epidemiology. No definitive data are available but 9% of first-episode psychoses can be diagnosed as a brief psychotic episode. More frequent in persons with pre-existing personality disorders or who have previously experienced major stressors, such as disasters or dramatic cultural changes. Onset is usually between 20 and 35 years of age, with a slightly higher incidence in women.

C. Etiology. Mood disorders are more common in the families of these patients. Psychosocial stress triggers the psychotic episode. Psychosis is understood as a defensive response in a person with inadequate coping mechanisms.

D. Diagnosis, signs, and symptoms. Similar to those of other psychotic disorders, with an increase in emotional volatility, strange or bizarre behavior, confusion, disorientation, and lability in mood ranging from elation to suicidality. See Table 10-9.

E. Differential diagnosis. Medical causes must be ruled out—in particular, drug intoxication and withdrawal. Seizure disorders must also be considered. Factitious disorders, malingering, schizophrenia, mood disorders, and transient psychotic episodes associated with borderline and schizotypal personality disorders must be ruled out.

F. Course and prognosis. By definition, course of the disorder is less than 1 month. Recovery is up to 80% with treatment. See Table 10-10.

G. Treatment
   1. Hospitalization. A patient who is acutely psychotic may need brief hospitalization for both evaluation and protection. Seclusion, physical restraints, or one-to-one monitoring of the patient may be necessary.

Table 10-10
Good Prognostic Features for Brief Psychotic Disorder

Good premorbid adjustment
Few premorbid schizoid traits
Severe precipitating stressor
Sudden onset of symptoms
Affective symptoms
Confusion and perplexity during psychosis
Little affective blunting
Short duration of symptoms
Absence of schizophrenic relatives

    2. Pharmacotherapy. The two major classes of drugs to be considered in the treatment of brief psychotic disorder are the antipsychotic drugs (i.e., haloperidol or ziprasidone) and the benzodiazepines. Anxiolytic medications are often used during the first 2 to 3 weeks after the resolution of the psychotic episode. Long-term use of any medication should be avoided.

    3. Psychotherapy. Psychotherapy is of use in providing an opportunity to discuss the stressors and the psychotic episode. An individualized treatment strategy based on increasing problem-solving skills while strengthening the ego structure through psychotherapy appears to be the most efficacious. Family involvement in the treatment process may be crucial to a successful outcome.

V. Shared Psychotic Disorder

    A. Definition. Delusional system shared by two or more persons; previously called *induced paranoid disorder* and *folie à deux.* In DSM-5, this disorder is referred to as "Delusional Symptoms in Partner of Individual with Delusional Disorder."

    B. Epidemiology. The disorder is rare; more common in women and in persons with physical disabilities that make them dependent on another person. Family members, usually two sisters, are involved in 95% of cases.

    C. Etiology. The cause is primarily psychological; however, a genetic influence is possible because the disorder most often affects members of the same family. The families of persons with this disorder are at risk for schizophrenia. Psychological or psychosocial factors include a socially isolated relationship in which one person is submissive and dependent and the other is dominant with an established psychotic system.

    D. Psychodynamic factors. The dominant psychotic personality maintains some contact with reality through the submissive person, whereas the submissive personality is desperately anxious to be cared for and accepted by the dominant person. The two often have a strongly ambivalent relationship.

    E. Diagnosis, signs, and symptoms. Persecutory delusions are most common, and the key presentation is the sharing and blind acceptance of these delusions between two people. Suicide or homicide pacts may be present. See Table 10-11.

Table 10-11
Signs and Symptoms of Shared Psychotic Disorder (Delusional Symptoms in Partner of Individual With Delusional Disorder)

A. Transfer of delusions from one person to another

 B. Persons are closely associated and typically live together in relative social isolation

 C. The individual who first has the delusion (the primary case) is often chronically ill

 D. The delusion is attributed to the strong influence of the more dominant member

 E. The disorder is not secondary to a medical condition, another psychotic disorder, or effect of a substance

F. Differential diagnosis. Rule out personality disorders, malingering, and factitious disorders in the submissive patient. Medical causes must always be considered.

G. Course and prognosis. Recovery rates vary; some are as low as 10% to 40%. Traditionally, the submissive partner is separated from the dominant, psychotic partner, with the ideal outcome being a rapid diminution in the psychotic symptoms. If symptoms do not remit, the submissive person may meet the criteria for another psychotic disorder, such as schizophrenia or delusional disorder.

H. Treatment. Separate the persons and help the more submissive, dependent partner develop other means of support to compensate for the loss of the relationship. Antipsychotic medications are beneficial for both persons.

 CLINICAL HINT:
The risk of infanticide remains high even if caregivers are in the home.
Careful supervision of mother–infant interaction can provide important clues
about hostile or loving feelings.

VI. Psychotic Disorder Not Otherwise Specified
A variety of clinical presentations that do not fit within current diagnostic rubrics. It includes psychotic symptomatology (i.e., delusions, hallucinations, disorganized speech, grossly disorganized or catatonic behavior) about which there is inadequate information to make a specific diagnosis or about which there is contradictory information. It includes:

A. Autoscopic psychosis. The characteristic symptom includes a visual hallucination of all or part of the person's own body. It is called a phantom, is colorless and transparent, and tends to appear suddenly and without warning. Hypothesis includes abnormal, episodic activity in the temporoparietal lobes. Patients usually respond to antianxiety medication. In severe cases, antipsychotic medications may be needed.

B. Motility psychosis. It is probably a variant of brief psychotic disorder. The two forms of motility psychosis are akinetic and hyperkinetic. The clinical presentation of akinetic is similar to catatonic stupor while hyperkinetic resembles manic or catatonic excitement.

C. Postpartum psychosis. Postpartum psychosis (sometimes called puerperal psychosis) is an example of psychotic disorder not otherwise specified that occurs in women who have recently delivered a baby; the syndrome is most often characterized by the mother's depression, delusions, and thoughts of harming either her infant or herself.

D. Signs and symptoms. See Table 10-12.

VII. Catatonic Disorder
Catatonia is a new diagnostic category introduced in DSM-5 because it can occur over a broad spectrum of mental disorders, most often in severe

Table 10-12
Signs and Symptoms of Psychotic Disorder Not Otherwise Specified

1. Hallucinations
2. Delusions
3. Disorganized speech and disorganized behavior
4. Clinical presentations that do not fit within current diagnostic rubrics
5. Psychotic symptoms that do not meet the criteria for any specific psychotic disorder
6. Ongoing symptoms lasting more than a month with exclusion of brief psychotic disorder

psychotic and mood disorders. It can also be caused by an underlying medical condition or induced by a substance.

A. Diagnosis, signs, and symptoms. Striking behavioral abnormalities that may include motoric immobility or excitement, profound negativism, or echolalia (mimicry of speech) or echopraxia (mimicry of movement). See Table 10-13.

Table 10-13
Signs and Symptoms of Catatonic Disorder

1. Stupor
2. Catalepsy
3. Waxy flexibility
4. Mutism
5. Negativism
6. Posturing
7. Mannerism
8. Stereotypy
9. Agitation
10. Grimacing
11. Echolalia
12. Echopraxia

B. Epidemiology. An uncommon condition mostly related to mood disorders and in 10% of patients with schizophrenia.

C. Etiology. Neurologic conditions (nonconvulsive status epilepticus and head trauma), infections (encephalitis), and metabolic (hepatic encephalopathy and hyponatremia).

D. Differential diagnosis. Includes hypoactive delirium, end-stage dementia, and akinetic mutism, as well as catatonia due to a primary psychiatric disorder.

E. Course and treatment. In most this requires hospitalization. Fluid and nutrient intake must be maintained, often with intravenous lines or feeding tubes. The primary treatment modality is identifying and correcting the underlying medical or pharmacologic cause. Offending substances must be removed or minimized.

VIII. Culture-Bound Syndromes
See Table 10-14.

Table 10-14
Example of Culture-Bound Syndromes

amok
Periods of dissociation
Violent and aggressive behavior following a period of brooding
Homicidal behavior directed at persons and objects
Triggered by an apparent insult
Predominantly affects men
May experience persecutory ideas, automatism, and amnesia
Return to normal functioning following the episode
Occurs especially in Malay culture but also seen in the Philippines, Polynesia (*cafard* or *cathard*),
    Laos, Puerto Rico (*mal de pelea*), Papua New Guinea, and among the Navajo (*iich'aa*)

ataque de nervios
Expression of distress
Primarily among Latinos from the Caribbean and Latin Mediterranean groups
Symptoms include attacks of crying, trembling, uncontrollable shouting, heat in the chest rising into
    the head, and verbal or physical aggression
Dissociative episodes
Seizure or fainting episodes
Sense of being out of control
Stressful occurrences (e.g., death, divorce, or conflicts in the family)
Amnesia during the *episode*
Rapid return to normal functioning

bilis and colera (*muina*)
Underlying anger or rage
Primarily among Latinos
Symptoms include headache, screaming, trembling, stomach disturbances, acute nervous tension,
    and loss of consciousness

bouffée délirante
Occurs in West Africa and Haiti
Sudden outburst with agitation and aggressive behavior
Confusion and psychomotor excitement
Visual and auditory hallucinations
Similar to brief psychotic disorder

brain fag
A terminology used to describe a stressful condition in young adults of West Africa
Usually in response to stress of schooling
Symptoms are difficulties in concentrating, remembering, and thinking
Described as brains being "fatigued"
Somatic symptoms include pain, pressure or tightness, blurring of vision, heat, or burning

dhat
A term used in India to describe severe anxiety related to discharge of semen, whitish discoloration
    of the urine, with weakness and exhaustion

falling-out or blackout
Mostly limited to southern United States and Caribbean
Feelings of dizziness and sudden collapse
Complaints of inability to see despite the person's eyes being open
Person can hear and understand but feel unable to move
Similar to conversion disorder or a dissociative disorder

ghost sickness
Mostly among American Indian tribes
Preoccupation with death and the dead
Symptoms include feeling of danger, bad dreams, weakness, loss of consciousness, feelings of futility,
    hallucinations, dizziness, loss of appetite, confusion, fear, and anxiety

(continued)

Table 10-14
Example of Culture-Bound Syndromes *(Continued)*

hwa-byung (also known as *wool-hwa-byung*)
Seen in Korean culture and means "anger syndrome"
Related to suppression of anger
Symptoms include panic, fear of impending death, insomnia, fatigue, anorexia, indigestion, feeling of a mass in the epigastrium, generalized aches and pains dyspnea, and palpitations

koro
A delusional syndrome, manifesting as sudden and intense anxiety that the genitals (penis or, in women, the vulva and nipples) will shrink into the body and cause death
The syndrome occurs in South and East Asia, and is also known as *shuk yang, shook yong,* and *suo yang* (Chinese); *jinjinia bemar* (Assamese); or *rok-joo* (Thai)

latah
Occurs in many parts of the world but the term is of Malaysian or Indonesian origin
Experienced as sudden reaction to fear with symptoms of echolalia, echopraxia and dissociative behavior
More prevalent in middle-aged women
Other names include *amurakh, irkunil, ikota, olan, myriachit, menkeiti* (Siberian groups); *bah tschi, bah-tsi, baah-ji* (Thailand); *imu* (Ainu, Sakhalin, Japan); and *mali-mali* and *silok* (Philippines)

locura
It is a form of chronic and severe psychoses
The term is described by Latinos
Symptoms include agitation, incoherence, auditory and visual hallucinations, unpredictability, and possibly violence

mal de ojo
Mostly in Mediterranean cultures but worldwide
Means "evil eye" in English
Children are especially at risk
Symptoms include diarrhea, vomiting, fever with disturbed sleep, and crying without an obvious cause
Women and children are at higher risk

nervios
More prevalent in Latinos
Frequent cause of distress
General state of vulnerability
Triggered by difficult life circumstances
Symptoms are emotional distress, somatic disturbance, and inability to function
Common symptoms include irritability, easy tearfulness, inability to concentrate, stomach disturbances, sleep difficulties, headaches and brain aches, nervousness, tingling sensations, and trembling

piblokto
Sudden dissociative episode
Extreme excitement that may last up to 30 minutes
Seizures and coma up to 12 hrs
Usually seen in Arctic and subarctic Eskimo population
Other symptoms include being withdrawn, irritable, and amnesia for the attack
Destruction of property, eat feces, scream obscenities, and engage in dangerous behavior

qigong psychotic reactions
Time-limited episodes of psychotic or nonpsychotic symptoms
Occurs after engaging in *qigong* (exercise of vital energy)

rootwork
Cultural belief that perceives illness as sorcery, witchcraft, hexing, or an evil influence
Symptoms include generalized anxiety, nausea, vomiting, diarrhea, weakness, dizziness, and fear of being killed (voodoo death)
Rootwork is found in the southern United States
It is also known as *mal puesto* or *brujeria* in Latino societies

(continued)

Table 10-14
Example of Culture-Bound Syndromes *(Continued)*

sangue dormido ("sleeping blood")
Most common among Portuguese Cape Verde Islanders
Symptoms are pain, numbness, tremor, paralysis, convulsions, stroke, blindness, heart attack, infection, and miscarriages

***shenjing shuariuo* ("neurasthenia")**
This syndrome is found in China
Symptoms include physical and mental fatigue, dizziness, headaches, poor concentration, sleep disturbance, and memory loss
Other symptoms include sexual dysfunction, excitability, gastrointestinal problems, and irritability

shen-k'uei (Taiwan); ***shenkui*** (China)
Syndrome marked by anxiety and panic symptoms as well as somatic complaints
There is no physical cause to explain the symptoms
Symptoms include fatigue, weakness, insomnia, sexual dysfunction, dizziness, backache, and impotence
The cause is related to excessive semen loss with the belief that it represents the loss of one's vital essence and can therefore be life-threatening

shin-byung
This syndrome is a Korean folk label characterized by anxiety and somatic complaints including weakness, dizziness, fear, anorexia, insomnia, and gastrointestinal problems
There may be dissociation and possession by ancestral spirits

spell
Considered a trance state in which persons "communicate" with deceased relatives or spirits
It is seen mostly among African Americans and European Americans from the southern United States

susto (*frigh* or "soul loss")
Most prevalent among Latinos in the United States and in Mexico, Central America, and South America
It is also known by *espanto, pasmo, tripa ida, perdida del alma,* or *chibih*
A terrifying and scary event makes the soul leave the body leading to sadness and sickness
The time lag for symptoms to develop can be days to years
Susto may result in death
Symptoms include insufficient, excessive, or disturbed sleep, appetite disturbances, lack of motivation, feelings of sadness, and low self-worth
Somatic symptoms include muscle aches and pains, headache, stomachache, and diarrhea

taijin kyofusho
Similar to social phobia
Common in Japan
An intense fear that one's body, its parts, or its functions displease, embarrass, or are offensive to other people in appearance, odor, facial expressions, or movements

zar
Refers to the spirits possessing the person
Seen in Ethiopia, Somalia, Egypt, Sudan, Iran, and other North African and Middle Eastern societies
Affected individuals may experience dissociative episodes that may include shouting, laughing, hitting the head against a wall, singing, or weeping
Symptoms include apathy and withdrawal, refusing to eat or carry out daily tasks or may develop a long-term relationship with the possessing spirit

For more detailed discussion of this topic, see Chapter 12, Schizophrenia and Other Psychotic Disorders, Section 12.17, p. 1574, in CTP/X.

11

Mood Disorders

I. Introduction

Disorders of mood—sometimes called affective disorders encompass a large spectrum of disorders in which pathologic mood disturbances dominate the clinical picture. They include the following:

1. Major depressive disorder
2. Persistent depressive disorder (Dysthymia)
3. Cyclothymic disorder
4. Disruptive mood dysregulation disorder
5. Premenstrual dysphoric disorder
6. Bipolar (I and II) and related disorders
7. Mood disorders (depressive and bipolar related) due to another medical condition
8. Substance/Medication-induced mood (depressive and bipolar related) disorder
9. The general category of unspecified depressive and bipolar and related disorders

Mood is a pervasive and sustained feeling tone that is experienced internally and that influences a person's behavior and perception of the world. Affect is the external expression of mood. Mood can be normal, elevated, or depressed. Healthy persons experience a wide range of moods and have an equally large repertoire of affective expressions; they feel in control of their moods and affects.

II. Epidemiology

A. Incidence and prevalence. Mood disorders are common. In the most recent surveys, major depressive disorder has the highest lifetime prevalence (almost 17%) of any psychiatric disorder. The annual incidence (number of new cases) of a major depressive episode is 1.59% (women, 1.89%; men, 1.10%). The annual incidence of bipolar illness is less than 1%, but it is difficult to estimate because milder forms of bipolar disorder are often missed (Tables 11-1 and 11-2).

B. Sex. Major depression is more common in women; bipolar I disorder is equal in women and men. Manic episodes are more common in women, and depressive episodes are more common in men.

C. Age. The age of onset for bipolar I disorder is usually about age 30. However, the disorder also occurs in young children as well as older adults.

D. Sociocultural. Depressive disorders are more common among single and divorced persons compared to married persons. No correlation with socioeconomic status. No difference between races or religious groups.

Table 11-1
Lifetime Prevalence Rates of Depressive Disorders

	Type	Lifetime (%)
Major depressive episode	Range	5–17
	Average	12
Dysthymic disorder	Range	3–6
	Average	5
Minor depressive disorder	Range	10
	Average	—
Recurrent brief depressive disorder	Range	16

Adapted from Rihmer Z, Angst A. Mood disorders: Epidemiology. In: Sadock BJ, Sadock VA, eds. *Comprehensive Textbook of Psychiatry.* 8th ed. Baltimore, MD: Lippincott Williams & Wilkins; 2004.

III. Etiology

A. Neurotransmitters

1. **Serotonin.** Serotonin has become the biogenic amine neurotransmitter most commonly associated with depression. Serotonin depletion occurs in depression; thus, serotonergic agents are effective treatments. The identification of multiple serotonin receptor subtypes may lead to even more specific treatments for depression. Some patients with suicidal impulses have low cerebrospinal fluid (CSF) concentrations of serotonin metabolites (5-hydroxyindole acetic acid [5-HIAA]) and low concentrations of serotonin uptake sites on platelets.

2. **Norepinephrine.** Abnormal levels (usually low) of norepinephrine metabolites (3-methoxy-4-hydroxyphenylglycol [MHPG]) are found in blood, urine, and CSF of depressed patients. Venlafaxine (Effexor) increases both serotonin and norepinephrine levels and is used in depression for that reason.

3. **Dopamine.** Dopamine activity may be reduced in depression and increased in mania. Drugs that reduce dopamine concentrations (e.g., reserpine [Serpasil]) and diseases that reduce dopamine concentrations (e.g., Parkinson's disease) are associated with depressive symptoms. Drugs that increase dopamine concentrations, such as tyrosine, amphetamine, and bupropion (Wellbutrin), reduce the symptoms of depression. Two recent theories about dopamine and depression are

Table 11-2
Lifetime Prevalence Rates of Bipolar I Disorder, Bipolar II Disorder, Cyclothymic Disorder, and Hypomania

	Lifetime Prevalence (%)
Bipolar I disorder	0–2.4
Bipolar II disorder	0.3–4.8
Cyclothymia	0.5–6.3
Hypomania	2.6–7.8

Adapted from Rihmer Z, Angst A. Mood disorders: Epidemiology. In: Sadock BJ, Sadock VA, eds. *Comprehensive Textbook of Psychiatry.* 8th ed. Baltimore, MD: Lippincott Williams & Wilkins; 2004.

that the mesolimbic dopamine pathway may be dysfunctional in depression and that the dopamine D_1 receptor may be hypoactive in depression.

B. Psychosocial

1. **Psychoanalytic.** Freud described internalized ambivalence toward a love object (person), which can produce a pathologic form of mourning if the object is lost or perceived as lost. This mourning takes the form of severe depression with feelings of guilt, worthlessness, and suicidal ideation. Symbolic or real loss of love object is perceived as rejection. Mania and elation are viewed as defense against underlying depression. Rigid superego serves to punish person with feelings of guilt about unconscious sexual or aggressive impulses.

2. **Psychodynamics.** In depression, introjection of ambivalently viewed lost objects leads to an inner sense of conflict, guilt, rage, pain, and loathing; a pathologic mourning becomes depression as ambivalent feelings meant for the introjected object are directed at the self. In mania, feelings of inadequacy and worthlessness are converted by means of denial, reaction formation, and projection to grandiose delusions.

3. **Cognitive.** Cognitive triad of Aaron Beck: (1) negative self-view ("things are bad because I'm bad"); (2) negative interpretation of experience ("everything has always been bad"); (3) negative view of future (anticipation of failure).

4. **Learned helplessness.** A theory that attributes depression to a person's inability to control events. Theory is derived from observed behavior of animals experimentally given unexpected random shocks from which they cannot escape.

5. **Stressful life events.** Often precede first episodes of mood disorders. Such events may cause permanent neuronal changes that predispose a person to subsequent episodes of a mood disorder. Losing a parent before age 11 is the life event most associated with later development of depression.

IV. Laboratory, Brain Imaging, and Psychological Tests

A. **Dexamethasone suppression test.** Nonsuppression (positive test result) represents hyper secretion of cortisol secondary to hyperactivity of hypothalamic–pituitary–adrenal axis. Abnormal in 50% of patients with major depression but is of limited clinical usefulness owing to frequency of false-positives and false-negatives. Diminished release of TSH in response to thyrotropin-releasing hormone (TRH) reported in both depression and mania. Prolactin release decreased in response to tryptophan. Tests are not definitive.

B. **Brain imaging.** No gross brain changes. Enlarged cerebral ventricles on computed tomography (CT) in some patients with mania or psychotic depression; diminished basal ganglia blood flow in some depressive patients. Magnetic resonance imaging (MRI) studies have also indicated that patients with major depressive disorder have smaller caudate nuclei and smaller frontal lobes than do control subjects. Magnetic resonance spectroscopy (MRS) studies of patients with bipolar I disorder have produced data consistent with the hypothesis that the pathophysiology of the disorder may involve an abnormal regulation of membrane phospholipid metabolism.

C. Psychological tests
1. **Rating scales.** Can be used to assist in diagnosis and assessment of treatment efficacy. The Beck Depression Inventory (BDI) and Zung Self-rating Scale are scored by patients. The Hamilton Rating Scale for Depression (HAM-D), Montgomery Asberg Depression Rating Scale (MADRS), and Young Manic Rating Scale are scored by the examiner.
2. **Rorschach test.** Standardized set of 10 inkblots scored by examiner— few associations, slow response time in depression.
3. **Thematic apperception test (TAT).** Series of 30 pictures depicting ambiguous situations and interpersonal events. Patient creates a story about each scene. Depressives will create depressed stories, manics more grandiose and dramatic ones.

V. Bipolar Disorder
There are two types of bipolar disorder: bipolar I characterized by the occurrence of manic episodes with or without a major depressive episode and bipolar II characterized by at least one depressive episode with or without a hypomanic episode.

 CLINICAL HINT:
If there is a history of a single full-blown manic episode, the diagnosis will always be bipolar I; a history of a major depressive episode is always present in bipolar II.

A. Depression (major depressive episode). See Table 11-3.
1. Information obtained from history
   a. Depressed mood: subjective sense of sadness, feeling "blue" or "down in the dumps" for a prolonged period of time.

 Table 11-3
Signs and Symptoms of Major Depressive Episode

1. A depressed mood and a loss of interest or pleasure
2. Feeling blue, hopeless, in the dumps, or worthless
3. Trouble sleeping, especially early morning awakening or hypersomnia
4. Decreased appetite and weight loss, or increased appetite and weight gain
5. Inability to concentrate and impairments in thinking
6. Depressed mood most of the day, and nearly every day
7. Psychomotor agitation or retardation
8. Fatigue and decreased energy
9. Feeling worthless with guilt
10. Suicidal and recurrent morbid thoughts

   b. Anhedonia: inability to experience pleasure.
   c. Social withdrawal.
   d. Lack of motivation, little tolerance of frustration.
   e. Vegetative signs.
      (1) Loss of libido.
      (2) Weight loss and anorexia.
      (3) Weight gain and hyperphagia.
      (4) Low-energy level; fatigability.
      (5) Abnormal menses.
      (6) Early morning awakening (terminal insomnia); approximately 75% of depressed patients have sleep difficulties, either insomnia or hypersomnia.
      (7) Diurnal variation (symptoms worse in morning).
   f. Constipation.
   g. Dry mouth.
   h. Headache.
2. **Information obtained from mental status examination**
   a. General appearance and behavior. Psychomotor retardation or agitation, poor eye contact, tearful, downcast, inattentive to personal appearance.
   b. Affect. Constricted or labile.
   c. Mood. Depressed, irritable, frustrated, sad.
   d. Speech. Little or no spontaneity; monosyllabic; long pauses; soft, low monotone.
   e. Thought content. Suicidal ideation affects 60% of depressed patients, and 15% commit suicide; obsessive rumination; pervasive feelings of hopelessness, worthlessness, and guilt; somatic preoccupation; indecisiveness; poverty of thought content and paucity of speech; mood-congruent hallucinations and delusions.
   f. Cognition. Distractible, difficulty concentrating, complaints of poor memory, apparent disorientation; abstract thought may be impaired.
   g. Insight and judgment. Impaired because of cognitive distortions of personal worthlessness.
3. **Associated features**
   a. Somatic complaints may mask depression: in particular, cardiac, gastrointestinal, and genitourinary symptoms; low back pain, other orthopedic complaints.
   b. Content of delusions and hallucinations, when present, tends to be congruent with depressed mood; most common are delusions of guilt, poverty, and deserved persecution, in addition to somatic and nihilistic (end of the world) delusions. Mood-incongruent delusions are those with content not apparently related to the predominant mood (e.g., delusions of thought insertion, broadcasting, and control, or persecutory delusions unrelated to depressive themes).

4. **Age-specific features.** Depression can present differently at different ages.

   a. **Prepubertal.** Somatic complaints, agitation, single-voice auditory hallucinations, anxiety disorders, and phobias.

   b. **Adolescence.** Substance abuse, antisocial behavior, restlessness, truancy, school difficulties, promiscuity, increased sensitivity to rejection, poor hygiene.

   c. **Elderly.** Cognitive deficits (memory loss, disorientation, confusion); pseudodementia or the dementia syndrome of depression, apathy, and distractibility.

B. **Mania (manic episode).** Persistent elevated expansive mood. See Table 11-4.

   1. **Information obtained from history**

      a. Erratic and disinhibited behavior.

         (1) Excessive spending or gambling.

         (2) Impulsive travel.

         (3) Hypersexuality, promiscuity.

      b. Overextended in activities and responsibilities.

      c. Low frustration tolerance with irritability, outbursts of anger.

      d. Vegetative signs.

         (1) Increased libido.

         (2) Weight loss, anorexia.

         (3) Insomnia (expressed as no need to sleep).

         (4) Excessive energy.

   2. **Information obtained from mental status examination**

      a. **General appearance and behavior.** Psychomotor agitation; seductive, colorful clothing; excessive makeup; inattention to personal appearance or bizarre combinations of clothes; intrusive; entertaining; threatening; hyperexcited.

      b. **Affect.** Labile, intense (may have rapid depressive shifts).

      c. **Mood.** Euphoric, expansive, irritable, demanding, flirtatious.

      d. **Speech.** Pressured, loud, dramatic, exaggerated; may become incoherent.

      e. **Thought content.** Highly elevated self-esteem, grandiose, extremely egocentric; delusions and less frequently hallucinations (mood-congruent themes of inflated self-worth and power, most often grandiose and paranoid).

Table 11-4
Signs and Symptoms of Manic Episode

1. An elevated, expansive, or irritable mood
2. Increased self-esteem or grandiosity
3. Less need for sleep (2–3 hours)
4. Very talkative and desire to keep talking
5. Racing thoughts
6. Easily distracted and unable to focus
7. Excessive spending and engaging in pleasurable activities (sex and gambling)
8. Severe impairment in occupational and social functioning

Table 11-5
Signs and Symptoms of Hypomanic Episode

1. An expansive, elevated, or irritable mood, but of lesser duration than mania
2. Increased self-esteem or grandiosity
3. Less need for sleep
4. Very talkative and desire to keep talking
5. Racing thoughts
6. Easily distracted and unable to focus
7. Excessive spending and engaging in pleasurable activities (sex and gambling)
8. Less severe than mania and with no significant change in daily functioning

    f. Thought process. Flight of ideas (if severe, can lead to incoherence); racing thoughts, neologisms, clang associations, circumstantiality, tangentially.

    g. Sensorium. Highly distractible, difficulty concentrating; memory, if not too distracted, generally intact; abstract thinking generally intact.

    h. Insight and judgment. Extremely impaired; often total denial of illness and inability to make any organized or rational decisions.

C. Other types of bipolar disorders

    1. Rapid-cycling bipolar disorder. Four or more depressive, manic, or mixed episodes within 12 months. Bipolar disorder with mixed or rapid-cycling episodes appears to be more chronic than bipolar disorder without alternating episodes.

    2. Hypomania. Elevated mood associated with decreased need for sleep, hypoactivity, and hedonic pursuits. Less severe than mania with no psychotic features (see Table 11-5).

D. Depressive disorders

    1. Major depressive disorder. Can occur alone or as part of bipolar disorder. When it occurs alone it is also known as *unipolar depression*. Symptoms must be present for at least 2 weeks and represent a change from previous functioning. More common in women than in men by 2:1. Precipitating event occurs in at least 25% of patients. Diurnal variation, with symptoms worse early in morning. Psychomotor retardation or agitation is present. Associated with vegetative signs. Mood-congruent delusions and hallucinations may be present. Median age of onset is 40 years, but can occur at any time. Genetic factor is present. Major depressive disorder may occur as a single episode in a person's life or may be recurrent (see Table 11-3).

    2. Other types of major depressive disorder

        a. Melancholic. Severe and responsive to biologic intervention. See Table 11-6.

        b. Seasonal pattern. Depression that develops with shortened daylight in winter and fall and disappears during spring and summer; also known as *seasonal affective disorder*. Characterized by hypersomnia, hyperphagia, and psychomotor slowing. Related to abnormal melatonin metabolism. Treated with exposure to bright,

Table 11-6
Signs and Symptoms: Melancholic Features Specifier

1. Lack of interest and pleasure in usual and all activities
2. Poor response to enjoyable activities
3. Depressed mood is different than usual reaction to stressful events
4. Mood is worse in the morning
5. Disturbed sleep with early morning arousal
6. Loss of appetite and weight loss
7. Inappropriate self-blame and remorse

artificial light for 2 to 6 hours daily. May also occur as part of bipolar I and II disorders.

c. **Peripartum onset.** Severe depression beginning within 4 weeks of giving birth. Most often occurs in women with underlying or pre-existing mood or other psychiatric disorder. Symptoms range from marked insomnia, liability, and fatigue to suicide. Homicidal and delusional beliefs about the baby may be present. Can be psychiatric emergency, with both mother and baby at risk. Also applies to manic or mixed episodes or to brief psychotic disorder.

d. **Atypical features.** Sometimes called *hysterical dysphoria*. Major depressive episode characterized by weight gain and hypersomnia rather than weight loss and insomnia. More common in women than in men by 2:1 to 3:1. Common in major depressive disorder with seasonal pattern. May also occur as part of depression in bipolar I or II disorder and dysthymic disorder (see Table 11-7).

e. **Catatonic.** Stuporous, blunted affect, extreme withdrawal, negativism, pyschomotor retardation with posturing and waxy flexibility. Responds to electroconvulsive therapy (ECT).

f. **Pseudodementia.** Though not mentioned in DSM-5, this category is clinical relevant and clinicians should be aware of this specifier of major depressive disorder presenting as cognitive dysfunction resembling dementia. Occurs in elderly persons, and more often in patients with previous history of mood disorder. Depression is primary and preeminent, antedating cognitive deficits. Responsive to ECT or antidepressant medication.

g. **Depression in children.** This is also not mentioned in DSM-5 but is not uncommon and clinically relevant. Signs and symptoms similar to those in adults. Masked depression seen in somatic symptoms, running away from home, school phobia, and substance abuse. Suicide may occur.

Table 11-7
Signs and Symptoms: Atypical Features Specifier

1. Positive mood changes in happy environment
2. Increased appetite and weight gain
3. Increased sleep
4. Feeling exhausted with sense of heavy limbs
5. Feeling easily rejected by others

h. **Double depression.** Development of superimposed major depressive disorder in dysthymic patients (about 10% to 15%).

i. **Depressive disorder not otherwise specified.** This is a separate category is DSM-5 and called unspecified depressive disorder that does not meet the criteria for a specific mood disorder (e.g., minor depressive disorder and recurrent brief depressive disorder).

j. **Psychotic features.** Hallucinations or delusions associated with depression.

k. **With anxious distress.** Feeling tense, restless, with poor focus, concentration and worry about something dreadful happening in the future.

l. **With mixed features.** Symptoms of mania with euphoria or elevated, irritable mood, increased self-esteem, hyperverbal, racing thoughts, decreased need for sleep among others.

m. **With catatonic features.** The symptoms should be present for a major part of the depressive episode. The hallmark symptoms of catatonia are stuporousness, blunted affect, extreme withdrawal, negativism, and marked psychomotor retardation.

 CLINICAL HINT:
If delusions are mood incongruent, diagnosis is more likely to be schizophrenia.

---

3. **Persistent depressive disorder (Dysthymia).** Previously known as *depressive neurosis*. Less severe than major depressive disorder. More common and chronic in women than in men. Insidious onset. Occurs more often in persons with history of long-term stress or sudden losses; often coexists with other psychiatric disorders (e.g., substance abuse, personality disorders, obsessive-compulsive disorder). Symptoms tend to be worse later in the day. Onset generally between ages of 20 and 35, although an early-onset type begins before age 21. More common among first-degree relatives with major depressive disorder. Symptoms should include at least two of the following: poor appetite, overeating, sleep problems, fatigue, low self-esteem, poor concentration or difficulty making decisions, and feelings of hopelessness (see Table 11-8).

 Table 11-8
Signs and Symptoms of Persistent Depressive Disorder (Dysthymia)

1. Easily depressed
2. Little joy in living
3. Inclined to be gloomy and morbid
4. Pessimistic, self-deprecatory
5. Low self-esteem
6. Fearful of disapproval, indecisive
7. May be suspicious of others

Table 11-9
Signs and Symptoms of Cyclothymic Disorder

1. Numerous episodes of hypomania and depression for 2 years
2. No major depressive or manic episode during the time
3. Symptoms have persisted for majority of the time and absent for no more than 2 months at a time

4. **Cyclothymic disorder.** Less severe disorder, with alternating periods of hypomania and moderate depression. The condition is chronic and nonpsychotic. Symptoms must be present for at least 2 years. Equally common in men and women. Onset usually is insidious and occurs in late adolescence or early adulthood. Substance abuse is common. Major depressive disorder and bipolar disorder are more common among first-degree relatives than among the general population. Recurrent mood swings may lead to social and professional difficulties. May respond to lithium (see Table 11-9).

5. **Disruptive mood dysregulation disorder.** The disorder is a new category included in the DSM-5 to prevent over diagnosis of bipolar disorder in children. The pertinent symptoms include; acute and recurrent angry outbursts that are inconsistent with the developmental age and manifest as irritability, anger, and occur frequently three or more times a week. Of note the diagnosis should not be made before age 6 or after 18 years.

6. **Premenstrual dysphoric disorder.** This disorder has been reclassified in DSM-5 and categorized under depressive disorders. Is a distinct condition that responds to treatment that begins after ovulation and remits early in the menstruation phase. The hallmark symptoms are; begins in the final week of menstrual cycle, with mood lability (ups and downs, sudden tearfulness, and sense of rejection), irritability, depressed mood, hopelessness, anxiety, poor concentration, fatigue, changes in appetite, changes in sleep pattern and physical symptoms (breast tenderness, swelling, and bloating).

VI. Differential Diagnosis

Table 11-10 lists the clinical differences between depression and mania.

A. **Mood disorder resulting from general medical condition.** Depressive, manic, or mixed features or major depressive-like episode secondary to medical illness (e.g., brain tumor, metabolic illness, HIV disease, Parkinson's disease, Cushing's syndrome) (Table 11-11). Cognitive deficits are common.

1. **Myxedema madness.** Hypothyroidism associated with fatigability, depression, and suicidal impulses. May mimic schizophrenia, with thought disorder, delusions, hallucinations, paranoia, and agitation. More common in women.

2. **Mad hatter's syndrome.** Chronic mercury intoxication (poisoning) produces manic (and sometimes depressive) symptoms.

Table 11-10
Clinical Differences Between Depression and Mania

	Depressive Syndrome	**Mania Syndrome**
Mood	Depressed, irritable, or anxious (the patient may, however, smile or deny subjective mood change and instead complain of pain or other somatic distress)	Elated, irritable, or hostile
	Crying spells (the patient may, however, complain of inability to cry or experience emotions)	Momentary tearfulness (as part of mixed state)
Associated psychological manifestations	Lack of self-confidence; low self-esteem; self-reproach	Inflated self-esteem; boasting; grandiosity
	Poor concentration; indecisiveness	Racing thoughts; clang associations (new thoughts triggered by word sounds rather than meaning); distractibility
	Reduction in gratification; loss of interest in usual activities; loss of attachments; social withdrawal	Heightened interest in new activities, people, creative pursuits; increased involvement with people (who are often alienated because of the patient's intrusive and meddlesome behavior); buying sprees; sexual indiscretions; foolish business investment
	Negative expectations; hopelessness; helplessness; increased dependency	
	Recurrent thoughts of death and suicide	
Somatic manifestations	Psychomotor retardation; fatigue Agitation	Pyschomotor acceleration; eutonia (increased sense of physical well-being)
	Anorexia and weight loss, or weight gain	Possible weight loss from increased activity and inattention to proper dietary habits
	Insomnia or hypersomnia	Decreased need for sleep
	Menstrual irregularities; amenorrhea	
	Anhedonia; loss of sexual desire	Increased sexual desire
Psychotic symptoms	Delusions of worthlessness and sinfulness	Grandiose delusions of exceptional talent
	Delusions of reference and persecution	Delusions of assistance; delusions of reference and persecution
	Delusion of ill health (nihilistic, somatic, or hypochondriacal)	Delusions of exceptional mental and physical fitness
	Delusions of poverty	Delusions of wealth, aristocratic ancestry, or other grandiose identity
	Depressive hallucinations in the auditory, visual, and (rarely) olfactory spheres	Fleeting auditory or visual hallucinations

From Berkow R, ed. *Merck Manual.* 15th ed. Rahway, NJ: Merck Sharp & Dohme Research Laboratories, 1987:1518, with permission.

B. Substance-induced mood disorder. See Table 11-12. Mood disorders caused by a drug or toxin (e.g., cocaine, amphetamine, propranolol [Inderal], steroids). Must always be ruled out when patient presents with depressive or manic symptoms. Mood disorders often occur simultaneously with substance abuse and dependence.

C. Schizophrenia. Schizophrenia can look like a manic, major depressive, or mixed episode with psychotic features. To differentiate, rely on such factors as family history, course, premorbid history, and response to medication.

Table 11-11
Neurologic and Medical Causes of Depressive (and Manic) Symptoms

Neurologic	Infectious and inflammatory
Cerebrovascular diseases	AIDS[a]
Dementias (including dementia of the Alzheimer's type with depressed mood)	Chronic fatigue syndrome
	Mononucleosis
Epilepsy[a]	Pneumonia—viral and bacterial
Fahr's disease[a]	Rheumatoid arthritis
Huntington's disease[a]	Sjögren's arteritis
Hydrocephalus	Systemic lupus erythematosus[a]
Infections (including HIV and neurosyphilis)[a]	Temporal arthritis
Migraines[a]	Tuberculosis
Multiple sclerosis[a]	**Miscellaneous medical**
Narcolepsy	Cancer (especially pancreatic and other gastrointestinal)
Neoplasms[a]	
Parkinson's disease	Cardiopulmonary disease
Progressive supranuclear palsy	Porphyria
Sleep apnea	Uremia (and other renal diseases)[a]
Trauma[a]	Vitamin deficiencies (B$_{12}$, folate, niacin, thiamine)[a]
Wilson's disease[a]	
Endocrine	
Adrenal (Cushing's, Addison's diseases)	
Hyperaldosteronism	
Menses-related[a]	
Parathyroid disorders (hyper- and hypo-)	
Postpartum[a]	
Thyroid disorders (hypothyroidism and apathetic hyperthyroidism)[a]	

[a]These conditions are also associated with manic symptoms.

Depressive-like or manic-like episode with presence of mood-incongruent psychotic features suggests schizophrenia. Thought insertion and broadcasting, loose associations, poor reality testing, or bizarre behavior may also suggest schizophrenia. Bipolar disorder with depression or mania more often is associated with mood-congruent hallucinations or delusions.

D. Grief. Not a true disorder. Known as *bereavement* in *DSM-5*. Profound sadness secondary to major loss. Presentation may be similar to that of major depressive disorder, with anhedonia, withdrawal, and vegetative signs. Remits with time. Differentiated from major depressive disorder by absence of suicidal ideation or profound feelings of hopelessness and worthlessness. Usually resolves within a year. May develop into major depressive episode in predisposed persons.

E. Personality disorders. Lifelong behavioral pattern associated with rigid defensive style; depression may occur more readily after stressful life event because of inflexibility of coping mechanisms. Manic episode may also occur more readily in predisposed people with pre-existing personality disorder. A mood disorder may be diagnosed on Axis I simultaneously with a personality disorder on Axis II.

F. Schizoaffective disorder. Signs and symptoms of schizophrenia accompany prominent mood symptoms. Course and prognosis are between those of schizophrenia and mood disorders.

Table 11-12
Pharmacologic Causes of Depression and Mania

Pharmacologic Causes of Depression		Pharmacologic Causes of Mania
Cardiac and antihypertensive drugs		
Bethanidine	Digitalis	Amphetamines
Clonidine	Prazosin	Antidepressants
Guanethidine	Procainamide	Baclofen
Hydralazine	Veratrum	Bromide
Methyldopa	Lidocaine	Bromocriptine
Propranolol	Oxprenolol	Captopril
Reserpine	Methoserpidine	Cimetidine
Sedatives and hypnotics		Cocaine
Barbiturates	Benzodiazepines	Corticosteroids (including corticotropin)
Chloral hydrate	Chlormethiazole	Cyclosporine
Ethanol	Clorazepate	Disulfiram
Steroids and hormones		Hallucinogens (intoxication and flashbacks)
Corticosteroids	Triamcinolone	Hydralazine
Oral contraceptives	Norethisterone	Isoniazid
Prednisone	Danazol	Levodopa
Stimulants and appetite suppressants		Methylphenidate
Amphetamine	Diethylpropion	Metrizamide (following myelography)
Fenfluramine	Phenmetrazine	Opioids
Psychotropic drugs		Phencyclidine
Butyrophenones	Phenothiazines	Procarbazine
Neurologic agents		Procyclidine
Amantadine	Baclofen	Yohimbine
Bromocriptine	Carbamazepine	
Levodopa	Methosuximide	
Tetrabenazine	Phenytoin	
Analgesics and anti-inflammatory drugs		
Fenoprofen	Phenacetin	
Ibuprofen	Phenylbutazone	
Indomethacin	Pentazocine	
Opioids	Benzydamine	
Antibacterial and antifungal drugs		
Ampicillin	Griseofulvin	
Sulfamethoxazole	Metronidazole	
Clotrimazole	Nitrofurantoin	
Cycloserine	Nalidixic acid	
Dapsone	Sulfonamides	
Ethionamide	Streptomycin	
Tetracycline	Thiocarbanilide	
Antineoplastic drugs		
C-Asparaginase	6-Azauridine	
Mithramycin	Bleomycin	
Vincristine	Trimethoprim	
	Zidovudine	
Miscellaneous drugs		
Acetazolamide	Anticholinesterases	
Choline	Cimetidine	
Cyproheptadine	Diphenoxylate	
Disulfiram	Lysergide	
Methysergide	Mebeverine	
Meclizine	Metoclopramide	
Pizotifen	Salbutamol	

Adapted from Cummings JL. *Clinical Neuropsychiatry.* Orlando, FL: Grune & Stratton; 1985:187.

G. Adjustment disorder with depressed mood. Moderate depression in response to clearly identifiable stress, which resolves as stress diminishes. Considered a maladaptive response resulting from either impairment in functioning or excessive and disproportionate intensity of symptoms. Persons with personality disorders or cognitive deficits may be more vulnerable.

H. Primary sleep disorders. Can cause anergy, dyssomnia, irritability. Distinguish from major depression by assessing for typical signs and symptoms of depression and occurrence of sleep abnormalities only in the context of depressive episodes. Consider obtaining a sleep laboratory evaluation in cases of refractory depression.

I. Other mental disorders. Eating disorders, somatoform disorders, and anxiety disorders are all commonly associated with depressive symptoms and must be considered in the differential diagnosis of a patient with depressive symptoms. Perhaps the most difficult differential is that between anxiety disorders with depression and depressive disorders with marked anxiety.

VII. Course and Prognosis

Fifteen percent of depressed patients eventually commit suicide. An untreated, average depressed episode lasts about 10 months. At least 75% of affected patients have a second episode of depression, usually within the first 6 months after the initial episode. The average number of depressive episodes in a lifetime is five. The prognosis generally is good: 50% recover, 30% partially recover, 20% have a chronic course. About 20% to 30% of dysthymic patients develop, in descending order of frequency, major depressive disorder (called *double depression*), bipolar II disorder, or bipolar I disorder. A major mood disorder, usually bipolar II disorder, develops in about 30% of patients with cyclothymic disorder. Forty-five percent of manic episodes recur. Untreated, manic episodes last 3 to 6 months, with a high rate of recurrence (average of 10 recurrences). Some 80% to 90% of manic patients eventually experience a full depressive episode. The prognosis is fair: 15% recover, 50% to 60% partially recover (multiple relapses with good interepisodic functioning), and one-third have some evidence of chronic symptoms and social deterioration.

 CLINICAL HINT:
Depressed patients with suicidal ideation should be hospitalized if there is any doubt in the clinician's mind about the risk. If the clinician cannot sleep because of worry about a patient, that patient belongs in a hospital.

VIII. Treatment

A. Depressive disorders. Major depressive episodes are treatable in 70% to 80% of patients. The most effective approach is to integrate pharmacotherapy with psychotherapeutic interventions.

   1. Psychopharmacologic.
      a. Most clinicians begin treatment with a selective serotonin reuptake inhibitor (SSRI). Early transient side effects include anxiety,

gastrointestinal upset, and headache. Educating patients about the self-limited nature of these effects can enhance compliance. Sexual dysfunction is often a persistent, common side effect that may respond to a change in drug or dosage, or adjunctive therapy with an agent such as bupropion (Wellbutrin) or buspirone (BuSpar). The early anxiogenic effects of SSRIs may aggravate suicidal ideation and can be managed by either reducing the dose or adding an anxiolytic (e.g., 0.5 mg of clonazepam [Klonopin] in the morning and at night). Insomnia can be managed with a benzodiazepine, zolpidem (Ambien), trazodone (Desyrel), or mirtazapine (Remeron). Patients who do not respond to or who cannot tolerate one SSRI may respond to another. Some clinicians switch to an agent with a different mechanism of action, such as bupropion, venlafaxine (Effexor), desvenlafaxine (pristiq), duloxetine (Cymbalta), mirtazapine (Remeron), a tricyclic, or a monoamine oxidase inhibitor (MAOI). The tricyclics and MAOIs are generally considered as second- or third-line agents because of their side effects and potential lethality in overdose.

 CLINICAL HINT:
There is an increased risk of suicide as suicidally depressed patients begin to improve. They have the physical energy to carry out the act whereas, before, they lacked the will to do so. Known as paradoxical suicide.

---

b. Bupropion is a noradrenergic, dopaminergic drug with stimulant like properties. It comes in three formulations (Regular, SR, and XL) the difference being in the half-life and subsequently the dosing frequency. It is generally well tolerated and may be particularly useful for depression marked by anergy and psychomotor retardation. It is also devoid of sexual side effects. It may exacerbate anxiety and agitation. Its dopaminergic properties have the potential to exacerbate psychosis. Prior concerns about its tendency to cause seizures have been mitigated by the availability of a sustained-release formulation that carries the same risk for seizure as the SSRIs (0.1%). The average dose is 150 to 300 mg/day but some patients require doses up to 450 mg.

c. Venlafaxine, desvenlafaxine, and duloxetine are serotonin–norepinephrine reuptake inhibitors that may be particularly effective in severe or refractory cases of depression. Response rates increase with higher doses. Side effects are similar to those of SSRIs. The average dose of venlafaxine is 75 to 375 mg/day, desvenlafaxine is 50 to 100 mg, and of duloxetine is 20 to 60 mg/day.

d. Nefazodone is a drug with serotoninergic properties. Its main mechanism of action is postsynaptic 5-HT$_2$ blockade. As a result, it produces beneficial effects on sleep and has a low rate of sexual side effects. It has been associated with liver toxicity and should be used with caution in patients with suspected liver damage. The average dose is 300 to 600 mg/day. It is only available only as a generic preparation.

e. Mirtazapine has antihistamine, noradrenergic, and serotoninergic actions. It specifically blocks 5-HT₂ and 5-HT₃ receptors, so that the anxiogenic, sexual, and gastrointestinal side effects of serotoninergic drugs are avoided. At low doses, it can be highly sedating and cause weight gain. At higher dosages, it becomes more noradrenergic relative to its antihistamine effects and so a more activating drug. Average dose is 15 to 30 mg/day.

f. The tricyclics are highly effective but require dose titration. Side effects include anticholinergic effects in addition to potential cardiac conduction delay and orthostasis. The secondary amines, such as nortriptyline, are often better tolerated than the tertiary amines, such as amitriptyline (Elavil). Blood levels can be helpful in determining optimal dosage and adequacy of a therapeutic trial. Lethality in overdose remains a concern.

g. Augmentation strategies in treatment-resistant or partially responsive patients include liothyronine (Cytomel), lithium, amphetamines, buspirone, or antidepressant combinations such as bupropion added to an SSRI.

h. If symptoms still do not improve, try an MAOI. An MAOI is safe with reasonable dietary restriction of tyramine-containing substances. Major depressive episodes that have atypical features or psychotic features or that are related to bipolar I disorder may preferentially respond to MAOIs. MAOIs must not be administered for 2 to 5 weeks after discontinuation of an SSRI or other serotoninergic drugs (e.g., 5 weeks for fluoxetine [Prozac], 2 weeks for paroxetine [Paxil]). An SSRI or other serotoninergic drug (e.g., clomipramine [Anafranil]) must not be administered for 2 weeks after discontinuation of an MAOI. Serotoninergic-dopamine antagonists are also of use in depression with psychotic features.

i. Maintenance treatment for at least 5 months with antidepressants helps to prevent relapse. Long-term treatment may be indicated in patients with recurrent major depressive disorder. The antidepressant dosage required to achieve remission should be continued during maintenance treatment. For an extensive list of medications used in the treatment of depression see Table 11-13.

 CLINICAL HINT:
An extensive NIH study (STAR*D) developed a pharmacologic protocol for the treatment of depression. Clinicians can follow the protocol or vary it depending on the clinical situation and their experience.

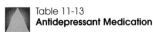

Table 11-13
Antidepressant Medication

Generic (Brand) Name	Usual Daily Dose (mg)	Common Side Effects	Clinical Caveats
NE reuptake inhibitors			
Desipramine (Norpramin, Pertofrane)	75–300	Drowsiness, insomnia, OSH, agitation, CA, weight ↑, anticholinergic[a]	Overdose may be fatal. Dose titration is needed.
Protriptyline (Vivactil)	20–60	Drowsiness, insomnia, OSH, agitation, CA, anticholinergic[a]	Overdose may be fatal. Dose titration is needed.
Nortriptyline (Aventyl, Pamelor)	40–200	Drowsiness, OSH, CA, weight ↑, anticholinergic[a]	Overdose may be fatal. Dose titration is needed.
Maprotiline (Ludiomil)	100–225	Drowsiness, CA, weight ↑, anticholinergic[a]	Overdose may be fatal. Dose titration is needed.
5-HT reuptake inhibitors			
Citalopram (Celexa)	20–60	All SSRIs may cause insomnia, agitation, sedation, GI distress, and sexual dysfunction	Many SSRIs inhibit various cytochrome P450 isoenzymes. They are better tolerated than tricyclics and have high safety in overdose. Shorter half-life SSRIs may be associated with discontinuation symptoms when abruptly stopped.
Escitalopram (Lexapro)	10–20		
Fluoxetine (Prozac)	10–40		
Fluvoxamine (Luvox)[b]	100–300		
Paroxetine (Paxil)	20–50		
Sertraline (Zoloft)	50–150		
Vortioxetine (Trintellix)	10–20		
NE and 5-HT reuptake inhibitors			
Amitriptyline (Elavil, Endep)	75–300	Drowsiness, OSH, CA, weight ↑, anticholinergic[a]	Overdose may be fatal. Dose titration is needed.
Doxepin (Triadapin, Sinequan)	75–300	Drowsiness, OSH, CA, weight ↑, anticholinergic[a]	Overdose may be fatal.
Imipramine (Tofranil)	75–300	Drowsiness, insomnia and agitation, OSH, CA, GI distress, weight ↑, anticholinergic[a]	Overdose may be fatal. Dose titration needed.
Trimipramine (Surmontil)	75–300	Drowsiness, OSH, CA, weight ↑, anticholinergic[a]	—
Venlafaxine (Effexor)	150–375	Sleep changes, GI distress, discontinuation syndrome	Higher doses may cause hypertension. Dose titration is needed. Abrupt discontinuation may result in discontinuation symptoms.
Duloxetine (Cymbalta)	30–60	GI distress, discontinuation syndrome	
Pre- and postsynaptic active agents			
Nefazodone	300–600	Sedation	Dose titration is needed. No sexual dysfunction.
Mirtazapine (Remeron)	15–30	Sedation, weight ↑	No sexual dysfunction.
Dopamine reuptake inhibitor			
Bupropion (Wellbutrin)	200–400	Insomnia or agitation, GI distress	Twice-a-day dosing with sustained release. No sexual dysfunction or weight gain.

(continued)

Table 11-13
Antidepressant Medication *(Continued)*

Generic (Brand) Name	Usual Daily Dose (mg)	Common Side Effects	Clinical Caveats
Mixed action agents			
Amoxapine (Asendin)	100–600	Drowsiness, insomnia or agitation, CA, weight ↑, OSH, anticholinergic[a]	Movement disorders may occur. Dose titration is needed.
Clomipramine (Anafranil)	75–300	Drowsiness, weight ↑	Dose titration is needed.
Trazodone (Desyrel)	150–600	Drowsiness, OSH, CA, GI distress, weight ↑	Priapism is possible.

[a]Dry mouth, blurred vision, urinary hesitancy, and constipation.
[b]Not approved as an antidepressant in the United States by the U.S. Food and Drug Administration.
Note: Dose ranges are for adults in good general medical health, taking no other medications, and ages 18–60 years. Doses vary depending on the agent, concomitant medications, the presence of general medical or surgical conditions, age, genetic constitution, and other factors. Brand names are those used in the United States.
CA, cardiac arrhythmia; 5-HT, serotonin; GI, gastrointestinal; NE, norepinephrine; OSH, orthostatic hypotension; SSRI, selective serotonin reuptake inhibitor.

j. ECT is useful in refractory major depressive disorder and major depressive episodes with psychotic features; ECT also is indicated when a rapid therapeutic response is desired or when side effects of antidepressant medications must be avoided. (ECT is underused as a first-line antidepressant treatment.)

k. Lithium can be a first-line antidepressant in treating the depression of bipolar disorder. A heterocyclic antidepressant or MAOI may be added as necessary, but monitor the patient carefully for emergence of manic symptoms.

l. Repetitive transcranial magnetic stimulation (rTMS) is currently experimental. Shows promise as a treatment for depression. rTMS uses magnetic fields to stimulate specific brain regions (e.g., left prefrontal cortex) believed to be involved in the pathophysiology of specific disorders.

m. Vagus nerve stimulation with implanted electrodes has been successful in some cases of depression and is being studied.

2. Psychological. Psychotherapy in conjunction with antidepressants is more effective than either treatment alone in the management of major depressive disorder.

a. Cognitive. Short-term treatment with interactive therapist and assigned homework aimed at testing and correcting negative cognitions and the unconscious assumptions that underlie them; based on correcting chronic distortions in thinking that lead to depression, in particular the cognitive triad of feelings of helplessness and hopelessness about one's self, one's future, and one's past.

b. Behavioral. Based on learning theory (classic and operant conditioning). In general, short-term and highly structured; aimed at specific, circumscribed undesired behaviors. The operant conditioning technique of positive reinforcement may be an effective adjunct in the treatment of depression.

c. **Interpersonal.** Developed as a specific short-term treatment for nonbipolar, nonpsychotic depression in outpatients. Emphasis on ongoing, current interpersonal issues as opposed to unconscious, intrapsychic dynamics.

d. **Psychoanalytically oriented.** Insight-oriented therapy of indeterminate length aimed at achieving understanding of unconscious conflicts and motivations that may be fueling and sustaining depression.

e. **Supportive.** Therapy of indeterminate length with the primary aim of providing emotional support. Indicated particularly in acute crisis, such as grief, or when the patient is beginning to recover from a major depressive episode but cannot yet engage in more demanding, interactive therapy.

f. **Group.** Not indicated for acutely suicidal patients. Other depressed patients may benefit from support, ventilation, and positive reinforcement of groups, and from interpersonal interaction and immediate correction of cognitive and transference distortions by other group members.

g. **Family.** Particularly indicated when patient's depression is disrupting family stability, when depression is related to family events, or when it is supported or maintained by family patterns.

B. Bipolar disorders

1. Biologic

a. Lithium, divalproex (Depakote), and olanzapine (Zyprexa) are first-line treatments for the manic phase of bipolar disorder, but carbamazepine (Tegretol) is also a well-established treatment. Gabapentin (Neurontin) and lamotrigine (Lamictal) are also of use. Topiramate (Topamax) is another anticonvulsant showing benefit in bipolar patients. ECT is highly effective in all phases of bipolar disorder. Carbamazepine, divalproex, and valproic acid (Depakene) may be more effective than lithium in the treatment of mixed or dysphoric mania, rapid cycling, and psychotic mania, and in the treatment of patients with a history of multiple manic episodes or comorbid substance abuse.

b. Treatment of acute manic episodes often requires adjunctive use of potent sedative drugs. Drugs commonly used at the start of treatment include clonazepam (1 mg every 4 to 6 hours) and lorazepam (Ativan) (2 mg every 4 to 6 hours). Haloperidol (Haldol) (2 to 10 mg/day), olanzapine (2.5 to 10 mg/day), and risperidone (Risperdal) (0.5 to 6 mg/day) are also of use. Bipolar patients may be particularly sensitive to the side effects of typical antipsychotics. The atypical antipsychotics (e.g., olanzapine [Zyprexa] [10 to 20 mg/day]) are often used as monotherapy for acute control and may have intrinsic antimanic properties. Physicians should attempt to taper these adjunctive agents when the patient stabilizes.

c. Lithium remains a mainstay of treatment in bipolar disorders. A blood level of 0.8 to 1.2 mEq/L is usually needed to control acute symptoms. A complete trial should last at least 4 weeks, with 2 weeks at therapeutic levels. Prelithium workup includes a complete blood cell count, electrocardiogram (ECG), thyroid function tests, measurement of blood urea nitrogen and serum creatinine, and a pregnancy test. Lithium has a narrow therapeutic index, and levels can become toxic quickly when a patient is dehydrated. A level of 2.0 mEq or higher is toxic. Lithium treatment can be initiated at 300 mg three times per day but can be given as a single nightly dose. A level should be checked after 5 days and the dose titrated accordingly. The clinical response may take 4 days after a therapeutic level has been achieved. Typical side effects include thirst, polyuria, tremor, metallic taste, cognitive dulling, and gastrointestinal upset. Lithium can induce hypothyroidism and, in rare cases, renal toxicity. Lithium is a first-line treatment for bipolar depression and achieves an antidepressant response in 50% of patients. Lithium is most effective for prophylaxis of further mood episodes at levels of 0.8 to 1.2 mEq/L. However, in many patients, remission can be maintained at lower levels, which are better tolerated and thereby promote enhanced compliance. Patients with depressive breakthrough on lithium should be assessed for lithium-induced hypothyroidism. Lithium is excreted unchanged by the kidneys and must be used with caution in patients with renal disease. Because lithium is not metabolized by the liver, it may be the best choice for treating bipolar disorder in patients with hepatic impairment.

d. Valproic acid and divalproex have a broad therapeutic index and appear effective at levels of 50 to 125 mcg/mL. Pretreatment workup includes a complete blood cell count and liver function tests. A pregnancy test is needed because this drug can cause neural tube defects in developing fetuses. It can cause thrombocytopenia and increased transaminase levels, both of which are usually benign and self-limited but require increased blood monitoring. Fatal hepatic toxicity has been reported only in children under age 10 who received multiple anticonvulsants. Typical side effects include hair loss (which can be treated with zinc and selenium), tremor, weight gain, and sedation. Gastrointestinal upset is common but can be minimized by using enteric-coated tablets (Depakote) and titrating gradually. Valproic acid can be loaded for acute symptom control by administering at 20 mg/kg in divided doses. This strategy also produces a therapeutic level and may improve symptoms within 7 days. For outpatients, more physically brittle patients, or less severely ill patients, medication can be started at 250 to 750 mg/day and gradually titrated to a therapeutic level. Blood levels can be checked after 3 days at a particular dosage.

e. Carbamazepine is usually titrated to response rather than blood level, although many clinicians titrate to reach levels of 4 to 12 mcg/mL. Pretreatment evaluation should include liver function tests and a complete blood cell count as well as ECG, electrolytes, reticulocytes, and pregnancy test. Side effects include nausea, sedation, and ataxia. Hepatic toxicity, hyponatremia, or bone marrow suppression may rarely occur. Rash occurs in 10% of patients. Exfoliative rashes (Stevens–Johnson syndrome) are rare but potentially fatal. The drug can be started at 200 to 600 mg/day, with adjustments every 5 days based on clinical response. Improvement may be seen 7 to 14 days after a therapeutic dose has been achieved. Drug interactions complicate carbamazepine use and probably relegate it to second-line status. It is a potent enzyme inducer and can lower levels of other psychotropics, such as haloperidol. Carbamazepine induces its own metabolism (autoinduction), and the dosage often needs to be increased during the first few months of treatment to maintain a therapeutic level and clinical response.

f. Lamotrigine and gabapentin are anticonvulsants that may have antidepressant, antimanic, and mood-stabilizing properties. They do not require blood monitoring. Gabapentin is excreted exclusively by the kidneys. It has a benign side-effect profile that can include sedation or activation, dizziness, and fatigue. It does not interact with other drugs. Dose reduction in patients with renal insufficiency is required. Gabapentin can be titrated aggressively, and therapeutic response has been reported at dosages of 300 to 3,600 mg/day. It has a short half-life, and dosing to three times a day is required. Lamotrigine requires gradual titration to decrease the risk for rash, which occurs in 10% of patients. Stevens–Johnson syndrome occurs in 0.1% of patients treated with lamotrigine. Other side effects include nausea, sedation, ataxia, and insomnia. Dosage can be initiated at 25 to 50 mg/day for 2 weeks and then increased slowly to 150 to 250 mg twice daily. Valproate raises lamotrigine levels. In the presence of valproate, lamotrigine titration should be slower and dosages lower (e.g., 25 mg orally four times daily for 2 weeks, with 25-mg increases every 2 weeks to a maximum of 150 mg/day).

Topiramate has shown efficacy in bipolar disorders. Its side effects include fatigue and cognitive dulling. This drug has the unique property of causing weight loss. One series of overweight patients with bipolar disorder lost an average of 5% of their body weight while taking topiramate as an adjunct to other medications. The starting dosage is usually 25 to 50 mg/day to a maximum of 400 mg/day.

g. Maintenance treatment is required in patients with recurrent illness. During long-term treatment, laboratory monitoring is required for lithium, valproic acid, and carbamazepine. These requirements are outlined in Chapter 25.

h. Patients who do not respond adequately to one mood stabilizer may do well with combination treatment. Lithium and valproic acid are commonly used together. Increased neurotoxicity is a risk, but the combination is safe. Other combinations include lithium plus carbamazepine, carbamazepine plus valproic acid (requires increased laboratory monitoring for drug interactions and hepatic toxicity), and combinations with the newer anticonvulsants.

i. Other agents used in bipolar disorder include verapamil (Isoptin, Calan), nimodipine (Nimotop), clonidine (Catapres), clonazepam, and levothyroxine (Levoxyl, Levothroid, Synthroid). Atypical, second-generation antipsychotics may also be of use in bipolar patients. Quetiapine (Seroquel) has been approved for use and risperidone (Risperdal) and clozapine (Clozaril) have been shown to have antimanic and mood-stabilizing properties. Table 11-13 lists the drugs used in the treatment of depression and Table 11-14 lists the drugs used in the treatment of mania.

j. ECT should be considered in refractory or emergent cases. See Chapter 30 for further discussion.

2. Psychological. Psychotherapy in conjunction with antimanic drugs (e.g., lithium) is more effective than either treatment alone. Psychotherapy is not indicated when a patient is experiencing a manic episode. In this situation, the safety of the patient and others must be paramount, and pharmacologic and physical steps must be taken to protect and calm the patient.

a. Cognitive. Has been studied in relation to increasing compliance with lithium therapy among patients with bipolar disorder.

b. Behavioral. Can be most effective during inpatient treatment of manic patients. Helps to set limits on impulsive or inappropriate behavior through such techniques as positive and negative reinforcement and token economies.

c. Psychoanalytically oriented. Can be beneficial in the recovery and stabilization of manic patients if patient is capable of and desires insight into underlying conflicts that may trigger and fuel manic episodes. Can also help patients understand resistance to medication and thus increase compliance.

d. Supportive. Indicated particularly during acute phases and in early recompensation. Some patients can tolerate only supportive therapy, whereas others can tolerate insight-oriented therapy. Supportive therapy more often is indicated for patients with chronic bipolar disorder, who may have significant interepisodic residual symptoms and experience social deterioration.

e. Group. Can be helpful in challenging denial and defensive grandiosity of manic patients. Useful in addressing such common issues among manic patients as loneliness, shame, inadequacy, fear of

Table 11-14
Antimanic Medications

This table lists medications for which there are data supporting their use in the treatment of acute mania

Drug	Usual Adult Daily Dose	Starting Dose and Titration	Maximum Recommended Dose or Blood Level	Common Side Effects	Monitoring	Warnings
Lithium and anticonvulsants						
Lithium	Target level 0.6–1.2 mEq/L	300–900 mg: increase by 300 mg/day	1.2 mEq/L plasma level	Nausea, vomiting, diarrhea, sedation, tremor, polyuria, polydipsia, weight gain, acne, cognitive slowing	Lithium level 12 hours after last dose and every week while titrating, then every 2 months	Lithium toxicity
Carbamazepine	800–1,000 mg: titrate to clinical response (target level 4–12 mcg/mL)	Start 200 mg at night, BID, or TID; increase by 200 mg/day	1,600 mg/day, Level of 12 mcg/mL	Sedation, dizziness, nausea, cognitive impairment, LFT elevation, dyspepsia, ataxia	CBC, LFT, drug level every 7–14 days while titrating, then monthly for 4 months, then every 6–12 months	Aplastic anemia, agranulocytosis, seizures, myocarditis
Carbamazepine Extended Release	800–1,000 mg: titrate to clinical response (target level 4–12 mcg/mL)	400 mg/day	1,600 mg/ day; Level of 12 mcg/mL	Sedation, dizziness, nausea, cognitive impairment, LFT elevation, dyspepsia, ataxia	CBC, LFT, drug level every 7–14 days while titrating, then monthly for 4 months, then every 6–12 months	Aplastic anemia, agranulocytosis, seizures, myocarditis
Divalproex	Titrate to 50–150 mg	Start 250–500 at night for 2 days; increase by 250 mg/day. Alternative: orally load 20–30 mg/kg/day to start	Level of 150 mEq/L	Nausea, vomiting, sedation, weight gain, hair loss	CBC with increased platelets, LFT level weekly until stable, then monthly for 6 months, then every 6–12 months	Hepatoxicity, teratogenicity, pancreatitis
Oxcarbazepine	600–2,400 dosed BID or TID	Start 300 mg BID; increase by 300 mg QOD	2,500 mg	Fatigue, nausea/vomiting, dizziness, sedation, diplopia, hyponatremia	Electrolytes (sodium)	None
Atypical antipsychotics						
Aripiprazole	15–30 mg	5–15 mg/day increase by 10 mg/wk	30 mg	Nausea, dyspepsia, somnolence, vomiting, akathisia	None	None

(continued)

Table 11-14
Antimanic Medications (Continued)

Drug	Usual Adult Daily Dose	Starting Dose and Titration	Maximum Recommended Dose or Blood Level	Common Side Effects	Monitoring	Warnings
Clozapine	100–900 mg dosed BID or QD	12.5–25 mg BID; increase by 25–50 mg/day	900 mg	Sedation, salivation, sweating, tachycardia, hypotension, constipation, fever, weight gain, diabetes mellitus	CBC with differential every week for 6 months (more frequent if WBC <3,500 or substantial decrease from baseline); then every other week indefinitely, weight, glucose	Agranulocytosis, seizure, myocarditis, other adverse cardiovascular and respiratory effects (orthostatic hypotension)
Olanzapine	10–20 mg dosed QD or BID	5–10 mg at night; also available in dissolving wafer	40 mg	Somnolence, dry mouth, dizziness, asthenia, weight gain	Weight, glucose	None
Quetiapine	200–800 mg dosed QD or BID	25–200 mg at night; increase by 25–50 mg/week	800 mg	Somnolence, dry mouth, weight gain, dizziness	Weight, glucose	None
Risperidone	3 mg	0.5–1 mg, every 1–2 days	6 mg	Somnolence, hyperkinesia, dyspepsia, nausea	Prolactin	None
Ziprasidone	40–160 mg dosed QD or BID	20–40 mg BID; also available in IM form: 10 mg up to every 2 hours or 20 mg up to every 4 hours, max 40 mg	160 mg	Somnolence, dizziness, hypertonia, akathisia, EPS	EKG	None
Lurasidone (bipolar depression)	20–120 mg dosed qhs With 350 calories of food	20 mg single dose available in Po form; increase by 20 mg every week	120 mg	Somnolence, drowsiness akathisia, rigidity	None	None
Asenapine	5–10 mg dosed BID	5–20 mg dosed twice daily or as qhs; available in sublingual tablet (no food or drink for 10 minutes post administration). Dose can be increased by 2.5–5 mg every few days.		Constipation, sedation, akathisia, somnolence, oral hypoesthesia	None	None

Adapted from data by RMA Hirschfeld HD, RH Perlis MD and LA Vornik, MSc.

mental illness, and loss of control. Helpful in reintegrating patients socially.

f. **Family.** Particularly important with bipolar patients because their disorder is strongly familial (22% to 25% of first-degree relatives) and because manic episodes are so disruptive to patients' interpersonal relationships and jobs. During manic episodes, patients may spend huge amounts of family money or act with sexual inappropriateness; residual feelings of anger, guilt, and shame among family members must be addressed. Ways to help with compliance and recognizing triggering events can be explored.

For more detailed discussion of this topic, see Chapter 13, Mood Disorders, Section 13.17, p. 1599, in CTP/X.

12
Anxiety Disorders

I. Introduction

Anxiety disorders can be viewed as a family of related but distinct mental disorders, which include (1) panic disorder, (2) agoraphobia, (3) specific phobia, (4) social anxiety disorder or phobia, and (5) generalized anxiety disorder. It influences cognition and tends to produce distortions of perception. It is differentiated from fear, which is an appropriate response to a known threat; anxiety is a response to a threat that is unknown, vague, or conflictual. Table 12-1 lists the signs and symptoms of anxiety disorders. Most of the effects of anxiety are dread accompanied by somatic complaints that indicate a hyperactive autonomic nervous system such as palpitations and sweating.

II. Classification

There are 11 diagnostic types of anxiety disorders ranging in the fifth edition of *Diagnostic Statistical Manual of Mental Disorders* (DSM-5) from separation anxiety disorder to unspecified anxiety disorder. They are among the most common groups of psychiatric disorders. Each disorder is discussed separately below.

A. **Separation anxiety disorder.** Fears of separation from loved ones (not commensurate with appropriate development) (at least 3 of the following for >1 month if under 18, and >6 months if an adult):

Anxiety when
- separating from home or loved ones
- leaving the home because it will entail such separation
- sleeping away (different room) from loved ones

Along with feelings of
- worry about harm to loved ones
- worry about separation (even if not impending) from loved ones
- fear about isolation from loved ones

Including
- nightmares
- physical symptoms

B. **Selective mutism.** Inability to speak in certain social situations despite the ability to speak in others (occurring for at least 1 month in the absence of a separate disorder and impeding social/educational/occupational functioning).

Specific phobia. Marked and disproportionate anxiety about a specific thing (e.g., horses, heights, needles) or situation. See Table 12-2. This fear must be consistently and persistently present. The person experiences massive anxiety when exposed to the feared object and tries to avoid it

Table 12-1
Signs and Symptoms of Anxiety Disorders

Physical Signs	Psychological Symptoms
Trembling, twitching, feeling shaky	Feeling of dread
Backache, headache	Difficulty concentrating
Muscle tension	Hypervigilance
Shortness of breath, hyperventilation	Insomnia
Fatigability	Decreased libido
Startle response	"Lump in the throat"
Autonomic hyperactivity	Upset stomach ("butterflies")
Flushing and pallor	
Tachycardia, palpitations	
Sweating	
Cold hands	
Diarrhea	
Dry mouth (xerostomia)	
Urinary frequency	
Paresthesia	
Difficulty swallowing	

at all costs. Up to 25% of the population has specific phobias. See Table 12-3. More common in females. See Table 12-4 for psychodynamic factors in phobias.

C. **Social anxiety disorder (social phobia).** Social anxiety disorder is an irrational fear of public situations (e.g., speaking in public, eating in public, using public bathrooms [shy bladder]). May be associated with panic attacks. It usually occurs during early teens but can develop during childhood. Effects up to 13% of persons. Equally common in men and women. See Tables 12-5 and 12-6.

D. **Panic disorder.** Panic disorder is characterized by spontaneous panic attacks (Table 12-7). It may occur alone or be associated with agoraphobia (fear of being in open spaces, outside the home alone, or in a crowd). Panic may evolve in stages: subclinical attacks, full panic attacks, anticipatory anxiety, phobic avoidance of specific situations, and agoraphobia. It can lead to alcohol or drug abuse, depression, and occupational and social restrictions. Agoraphobia can occur alone, although patients usually have associated panic attacks. Anticipatory anxiety is characterized by the fear

Table 12-2
Phobias

Acrophobia	Fear of heights
Agoraphobia	Fear of open places
Ailurophobia	Fear of cats
Hydrophobia	Fear of water
Claustrophobia	Fear of closed spaces
Cynophobia	Fear of dogs
Mysophobia	Fear of dirt and germs
Pyrophobia	Fear of fire
Xenophobia	Fear of strangers
Zoophobia	Fear of animals

Table 12-3
Lifetime Prevalence Rates of Specific Phobia

Site	Men (%)	Women (%)	Total (%)
United States (National Comorbidity Survey)	6.7	15.7	11.3
United States (Epidemiological Catchment Area Study)	7.7	14.4	11.2
Puerto Rico	7.6	9.6	8.6
Edmonton, Canada	4.6	9.8	7.2
Korea	2.6	7.9	5.4
Zurich, Switzerland	5.2	16.1	10.7
The Netherlands	6.6	13.6	10.1

Table 12-4
Psychodynamic Themes in Phobias

- Principal defense mechanisms include displacement, projection, and avoidance.
- Environmental stressors, including humiliation and criticism from an older sibling, parental fights, or loss and separation from parents, interact with a genetic-constitutional diathesis.
- A characteristic pattern of internal object relations is externalized in social situations in the case of social phobia.
- Anticipation of humiliation, criticism, and ridicule is projected onto individuals in the environment.
- Shame and embarrassment are the principal affect states.
- Family members may encourage phobic behavior and serve as obstacles to any treatment plan.
- Self-exposure to the feared situation is a basic principle of all treatment.

Table 12-5
Lifetime Prevalence Rates of Social Anxiety Disorder

Site	Men (%)	Women (%)	Total (%)
United States (National Comorbidity Survey)	11.1	15.5	13.3
United States (Epidemiological Catchment Area Study)	2.1	3.1	2.6
Edmonton, Canada	1.3	2.1	1.7
Puerto Rico	0.8	1.1	1.0
Korea	0.1	1.0	0.5
Zurich, Switzerland	3.7	7.3	5.6
Taiwan	0.2	1.0	0.6
The Netherlands	5.9	9.7	7.8

Table 12-6
Signs and Symptoms Upon Exposure to the Phobic Situation

Anxiety
Fatigue
Palpitations
Nausea
Tremor
Sweating
Panic attack
Urinary frequency
Withdrawal from feared situation

Table 12-7
Signs and Symptoms of Panic Disorder

Recurrent unexpected panic attacks (focal fear lasting a few minutes) with ≥4 of:
1. Palpable heart pulsations or tachycardia.
2. Diaphoresis.
3. Jitteriness.
4. Sensations of shortness of breath or smothering.
5. Suffocating feelings.
6. Chest pain.
7. Queasy, upset stomach.
8. Dizziness or vertigo.
9. Hot flushes or chilliness.
10. Numbness or tingling.
11. Detachment from oneself or reality.
12. Worries about losing control ("freaking out").
13. Worries about death.
These attacks must cause either persistent worry about future attacks or a maladaptive behavioral change to evade future attacks.
(Panic attacks can be present in anxiety and other disorders. In panic disorder, they are otherwise unprovoked.)

that panic, with helplessness or humiliation, will occur. See Table 12-8. Patients with panic disorder often have multiple somatic complaints related to autonomic nervous system dysfunction, with a higher risk in females. See Table 12-9. Medications are often necessary and are the mainstay of the treatment. See Table 12-10.

E. Agoraphobia. Anxiety about being in places or situations such as in a crowd or in open spaces, outside the home, from which escape or egress is feared to be impossible. The situation is avoided or endured with marked distress, sometimes including the fear of having a panic attack. Agoraphobic patients may become housebound and never leave the home or go outside only with a companion. See Table 12-11.

F. Generalized anxiety disorder. Involves excessive worry about everyday life circumstances, events, or conflicts. The symptoms may fluctuate and overlap with other medical and psychiatric disorders (depressive and other anxiety disorders). The anxiety is difficult to control, is subjectively distressing, and produces impairments in important areas of a person's life. Occurs in children and adults with a lifetime prevalence of 45%. Ratio of women to men is 2:1. See Table 12-12.

Table 12-8
Psychodynamic Themes in Panic Disorder

1. Difficulty tolerating anger
2. Physical or emotional separation from significant person both in childhood and in adult life
3. May be triggered by situations of increased work responsibilities
4. Perception of parents as controlling, frightening, critical, and demanding
5. Internal representations of relationships involving sexual or physical abuse
6. A chronic sense of feeling trapped
7. Vicious cycle of anger at parental rejecting behavior followed by anxiety that the fantasy will destroy the tie to parents
8. Failure of signal anxiety function in ego related to self-fragmentation and self-other boundary confusion
9. Typical defense mechanisms: reaction formation, undoing, somatization, and externalization

Table 12-9
Differential Diagnosis for Panic Disorder

Cardiovascular diseases	
Anemia	Hypertension
Angina	Mitral valve prolapse
Congestive heart failure	Myocardial infarction
Hyperactive β-adrenergic state	Paradoxical atrial tachycardia

Pulmonary diseases	
Asthma	Pulmonary embolus
Hyperventilation	

Neurologic diseases	
Cerebrovascular disease	Migraine
Epilepsy	Multiple sclerosis
Huntington's disease	Transient ischemic attack
Infection	Tumor
Ménière's disease	Wilson's disease

Endocrine diseases	
Addison's disease	Hypoglycemia
Carcinoid syndrome	Hyperparathyroidism
Cushing's syndrome	Menopausal disorders
Diabetes	Pheochromocytoma
Hyperthyroidism	Premenstrual syndrome

Drug intoxications	
Amphetamine	Hallucinogens
Amyl nitrite	Marijuana
Anticholinergics	Nicotine
Cocaine	Theophylline

Drug withdrawal	
Alcohol	Opiates and opioids
Antihypertensives	Sedative-hypnotics

Other conditions	
Anaphylaxis	Systemic infections
B$_{12}$ deficiency	Systemic lupus erythematosus
Electrolyte disturbances	Temporal arteritis
Heavy metal poisoning	Uremia

G. **Substance/medication-induced anxiety disorder.** Panic attacks or anxiety developing during or soon after intoxication of or withdrawal from a substance/medication that is known to produce such symptoms.

(Red flags include delirium and panic attacks at baseline.) A wide range of substances can cause anxiety symptoms that are often associated with intoxication or withdrawal states. Most common contributing drugs include amphetamine, cocaine, and caffeine, as well as LSD and MDMA. Primary treatment includes removal of casually involved substance. See Table 12-13.

H. **Anxiety disorder due to another medical condition.** Many medical disorders are associated with anxiety. It is fairly a common condition and DSM-5 suggests that clinicians specify whether the disorder is characterized by symptoms of generalized anxiety or panic attacks. A wide range of medical and neurologic conditions can cause anxiety symptoms. See Tables 12-14 and 12-15.

Table 12-10
Recommended Dosages for Commonly Used Antipanic Drugs (Daily Unless Indicated Otherwise)

Drug	Starting (mg)	Maintenance (mg)
SSRIs		
Paroxetine	5–10	20–60
Paroxetine CR	12.5–25	62.5
Fluoxetine	2–5	20–60
Sertraline	12.5–25	50–200
Fluvoxamine	12.5	100–150
Citalopram	10	20–40
Escitalopram	10	20
Tricyclic antidepressants		
Clomipramine	5–12.5	50–125
Imipramine	10–25	150–500
Desipramine	10–25	150–200
Benzodiazepines		
Alprazolam	0.25–0.5 tid	0.5–2 tid
Clonazepam	0.25–0.5 bid	0.5–2 bid
Diazepam	2–5 bid	5–30 bid
Lorazepam	0.25–0.5 bid	0.5–2 bid
MAOIs		
Phenelzine	15 bid	15–45 bid
Tranylcypromine	10 bid	10–30 bid
RIMAs		
Moclobemide	50	300–600
Brofaromine	50	150–200
Atypical antidepressants		
Venlafaxine	6.25–25	50–150
Venlafaxine XR	37.5	150–225
Other agents		
Valproic acid	125 bid	500–750 bid
Inositol	6,000 bid	6,000 bid

bid, twice a day; MAOI, monoamine oxidase inhibitors; RIMA, reversible inhibitor of monoamine oxidase type A; SSRIs, selective serotonin reuptake inhibitor; tid, three times a day.

I. Other specified anxiety disorder. Anxiety disorder not meeting full criteria (e.g., short duration, culturally specific symptoms, etc.).

J. Unspecified anxiety disorder. This condition does not meet criteria for any of the above-listed anxiety disorders despite resulting in significant social and occupational dysfunction. There is incomplete information for diagnoses. This may include the following conditions.

Table 12-11
Signs and Symptoms of Agoraphobia

Excessive and disproportionate anxiety about ≥2 of the following:
1. Public transport
2. Open public spaces
3. Enclosed public places
4. Queues or crowds
5. Being alone outside of the house
This fear must be consistently and persistently present.
Anxiety/avoidance of these situations occurs because of thoughts of the futility of escape.
(Can be diagnosed independently of or alongside panic disorder.)

Table12–12
Signs and Symptoms of Generalized Anxiety Disorder

Extreme anxiety about various activities, along with ≥3 of the following for more than half the days for ≥6 mos:
1. Fidgetiness and unease
2. Exhaustion
3. Inattention
4. Moodiness
5. Muscle stiffness
6. Sleep problems (either going to sleep or remaining asleep)
(Only 1 is necessary for pediatric diagnoses.)

1. **Adjustment disorder with anxiety.** This applies to the patient with an obvious stressor in whom excessive anxiety develops within 3 months and is expected to last no longer than 6 months. It may occur as a reaction to illness, rejection, or loss of a job, especially if it is experienced as a defeat or failure.

2. **Anxiety secondary to another psychiatric disorder.** Seventy percent of depressed patients have anxiety. Patients with psychoses—schizophrenia, mania, or brief psychotic disorder—often exhibit anxiety (psychotic anxiety). Anxiety is common in delirium and in dementia (catastrophic reaction).

3. **Situational anxiety.** Effects of a stressful situation temporarily overwhelm the ability to cope. This may occur in minor situations if it brings to mind past overwhelming stress.

4. **Existential anxiety.** This involves fears of helplessness, aging, loss of control, and loss of others in addition to the fear of death and dying.

5. **Separation anxiety and stranger anxiety.** Regressed adults, including some who are medically ill, may manifest anxiety when separated from loved ones or when having to react to staff in a hospital. Separation anxiety disorder occurs in some young children when going to school for the first time. It is a normal reaction in infants and children until about 2½ years of age.

6. **Anxiety related to loss of self-control.** In circumstances in which control must be surrendered, such as medical illness or hospitalization,

Table 12-13
Some Substances That May Cause Anxiety

Intoxication	Withdrawal
Amphetamines and other sympathomimetics	Alcohol
Amyl nitrite	Antihypertensives
Anticholinergics	Caffeine
Caffeine	Opioids
Cannabis	
Sedative–hypnotics	
Cocaine	
Hallucinogens	
Theophylline	
Yohimbine	

Table 12-14
Medical and Neurologic Causes of Anxiety

Neurologic disorders
  Cerebral neoplasms
  Cerebral trauma and postconcussive syndromes
  Cerebrovascular disease
  Subarachnoid hemorrhage
  Migraine
  Encephalitis
  Cerebral syphilis
  Multiple sclerosis
  Wilson's disease
  Huntington's disease
  Epilepsy

Systemic conditions
  Hypoxia
  Cardiovascular disease
  Pulmonary insufficiency
  Anemia

Endocrine disturbances
  Pituitary dysfunction
  Thyroid dysfunction
  Parathyroid dysfunction
  Adrenal dysfunction
  Pheochromocytoma
  Female virilization disorders

Inflammatory disorders
  Lupus erythematosus
  Rheumatoid arthritis
  Polyarteritis nodosa
  Temporal arteritis

Deficiency states
  Vitamin B_{12} deficiency
  Pellagra

Miscellaneous conditions
  Hypoglycemia
  Carcinoid syndrome
  Systemic malignancies
  Premenstrual syndrome
  Febrile illnesses and chronic infections
  Porphyria
  Infectious mononucleosis
  Posthepatitis syndrome
  Uremia

Toxic conditions
  Alcohol and drug withdrawal
  Vasopressor agents
  Penicillin
  Sulfonamides
  Mercury
  Arsenic
  Phosphorus
  Organophosphates
  Carbon disulfide
  Benzene
  Aspirin intolerance

Adapted from Cummings JL. *Clinical Neuropsychiatry.* Orlando, FL: Grune & Stratton, 1985:214.

patients with a need to feel in control may be very threatened. Loss of autonomy at work can precipitate anxiety.

7. **Anxiety related to dependence or intimacy.** If past dependency needs were not met or resolved, a patient can be anxious being in a close relationship, which involves some dependence, or being a patient in a hospital, which involves giving up control.

Table 12-15
Differential Diagnosis of Common Medical Conditions Mimicking Anxiety

Angina pectoris/ myocardial infarction (MI)	Electrocardiogram with ST depression in angina; cardiac enzymes in MI. Crushing chest pain usually associated with angina/MI. Anxiety pains usually sharp and more superficial.
Hyperventilation syndrome	History of rapid, deep respirations; circumoral pallor; carpopedal spasm; responds to rebreathing in paper bag.
Hypoglycemia	Fasting blood sugar usually under 50 mg/dL; signs of diabetes mellitus—polyuria, polydypsia, olyphagia.
Hyperthyroidism	Elevated triiodothyronine (T_3), thyroxine (T_4); exophthalmos in severe cases.
Carcinoid syndrome	Hypertension accompanies anxiety; elevated urinary catecholamines (5-hydroxyindoleacetic acid (5-HIAA)).

Table 12-16
Epidemiology of Anxiety Disorders

	Panic Disorder	**Phobia**	**Obsessive–Compulsive Disorder**	**Generalized Anxiety Disorder**	**Posttraumatic Stress Disorder**
Lifetime prevalence	1.5–4% of population	Most common anxiety disorder: 10% of population	2–3% of population	3–8% of population	1–3% of population: 30% of Vietnam veterans
Male-to-female ratio	1:1 (without agoraphobia) 1:2 (with agoraphobia)	1:2	1:1	1:2	1:2
Age of onset	Late 20s	Late childhood	Adolescence or early adulthood	Variable: early adulthood	Any age, including childhood
Family history	20% of first-degree relatives of agoraphobic patients have agoraphobia	May run in families, especially blood injec-tion, injury type	35% in first-degree relatives	25% of first-degree relatives affected	—
Twin studies	Higher con-cordance in monozygotic (MZ) twins than in dizygotic (DZ) twins	—	Higher con-cordance in MZ twins than in DZ twins	80–90% concor-dance in MZ twins; 10–15% in DZ twins	—

8. **Anxiety related to guilt and punishment.** If a patient expects punish-ment for imagined or real misdeeds, he or she may feel anxiety and the punishment may be actively sought or even self-inflicted.

K. **Mixed anxiety–depressive disorder.** This disorder describes patients with both anxiety and depressive symptoms that do not meet the diagnos-tic criteria for either an anxiety disorder or a mood disorder. The diagnosis is sometimes used in primary care settings and is used in Europe; some-times called *neurasthenia*.

III. **Epidemiology**

The anxiety disorders make up the most common group of psychiatric disor-ders. One in four persons has met the diagnostic criteria for at least one of the above-listed anxiety disorders, and there is a 12-month prevalence rate of about 17%. Women are more likely to have an anxiety disorder than are men. The prevalence of anxiety disorders decreases with higher socioeconomic status. An epidemiologic overview of anxiety disorders as well as obsessive–compul-sive disorder and posttraumatic stress disorder is given in Table 12-16.

IV. **Etiology**

A. **Biologic**

1. Anxiety involves an excessive autonomic reaction with increased sym-pathetic tone.

2. The release of catecholamines is increased with the increased production of norepinephrine metabolites (e.g., 3-methoxy-4-hydroxyphenylglycol).
3. Decreased rapid eye movement (REM) latency and stage IV sleep (similar to depression) may develop.
4. Decreased levels of γ-aminobutyric acid (GABA) cause central nervous system (CNS) hyperactivity (GABA inhibits CNS irritability and is widespread throughout the brain).
5. Alterations in serotonergic system and increased dopaminergic activity are associated with anxiety.
6. Activity in the temporal cerebral cortex is increased.
7. The locus coeruleus, a brain center of noradrenergic neurons, is hyperactive in anxiety states, especially panic attacks.
8. Recent studies also suggest a role for neuropeptides (substance P, CRF, and cholecystokinin), but currently there are no agents available for these targets.
9. Hyperactivity and dysregulation in the amygdala may be associated with social anxiety.

B. Psychoanalytic. According to Freud, unconscious impulses (e.g., sex or aggression) threaten to burst into consciousness and produce anxiety. Anxiety is related developmentally to childhood fears of disintegration that derive from the fear of an actual or imagined loss of a love object or the fear of bodily harm (e.g., castration). Freud used the term *signal anxiety* to describe anxiety not consciously experienced but that triggers defense mechanisms used by the person to deal with a potentially threatening situation. See Table 12-17.

C. Learning theory
1. Anxiety is produced by continued or severe frustration or stress. The anxiety then becomes a conditioned response to other situations that are less severely frustrating or stressful.

Table 12-17
Psychodynamics of Anxiety Disorders

Disorder	Defense	Comment
Phobia	Displacement Symbolization	Anxiety detached from idea or situation and displaced on some other symbolic object or situation.
Agoraphobia	Projection Displacement	Repressed hostility, rage, or sexuality projected on environment, which is seen as dangerous.
Obsessive–compulsive disorder	Undoing Isolation Reaction formation	Severe superego acts against impulses about which patient feels guilty; anxiety controlled by repetitious act or thought.
Anxiety	Regression	Repression of forbidden sexual, aggressive, or dependency strivings breaks down.
Panic	Regression	Anxiety overwhelms personality and is discharged in panic state. Total breakdown of repressive defense and regression occurs.
Posttraumatic stress disorder	Regression Repression Denial Undoing	Trauma reactivates unconscious conflicts; ego relives anxiety and tries to master it.

2. It may be learned through identification and imitation of anxiety patterns in parents (social learning theory).
3. Anxiety is associated with a naturally frightening stimulus (e.g., accident). Subsequent displacement or transference to another stimulus through conditioning produces a phobia to a new and different object or situation.
4. Anxiety disorders involve faulty, distorted, or counterproductive patterns of cognitive thinking.

D. Genetic studies
1. Half of patients with panic disorder have one affected relative.
2. About 5% of persons with high levels of anxiety have a polymorphic variant of the gene associated with serotonin transporter metabolism.

V. Psychological Tests
A. Rorschach test
1. Anxiety responses include animal movements, unstructured forms, and heightened color.
2. Phobic responses include anatomic forms or bodily harm.
3. Obsessive–compulsive responses include over attention to detail.

B. Thematic apperception test
1. Increased fantasy productions may be present.
2. Themes of aggression and sexuality may be prominent.
3. Feelings of tension may be evident.

C. Bender–Gestalt
1. No changes indicative of brain damage are apparent.
2. Use of small area may be manifested in obsessive–compulsive disorder.
3. Productions may spread out on the page in anxiety states.

D. Draw-a-Person
1. Attention to head and general detailing may be noted in obsessive–compulsive disorder.
2. Body image distortions may be present in phobias.
3. Rapid drawing may be evident in anxiety disorders.

E. Minnesota Multiphasic Personality Inventory-2. High hypochondriasis, psychasthenia, hysteria scales in anxiety.

VI. Laboratory Tests
A. No specific laboratory tests for anxiety.
B. Experimental infusion of lactate increases norepinephrine levels and produces anxiety in patients with panic disorder.

VII. Pathophysiology and Brain-Imaging Studies
A. No consistent pathognomonic changes.
B. In obsessive–compulsive disorder, positron emission tomography (PET) reveals decreased metabolism in the orbital gyrus, caudate nuclei, and cingulate gyrus.

C. In generalized anxiety disorder and panic states, PET reveals increased blood flow in the right parahippocampus in the frontal lobe.

D. Magnetic resonance imaging (MRI) has shown increased ventricular size in some cases, but findings are not consistent.

E. Right temporal atrophy is seen in some panic disorder patients, and cerebral vasoconstriction is often present in anxiety.

F. Mitral valve prolapse is present in 50% of patients with panic disorder, but clinical significance unknown.

G. Nonspecific electroencephalogram (EEG) changes may be noted.

H. Dexamethasone suppression test does not suppress cortisol in some obsessive–compulsive patients.

I. Panic-inducing substances include carbon dioxide, sodium lactate, methyl-chlorophenyl-piperazine (mCPP), carbolines, $GABA_B$ receptor antagonists, caffeine, isoproterenol, and yohimbine (Yocon).

VIII. Differential Diagnosis

A. Depressive disorders. Fifty percent to 70% of depressed patients exhibit anxiety or obsessive brooding; 20% to 30% of primarily anxious patients also experience depression.

B. Schizophrenia. Schizophrenic patients may be anxious and have severe obsessions in addition to or preceding the outbreak of hallucinations or delusions.

C. Bipolar I disorder. Massive anxiety may occur during a manic episode.

D. Atypical psychosis (psychotic disorder not otherwise specified). Massive anxiety is present, in addition to psychotic features.

E. Adjustment disorder with anxiety. Patient has a history of a psychosocial stressor within 3 months of onset.

F. Medical and neurologic conditions. A secondary anxiety disorder is caused by a specific medical or biologic factor. Undiagnosed hyperthryroidism is a frequent cause. Other causes are listed in Table 12-18.

G. Substance-related disorders. Panic or anxiety is often associated with intoxication (especially caffeine, cocaine, amphetamines, hallucinogens) and withdrawal states (see Table 12-13).

H. Cognitive disorder. Severe anxiety may interfere with cognition and impairments may occur; however, they remit when the anxiety is diminished, unlike the cognitive defects in dementia.

IX. Course and Prognosis

A. Separation anxiety disorder

1. Starts as early as 1 year of age.
2. Periods of exacerbations and remissions.
3. Adults may have social and occupational dysfunction.
4. Overall good prognosis with 96% remission.

B. Selective mutism

1. Shy, anxious, and risk for depression.
2. Academic difficulties.

Table 12-18
Disorders Associated with Anxiety

Neurologic disorders	Deficiency states
Cerebral neoplasms	Vitamin B_{12} deficiency
Cerebral trauma and postconcussive syndromes	Pellagra
Cerebrovascular disease	Miscellaneous conditions
Subarachnoid hemorrhage	Hypoglycemia
Migraine	Carcinoid syndrome
Encephalitis	Systemic malignancies
Cerebral syphilis	Premenstrual syndrome
Multiple sclerosis	Febrile illnesses and chronic infections
Wilson's disease	Porphyria
Huntington's disease	Infectious mononucleosis
Epilepsy	Posthepatitic syndrome
Systemic conditions	Uremia
Hypoxia	Toxic conditions
Cardiovascular disease	Alcohol and drug withdrawal
Cardiac arrhythmias	Amphetamines
Pulmonary insufficiency	Sympathomimetic agents
Anemia	Vasopressor agents
Endocrine disturbances	Caffeine and caffeine withdrawal
Pituitary dysfunction	Penicillin
Thyroid dysfunction	Sulfonamides
Parathyroid dysfunction	Cannabis
Adrenal dysfunction	Mercury
Pheochromocytoma	Arsenic
Virilization disorders of females	Phosphorus
Inflammatory disorders	Organophosphates
Lupus erythematosus	Carbon disulfide
Rheumatoid arthritis	Benzene
Polyarteritis nodosa	Aspirin intolerance
Temporal arteritis	

Adapted from Cumming JL. *Clinical Neuropsychiatry.* Orlando, FL: Grune & Stratton; 1985:214.

    3. Increased risk for comorbid anxiety disorders.

    4. Good treatment response to SSRIs.

C. Specific phobia

    1. The course tends to be chronic.

    2. Phobias may worsen or spread if untreated.

    3. Agoraphobia is the most resistant of all phobias.

    4. Prognosis is good to excellent with therapy.

D. Social anxiety disorder (social phobia)

    1. Onset in late childhood or early adolescence.

    2. Chronic but symptoms may remit.

    3. Disruption in the individual's life.

    4. Good prognosis with pharmacotherapy and psychotherapy.

E. Panic disorder

    1. The course is chronic, with remissions and exacerbations.

    2. Panic attacks tend to recur two to three times a week.

    3. Patients with panic disorder may be at increased risk for committing suicide.

    4. The prognosis is good with combined pharmacotherapy and psychotherapy.

F. Agoraphobia

1. Frequently caused by panic disorder.
2. Without panic disorder is chronic and incapacitating.
3. Comorbid alcohol dependence and depressive symptoms.
4. Treatment approach requires pharmacotherapy with CBT and virtual therapy.

G. Generalized anxiety disorder

1. Course is chronic; symptoms may diminish, as the patient gets older.
2. With time, secondary depression may develop. This is not uncommon if the condition is left untreated.
3. With treatment, prognosis is good; over 70% of patients improve with pharmacologic therapy; best when combined with psychotherapy.

X. Treatment

The treatment of anxiety disorders involves both a psychopharmacologic approach as well as psychotherapy (CBT, psychodynamic, time-limited, group, and family therapies).

A. Pharmacologic.

1. **Benzodiazepines.** These drugs are effective in reducing anxiety generally. In panic disorder, they reduce both the number and intensity of attacks. They are also useful in social and specific phobia. Because of concern about physical dependence, benzodiazepines are not prescribed by physicians as often as they should be. With proper psychotherapeutic monitoring, however, they can be used safely for long periods of time without being abused. Discontinuation (withdrawal) syndromes may occur in patients who use these drugs for long periods, but, if the medication is properly withdrawn, signs and symptoms of withdrawal are easily managed. Commonly used drugs in this class include alprazolam (Xanax), clonazepam (Klonopin), diazepam (Valium), and lorazepam (Ativan). Alprazolam is effective in panic disorder and anxiety associated with depression. Alprazolam has been associated with a discontinuation syndrome after as little as 6 to 8 weeks of treatment.

2. **Selective serotonin reuptake inhibitors (SSRIs).** There are six SSRIs available in the United States that are effective in anxiety disorder: fluoxetine (Prozac), citalopram (Celexa), escitalopram (Lexapro), paroxetine(Paxil), sertraline (Zoloft), and venlafaxine (Effexor). Paroxetine is especially useful for the treatment of panic disorder. SSRIs are safer than the tricyclic drugs because they lack anticholinergic effects and are not as lethal if taken in overdose. The most common side effects are transient nausea, headache, and sexual dysfunction. Some patients, especially those with panic disorder, report an initial increase in anxiety after starting these drugs, which can be controlled with benzodiazepines until the full SSRI effect is felt, usually within 2 to 4 weeks. SSRIs are used with extreme caution in children and adolescents because of reports of agitation and impulsive suicidal acts as side effects of the medication in that population.

3. **Tricyclics.** Drugs in this class reduce the intensity of anxiety in all the anxiety disorders. Because of their side effect profile (e.g., anticholinergic effects, cardiotoxicity, and potential lethality in overdose [10 times the daily recommended dose can be fatal]), they are not first-line agents. Typical drugs in this class include imipramine (Tofranil), nortryptaline (Aventyl, Pamelor), and clomipramine (Anafranil).

4. **Monoamine oxidase inhibitors (MAOIs).** MAOIs are effective for the treatment of panic and other anxiety disorders; however, they are not first-line agents because of a major adverse side effect, which is the occurrence of a hypertensive crisis secondary to ingestion of foods containing tyramine. Certain medications such as sympathomimetics and opioids (especially meperidine [Demerol]) must be avoided because if combined with MAOIs, death may ensue. Common drugs in this class include phenelzine (Nardil) and tranylcypromine (Parnate).

5. **Other drugs used in anxiety disorders**

a. **Adrenergic receptor antagonists (beta blockers).** Drugs in this class include propranolol (Inderal) and atenolol (Tenormin), which act to suppress the somatic signs of anxiety, particularly panic attacks. They have been reported to be particularly effective in blocking the anxiety of social phobia (e.g., public speaking) when taken as a single dose about 1 hour before the phobic event. Adverse effects include bradycardia, hypotension, and drowsiness. They are not useful in chronic anxiety, unless it is caused by a hypersensitive adrenergic state.

 CLINICAL HINT:
Do not use beta blockers if the patient has a history of asthma, congestive heart failure, or diabetes.

---

b. **Venlafaxine (Effexor).** This drug has been found to be effective in the treatment of both generalized anxiety disorder and panic disorder. Because it also acts as an antidepressant, it is of use in mixed states. Its major indication is for the treatment of depression.

c. **Buspirone (Buspar).** This drug has mild serotonergic effects and is most effective in generalized anxiety disorder rather than in acute states. It is not cross-tolerant with benzodiazepines and cannot be used to treat discontinuation syndromes. It has a slow level of onset and may produce dizziness and headache in some patients.

d. **Anticonvulsant anxiolytics.** Typical drugs in this class used in the treatment of anxiety disorders include gabapentin (Neurontin), tiagabine (Gabitril), and valproate (Depakene, Depakote). Reports of their efficacy are few and anecdotal; however, they deserve consideration in the treatment of these disorders, especially if panic attacks are present.

Table 12-19 summarizes dosages for drugs used in anxiety disorders.

Table 12-19
Dosages for Drugs Used in Anxiety Disorders

	Starting (mg)	Maintenance (mg)	High Dosage (mg)	Side Effects
SSRIs				
Paroxetine	5–10	20–60	>60	Nausea, vomiting, dry mouth, headache, somnolence, insomnia, sweating, tremor, diarrhea, sexual dysfunction, syndrome of inappropriate antidiuretic hormone, cytochrome P-450 2D6 substrate elevation due to enzyme inhibition (paroxetine especially; citalopram and escitalopram are not significant inhibitors), discontinuation effects (fatigue, dysphoria, psychomotor changes)
Fluoxetine	2–5	20–60	>80	
Sertaline	12.5–25	50–200	>300	
Citalopram	10	20–40	>60	
Escitalopram	5	10–30	>30	
Tricyclic antidepressants				
Clomipramine	5–12.5	50–125	>200	Orthostasis, conduction defects, ventricular arrhythmias, reflex tachycardia, anticholinergic effects, weight gain, potential lethality in overdose
Imipramine	10–25	150–500	>300	
Desipramine	10–25	150–200	>300	
Benzodiazepines				
Alprazolam	0.25–0.5 tid	0.5–2 tid	>8	Orthostasis, conduction defects, ventricular arrhythmias, reflex tachycardia, anticholinergic effects, weight gain, potential lethality in overdose
Clonazepam	0.25–0.5 bid	0.5–2 bid	>4	
Diazepam	2–5 bid	5–30 bid	>80	
Lorazepam	0.25–0.5 bid	0.5–2 bid	>8	
MAOIs				
Phenelzine	15 bid	15–45 bid	>15	Orthostatic hypotension, insomnia, weight gain, edema, sexual dysfunction, hypertensive crisis with tyramine-containing foods
Tranylcypromine	10 bid	10–30 bid	>70	
SNRIs				
Venlafaxine (Effexor)	6.25–25	50–150	>375	Nausea, somnolence, dizziness, dry mouth, nervousness, tremor, insomnia, constipation, sexual dysfunction, sweating, anorexia, blood pressure elevation, orthostasis, conduction defects, ventricular arrhythmias, discontinuation effects (fatigue, dysphoria, psychomotor changes); half usual dose used in moderate hepatic or renal impairment
Venlataxine XR (Effexor XR)	37.5	37.5	>225	
Other agents				
Valproic acid	125 bid	500–750 bid	>2,000	Nausea, vomiting, indigestion
Gabapentin	100–200	600–3,400	>3,400	Somnolence, ataxia, nausea
BuSpar	5–10	10	>60	Dizziness, fatigue, nausea

Table 12-20
Common Medications for the Treatment of Recurrent Anxiety

Medication	Brand Name	Recommended Initial Dose	Daily Dose (mg)[a]
Antidepressants[b]			
Fluoxetine	Prozac	5 mg/day	20–80
Fluvoxamine	Luvox	50 mg/day	100–300
Paroxetine	Paxil	10 mg/day	20–50
	Paxil CR	12.5 mg/day	25–75
Sertraline	Zoloft	25–50 mg/day	50–200
Citalopram	Celexa	10 mg/day	20–60
Escitalopram	Lexapro	5 mg/day	10–30
Venlafaxine	Effexor XR	37.5 mg/day	75–225
Phenelzine	Nardil	15 mg/day	45–90
Benzodiazepines[c]			
Alprazolam	Xanax	0.25 mg tid	1–4[e]
Clonazepam	Klonopin	0.25 mg bid	1–3
Lorazepam	Ativan	0.5 mg tid	2–6[e]
Azapirone[d]			
Buspirone	BuSpar	7.5 mg bid	30–60

[a]Some individuals will require higher or lower doses than those listed here.
[b]Useful as a primary treatment for panic disorder (in which lower starting doses are usually used) with or without agoraphobia, generalized anxiety disorder, generalized social anxiety disorder, and posttraumatic stress disorder.
[c]Useful as a primary treatment for panic disorder with or without agoraphobia, generalized anxiety disorder, and generalized social anxiety disorder. May be a useful adjunct to antidepressants in the treatment of posttraumatic stress disorder or obsessive–compulsive disorder.
[d]Useful as a primary treatment for generalized anxiety disorder.
[e]Total daily dose is divided across 2–4 doses per day.
bid, twice daily; tid, three times daily. All except phenelzine are useful as a primary treatment for obsessive–compulsive disorder.

See Table 12-20 for medications used for treatment of recurrent anxiety.

B. Psychological. The following information can be viewed as an introduction to the topic discussed in greater detail in Chapter 24.

1. **Supportive psychotherapy.** This approach involves the use of psychodynamic concepts and a therapeutic alliance to promote adaptive coping. Adaptive defenses are encouraged and strengthened, and maladaptive ones are discouraged. The therapist assists in reality testing and may offer advice regarding behavior.

2. **Insight-oriented psychotherapy.** The goal is to increase the patient's development of insight into psychological conflicts that, if unresolved, can manifest as symptomatic behavior (e.g., anxiety and phobias). This modality is particularly indicated if (1) anxiety symptoms are clearly secondary to an underlying unconscious conflict, (2) anxiety continues after behavioral or pharmacologic treatments are instituted, (3) new anxiety symptoms develop after the original symptoms have resolved (symptom substitution), or (4) the anxieties are more generalized and less specific.

3. Behavior therapy. The basic assumption is that change can occur without the development of psychological insight into underlying causes. Techniques include positive and negative reinforcement, systematic desensitization, flooding, implosion, graded exposure, response prevention, stop-thought, relaxation techniques, panic control therapy, self-monitoring, and hypnosis. Virtual Therapy Treatment (VRT) uses augmented reality and virtual immersion experience to desensitize the patient against anxiety.

 CLINICAL HINT:

Some patients may carry a single anxiolytic pill such as 5 mg of diazepam to use if they think they are going to have an anxiety attack. Knowing they have the pill to use in that situation often aborts the attack since they have become conditioned to associate the pill with anxiety reduction.

    a. Behavior therapy is indicated for clearly delineated, circumscribed, maladaptive behaviors (e.g., panic attacks and phobias).
    b. Most current strategies for the treatment of anxiety disorders include a combination of pharmacologic and behavioral interventions.
    c. Current thinking generally maintains that although drugs can reduce anxiety early, treatment with drugs alone leads to equally early relapse. The response of patients who are also treated with cognitive and behavioral therapies appears to be significantly and consistently better than the response of those who receive drugs alone.

4. Cognitive therapy. This is based on the premise that maladaptive behavior is secondary to distortions in how people perceive themselves and in how others perceive them. Treatment is short-term and interactive, with assigned homework and tasks to be performed between sessions that focus on correcting distorted assumptions and cognitions. The emphasis is on confronting and examining situations that elicit interpersonal anxiety and associated mild depression.

5. Group therapy. Groups range from those that provide only support and an increase in social skills to those that focus on relief of specific symptoms to those that are primarily insight-oriented. Groups may be heterogeneous or homogeneous in terms of diagnosis. Homogeneous groups are commonly used in the treatment of such diagnoses as post-traumatic stress disorder, in which therapy is aimed at education about dealing with stress.

For more detailed discussion of this topic, see Chapter 14, Anxiety Disorders, p. 1720, in CTP/X.

13

Obsessive–Compulsive and Related Disorders

I. Obsessive–Compulsive Disorder

Obsessive–compulsive disorder (OCD) is represented by a diverse group of symptoms that include intrusive thoughts, rituals, preoccupations, and compulsions. An obsession is a recurrent and intrusive thought, feeling, idea, or sensation. In contrast to an obsession, which is a mental event, a compulsion is a behavior. Specifically, a compulsion is a conscious, standardized, recurrent behavior, such as counting, checking, or avoiding. These recurrent obsessions or compulsions cause severe distress to the person. The obsessions or compulsions are time-consuming and interfere significantly with the person's normal routine, occupational functioning, usual social activities, or relationships. A patient with OCD may have an obsession, a compulsion, or both.

A variety of related disorders including hoarding, hair pulling and skin picking are described in this chapter.

A. Epidemiology

The lifetime prevalence of OCD in the general population is estimated at 1% to 3%. OCD is the fourth most common psychiatric diagnosis and among adults, men and women are equally affected with a slight trend toward women, but among adolescents, boys are more commonly affected than girls. The mean age of onset is about 20 years.

B. Comorbidity

Persons with OCD have high comorbidity with lifetime prevalence for major depressive disorder around 67% and for social phobia is about 25%. Other conditions include alcohol use disorders, generalized anxiety disorder, specific phobia, panic disorder, eating disorders, and personality disorders. The incidence of Tourette's disorder in patients with OCD is 5% to 7%, and 20% to 30% of patients with OCD have a history of tics.

C. Etiology

1. Biologic factors

a. Neurotransmitters

Numerous clinical drug trials support the hypothesis that dysregulation of serotonin is involved in the symptom formation of obsessions and compulsions in the disorder. Serotonergic drugs are more effective in treating OCD, but whether serotonin is involved in the cause of OCD is not clear.

Some interest exists in a positive link between streptococcal infection and OCD.

b. Brain-imaging studies

Various functional brain-imaging studies have shown increased activity (e.g., metabolism and blood flow) in the frontal lobes, the basal ganglia (especially the caudate), and the cingulum of patients with OCD. Pharmacologic and behavioral treatments reportedly reverse these abnormalities. Computed tomographic (CT) and magnetic resonance imaging (MRI) studies have found bilaterally smaller caudates in patients with OCD.

c. Genetics

Available genetic data on OCD support the hypothesis that the disorder has a significant genetic component. Relatives of probands with OCD consistently have a threefold to fivefold higher probability of having OCD or obsessive–compulsive features than families of control probands. Studies show increased rates of a variety of conditions among relatives of OCD probands, including generalized anxiety disorder, tic disorders, body dysmorphic disorder, hypochondriasis, eating disorders, and habits such as nail-biting.

A higher rate of OCD, Tourette's disorder, and chronic motor tics are found in relatives of patients with Tourette's disorder.

2. Psychosocial factors

OCD differs from obsessive–compulsive personality disorder, which is associated with an obsessive concern for details, perfectionism, and other similar personality traits.

Research suggests that OCD may be precipitated by a number of environmental stressors, especially those involving pregnancy, childbirth, or parental care of children.

D. Diagnosis and clinical features

The diagnostic criteria for OCD include recurrent and persistent thoughts (obsessions) or repetitive behaviors (compulsions). See Table 13-1. In addition, clinicians can indicate whether the patient's OCD is characterized by good or fair insight, poor insight, or absent insight.

Patients with OCD often take their complaints to physicians rather than psychiatrists (Table 13-2). Obsessions and compulsions are the essential features of OCD. Typical obsessions associated with OCD include thoughts about contamination ("My hands are dirty") or doubts ("I forgot to turn off the stove").

Table 13-1
Signs and Symptoms of Obsessive–Compulsive Disorder

Obsessive–Compulsive Disorder
- Must have obsessions, compulsions, or both.
- *Obsessions* are thoughts or urges that are so pervasive and undesirable they prompt some suppressive thought or action (usually a *compulsion*).
- *Compulsions* are behaviors that an individual feels he or she must perform (*obsessively*) in a particular manner to reduce stress, in spite of the fact that they have no logical basis.
- These propensities must cause distress or extreme distraction from conventional activities.

(Cannot be better explained by another disorder or medication/substances, though *tic-related OCD* may be specified.)

Table 13-2
Nonpsychiatric Clinical Specialists Likely to See Obsessive–Compulsive Disorder Patients

Specialist	Presenting Problem
Dermatologist	Chapped hands, eczematoid appearance
Family practitioner	Family member washing excessively, may mention counting or checking compulsions
Oncologist, infectious disease internist	Insistent belief that person has acquired immune deficiency syndrome
Neurologist	Obsessive-compulsive disorder associated with Tourette's disorder, head injury, epilepsy, choreas, other basal ganglia lesions or disorders
Neurosurgeon	Severe, intractable obsessive–compulsive disorder
Obstetrician	Postpartum obsessive–compulsive disorder
Pediatrician	Parent's concern about child's behavior, usually excessive washing
Pediatric cardiologist	Obsessive-compulsive disorder secondary to Sydenham's chorea
Plastic surgeon	Repeated consultations for "abnormal" features
Dentist	Gum lesions from excessive teeth cleaning

From Rapoport JL. The neurobiology of obsessive-compulsive disorder. *JAMA.* 1988;260:2889, with permission.

1. Symptom patterns

The presentation of obsessions and compulsions is heterogeneous in adults (Table 13-3) and in children and adolescents (Table 13-4). The symptoms of an individual patient can overlap and change with time.

Table 13-3
Obsessive–Compulsive Symptoms in Adults

Variable	%
Obsessions (*N* = 200)	
Contamination	45
Pathologic doubt	42
Somatic	36
Need for symmetry	31
Aggressive	28
Sexual	26
Other	13
Multiple obsessions	60
Compulsions (*N* = 200)	
Checking	63
Washing	50
Counting	36
Need to ask or confess	31
Symmetry and precision	28
Hoarding	18
Multiple comparisons	48
Course of illness (*N* = 100)[a]	
Type	
Continuous	85
Deteriorative	10
Episodic	2
Not present	71
Present	29

[a]Age at onset: men, 17.5 ± 6.8 years; women, 20.8 ± 8.5 years.
From Rasmussen SA, Eiser JL. The epidemiology and differential diagnosis of obsessive compulsive disorder. *J Clin Psychiatry.* 1992;53(4 Suppl):6, with permission.

Table 13-4
Reported Obsessions and Compulsions for 70 Consecutive Child and Adolescent Patients

Major Presenting Symptom	No. (%) of Reporting Symptom at Initial Interview[a]
Obsession	
Concern or disgust with bodily wastes or secretions (urine, stool, saliva), dirt, germs, environmental toxins	30 (43)
Fear something terrible may happen (fire, death or illness of loved one, self, or others)	18 (24)
Concern or need for symmetry, order, or exactness	12 (17)
Scrupulosity (excessive praying or religious concerns out of keeping with patient's background)	9 (13)
Lucky and unlucky numbers	6 (8)
Forbidden or perverse sexual thoughts, images, or impulses	3 (4)
Intrusive nonsense sounds, words, or music	1 (1)
Compulsion	
Excessive or ritualized hand washing, showering, bathing, tooth brushing, or grooming	60 (85)
Repeating rituals (e.g., going in and out of door, up and down from chair)	36 (51)
Checking doors, locks, stove, appliances, car brakes	32 (46)
Cleaning and other rituals to remove contact with contaminants	16 (23)
Touching	14 (20)
Ordering and arranging	12 (17)
Measures to prevent harm to self or others (e.g., hanging clothes a certain way)	11 (16)
Counting	13 (18)
Hoarding and collecting	8 (11)
Miscellaneous rituals (e.g., licking, spitting, special dress pattern)	18 (26)

[a]Multiple symptoms recorded, so total exceeds 70.
From Rapoport JL. The neurobiology of obsessive-compulsive disorder. *JAMA.* 1988;260:2889, with permission.

a. Contamination

The most common pattern is an obsession of contamination, followed by washing or accompanied by compulsive avoidance of the presumably contaminated object.

b. Pathologic doubt

The second most common pattern is an obsession of doubt, followed by a compulsion of checking.

c. Intrusive thoughts

In the third most common pattern, there are intrusive obsessional thoughts without a compulsion. Suicidal ideation may also be obsessive; but a careful suicidal assessment of actual risk must always be done.

d. Symmetry

The fourth most common pattern is the need for symmetry or precision, which can lead to a compulsion of slowness. Patients can literally take hours to eat a meal or shave their faces.

e. Other symptom patterns

Religious obsessions and compulsive hoarding are common in patients with OCD. Compulsive hair pulling and nail biting are behavioral patterns related to OCD. Masturbation may also be compulsive.

E. Differential diagnosis

1. Medical conditions

A number of primary medical disorders can produce symptoms similar to OCD. The concept of OCD as a disorder of the basal ganglia derives from the phenomenologic similarity between idiopathic OCD and OCD-like disorders that are associated with basal ganglia diseases, such as Sydenham's chorea and Huntington's disease. It should also be noted that OCD frequently develops before age 30 years, and new-onset OCD in an older individual should raise questions about potential neurologic contributions to the disorder.

2. Tourette's disorder

OCD is closely related to Tourette's disorder, as the two conditions frequently co-occur, both in individuals over time and within families. About 90% of persons with Tourette's disorder have compulsive symptoms, and as many as two thirds meet the diagnostic criteria for OCD.

3. Other psychiatric conditions

OCD exhibits a superficial resemblance to obsessive–compulsive personality disorder, which is associated with an obsessive concern for details, perfectionism, and other similar personality traits. The conditions are easily distinguished in that only OCD is associated with a true syndrome of obsessions and compulsions.

Psychotic symptoms often lead to obsessive thoughts and compulsive behaviors. Similarly, OCD can be difficult to differentiate from depression because the two disorders often occur comorbidly, and major depression is often associated with obsessive thoughts that, at times, border on true obsessions such as those that characterize OCD.

F. Course and prognosis

More than half of patients with OCD have a sudden onset of symptoms. The onset of symptoms for about 50% to 70% of patients occurs after a stressful event, such as a pregnancy, a sexual problem, or the death of a relative. The course is usually long but variable; some patients experience a fluctuating course, and others experience a constant one.

About 20% to 30% of patients have significant while 20% to 40% of patients either remain ill or their symptoms worsen.

Suicide is a risk for all patients with OCD.

G. Treatment

Many patients with OCD tenaciously resist treatment efforts. Well-controlled studies have found that pharmacotherapy, behavior therapy, or a combination of both is effective in significantly reducing the symptoms of patients with OCD.

1. Pharmacotherapy

The efficacy of pharmacotherapy in OCD has been proved in many clinical trials and drugs, some of which are used to treat depressive disorders or other mental disorders, can be given in their usual dosage ranges. Initial effects are generally seen after 4 to 6 weeks of treatment, although 8 to 16 weeks are usually needed to obtain maximal therapeutic benefit.

The standard approach is to start treatment with an selective serotonin reuptake inhibitor (SSRI) or clomipramine and then move to other pharmacologic strategies if the serotonin-specific drugs are not effective.

a. Selective serotonin reuptake inhibitors

Each of the SSRIs available in the United States—fluoxetine (Prozac), fluvoxamine (Luvox), paroxetine (Paxil), sertraline (Zoloft), citalopram (Celexa)—has been approved by the U.S. Food and Drug Administration (FDA) for the treatment of OCD. Higher dosages have often been necessary for a beneficial effect, such as 80 mg a day of fluoxetine. Although the SSRIs can cause sleep disturbance, nausea and diarrhea, headache, anxiety, and restlessness, these adverse effects are often transient and are generally less troubling than the adverse effects associated with tricyclic drugs, such as clomipramine. The best clinical outcomes occur when SSRIs are used in combination with behavioral therapy.

b. Clomipramine

Of all the tricyclic and tetracyclic drugs, clomipramine is the most selective for serotonin reuptake versus norepinephrine reuptake, and is exceeded in this respect only by the SSRIs. Its dosing must be titrated upward over 2 to 3 weeks to avoid gastrointestinal adverse effects and orthostatic hypotension. It causes significant sedation and anticholinergic effects, including dry mouth and constipation.

c. Other drugs

If treatment with clomipramine or an SSRI is unsuccessful, many therapists augment the first drug by the addition of valproate (Depakene), lithium (Eskalith), or carbamazepine (Tegretol). Other drugs that can be tried in the treatment of OCD are venlafaxine (Effexor), pindolol (Visken), and the monoamine oxidase inhibitors (MAOIs), especially phenelzine (Nardil). Other pharmacologic agents for the treatment of unresponsive patients include buspirone (BuSpar), 5-hydroxytryptamine (5-HT), L-tryptophan, and clonazepam (Klonopin). Adding an atypical antipsychotic such as risperidone (Risperdal) has helped in some cases.

2. Behavior therapy

Behavior therapy is as effective as pharmacotherapies in OCD, and some data indicate that the beneficial effects are longer lasting with behavior therapy. The principal behavioral approaches in OCD are exposure and response prevention. Desensitization, thought-stopping, flooding, implosion therapy, and aversive conditioning have also been used in patients with OCD.

3. Other therapies

Family therapy is often useful in supporting the family, helping reduce marital discord resulting from the disorder, and group therapy is useful as a support system for some patients.

For extreme cases, electroconvulsive therapy (ECT) and psycho-surgery are considerations. A psychosurgical procedure for OCD is cingulotomy, which may be successful in treating otherwise severe and treatment-unresponsive patients.

4. Deep brain stimulation (DBS)

Nonablative surgical techniques involving indwelling electrodes in various basal ganglia nuclei are under investigation to treat both OCD and Tourette's disorder. DBS is performed using MRI-guided stereotactic techniques in which electrodes are implanted in the brain.

II. Obsessive–Compulsive or Related Disorder Due to Another Medical Condition

Many medical conditions can result in obsessive–compulsive symptoms (i.e., hair pulling, skin picking). OCD-like symptoms have been reported in children following group A β-hemolytic streptococcal infection and have been called *pediatric autoimmune neuropsychiatric disorders associated with streptococcus* (PANDAS). They are believed to result from an autoimmune process that leads to inflammation of the basal ganglia that disrupts cortical–striatal–thalamic axis functioning

III. Substance-Induced Obsessive–Compulsive or Related Disorder

Substance-induced obsessive–compulsive or related disorder is characterized by the emergence of obsessive–compulsive or related symptoms as a result of a substance, including drugs, medications, and alcohol.

IV. Other Specified Obsessive–Compulsive or Related Disorder

This category is for patients who have symptoms characteristic of obsessive–compulsive and related disorder but do not meet the full criteria for any specific obsessive-compulsive or related disorder.

A. Olfactory reference syndrome

Olfactory reference syndrome is characterized by a false belief by the patient that he or she has a foul body odor that is not perceived by others. The preoccupation leads to repetitive behaviors such as washing the body or changing clothes. The syndrome is predominant in males and single status. The mean age of onset is 25 years of age. Olfactory reference syndrome is included in the "other specified" designation for obsessive–compulsive and related disorder of DSM-5.

B. Body dysmorphic disorder

1. Definition. Imagined belief (not of delusional proportions) that a defect in the appearance of all or a part of the body is present.

2. Epidemiology. Onset from adolescence through early adulthood. Men and women are affected equally.

3. Etiology. Unknown

a. Biologic. Responsiveness to serotonergic agents suggests involvement of serotonin or relation to another mental disorder.

b. Psychological. Unconscious conflict relating to a distorted body part may be present.

Table 13-5
Signs and Symptoms of Body Dysmorphic Disorder

- An obsession with imagined flaws in physical appearance...
  - prompting compulsive behaviors or thoughts about said appearance
- Excluding body fat dysmorphia if an eating disorder can be diagnosed but including muscle dysmorphia.

    c. Psychodynamics. Defense mechanisms involved include repression (of unconscious conflict), distortion and symbolization (of body part), and projection (belief that other persons also see imagined deformity).

4. **Laboratory and psychological tests.** Draw-a-Person test shows exaggeration, diminution, or absence of affected body part.

5. **Pathophysiology.** No known pathologic abnormalities. Minor body deficits may actually exist upon which imagined belief develops.

6. **Diagnosis, signs, and symptoms.** Patient complains of defect (e.g., wrinkles, hair loss, small breasts or penis, age spots, stature). Complaint is out of proportion to objective abnormality. If a slight physical anomaly is present, the person's concern is grossly excessive; however, the belief is not of delusional intensity. The person can acknowledge the possibility that he or she may be exaggerating the extent of the defect or that there may be no defect at all. In delusional disorder, the belief is fixed and not subject to reality testing. See Table 13-5.

7. **Differential diagnosis.** Distorted body image can also occur in schizophrenia, mood disorders, medical disorders, anorexia nervosa, bulimia nervosa, OCD, gender identity disorder, and so-called, specific "culture-bound syndromes" (e.g., *koro,* worry that penis is shrinking into abdomen).

8. **Course and prognosis.** Chronic course with repeated visits to doctors, plastic surgeons, or dermatologists. Secondary depression may occur. In some cases, imagined body distortion progresses to delusional belief.

9. **Treatment**
       a. Pharmacologic. Serotoninergic drugs (e.g., fluoxetine [Prozac], clomipramine [Anafranil]) effectively reduce symptoms in at least 50% of patients. Treatment with surgical, dermatologic, and dental procedures is rarely successful.
       b. Psychological. Psychotherapy is useful; uncovers conflicts relating to symptoms, feelings of inadequacy.

V. Hoarding Disorder
    Compulsive hoarding is characterized by acquiring and not discarding things that are deemed to be of little or no value resulting in excessive clutter of living spaces. Hoarding may result in health with impairment in such functions as eating, sleeping, and grooming. The disorder was originally considered a subtype of OCD, but is now considered to be a separate diagnostic entity.

Table 13-6
Signs and Symptoms of Hoarding Disorder

- Difficulty eliminating possessions, regardless of value.
- Distress when discarding possessions or obsession with retaining them
- Clutter from the retention of many unnecessary possessions

An excessive acquisition specifier exists
(Diagnosable if not the sequelae of another disorder.)

A. **Epidemiology**

Hoarding is believed to occur in approximately 2% to 5% of the population, and as high as 14%, equally among men and women, is more common in single persons and is associated with social anxiety, withdrawal, and dependent personality traits. Hoarding usually begins in early adolescence and persists throughout the life span.

B. **Comorbidity**

Significant comorbidity with OCD and strong association between hoarding and compulsive buying. Associated with high rates of personality disorders including dependent, avoidant, schizotypal, and paranoid types. Hoarding disorder has high rates of ADHD with 10 times higher rate of developing ADHD than those without. It is common among schizophrenic patients as well as dementia and brain injury patients.

C. **Etiology**

There is a familial aspect to hoarding disorder with about 80% of hoarders reporting at least one first-degree relative with hoarding behavior.

D. **Diagnosis**

Hoarding disorder is characterized by (1) the acquiring of and failure to discard a large amount of possessions that are deemed useless or of little value; (2) greatly cluttered living areas precluding normal activities; and (3) significant distress and impairment in functioning due to hoarding. DSM-5 includes diagnostic specifiers that relate to insight which may be poor, fair, or good (see Table 13-6).

E. **Clinical features**

Most hoarders do not perceive their behavior to be a problem. Most hoarding patients accumulate possessions passively rather than intentionally, thus clutter accumulates gradually over time. Common hoarded items include newspapers, mail, magazines, old clothes, bags, books, lists, and notes. Hoarding poses risks to not only the patient, but to those around them.

Patients with hoarding disorder also overemphasize the importance of recalling information and possessions.

F. **Differential diagnosis**

The diagnosis of hoarding disorder should not be made if the excessive acquisition and inability to discard of possessions is better accounted for by another medical or psychiatric condition. Hoarding was considered to be a symptom of OCD but there are some major differences. Hoarding disorder patients do not display some of the classic symptoms of OCD such as recurring intrusive thoughts or compulsive rituals and symptoms worsen over time. Hoarding behavior is seldom repetitive and is not viewed as intrusive or distressing to the hoarder.

Some case reports show the onset of this behavior in patients after suffering brain lesions. It is a common symptom in moderate to severe dementia. It is also seen in schizophrenia.

G. Course and prognosis

The disorder is a chronic condition with a treatment-resistant course. Symptoms may fluctuate throughout the course of the disorder, but full remission is rare. Patients have very little insight into their behavior and usually seek treatment under pressure from others. Those with an earlier age of onset run a longer and more chronic course.

H. Treatment

Hoarding disorder is difficult to treat. Although it shows similarities to OCD, effective treatments for OCD have shown little benefit for patients with hoarding disorder. In one study, only 18% of patients responded to medication and cognitive–behavioral therapy (CBT).

The most effective treatment for the disorder is a cognitive–behavioral model that includes training in decision making and categorizing; exposure and habituation to discarding; and cognitive restructuring. Pharmacologic treatment studies using SSRIs have shown mixed results.

VI. Hair-Pulling Disorder (Trichotillomania)

Hair-pulling disorder is a chronic disorder characterized by repetitive hair pulling that leads to variable hair loss that may be visible to others. It is also known as trichotillomania. The disorder is similar to OCD and impulse control disorders.

A. Epidemiology

The prevalence of hair-pulling disorder may be underestimated and the diagnosis encompasses at least two categories of hair pulling that differ in incidence, severity, age of presentation, and gender ratio. Other subsets may exist.

The lifetime prevalence ranges from 0.6% to as high as 3.4% in general populations and with female to male ratio as high as 10 to 1. A childhood type of hair-pulling disorder occurs approximately equally in girls and boys. An estimated 35% to 40% of patients with hair-pulling disorder chew or swallow the hair that they pull out at one time or another.

B. Comorbidity

Significant comorbidity is found between hair-pulling disorder and OCD; anxiety disorders; Tourette's syndrome; depressive disorders; eating disorders; and various personality disorders—particularly obsessive–compulsive, borderline, and narcissistic personality disorders.

C. Etiology

Although hair-pulling disorder is regarded as multi-determined, its onset has been linked to stressful situations in more than one-fourth of all cases. Family members of hair-pulling disorder patients often have a history of tics, impulse-control disorders, and obsessive–compulsive symptoms, further supporting a possible genetic predisposition.

D. Diagnosis and clinical features

The fifth edition of the *Diagnostic and Statistical Manual of Mental Disorders* (DSM-5) diagnostic criteria from hair-pulling disorder requires that hair pulling results in hair loss. All areas of the body may be affected, most commonly the scalp. Other areas involved are eyebrows, eyelashes, and beard; trunk, armpits, and pubic area are less commonly involved.

Two types of hair pulling include *focused pulling* (intentional act) and *automatic pulling* (outside the person's awareness). Patients usually deny the behavior and often try to hide the resultant alopecia. Head banging, nail biting, scratching, gnawing, excoriation, and other acts of self-mutilation may be present.

E. Differential diagnosis

Unlike those with OCD, patients with hair-pulling disorder do not experience obsessive thoughts, and the compulsive activity is limited to one act, hair pulling. Other conditions to consider include factitious disorder and patients who malinger or who have factitious disorder may mutilate themselves to get medical attention.

F. Course and prognosis

The mean age at onset of hair-pulling disorder is in the early teens, most frequently before age 17, but onset has been reported much later in life. Late onset (after age 13) is associated with an increased likelihood of chronicity and poorer prognosis than the early-onset form.

G. Treatment

Treatment usually involves psychiatrists and dermatologists in a joint endeavor. Psychopharmacologic methods include topical steroids and hydroxyzine hydrochloride (Vistaril), an anxiolytic with antihistamine properties; antidepressants; and antipsychotics. Patients who respond poorly to SSRIs may improve with augmentation with pimozide (Orap), a dopamine receptor antagonist. Other medications include fluvoxamine (Luvox), citalopram (Celexa), venlafaxine (Effexor), naltrexone (ReVia), and lithium.

Successful treatment has been reported with biofeedback, self-monitoring, desensitization, and habit reversal.

VII. Excoriation (Skin-Picking) Disorder

Excoriation or skin-picking disorder is characterized by the compulsive and repetitive picking of the skin. It can lead to severe tissue damage and result in the need for various dermatologic treatments. It was also known as skin-picking syndrome, emotional excoriation, nervous scratching artifact, epidermotillomania, and para-artificial excoriation.

A. Epidemiology

Skin-picking disorder has lifetime prevalence between 1% and 5% in the general population, about 12% in the adolescent psychiatric population, and occurs in 2% of patients with other dermatologic disorders. It is more prevalent in women than in men.

B. Comorbidity

The repetitive nature of skin-picking behavior is similar to OCD and is associated with high rates of OCD. Other comorbid conditions include hair-pulling disorder (trichotillomania, 38%), substance dependence (38%), major depressive disorder (32% to 58%), anxiety disorders (23% to 56%), and body dysmorphic disorder (27% to 45%).

C. Etiology

The cause of skin picking is unknown. Some theorists speculate that skin-picking behavior is a manifestation of repressed rage at authoritarian parents. Abnormalities in serotonin, dopamine, and glutamate metabolism have been theorized to be an underlying neurochemical cause of the disorder, but further research is needed.

D. Diagnosis

The fifth edition of the *Diagnostic and Statistical Manual of Mental Disorders* (DSM-5) diagnostic criteria for skin-picking disorder requires recurrent skin picking resulting in skin lesions and repeated attempts to decrease or stop picking. The skin picking must cause clinically relevant distress or impairment in functioning. The skin-picking behavior cannot be attributed to another medical or mental condition and cannot be a result of a substance use disorder (e.g., cocaine or methamphetamine use).

E. Clinical features

The face is the most common site of skin picking. Other common sites are legs, arms, torso, hands, cuticles, fingers, and scalp. In severe cases, skin picking can result in physical disfigurement and medical consequences that require medical or surgical interventions (e.g., skin grafts or radio-surgery).

Many report picking as a means to relieve stress, tension, and other negative feelings of skin-picking patients, 15% report suicidal ideation due to their behavior and about 12% have attempted suicide.

F. Differential diagnosis

The diagnosis of skin-picking disorder cannot be made if the behavior can be better accounted for by another medical or psychological condition. Many medical and dermatologic conditions may result in urges to itch and pick at the skin including eczema, psoriasis, diabetes, liver or kidney disease, Hodgkin's disease, polycythemia vera, or systemic lupus. A thorough physical examination is crucial prior to psychiatric diagnosis.

Skin picking is commonly seen in body dysmorphic disorder. In one study, 45% of body dysmorphic patients report lifetime skin picking disorder and 37% report having skin picking disorder secondary to body dysmorphic disorder. Methamphetamine and cocaine use may result in the sensation something crawling on the body or under skin (formication) which can result in skin picking.

VIII. Factitious Dermatitis

Factitious dermatitis or *dermatitis artefacta* is a disorder in which skin picking is the target of self-inflicted injury and the patient uses more elaborate methods than simple excoriation to self-induced skin lesions. It is seen in 0.3% of dermatology patients and has a female to male ratio of 8:1. It can present at any age, but occurs most frequently in adolescents and young adults. Presence of completely normal, unaffected skin adjacent to the horrific-looking lesions is a clue to the diagnosis of factitious dermatitis.

A. Course and prognosis

The onset of skin-picking disorder is either in early adulthood or between 30 and 45 years of age. The mean age of onset is between 12 and 16 years of age. Typically, symptoms wax and wane over the course of the patient's life. Approximately 44% of women report that amount of picking coincides with their menstrual cycle.

B. Treatment

Skin-picking disorder is difficult to treat and there is little data on effective treatments. There is support for the use of SSRIs. Studies comparing fluoxetine (Prozac) against placebo has shown to fluoxetine to be superior in reducing skin picking. The opioid antagonist naltrexone has proven to reduce the urge to pick, particularly in patients who experience pleasure from the behavior. Glutamatergic agents and lamotrigine (Lamictal) have also shown efficacy. Nonpharmacologic treatments include habit reversal and brief CBT.

For more detailed discussion of this topic, see Chapter 15, Obsessive-Compulsive and Related Disorders, p. 1785, in CTP/X.

14
Trauma- and Stressor-Related Disorders

I. Posttraumatic Stress Disorder and Acute Stress Disorder

Both posttraumatic stress disorder (PTSD) and acute stress disorder are marked by increased stress and anxiety following exposure to a traumatic or stressful event. Traumatic or stressful events may include being a witness to or being involved in a violent accident or crime, military combat, or assault, being kidnapped, being involved in a natural disaster or experiencing systematic physical or sexual abuse. The person reacts to the experience with fear and helplessness, persistently relives the event, and tries to avoid being reminded of it.

The stressors causing both acute stress disorder and PTSD are sufficiently overwhelming to affect almost everyone. Persons re-experience the traumatic event in their dreams and their daily thoughts (flashbacks); they are determined to avoid anything that brings the event to mind and they undergo a numbing of responsiveness along with a state of hyperarousal. Other symptoms are depression, anxiety, and cognitive difficulties such as poor concentration.

A link between acute mental syndromes and traumatic events has been recognized for more than 200 years. Moreover, increasing documentation of mental reactions to the Holocaust, to a series of natural disasters, and to assault contributed to the growing recognition of a close relation between trauma and psychopathology.

A. Epidemiology

The lifetime incidence of PTSD is estimated to be 9% to 15% and the lifetime prevalence of PTSD is estimated to be about 8% of the general population, although an additional 5% to 15% may experience subclinical forms of the disorder. The lifetime prevalence rate is 10% in women and 4% in men. Among veterans of the Iraq and Afghanistan wars, 13% received the diagnosis of PTSD.

It is most prevalent in young adults though children can also have the disorder. The disorder is most likely to occur in those who are single, divorced, widowed, socially withdrawn, or of low socioeconomic level, but anyone can be effected. The risk factors are severity, duration, and proximity of a person's exposure to the actual trauma. A familial pattern exists and first-degree biologic relatives of persons with a history of depression have an increased risk for developing PTSD following a traumatic event.

B. Comorbidity

Comorbidity is high with about two-thirds having at least two other disorders. Common comorbid conditions include depressive disorders, substance-related disorders, anxiety disorders, and bipolar disorders. Comorbid disorders make persons more vulnerable to develop PTSD.

C. Etiology

1. Stressor

By definition, a stressor is the prime causative factor in the development of PTSD but not everyone experiences the disorder after a traumatic event. The stressor alone does not suffice to cause the disorder. Clinicians must also consider individual's pre-existing biologic and psychosocial factors and events that happened before and after the trauma.

2. Risk factors

Even when faced with overwhelming trauma, most persons do not experience PTSD symptoms. About 60% of males and 50% of females have experienced some significant trauma, whereas the reported lifetime prevalence of PTSD is only about 8%. Similarly, events that may appear mundane or less than catastrophic to most persons can produce PTSD in some. Evidence indicates of a dose–response relationship between the degree of trauma and the likelihood of symptoms. Table 14-1 summarizes vulnerability factors that appear to play etiologic roles in the disorder.

3. Biologic factors

Many neurotransmitter systems have been implicated and have led to theories about norepinephrine, dopamine, endogenous opioids, and benzodiazepine receptors and the hypothalamic–pituitary–adrenal (HPA) axis. Studies suggest that the noradrenergic and endogenous opiate systems, as well as the HPA axis, are hyperactive in at least some patients with PTSD. There is also increased activity and responsiveness of the autonomic nervous system, (elevated heart rates and blood pressure) and abnormal sleep architecture (e.g., sleep fragmentation and increased sleep latency).

4. Noradrenergic system

Soldiers with PTSD-like symptoms exhibit nervousness, increased blood pressure and heart rate, palpitations, sweating, flushing, and tremors. Studies show increased 24-hour urine epinephrine concentrations in veterans with PTSD and increased urine catecholamine concentrations in sexually abused girls. These findings are strong evidence for altered function in the noradrenergic system in PTSD.

5. Opioid system

Combat veterans with PTSD demonstrate a naloxone (Narcan)-reversible analgesic response to combat-related stimuli, raising the possibility of opioid system hyperregulation similar to that in the HPA axis.

Table 14-1
Predisposing Vulnerability Factors in Posttraumatic Stress Disorder

Presence of childhood trauma
Borderline, paranoid, dependent, or antisocial personality disorder traits
Inadequate family or peer support system
Being female
Genetic vulnerability to psychiatric illness
Recent stressful life changes
Perception of an external locus of control (natural cause) rather than an internal one (human cause)
Recent excessive alcohol intake

6. Corticotropin-releasing factor and the HPA axis

Studies show low plasma and urinary free cortisol concentrations in PTSD. There is hyperregulation of the HPA axis in PTSD and cortisol hypersuppression in trauma-exposed patients who develop PTSD, compared with patients exposed to trauma who do not develop PTSD, indicating that it might be specifically associated with PTSD and not just trauma.

D. Diagnosis

The fifth edition of the *Diagnostic and Statistical Manual of Mental Disorders* (DSM-5) criteria for PTSD includes symptoms of intrusion, avoidance, alternations of mood, cognitive difficulties, and hyperarousal (see Clinical Features below). In addition, symptoms must be present for at least 1 month. The DSM-5 diagnosis of PTSD allows the physician to specify if the symptoms occur in preschool-aged children or with dissociative (depersonalization/derealization) symptoms. For patients whose symptoms have been present less than 1 month, the appropriate diagnosis may be acute stress disorder.

E. Clinical features

Individuals with PTSD show symptoms in three domains: intrusion symptoms following the trauma, avoiding stimuli associated with the trauma, and experiencing symptoms of increased automatic arousal, such as an enhanced startle. Flashbacks represent a classic intrusion symptom. Other intrusion symptoms include distressing recollections or dreams and either physiologic or psychological stress reactions to stimuli linked to the trauma. An individual must exhibit at least one intrusion symptom to meet the criteria for PTSD. Symptoms of avoidance associated with PTSD include efforts to avoid thoughts or activities related to the trauma, anhedonia, reduced capacity to remember events related to the trauma, blunted affect, feelings of detachment or derealization, and a sense of a foreshortened future. Symptoms of increased arousal include insomnia, irritability, hypervigilance, and exaggerated startle (see Table 14-2).

1. Natural disasters

Natural disaster can cause PTSD. Over the years, we have witnessed various kinds including tsunamis in Indonesia, hurricanes in Florida, and

Table 14-2
Common Signs and Symptoms of PTSD

Intrusive memories of the event (flash backs)
Frightening dreams
Fear and avoidance of cues that relate to the event
Acute episodes of anxiety, fear, panic, or aggression triggered by cues
Insomnia
Startle reactions
Insomnia
Tendency toward substance abuse, e.g., alcohol
Detachment from others
Emotional blunting
Anhedonia
Sudden recollection or reliving of traumatic event

Table 14-3
Syndromes Associated with Toxic Exposure[a]

Syndrome	Characteristics	Possible Toxins
1	Impaired cognition	Insect repellant containing *N,N'*-diethyl-m-toluamide (DEET[b]) absorbed through skin
2	Confusion–ataxia	Exposure to chemical weapons (e.g., sarin)
3	Arthromyoneuropathy	Insect repellant containing DEET in combination with oral pyridostigmine[c]

[a]The three syndromes involved a relatively small group (N = 249) of veterans and are based on self-reported descriptions and selection. (Data are from R. W. Haley and T. L. Kurt.)
[b]DEET is a carbonate compound used as an insect repellant. Concentrations above 30% DEET are neurotoxic in children. The military repellant contains 75%. (DEET is available in 100% concentrations as an unregulated over-the-counter preparation usually sold in sport stores.)
[c]Most US troops took low-dose pyridostigmine (Mestinon, 30 mg every 8 hrs) for about 5 days in 1991 to protect against exposure to the nerve agent soman.

earthquakes in Haiti. Data show rates as high as 50% to 75% and many survivors continue to live in fear and show signs of PTSD.

F. Differential diagnosis

It is important to recognize treatable medical contributors to posttraumatic symptomatology, especially head injury during the trauma. Other organic considerations that can both cause and exacerbate the symptoms are epilepsy, alcohol-use disorders, and other substance-related disorders (Table 14-3). Acute intoxication or withdrawal from some substances may also present a clinical picture that is difficult to distinguish from the disorder.

Symptoms of PTSD can be difficult to distinguish from both panic disorder and generalized anxiety disorder, because all three syndromes are associated with prominent anxiety and autonomic arousal. Major depression is also a frequent concomitant of PTSD.

G. Course and prognosis

PTSD usually develops sometime after the trauma. The delay can be as short as 1 week or as long as 30 years. Symptoms fluctuate and may be most intense during periods of stress. Untreated, about 30% of patients recover completely, 40% have mild symptoms, 20% with moderate symptoms, and 10% remain unchanged or become worse. After 1 year, about 50% of patients will recover. For a list of good prognostic factors, see Table 14-4.

The very young and the very old have more difficulty with traumatic and about 80% of young children who sustain a burn injury show symptoms of PTSD 1 or 2 years after the initial injury; only 30% of adults who suffer such

Table 14-4
Good Prognostic Factors in PTSD

Rapid onset of the symptoms
Short duration of the symptoms (less than 6 mos)
Good premorbid functioning
Strong social supports
Absence of other psychiatric, medical, or substance-related disorders

Table 14-5
Predisposing Factors in PTSD

Young children (Inadequate coping mechanisms
Older persons (rigid coping mechanisms)
Physical disabilities in late life
Disabilities of the nervous system such as reduced cerebral blood flow
Compromised cardiovascular system (palpitations, and arrhythmias)
Pre-existing psychiatric disability
PTSD that is comorbid with other disorders is often more severe and perhaps more chronic and may be difficult to treat.

an injury have symptoms of PTSD after 1 year. For a list of predisposing factors, see Table 14-5. In general, patients who have a good network of social support are less likely to have the disorder and to experience it in its severe forms and are more likely to recover faster.

H. Treatment

When a patient has experienced a traumatic event in the past and has now developed PTSD, the emphasis should be on education about the disorder and its treatment, both pharmacologic and psychotherapeutic. To press a person who is reluctant to talk about a trauma into doing so is likely to increase rather than decrease the risk of developing PTSD. The use of sedatives and hypnotics can also be helpful in some cases. Additional support for the patient and the family can be obtained through local and national support groups for patients with PTSD.

1. Pharmacotherapy

Selective serotonin reuptake inhibitors (SSRIs), such as sertraline (Zoloft) and paroxetine (Paxil), are considered first-line treatments for PTSD, owing to their efficacy, tolerability, and safety ratings. SSRIs reduce symptoms from all PTSD symptom clusters and are effective in improving symptoms unique to PTSD. Buspirone (BuSpar) is serotonergic and may also be of use.

The efficacy of imipramine (Tofranil) and amitriptyline (Elavil), two tricyclic drugs, in the treatment of PTSD is supported by a number of well-controlled clinical trials. Other drugs that may be useful in the treatment of PTSD include the monoamine oxidase inhibitors (MAOIs) (e.g., phenelzine [Nardil]), trazodone (Desyrel), and the anticonvulsants (e.g., carbamazepine [Tegretol], valproate [Depakene]). Some studies have also revealed improvement in PTSD in patients treated with reversible monoamine oxidase inhibitors (RIMAs). Use of clonidine (Catapres) and propranolol (Inderal), which are antiadrenergic agents, is suggested by the theories about noradrenergic hyperactivity in the disorder.

2. Psychotherapy

Psychodynamic psychotherapy may be useful in the treatment of many patients with PTSD. In some cases, reconstruction of the traumatic events with associated abreaction and catharsis may be therapeutic, but psychotherapy must be individualized because re-experiencing the trauma overwhelms some patients.

Psychotherapeutic interventions for PTSD include behavior therapy, cognitive therapy, and hypnosis. Abreaction—experiencing the emotions associated with the event—may be helpful for some patients. When PTSD has developed, two major psychotherapeutic approaches can be taken. The first is exposure therapy, in which the patient re-experiences the traumatic event through imaging techniques or *in vivo* exposure. The second approach is to teach the patient methods of stress management, including relaxation techniques and cognitive approaches, to coping with stress.

Another psychotherapeutic technique that is relatively novel and somewhat controversial is eye movement desensitization and reprocessing (EMDR), in which the patient focuses on the lateral movement of the clinician's finger while maintaining a mental image of the trauma experience.

In addition, group and family therapies have been reported to be effective in cases of PTSD.

II. Trauma- or Stressor-Related Disorder Unspecified

In DSM-5, the category of "unspecified trauma- or stressor-related disorder" is used for patients who develop emotional or behavioral symptoms in response to an identifiable stressor but do not meet the full criteria of any other specified trauma- or stressor-related disorder (e.g., acute stress disorder, PTSD, or adjustment disorder). The symptoms cannot meet the criteria for another mental, medical disorder and is not an exacerbation of a pre-existing mental disorder. The symptoms also cannot be attributed to the direct physiologic effects of a substance.

A. Adjustment disorders

Adjustment disorders are characterized by an emotional response to a stressful event and are linked to the development of symptoms. Typically, the stressor involves financial issues, a medical illness, or relationship problem. The symptom complex must begin within 3 months of the stressor and includes anxious or depressive affect or may present with a disturbance of conduct. The subtypes of adjustment disorder include adjustment disorder with depressed mood, mixed anxiety and depressed mood, disturbance of conduct, mixed disturbance of emotions and conduct, acute stress disorder, bereavement, and unspecified type.

1. Epidemiology

The prevalence ranges from 2% to 8% in the general population. Women are diagnosed with the disorder twice as often as men, and single women are generally overly represented as most at risk. The disorders can occur at any age but are most frequently diagnosed in adolescents with boys and girls being equally diagnosed. Common precipitating stresses are school problems, parental rejection and divorce, and substance abuse. Among adults, common precipitating stresses are marital problems, divorce, moving to a new environment, and financial problems.

Adjustment disorders are extremely common among patients hospitalized for medical and surgical problems.

Table 14-6
Specific Developmental Stage Stressors

Often associated with adjustment disorders.
- Beginning school
- Leaving home
- Getting married
- Becoming a parent
- Failing to achieve occupational goals
- Having the last child leave home, and
- Retiring

---

2. Etiology

An adjustment disorder is precipitated by one or more stressors and the severity does not always predict the severity of the disorder. The loss of a parent is different for a child 10 years of age than for a person 40 years of age. Personality organization and cultural or group norms and values also contribute to the disproportionate responses to stressors.

Stressors may be single, or multiple as well as recurrent, or continuous. Adjustment disorders can occur in a group or community setting as in a natural disaster or in racial, social, or religious persecution. For specific developmental stage stressors, see Table 14-6.

a. Psychodynamic factors

A concurrent personality disorder or organic impairment may make a person vulnerable to adjustment disorders. Throughout early development, each child develops a unique set of defense mechanisms to deal with stressful events. Resilience is also crucially determined by the nature of children's early relationships with their parents. These factors may predispose or make an individual more resilient.

3. Diagnosis and clinical features

Although by definition adjustment disorders follow a stressor, up to 3 months may elapse between a stressor and the development of symptoms. The disorder can occur at any age, and its symptoms vary considerably, with depressive, anxious, and mixed features most common in adults. Manifestations may also include assaultive behavior and reckless driving, excessive drinking, defaulting on legal responsibilities, withdrawal, vegetative signs, insomnia, and suicidal behavior.

The clinical presentations of adjustment disorder can vary widely. DSM-5 lists six adjustment disorders: with depressed mood; with anxiety; with mixed anxiety and depression; with conduct disturbance; with conduct disturbance and disturbance of emotion; and an unspecified category.

a. Adjustment disorder with depressed mood

In adjustment disorder with depressed mood, the predominant manifestations are depressed mood, tearfulness, and hopelessness. This type must be distinguished from major depressive disorder and uncomplicated bereavement.

b. Adjustment disorder with anxiety

Symptoms of anxiety, such as palpitations, jitteriness, and agitation, are present in adjustment disorder with anxiety, which must be differentiated from anxiety disorders.

c. Adjustment disorder with mixed anxiety and depressed mood

In adjustment disorder with mixed anxiety and depressed mood, patients exhibit features of both anxiety and depression that do not meet the criteria for an already established anxiety disorder or depressive disorder.

d. Adjustment disorder with disturbance of conduct

In adjustment disorder with disturbance of conduct, the predominant manifestation involves conduct in which the rights of others are violated or age-appropriate societal norms and rules are disregarded. It must be differentiated from conduct disorder and antisocial personality disorder.

e. Adjustment disorder with mixed disturbance of emotions and conduct

A combination of disturbances of emotions and of conduct sometimes occurs. Clinicians are encouraged to try to make one or the other diagnosis in the interest of clarity.

f. Adjustment disorder unspecified

Adjustment disorder unspecified is a residual category for atypical maladaptive reactions to stress. Examples include inappropriate responses to the diagnosis of physical illness, such as massive denial, severe noncompliance with treatment, and social withdrawal, without significant depressed or anxious mood.

4. Differential diagnosis

In uncomplicated, the person's dysfunction remains within the expectable bounds of a reaction to the loss of a loved one and, thus, is not considered adjustment disorder. Other disorders from which adjustment disorder must be differentiated include major depressive disorder, brief psychotic disorder, generalized anxiety disorder, somatic symptom disorder, substance-related disorder, conduct disorder, and PTSD. Patients with an adjustment disorder are impaired in social or occupational functioning and show symptoms beyond the normal and expectable reaction to the stressor.

B. Acute and posttraumatic stress disorders

The presence of a stressor is a requirement in the diagnosis of adjustment disorder, PTSD, and acute stress disorder. PTSD and acute stress disorder have the nature of the stressor better characterized and are accompanied by a defined constellation of affective and autonomic symptoms while the stressor in adjustment disorder can be of any severity, with a wide range of possible symptoms.

1. Course and prognosis

With appropriate treatment, the overall prognosis of an adjustment disorder is generally favorable. Most patients return to their previous level of functioning within 3 months.

There is a risk of suicide in patients with adjustment disorder, especially in adolescent patients with adjustment disorder.

2. Treatment

a. Psychotherapy

Psychotherapy remains the treatment of choice for adjustment disorders. Group therapy can be particularly useful for patients who have had similar stresses. Individual psychotherapy offers the opportunity to explore the meaning of the stressor to the patient so that earlier traumas can be worked through.

b. Crisis intervention

Crisis intervention and case management are short-term treatments aimed at helping persons with adjustment disorders resolve their situations quickly by supportive techniques, suggestion, reassurance, environmental modification, and even hospitalization, if necessary.

c. Pharmacotherapy

No studies have assessed the efficacy of pharmacologic interventions in individuals with adjustment disorder, but it may be reasonable to use medication to treat specific symptoms for a brief time. The judicious use of medications can help patients with adjustment disorders, but they should be prescribed for brief periods. Depending on the type of adjustment disorder, a patient may respond to an antianxiety agent or to an antidepressant. Antipsychotic drugs may be used if there are signs of decompensation or impending psychosis. SSRIs have been found useful in treating symptoms of traumatic grief. Recently, there has been an increase in antidepressant use to augment psychotherapy in patients with adjustment disorders. Pharmacologic intervention in this population is most often used, however, to augment psychosocial strategies rather than serving as the primary modality.

For more detailed discussion of this topic, see Chapter 17, Posttraumatic Stress Disorder, p. 1812 and Chapter 25, Adjustment Disorders, p. 2116, in CTP/X.

15
Dissociative Disorders

I. General Introduction

Dissociation is defined as an unconscious defense mechanism involving the segregation of any group of mental or behavioral processes from the rest of the person's psychic activity. Dissociative disorders involve this mechanism so that there is a disruption in one or more mental functions, such as memory, identity, perception, consciousness, or motor behavior. The disturbance may be sudden or gradual, transient or chronic, and the signs and symptoms of the disorder are often caused by psychological trauma.

Dissociation usually happens in response to a traumatic event. There are four specific dissociative disorders: dissociative amnesia, dissociative fugue, dissociative identity disorder, and depersonalization/derealization disorder, as well as other specified or unspecified dissociative disorder.

II. Dissociative Amnesia

A. Definition. Dissociative phenomenon is specifically amnesic in that the patient is unable to recall an important memory which is usually traumatic or stressful, but retains the capacity to learn new material. There is no medical explanation for the occurrence, nor is the condition caused by a drug. The different types of dissociative amnesia are listed in Table 15-1.

B. Diagnosis. The *DSM-5* diagnostic criteria for dissociative amnesia emphasizes that the forgotten information is usually of traumatic or stressful nature (see Table 15-2). The forgotten memories are usually related to day-to-day information that is a routine part of conscious awareness (i.e., who a person is). Patients are capable of learning and remembering new information, and their general cognitive functioning and language capacity are usually intact. Onset of dissociative amnesia is often abrupt, and history usually shows a precipitating emotional trauma charged with painful emotions and psychological conflict. Patients are aware that they have lost their memories, and while some may be upset at the loss, others appear to be unconcerned or indifferent. Patients are usually alert before and after amnesia; however, some report a slight clouding of consciousness during the period immediately surrounding onset of amnesia. Depression and anxiety are common predisposing factors. Amnesia may provide a primary or a secondary gain (i.e., a woman who is amnestic about the birth of a dead infant). Dissociative amnesia may take one of several forms: localized amnesia (loss of memory for the events over a short time); generalized amnesia (loss of memory for a whole lifetime of experiences); and selective or systematized amnesia (inability to recall some but not all events over a short time). The amnesia is not

Table 15-1
Types of Dissociative Amnesia

Localized amnesia: Inability to recall events related to a circumscribed period of time
Selective amnesia: Ability to remember some, but not all, of the events occurring during a circumscribed period of time
Generalized amnesia: Failure to recall one's entire life
Continuous amnesia: Failure to recall successive events as they occur
Systematized amnesia: Failure to remember a category of information, such as all memories relating to one's family or to a particular person

the result of a general medical condition or the ingestion of a substance (see Table 15-3).

C. Epidemiology
   1. Most common dissociative disorder (2% to 6%).
   2. Occurs more often in women than in men.
   3. Occurs more often in adolescents and young adults than in older adults.
   4. Incidence increases during times of war and natural disasters.
D. Etiology
   1. Precipitating emotional trauma.
   2. Physical and sexual abuse.
   3. Rule out medical causes.
E. Psychodynamics
   1. Defenses include repression, denial, and dissociation.
   2. Memory loss is secondary to painful psychological conflict.
F. Differential diagnosis (see Table 15-4)
   1. Dementia or delirium. Amnesia is associated with many cognitive symptoms.
   2. Epilepsy. Sudden memory impairment associated with motor or electroencephalogram (EEG) abnormalities.
   3. Transient global amnesia. Associated with anterograde amnesia during episode; patients tend to be more upset and concerned about the symptoms and are able to retain personal identity; memory loss is generalized, and remote events are recalled better than recent events.
G. Course and prognosis. The symptoms of dissociative amnesia terminate abruptly. Recovery is complete with few recurrences. The condition may last a long time in some patients, especially in cases involving secondary gain. Patient's lost memories should be restored as soon as possible, or the repressed memory may form a nucleus in the unconscious mind where future amnestic episodes may develop. Recovery generally is spontaneous but is accelerated with treatment.

Table 15-2
Signs and Symptoms of Dissociative Amnesia

- Failure to remember personal information (often of stressful experiences) more extreme than forgetting
  - Can be with or without dissociative fugue (peregrination).

Table 15-3
Mental Status Examination Questions for Dissociative Amnesia

If answers are positive, ask the patient to describe the event.
Make sure to specify that the symptom does not occur during an episode of intoxication.
1. Do you ever have blackouts? Blank spells? Memory lapses?
2. Do you lose time? Have gaps in your experience of time?
3. Have you ever traveled a considerable distance without recollection of how you did this or where you went exactly?
4. Do people tell you of things you have said and done that you do not recall?
5. Do you find objects in your possession (such as clothes, personal items, groceries in your grocery cart, books, tools, equipment, jewelry, vehicles, weapons etc.) that you do not remember acquiring? Out-of-character items? Items that a child might have? Toys? Stuffed animals?
6. Have you ever been told or found evidence that you have talents and abilities that you did not know that you had? For example, musical, artistic, mechanical, literary, athletic, or other talents? Do your tastes seem to fluctuate a lot? For example, food preference, personal habits, taste in music or clothes, and so forth.
7. Do you have gaps in your memory of your life? Are you missing parts of your memory for your life history? Are you missing memories of some important events in your life? For example, weddings, birthdays, graduations, pregnancies, birth of children, and so on.
8. Do you lose track of or tune out conversations or therapy sessions as they are occurring? Do you find that, while you are listening to someone talk, you did not hear all or part of what was just said?
9. What is the longest period of time that you have lost? Minutes? Hours? Days? Weeks? Months? Years? Describe.

Adapted from Loewenstein RJ. An office mental status examination for chronic complex dissociative symptoms and multiple personality disorder. *Psychiatr Clin North Am.* 1991;14:567–604.

Table 15-4
Differential Diagnostic Considerations in Dissociative Amnesia

Dementia
Delirium
Ordinary forgetfulness and nonpathologic amnesia
Amnestic disorder due to a medical condition
   Anoxic amnesia
   Cerebral infections (e.g., herpes simplex affecting temporal lobes)
   Cerebral neoplasms (especially limbic and frontal)
   Epilepsy
   Metabolic disorders (e.g., uremia, hypoglycemia, hypertensive encephalopathy, porphyria)
   Postconcussion (posttraumatic) amnesia
   Postoperative amnesia
Electroconvulsive therapy (or other strong electric shock)
Substance-related amnesia (e.g., ethanol, sedative-hypnotics, anticholinergics, steroids, lithium, β-adrenergic receptor antagonists, pentazocine, phencyclidine, hypoglycemic agents, cannabis, hallucinogens, methyldopa)
Transient global amnesia
Wernicke–Korsakoff syndrome
Sleep-related amnesia (e.g., sleepwalking disorder)
Dissociative identity disorders
Other dissociative disorders
Posttraumatic amnesia
Posttraumatic stress disorder
Acute stress disorder
Somatoform disorders (somatization disorder, conversion disorder)
Malingering and factitious amnesia (especially when associated with criminal activity)

H. Treatment

1. **Psychotherapy.** Psychotherapy helps patients to incorporate the memories into their conscious state. Hypnosis is used primarily as a means to relax the patient sufficiently to recall forgotten information.
2. **Pharmacotherapy.** Drug-assisted interviews with short-acting barbiturates, such as thiopental (Pentothal) and sodium amobarbital (Amytal) given intravenously, and benzodiazepines may be used to help patients recover their forgotten memories.

III. Dissociative Fugue

A. Definition.
Dissociative fugue was deleted as a major diagnostic category in DSM-5 and is now diagnosed on a subtype (specifier) of dissociative amnesia. It is characterized by sudden, unexpected travel away from home, with the inability to recall some or all of one's past. This is accompanied by confusion about identity and, often, the assumption of an entirely new identity.

B. Diagnosis.
Memory loss is sudden and is associated with purposeful, unconfused travel, often for extended periods of time. Patients lose part or complete memory of their past life and are often unaware of the memory loss. They assume an apparently normal, nonbizarre new identity. However, perplexity and disorientation may occur. Once they suddenly return to their former selves, they recall the time antedating the fugue, but they are amnestic for the period of the fugue itself.

C. Epidemiology

1. Rare, with a prevalence rate of 0.2% in the general population.
2. Occurs most often during times of war, during natural disasters, and as a result of personal crises with intense internal conflict.
3. Sex ratio and age of onset are variable.

D. Etiology

1. Precipitating emotional trauma.
2. Psychosocial factors include marital, financial, occupational, and wartime stressors.
3. Predisposing factors include borderline, histrionic, schizoid personality disorders; alcohol abuse; mood disorders; organic disorders (especially epilepsy); and a history of head trauma.
4. Rule out medical causes.

E. Differential diagnosis

1. **Cognitive disorder.** Wandering is not as purposeful or complex.
2. **Temporal lobe epilepsy.** Generally, no new identity is assumed.
3. **Dissociative amnesia.** No purposeful travel or new identity.
4. **Malingering.** Difficult to distinguish; clear secondary gain should raise suspicion.
5. **Dissociative identity disorder.** Patients have multiple forms of complex amnesia and multiple identities.
6. **Bipolar disorder.** Patients are able to recall behavior during depressed or manic state.

7. **Schizophrenia.** Memory loss of events during wandering episodes is due to psychosis.
8. **General medical conditions, toxic and substance-related disorders, delirium, dementia.** Wandering behavior may occur and could be confused with fugue states; physical examination and laboratory tests may help rule out these conditions.

F. **Course and prognosis.** Fugues appear to be brief, lasting from hours to days. Most individuals recover, although refractory dissociative amnesia may persist in rare cases. Recovery is spontaneous and rapid. Recurrences are possible.

G. **Treatment.** Psychiatric interviews, drug-assisted interviews, and hypnosis help reveal to the clinician and the patient the psychological stressors that precipitated the fugue episode. Psychotherapy helps patients incorporate the precipitating stressors into their psyches in a healthy and integrated manner.

IV. **Dissociative Identity Disorder**

A. **Definition.** Formerly known as multiples personality disorder, dissociative identity disorder is usually the result of a traumatic event, often physical or sexual abuse in childhood. This disorder involves the manifestation of two or more distinct personalities, which, when present, will dominate the person's behaviors and attitudes as if no other personality existed.

B. **Diagnosis.** Diagnosis requires the presence of two distinct personality states. Original personality is generally amnestic for and unaware of other personalities. The median number of personalities ranges from 5 to 10, although data suggest an average of 8 personalities for men and 15 for women. Usually two or three identities are evident at diagnosis and others are recognized during the course of treatment (see Table 15-5).

Transition from one personality to another tends to be abrupt. During a personality state, patients are amnestic about other states and events that took place when another personality was dominant. Some personalities may be aware of aspects of other personalities; each personality may have its own set of memories and associations, and each generally has its own name or description. Different personalities may have different physiologic characteristics (e.g., different eyeglass prescriptions) and different responses to psychometric testing (e.g., different IQ scores). Personalities may be of different sexes, ages, or races. One or more of the personalities may exhibit signs of a coexisting psychiatric disorder (e.g., mood disorder, personality disorder). Signs of dissociative identity disorder are listed in Table 15-6.

C. **Epidemiology**
1. Occurs in 5% of psychiatric patients.
2. More common in females than males.
3. Most common in late adolescence and young adulthood, although symptoms may be present for 5 to 10 years before diagnosis.
4. More common in first-degree biologic relatives with the disorder.
5. As many as two-thirds of patients attempt suicide.

Table 15-5
Mental Status Examination Questions for Dissociative Identity Disorder Process Symptoms

If answers are positive, ask the patient to describe the event.
Make sure to specify that the symptom does not occur during an episode of intoxication

1. Do you act so differently in one situation compared to another situation that you feel almost like you were two different people?
2. Do you feel that there is more than one of you? More than one part of you? Side of you? Do they seem to be in conflict or in a struggle?
3. Does that part (those parts) of you have its (their) own independent way(s) of thinking, perceiving, and relating to the world and the self? Have its (their) own memories, thoughts, and feelings?
4. Does more than one of these entities take control of your behavior?
5. Do you ever have thoughts or feelings, or both, that come from inside you (outside you) that you cannot explain? That do not feel like thoughts or feelings that you would have? That seem like thoughts or feelings that are not under your control (passive influence)?
6. Have you ever felt that your body was engaged in behavior that did not seem to be under your control? For example, saying things, going places, buying things, writing things, drawing or creating things, hurting yourself or others, and so forth? That your body does not seem to belong to you?
7. Do you ever feel that you have to struggle against another part of you that seems to want to do or to say something that you do not wish to do or to say?
8. Do you ever feel that there is a force (pressure, part) inside you that tries to stop you from doing or saying something?
9. Do you ever hear voices, sounds, or conversations in your mind? That seem to be discussing you? Commenting on what you do? Telling you to do or not do certain things? To hurt yourself or others? That seem to be warning you or trying to protect you? That try to comfort, support, or soothe you? That provide important information about things to you? That argue or say things that have nothing to do with you? That have names? Men? Women? Children?
10. I would like to talk with that part (side, aspect, facet) of you (of the mind) that is called the "angry one" (the Little Girl, Janie, who went to Atlantic City last weekend and spend lots of money, etc.). Can that part come forward now, please?
11. Do you frequently have the experience of feeling like you are outside yourself? Inside yourself? Beside yourself, watching yourself as if you were another person?
12. Do you ever feel disconnected from yourself or your body as if you (your body) were not real?
13. Do you ever really experience the world around you as unreal? As if you are in a fog or daze? As if it were painted? Two-dimensional?
14. Do you ever looking in the mirror and not recognize who you see? See someone else there?

Adapted from Loewenstein RJ. An office mental status examination for a chronic complex dissociative symptoms and multiple personality disorder. *Psychiatr Clin North Am.* 1991;14:567.

D. Etiology

   1. Severe sexual and psychological abuse in childhood.

   2. Lack of support from significant others.

   3. Epilepsy may be involved.

   4. Rule out medical causes.

E. Psychodynamics. Severe psychological and physical abuse leads to a profound need to distance the self from horror and pain. Each personality expresses some necessary emotion or state (e.g., rage, sexuality, flamboyance, competence) that the original personality dares not express. During abuse, the child attempts to protect himself or herself from trauma by dissociating from the terrifying acts, becoming, in essence, another person or persons who are not experiencing abuse and who could not be subjected to abuse. The dissociated selves become a long-term, ingrained method of self-protection from perceived emotional threats.

Table 15-6
Signs and Symptoms of Dissociative Identity Disorder

1. Reports of time distortions, lapses, and discontinuities.
2. At least two distinct personality states (can be described/experienced as "being possessed by" another).
3. Discontinuous identity (e.g., dichotomies in memory, behavior, or consciousness).
4. Persistent gaps in memory and personal information.
5. Fantasy play in children is excluded.
6. Being recognized by others or called by another name by people whom the patient does not recognize.
7. Notable changes in the patient's behavior reported by a reliable observer: the patient may call himself or herself by a different name or refer to himself or herself in the third person.
8. Other personalities are elicited under hypnosis or during amobarbital interviews.
9. Use of the word "we" in the course of an interview.
10. Discovery of writings, drawings, or other productions or objects (e.g., identification cards, clothing) among the patient's personal belongings that are not recognized or cannot be accounted for.
11. Headaches.
12. Hearing voices originating from within and not identified as separate.
13. History of severe emotional or physical trauma as a child (usually before the age of 5 yrs).

From Cummings JL. Dissociative states, depersonalization, multiple personality, episodic memory lapses. In: Cummings JL, ed. *Clinical Neuropsychiatry*. Orlando, FL: Grune & Stratton, 1985: 122, with permission.

F. Differential diagnosis

1. **Schizophrenia.** Different identities are of delusional belief and patients have formal thought disorder and social deterioration.
2. **Malingering.** The most difficult differential diagnosis; clear secondary gain must raise suspicion. Drug-assisted interview may help.
3. **Borderline personality disorder.** Erratic mood, behavior, and interpersonal instability may mimic dissociative identity.
4. **Bipolar disorder with rapid cycling.** Discrete personalities are absent.
5. **Neurologic disorders.** The symptoms of complex partial epilepsy are the most likely to mimic those of dissociative identity disorder.

    For a list of differential diagnosis, see Table 15-7.

Table 15-7
Differential Diagnosis of Dissociative Identity Disorder

Comorbidity versus differential diagnosis
Affective disorders
Psychotic disorders
Anxiety disorders
Posttraumatic stress disorder
Personality disorders
Neurocognitive disorders
Neurologic and seizure disorders
Somatic symptom disorders
Factitious disorders
Malingering
Other dissociative disorders
Deep-trance phenomena

CLINICAL HINT:
Do not confuse imaginary companions which begin in childhood and may persist through adulthood with a multiple. The companion is recognized as a separate being that may or may not communicate with the patient; the companion is always known and never takes over the patient's personality.

G. **Course and prognosis.** The earlier the onset of dissociative identity disorder, the worse is the prognosis. It is the most chronic and severe of the dissociative disorders. Levels of impairment range from moderate to severe depending on the number, type, and chronicity of the various personalities. Recovery is generally incomplete. Individual personalities may have their own separate mental disorders, mood disorders, and personality disorders, with other dissociative disorders being the most common.

H. **Treatment**
   1. **Psychotherapy.** Insight-oriented psychotherapy, often with hypnotherapy or drug-assisted interviewing, is the most efficacious approach. Hypnotherapy is useful in obtaining additional history, identifying previously unrecognized identities, and fostering abreaction. Psychotherapeutic treatment begins by confirming the diagnosis and by identifying and characterizing the various personalities. Goals of therapy include reconciliation of disparate, split-off affects by helping the patient understand that the original reasons for the dissociation (overwhelming rage, fear, and confusion secondary to abuse) no longer exist, and that the affects can be expressed by one whole personality without the self being destroyed. Hospitalization may be necessary in some cases.
   2. **Pharmacotherapy.** Drug-assisted interviewing is helpful in obtaining additional history and identifying unrecognized identities. Antidepressant and antianxiety medications can be useful as adjuvants to psychotherapy. In selected patients, anticonvulsant medications, such as carbamazepine (Tegretol), have been helpful (see Table 15-8).

V. **Depersonalization/Derealization Disorder**
   A. **Definition.** Depersonalization is defined as the persistent or recurrent feeling of detachment or estrangement from one's self. The individual may report feeling like an automaton or watching himself or herself in a movie. Derealization is somewhat related and refers to feelings of unreality or of being detached from one's environment. The patient may describe his or her perception of the outside world as lacking lucidity and emotional coloring, as though dreaming or dead
   B. **Diagnosis.** A number of distinct components comprise the experience of depersonalization, including a sense of (1) bodily changes, (2) duality of self as observer and actor, (3) being cut off from others, and (4) being cut off from one's own emotions. Patients experiencing depersonalization often have great difficulty expressing what they are feeling. Trying to express

Table 15-8
Medications for Associated Symptoms in Dissociative Identity Disorder

Medications and somatic treatments for posttraumatic stress disorder (PTSD), affective disorders, anxiety disorders, and obsessive–compulsive disorder (OCD)
Selective serotonin reuptake inhibitors (no preferred agent, except for OCD symptoms)
Fluvoxamine (Luvox) (for OCD presentations)
Clomipramine (Anafranil) (for OCD presentations)
Tricyclic antidepressants
Monoamine oxidase inhibitors (if patient can reliably maintain diet safely)
Electroconvulsive therapy (for refractory depression with persistent melancholic features across all dissociative identity disorder alters)
Mood stabilizers (more useful for PTSD and anxiety than mood swings)
Divalproex (Depakote)
Lamotrigine (Lamictal)
Oral or intramuscular benzodiazepines
Medications for sleep problems
Low-dose trazodone (Desyrel)
Low-dose mirtazapine (Remeron)
Low-dose tricyclic antidepressants
Low-dose neuroleptics
Benzodiazepines (often less helpful for sleep problems in this population)
Zolpidem (Ambien)
Anticholinergic agents (diphenhydramine (Benadryl), hydroxyzine (Vistaril))
Medications for self-injury, addictions
Naltrexone (ReVia)

their subjective suffering with banal phrases, such as "I feel dead," "Nothing seems real," or "I'm standing outside of myself," depersonalized patients may not adequately convey to the examiner the distress they experience. While complaining bitterly about how this is ruining their life, they may nonetheless appear remarkably un-distressed (see Table 15-9).

C. Epidemiology

1. Occasional isolated depersonalization episodes are common and occur in 70% of a given population. Pathologic depersonalization is rare.
2. Occurs more often in women than in men.
3. Mean age of occurrence is 16 years. Rarely found in persons over the age of 40 years.

D. Etiology

1. Predisposing factors include anxiety, depression, and severe stress.
2. May be caused by a psychological, neurologic, or systemic disease.
3. Associated with an array of substances including alcohol, barbiturates, benzodiazepines, scopolamine, β-adrenergic antagonists, marijuana, and virtually any phencyclidine (PCP)-like or hallucinogenic substance.

Table 15-9
Signs and Symptoms of Depersonalization/Derealization Disorder

• Persistent feelings of depersonalization or derealization without loss of reality testing
• Depersonalization: feeling as though living outside one's body, disconnected from sensations, emotions, and actions
• Derealization: feeling detached from reality, as if in a dream

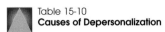 Table 15-10
Causes of Depersonalization

Neurologic disorders	**Idiopathic mental disorders**
Epilepsy	Schizophrenia
Migraine	Depressive disorders
Brain tumors	Manic episodes
Cerebrovascular disease	Conversion disorder
Cerebral trauma	Anxiety disorders
Encephalitis	Obsessive-compulsive disorder
General paresis	Personality disorders
Dementia of the Alzheimer's type	Phobic–anxiety depersonalization syndrome
Huntington's disease	
Spinocerebellar degeneration	**In normal persons**
	Exhaustion
Toxic and metabolic disorders	Boredom; sensory deprivation
Hypoglycemia	Emotional shock
Hypoparathyroidism	
Carbon monoxide poisoning	**In hemi-depersonalization**
Mescaline intoxication	Lateralized (usually right parietal) focal brain lesion
Botulism	
Hyperventilation	
Hypothyroidism	

Adapted from Cummings JL. Dissociative states, depersonalization, multiple personality, episodic memory lapses. In: Cummings JL, ed. *Clinical Neuropsychiatry*, Orlando, FL: Grune & Stratton, 1985:123.

4. Frequently associated with anxiety disorders, depressive disorders, and schizophrenia.

E. Differential diagnosis. Depersonalization as a symptom can occur in many syndromes, both psychiatric and medical. Mood disorders, anxiety disorders, schizophrenia, dissociative identity disorder, substance use, adverse effects of medication, brain tumors or injury, and seizure disorders (e.g., temporal lobe epilepsy) must be ruled out. Depersonalization disorder describes the condition in which depersonalization is predominant. Depersonalization is differentiated from psychotic disorders in that reality testing is intact (see Table 15-10).

F. Course and prognosis

1. Symptoms appear suddenly, most often between 15 and 30 years of age.

2. In more than 50% of cases, the disorder is long-lasting.

G. Treatment. Usually responds to anxiolytics and to both supportive and insight-oriented therapy. As anxiety is reduced, episodes of depersonalization decrease.

VI. Other Specified or Unspecified Dissociative Disorder

The category of dissociative disorder covers all of the conditions characterized by a primary dissociative response that do not meet diagnostic criteria for one of the other DSM-5 dissociative disorders.

A. Definition. Dissociative disorders not otherwise specified are disorders in which the predominant feature is a dissociative symptom, such as a disruption in consciousness or memory, but that does not meet the criteria for specific dissociative disorder. In order for a patient to be diagnosed with unspecified dissociative disorder one must fail to meet the criteria for acute stress disorder, PTSD, or somatization disorder, all of which include dissociative symptoms.

B. Epidemiology. Cases have been reported in a variety of cultures, but the overall frequency of such reports has declined with time. Men outnumber women by approximately 2 to 1. Three of Ganser's first four cases were convicts, leading some authors to consider it to be a disorder of penal populations and, thus, an indicator of potential malingering.

C. Etiology. Some case reports identify precipitating stressors, such as personal conflicts and financial reverses, whereas others note organic brain syndromes, head injuries, seizures, and medical or psychiatric illness. Psychodynamic explanations are common in the older literature, but organic etiologies are stressed in more recent case studies. It is speculated that the organic insults may act as acute stressors, precipitating the syndrome in vulnerable individuals. Some patients have reported significant histories of childhood maltreatment and adversity.

D. Examples

1. **Ganser's syndrome.** Giving approximate answers to questions (e.g., 2 + 2 = 5) or talking past the point; commonly associated with other symptoms (e.g., amnesia, disorientation, perceptual disturbances, fugue, conversion symptoms).

2. **Dissociative trance disorder.** Disturbances in consciousness, identity, or memory that are indigenous to particular locations and cultures (e.g., *amok* [rage reaction], *pibloktoq* [self-injurious behavior]). Trance states are altered states of consciousness with markedly diminished or selectively focused responsiveness to environmental stimuli. In children, such states may follow physical abuse or trauma. The dissociative trance state must not occur exclusively during the course of a psychotic disorder and is not the result of any substance use or general medical condition.

3. **Recovered memory syndrome.** The recovery of a memory of a painful experience or conflict during hypnosis or psychotherapy (e.g., sexual or physical abuse). The patient not only recalls the experience, but may also relive it with the appropriate affective response (a process called *abreaction*).

4. **Brainwashing.** Dissociated states in persons who have been subjected to periods of prolonged and intense coercive persuasion (e.g., brainwashing or indoctrination while the captive of terrorists or cultists). It implies that under conditions of adequate stress and duress, individuals can be made to comply with the demands of those in power, thereby undergoing major changes in their personality, beliefs, and behaviors. Persons subjected to such conditions can undergo considerable harm, including loss of health and life, and they typically manifest a variety of posttraumatic and dissociative symptoms.

E. Treatment. No systematic treatment studies have been conducted, given the rarity of this condition. In most case reports, the patient has been

Table 15-11
Summary of Dissociative Disorders

	Dissociative Amnesia	Dissociative Fugue	Dissociative Identity Disorder	Depersonalization Disorder
Signs and symptoms	Loss of memory, usually with abrupt onset Patient aware of loss Alert before and after loss	Purposeful wandering, often long distances Amnesia for past life Often unaware of loss of memory Often assumes new identity Normal behavior during fugue	More than one distinct personality within one person, each of which dominates person's behavior and thinking when it is present Sudden transition from one personality to another Generally amnesia for other personalities	Persistent sense of unreality about one's body and self Intact reality testing Ego-dynamic
Epidemiology	Most common dissociative disorder More common following disasters or during war Female > male Adolescence, young adulthood	Rare More common following disasters or during war Variable sex ratio and age of onset	Not nearly as rare as once thought Affects as many as 5% of psychiatric patients Adolescence–young adulthood (although may begin much earlier) Female > male Increased in first-degree relatives	Although pure disorder rare, intermittent episodes of depersonalization common Rare over age 40 May be more common in women
Etiology	Precipitating emotional trauma (e.g., domestic violence) Rule out medical causes	Precipitating emotional trauma Heavy alcohol abuse may predispose Borderline, histrionic, schizoid personality disorders predispose Rule out medical causes	Severe sexual and psychological abuse in childhood Lack of support from significant others Epilepsy may be involved Rule out medical causes	Severe stress, anxiety, depression predispose Rule out medical causes
Course and prognosis	Abrupt termination Few recurrences	Usually brief, hours or days Can last months and involve extensive travel Recovery generally spontaneous and rapid Recurrences rare	Most severe and chronic of dissociative disorders Incomplete recovery	Onset usually sudden Tends to be chronic

hospitalized and has been provided with a protective and supportive environment. In some instances, low doses of antipsychotic medications have been reported to be beneficial.

See Table 15-11 for an overview of all the dissociative disorders.

For more detailed discussion of this topic, see Chapter 20, Dissociative Disorders, Chapter 20, p. 1866, in CTP/X.

16
Somatic Symptom and Related Disorders

I. Somatic Symptoms Disorder

Somatic symptom disorder, also known as hypochondriasis, requires 6 or more months of a nondelusional preoccupation with fears of having, or that one has, a serious disease based on the misinterpretation of bodily symptoms. This causes significant distress and impairment in one's life, and is not accounted for by another psychiatric or medical disorder.

A. Epidemiology. In medical clinics, the 6-month prevalence is 4% to 6%, but it may be as high as 15%. Men and women are equally affected but women have more somatic complaints than men. Onset can occur at any age, but commonly appears at 20 to 30 years of age. Data indicate that it is more common among blacks, but social position, education level, gender, and marital status do not appear to affect the diagnosis. This disorder occurs in about 3% of medical students, usually in the first 2 years, but is generally transient.

B. Etiology. Persons augment and amplify their somatic sensations, and have low threshold and tolerance of physical discomfort. For example, person may perceive abdominal pressure as abdominal pain and misinterpret bodily sensations, becoming alarmed because of a faulty cognitive scheme.

In context of a social learning model, the person assumes the sick role and problems seemingly appear insurmountable and insolvable. The sick role allows a patient to avoid noxious obligations, and to be excused from usual duties and obligations.

About 80% of patients with this disorder may have coexisting depressive or anxiety disorders.

C. Diagnosis. According to the fifth edition of *Diagnostic and Statistical Manual of Mental Disorders* (DSM-5), the diagnostic criteria for somatic symptom disorder require that patients be preoccupied with the false belief that they have a serious disease, based on their misinterpretation of physical signs or sensations the belief must last at least 6 months, despite the absence of pathologic findings on medical and neurologic examinations. The diagnostic criteria also require that the belief cannot have the intensity of a delusion (more appropriately diagnosed as delusional disorder) and cannot be restricted to distress about appearance (more appropriately diagnosed as body dysmorphic disorder). The symptoms of somatic symptom disorder must be sufficiently intense to cause emotional distress or impair the patient's ability to function in important areas of life. Clinicians may specify the presence of poor insight; patients do not consistently recognize that their concerns about disease are excessive.

D. **Clinical features.** Patients believe that they have a serious disease that has not yet been detected and they cannot be persuaded to the contrary. They may maintain a belief that they have a particular disease despite negative laboratory results, the benign course of the alleged disease over time, and appropriate reassurances from physicians and as time progresses, they may transfer their belief to another disease. Symptoms of depression and anxiety may coexist.

DSM-5 specifies that the symptoms must be present for at least 6 months, but transient manifestations can occur after major stresses (death or serious illness of someone important to the patient or a serious life-threatening illness). Such states that last fewer than 6 months are diagnosed as "Other Specified Somatic Symptom and Related Disorders."

E. **Differential diagnosis.** Somatic symptom disorder must be differentiated from nonpsychiatric medical conditions with vague symptoms like acquired immunodeficiency syndrome (AIDS), endocrinopathies, myasthenia gravis, multiple sclerosis, degenerative diseases of the nervous system, systemic lupus erythematosus, and occult neoplastic disorders.

Somatic symptom disorder is differentiated from illness anxiety disorder, which is fear of having a disease rather than a concern about many symptoms. Patients with illness anxiety disorder are primarily concerned about being sick.

Conversion disorder is acute and transient, and involves a symptom rather than a particular disease. Somatic symptom disorder can also occur in patients with depressive and anxiety disorders, especially panic disorder. Careful questioning usually uncovers the symptoms of a panic attack. Delusional disorder can be by their delusional intensity and other psychotic symptoms. In addition, schizophrenic patients' somatic delusions tend to be bizarre.

Somatic symptom disorder is distinguished from factitious disorder and malingering in that patients actually experience and do not simulate the symptoms they report.

F. **Course and prognosis.** The course is usually episodic, lasting months to years with equally long quiescent periods. Psychosocial stressors may exacerbate the disorder, but one-third to one-half of all patients will improve significantly. Good prognostic signs are high socioeconomic status, treatment-responsive anxiety or depression, sudden onset of symptoms, absence of a personality disorder, and the absence of a nonpsychiatric medical condition.

G. **Treatment.** These patients usually resist psychiatric treatment, but some accept it in a medical setting with focus on stress reduction and coping with chronic illness. Group psychotherapy often benefits because it provides the social support and social interaction that reduce anxiety. Therapies like individual insight-oriented psychotherapy, behavior therapy, cognitive therapy, and hypnosis may be useful.

Regularly scheduled physical examinations help to reassure patients that their physicians are not abandoning them and that their complaints are being taken seriously. Invasive diagnostic procedures should only be done when objective evidence calls for them. Pharmacotherapy helps only in a drug-responsive condition, like anxiety or depressive disorder.

II. Illness Anxiety Disorder

Illness anxiety disorder is a new diagnosis in the fifth edition of DSM-5 that applies to those persons who are preoccupied with being sick or with developing a disease of some kind. It is a variant of somatic symptom disorder (hypochondriasis). The diagnosis may also be used for persons who do, in fact, have a medical illness but whose anxiety is out of proportion to their diagnosis and who assume the worst possible outcome imaginable.

A. **Epidemiology.** The prevalence is unknown aside from that related to hypochondriasis, which gives a prevalence of 4% to 6% in general medical clinics, while up to 15% of general population worry about becoming sick and incapacitated. There is no evidence that it is more common among different races or that gender, social position, education level, and marital status affect the diagnosis.

B. **Etiology.** The etiology is unknown. The social learning model may apply to this disorder with fear of illness viewed as a request to play the sick role under insurmountable and insolvable problems. It offers an escape that allows a patient to be excused from usual duties and obligations.

   The type of the fear may also be symbolic of unconscious conflicts that are reflected in the type of illness of which the person is afraid or the organ system selected (e.g., heart, kidney).

C. **Diagnosis.** The major DSM-5 diagnostic criteria for illness anxiety disorder are that patients be preoccupied with the false belief that they have or will develop a serious disease and there are few if any physical signs or symptoms. The belief must last at least 6 months, and there are no pathologic findings on medical or neurologic examinations. The belief cannot be a delusion as in delusional disorder or distress about appearance (more appropriately diagnosed as body dysmorphic disorder). The anxiety must be incapacitating and cause emotional distress and inability to function in important areas of life. Some persons with the disorder may visit physicians (care-seeking type) while others may not (care-avoidant type). The majority make repeated visits to health care providers.

D. **Clinical features.** Patients believe that they have a serious disease that has not yet been diagnosed, and they cannot be persuaded to the contrary. The belief may be about a particular disease or with time they may transfer their belief to another disease. Their convictions persist despite negative laboratory results, its benign course, and reassurances from physicians. This interferes in their daily interaction with others and they are often addicted to Internet searches about their feared illness.

E. **Differential diagnosis.** Illness anxiety disorder must be differentiated from other medical conditions. These patients are dismissed as "chronic complainers" and careful medical examinations are not performed. These patients are differentiated from those with somatic symptom disorder as they have fear of having a disease versus the emphasis in somatic symptom disorder on concern about many symptoms. Patients complain about fewer symptoms. Conversion disorder is acute, transient, and involves a symptom rather than a particular disease. Pain disorder is chronic, and limited to complaints of pain. The fear of illness can also occur in patients with depressive and anxiety disorders. Patients with panic can be ruled out by careful questioning that uncovers symptoms of a panic attack. Delusional beliefs can be differentiated by their delusional intensity and by the presence of other psychotic symptoms.

F. **Course and prognosis.** There are no reliable data about the prognosis but one may extrapolate from the course of somatic symptom disorder and episodes last months to years separated by equally long quiescent periods. Good prognosis is associated with high socioeconomic status, treatment-responsive anxiety or depression, sudden onset of symptoms, and the absence of a personality disorder.

G. **Treatment.** Patients usually resist psychiatric treatment but some accept it in a medical setting that focuses on stress reduction and education in coping with chronic illness. Group psychotherapy may be of helpful if the group is homogeneous with patients suffering from the same disorder. Other forms of psychotherapy, such as individual insight-oriented psychotherapy, behavior therapy, cognitive therapy, and hypnosis, may be useful.

Some patients may benefit from reassurance and that they do not have the illness. Others may be resistant to seeing a doctor or accepting the fact that there is nothing to worry about. Invasive diagnostic and therapeutic procedures should be done only when necessary.

Pharmacotherapy may be of help in alleviating the anxiety, but it is only ameliorative and cannot provide lasting relief. That can only come from an effective psychotherapeutic program that is acceptable to the patient and in which he or she is willing and able to participate.

III. Functional Neurologic Symptom Disorder (Conversion Disorder)

Conversion disorder, also called functional neurologic symptom disorder in the DSM-5, is an illness that affects voluntary motor or sensory functions, suggesting a medical condition, but is caused by psychological factors because it is preceded by conflicts or other stressors. The symptoms are not intentionally produced, are not caused by substance use, are not limited to pain or sexual symptoms, and the gain is primarily psychological and not social, monetary, or legal

A. **Epidemiology.** The incidence and prevalence are 10% of hospital inpatients and 5% to 15% of all psychiatric outpatients. Onset is in early adulthood, but can occur in middle or old age with twice as many women being affected. It is more frequent in family members and common in persons of low socioeconomic status, less well-educated persons, rural population, and military personnel who have been exposed to combat situations.

B. Etiology

1. Biologic factors. The symptoms may be caused by an excessive cortical arousal that sets off negative feedback loops between the cerebral cortex and the brainstem reticular formation. Elevated levels of corticofugal output, in turn, inhibit the patient's awareness of bodily sensation, which may explain the observed sensory deficits in some patients with conversion disorder. There is increased susceptibility in patients with frontal lobe trauma or other neurologic deficits.

2. Psychological factors. According to psychoanalytic theory, conversion disorder is caused by repression of unconscious intrapsychic conflict and conversion of anxiety into a physical symptom. Other factors are presence of personality disorder—avoidant, or histrionic and impulse (e.g., sex or aggression) that is unacceptable to ego and is disguised through symptoms.

3. Psychodynamics

   a. *La belle indifference* is a lack of concern about illness or obvious impairment and is present in some patients.

   b. *Primary gain* refers to the reduction of anxiety by repression of an unacceptable impulse. Symbolization of impulse onto symptom thus occurs (e.g., paralysis of arm prevents expression of aggressive impulse).

   c. *Secondary gain* refers to benefits of illness (e.g., compensation from lawsuit [compensation neurosis], avoidance of work, dependence on family). Patient usually lacks insight about this dynamic.

   Other defense mechanisms as source of symptoms: reaction formation, denial, and displacement.

4. Laboratory and psychological tests

   a. Evoked potentials show disturbed somatosensory perception; diminished or absent on side of defect.

   b. Mild cognitive impairment, attentional deficits, and visuoperceptual changes on Halstead–Reitan battery.

   c. Minnesota Multiphasic Personality Inventory-2 (MMPI-2) and Rorschach test show increased instinctual drives, sexual repression, inhibited aggression.

   d. Drug-assisted interview—intravenous amobarbital (Amytal) (100 to 500 mg) in slow infusion often causes conversion symptoms to abate. For example, patient with hysterical aphonia will begin to talk. Test can be used to aid in diagnosis but is not always reliable.

C. Pathophysiology. No changes; some brain imaging studies show hypometabolism in the dominant hemisphere and hypermetabolsim in the nondominant hemisphere.

D. Diagnosis. The DSM-5 limits the diagnosis to those symptoms that affect a voluntary motor or sensory function, that is, neurologic symptoms. The diagnosis of conversion disorder also excludes symptoms of pain and sexual dysfunction and symptoms that occur only in somatization disorder. DSM-5 describes several types of symptoms or deficits seen in conversion

Table 16-1
Common Symptoms of Conversion Disorder

Motor symptoms	Sensory deficits
Involuntary movements	Anesthesia, especially of extremities
Tics	Midline anesthesia
Blepharospasm	Blindness
Torticollis	Tunnel vision
Opisthotonos	Deafness
Seizures	**Visceral symptoms**
Abnormal gait	Psychogenic vomiting
Falling	Pseudocyesis
Astasia-abasia	Globus hystericus
Paralysis	Swooning or syncope
Weakness	Urinary retention
Aphonia	Diarrhea

Courtesy of Frederick G. Guggenheim, M.D.

disorder. These include weakness or paralysis; abnormal movements; attacks or seizures; swallowing or speech difficulties such as slurred speech; sensory symptoms and mixed symptoms. These are discussed below.

E. **Clinical features.** Paralysis, blindness, and mutism are the most common conversion disorder symptoms. Conversion disorder may be most commonly associated with passive-aggressive, dependent, antisocial, and histrionic personality disorders. Depressive and anxiety disorder symptoms often accompany the symptoms of conversion disorder, and affected patients are at risk for suicide. See Table 16-1.

F. **Differential diagnosis.** Patients should have thorough medical and neurologic workup since 25% to 50% are diagnosed with a medical disorder. The most common conditions are described below.

   1. **Paralysis.** It is inconsistent and does not follow motor pathways. Spastic paralysis, clonus, and cogwheel rigidity are also absent in conversion disorder.

   2. **Ataxia.** Movements are bizarre in conversion disorder. In organic lesions leg may be dragged and circumduction not possible. *Astasia–abasia* is an inconsistency patterned, unsteady gait that does not cause the patient with conversion disorder to fall or sustain injury.

   3. **Blindness.** No pupillary response is seen in true neurologic blindness (except note that occipital lobe lesions can produce cortical blindness with intact pupillary response). Tracking movements are also absent in true blindness. Monocular diplopia, triplopia, and tunnel vision can be conversion complaints. Ophthalmologists use tests with distorting prisms and colored lenses to detect hysterical blindness.

   4. **Deafness.** Loud noise will awaken sleeping patient with conversion disorder but not patient with organic deafness. Audiometric tests reveal varying responses in conversion.

   5. **Sensory.** On examination, reported sensory loss does not follow anatomic distribution of dermatomes, that is, hemisensory loss, which

Table 16-2
Factors Associated with Good and Poor Prognosis

Prognoses in Conversion Disorder
Good prognosis
Sudden onset
Clearly identifiable stress at onset
Short time between onset and treatment
Above-average IQ
Symptoms of paralysis, aphonia, blindness
Poor prognosis
Comorbid mental disorders
Ongoing litigation
Symptoms of tremor, seizures

stops at midline, or glove-and-stocking anesthesia in conversion disorder.

6. **Hysterical.** Pain most often relates to head, face, back, and abdomen. No organic cause for pain in evidence.

7. **Pseudoseizures.** Incontinence, loss of motor control, and tongue biting are rare in pseudoseizures; an aura usually is present in organic epilepsy. Look for abnormal electroencephalogram (EEG); however, EEG results are abnormal in 10% to 15% of the normal adult population. Babinski's sign occurs in organic seizure and postictal state but not in conversion seizures.

8. **Schizophrenia.** Thought disorder is present.

9. **Mood disorder.** Depression or mania from examination or history.

10. **Malingering and factitious disorder with physical symptoms.** Difficult to distinguish from conversion, but malingerers are aware that they are faking symptoms and have insight into what they are doing; patients with factitious disorder also are aware that they are faking, but they do so because they want to be patients and be in a hospital.

G. **Course and prognosis.** Tends to be recurrent. Episodes are separated by asymptomatic periods. Major concern is not to dismiss early neurologic symptom that subsequently progresses into full-blown syndrome (e.g., multiple sclerosis may begin with spontaneously remitting diplopia or hemiparesis). Table 16-2 lists factors associated with good and bad prognoses.

H. **Treatment.** Resolution of the conversion disorder symptom is usually spontaneous, although it is probably facilitated by insight-oriented supportive or behavior therapy.

1. **Pharmacologic.** These include benzodiazepines for anxiety and muscular tension; antidepressants or serotonergic agents for obsessive rumination about symptoms.

Psychological. Insight-oriented therapy is useful in helping the patient to understand the dynamic principles and conflicts behind symptoms. Patient learns to accept sexual or aggressive impulses and not to use conversion disorder as a defense. Other modalities include behavior therapy, hypnosis and narcoanalysis.

Table 16-3
Clues that Should Trigger Suspicion of Factitious Disorder

Unusual, dramatic presentation of symptoms that defy conventional medical or psychiatric understanding
Symptoms do not respond appropriately to usual treatment or medications
Emergence of new, unusual symptoms when other symptoms resolve
Eagerness to undergo procedures or testing or to recount symptoms
Reluctance to give access to collateral sources of information (i.e., refusing to sign releases of information or to give contact information for family and friends)
Extensive medical history or evidence of multiple surgeries
Multiple drug allergies
Medical profession
Few visitors
Ability to forecast unusual progression of symptoms or unusual response to treatment

From Dora L. Wang, M.D., Seth Powsner, M.D., and Stuart J. Eisendrath, M.D.

IV. Factitious Disorders

It is defined as intentional report and misrepresentation of symptoms, or self-infliction of physical signs of symptoms, of medical or mental disorders. The only apparent objective is to assume the role of a patient without an external incentive. Hospitalization is often a primary objective and a way of life. The disorders have a compulsive quality, but the behaviors are deliberate and voluntary, even if they cannot be controlled. See Table 16-3. Also known as *Munchausen syndrome*.

A. Epidemiology. Onset is usually in adulthood. It is more common in men than in women. Factitious illness, especially feigned fever, accounts for 5% to 10% of all hospital admissions. More common in health care workers.

B. Etiology. Early real illness coupled with parental abuse or rejection is typical. Patient recreates illness as an adult to gain loving attention from doctors. Can also express masochistic gratification for some patients who want to undergo surgical procedures. Others identify with an important past figure who had psychological or physical illness. No genetic or biologic etiologic factors have been identified.

C. Psychodynamics. Mechanisms of repression, identification with the aggressor, regression, symbolization may be present.

D. Diagnosis, signs, and symptoms

1. **With predominantly physical signs and symptoms.** This includes intentional production of physical symptoms—nausea, vomiting, pain, and seizures. Patients may intentionally put blood in feces or urine, artificially raise body temperature or take insulin to lower blood sugar. Gridiron abdomen sign is the result of scars from multiple surgical operations (Table 16-4).

2. **With predominantly psychological signs and symptoms.** This includes intentional production of psychiatric symptoms—hallucinations, delusions, depression, and bizarre behavior. Patients may make up a story that they suffered major life stress to account for symptoms. *Pseudologia fantastica* consists of making up extravagant lies that the patient

Table 16-4

Presentations of Factitious Disorder with Predominantly Physical Signs and Symptoms with Means of Simulation and Possible Methods of Detection

Presentation	Means of Simulation that Have Been Reported	Possible Methods of Detection
Autoimmune		
Goodpasture's syndrome	False history, adding blood to urine	Bronchoalveolar lavage negative for hemosiderin-laden cells
Systemic lupus erythematosus	Malar rash simulated through cosmetics, feigning joint pain	Negative antinuclear antibody test, removability of rash
Dermatologic		
Burns	Chemical agents such as oven cleaner	Unnatural shape of lesions, streaks left by chemicals, minor injury to fingers
Excoriations	Self-infliction	Found on accessible parts of the body, or a preponderance of left-sided lesions in a right-handed person
Lesions	Injection of exogenous material such as talc, milk, or gasoline	Puncture marks left by needles, discovery of syringes
Endocrine		
Cushing's syndrome	Steroid ingestion	Evidence of exogenous steroid use
Hyperthyroidism	Thyroxine or L-iodothyronine ingestion	The 24-hr I-131 uptake is suppressed in factitious disease and increased in Graves' disease
Hypoglycemia or insulinoma	1. Insulin injection 2. Ingestion of oral hypoglycemics	1. Insulin to C-peptide ratio greater than 1, detection of serum insulin antibodies 2. Serum levels of hypoglycemic medication
Pheochromocytomy	Epinephrine or metaraminol injection	Analysis of urinary catecholamines may reveal epinephrine only or other suspicious findings
Gastrointestinal		
Diarrhea	Phenolphthalein or castor oil ingestion	Testing of stool for laxatives, increased stool weight
Hemoptysis	Contamination of sputum sample, self-induced trauma such as cuts to tongue	Collect specimen under observation, examine mouth
Ulcerative colitis	Laceration of colon with knitting needle	
Hematologic		
Aplastic anemia	Self-administration of chemotherapeutic agents to suppress bone marrow	Hematology/oncology consultation
Anemia	Self-induced phlebotomy	Blood studies
Coagulopathy	Ingestion of warfarin or other anticoagulants	
Infectious disease		
Abdominal abscess	Injection of feces into abdominal wall	Unusual pathogens in microbiology tests
Acquired immuno-deficiency syndrome (AIDS)	False history	Collateral information
Neoplastic		
Cancer	False medical and family history, shaving head to simulate chemotherapy	Collateral information, examination
Neurologic		
Paraplegia or quadriplegia	Feigning, fictitious history	Imaging studies, electromyography
Seizures	Feigning, fictitious history	Video electroencephalogram

(continued)

254 POCKET HANDBOOK OF CLINICAL PSYCHIATRY

Table 16-4
Presentations of Factitious Disorder with Predominantly Physical Signs and Symptoms with Means of Simulation and Possible Methods of Detection (Continued)

Presentation	Means of Simulation that Have Been Reported	Possible Methods of Detection
Obstetrics/gynecology		
Antepartum hemorrhage	Vaginal puncture wounds, use of fake blood	Examination, test blood
Ectopic pregnancy	Feigning abdominal pain while self-injecting human chorionic gonadotropin	Ultrasound
Menorrhagia	Using stolen blood	Type blood
Placenta previa	Intravaginal use of hat pin	Examination
Premature labor	Feigned uterine contractions, manipulation of tocodynamometer	Examination
Premature rupture of membranes	Voiding urine into vagina	Examine fluid
Trophoblastic disease	Addition of human chorionic gonadotropin to urine	
Vaginal bleeding	Self-mutilation with fingernails, nail files, bleach, knives, tweezers, nutpicks, glass, pencils	Examination
Vaginal discharge	Applying cigarette ash to underwear	Examination
Systemic		
Fever	Warming thermometer against a lightbulb or other heat source, drinking hot fluids, friction from mouth or anal sphincter, false recordings, injection of pyrogens such as feces, vaccines, thyroid hormone, or tetanus toxoid	Simultaneous taking of temperature from two different locals (orally and rectally), recording the temperature of freshly voided urine, the appearance of cool skin despite high thermometer readings, normal white blood cell count, unusually high or inconsistent temperatures
Urinary		
Bacteriuria	Contamination of urethra or specimen	Unusual pathogen
Hematuria	Contamination of specimen with blood or meat, warfarin ingestion, foreign bodies in bladder (pins)	Collect specimen under observation
Proteinuria	Inserting egg protein into urethra	
Stones	Feigning of renal colic pain, bringing in stones made of exogenous materials or inserting them into urethra	Pathology report

Table by Dora L. Wang, M.D., Seth Powsner, M.D., and Stuart J. Eisendrath, M.D.

believes. Substance abuse, especially of opioids, is common in both types (Table 16-5).

3. **With combined physical and psychological signs and symptoms.** This includes intentional production of both physical and psychological symptoms.

4. **Factitious disorder not otherwise specified.** Includes disorders that do not meet criteria for factitious disorder (e.g., factitious disorder by

Table 16-5
Presentations in Factitious Disorder with Predominantly Psychological Signs and Symptoms

Bereavement	Eating Disorder
Depression	Amnesia
Posttraumatic stress disorder	Substance-related disorder
Pain disorder	Paraphilias
Psychosis	Hypersomnia
Bipolar I disorder	Transsexualism
Dissociative identity disorder	

Adapted from Feldman MD, Eisendrath SJ. *The Spectrum of Factitious Disorders.* Washington, DC: American Psychiatric Press; 1996.

proxy—intentionally feigning symptoms in another person who is under the person's care so as to assume the sick role indirectly). *Factitious disorder by proxy* is most common in mothers who feign an illness in their child but accounts for fewer than 1,000 of the almost 3 million cases of child abuse reported annually.

E. Differential diagnosis

1. **Physical illness.** Physical examination and laboratory workup should be performed; results will be negative. The nursing staff should observe carefully for deliberate elevation of temperature, alteration of body fluids.

2. **Somatoform disorder.** Symptoms are voluntary in factitious disorder and not caused by unconscious or symbolic factors. *La belle indifférence* is not present in factitious disorder. Hypochondriacs do not want to undergo extensive tests or surgery.

3. **Malingering.** It is a difficult differential diagnosis to make. Malingerers have specific goals (e.g., insurance payments, avoidance of jail term). Evidence of an intrapsychic need to maintain the sick role (e.g., to satisfy dependency needs) is more characteristic of factitious disorder.

4. **Ganser's syndrome.** Found in prisoners who give approximate answers to questions and talk past the point. Classified as a dissociative disorder not otherwise specified.

5. **Personality disorder.** Antisocial personalities are manipulative but do not usually feign illness or agree to invasive procedures or hospitalization. Borderline personalities usually have more chaotic lifestyles, parasuicidal behavior, and more disturbed interpersonal relationships.

F. Course and prognosis. Course is usually chronic. Begins in adulthood, but onset may be earlier. Frequent consultation with doctors and history of hospitalizations as patient seeks repeated care with high risk for substance abuse over time. Prognosis improves if associated depression or anxiety is present that responds to pharmacotherapy. Risk for death if patient undergoes multiple life-threatening surgical procedures.

G. Treatment. Avoid unnecessary laboratory tests or medical procedures. Confront patient with diagnosis of factitious disorder and feigned symptoms. Patients rarely enter psychotherapy because of poor motivation;

Table 16-6
Guidelines for Management and Treatment of Factitious Disorder

Active pursuit of a prompt diagnosis can minimize the risk of morbidity and mortality.
Minimize harm. Avoid unnecessary tests and procedures, especially if invasive. Treat according to clinical judgment, keeping in mind that subjective complaints may be deceptive.
Regular interdisciplinary meetings to reduce conflict and splitting among staff. Manage staff countertransference.
Consider facilitating healing by using the double-bind technique or face-saving behavioral strategies, such as self-hypnosis or biofeedback.
Steer the patient toward psychiatric treatment in an empathic, nonconfrontational, face-saving manner. Avoid aggressive direct confrontation.
Treat underlying psychiatric disturbances, such as Axis I disorders and Axis II disorders. In psychotherapy, address coping strategies and emotional conflicts.
Appoint a primary care provider as a gatekeeper for all medical and psychiatric treatment.
Consider involving risk management professionals and bioethicists from an early point.
Consider appointing a guardian for medical and psychiatric decisions.
Consider prosecution for fraud, as a behavioral disincentive.

however, working alliance with doctor is possible over time, and patient may gain insight into behavior. Good management, however, is more likely than a cure. A data-bank of patients with repeated hospitalizations for factitious illness is available in some areas of the United States.

Psychopharmacologic therapy is useful for associated anxiety or depression. Substance abuse should be treated if present.

Contact child welfare services if a child is at risk (e.g., with factitious disorder by proxy).

Guidelines for management and treatment are detailed in Tables 16-6 and 16-7.

V. Pain Disorder

Pain disorder is a preoccupation with pain in the absence of physical disease to account for its intensity. It does not follow a neuroanatomic distribution. Stress and conflict may closely correlate with the initiation or exacerbation of the pain.

Table 16-7
Interventions for Pediatric Factitious Disorder by Proxy

A pediatrician should serve as "gatekeeper" for medical care utilization. All other physicians should coordinate care with the gatekeeper.
Child protective services should be informed whenever a child is harmed.
Family psychotherapy and/or individual psychotherapy should be instituted for the perpetrating parent and the child.
Health insurance companies, school officials, and other nonmedical sources should be asked to report possible medical use to the physician gatekeeper. Permission of a parent or of child protective services must first be obtained.
The possibility should be considered of admitting the child to an inpatient or partial hospital setting to facilitate diagnostic monitoring of symptoms and to institute a treatment plan.
The child may require placement in another family. The perpetrating parent may need to be removed from the child through criminal prosecution and incarceration.

From Dora L. Wang, M.D., Seth Powsner, M.D., and Stuart J. Eisendrath, M.D.

A. **Epidemiology.** Onset can be at any age, but especially in the 30s and 40s. It is more common in women than in men and some evidence of first-degree biologic relatives having a high incidence of pain, depression, and alcoholism. The 6-month and lifetime prevalence is approximately 5% and 12%.

B. **Etiology**

1. **Behavioral.** Pain behaviors are reinforced when rewarded (e.g., pain symptoms may become intense when followed by attentive behavior from others or avoidance of disliked activity).

2. **Interpersonal.** Pain is a way to manipulate and gain advantage in a relationship (e.g., to stabilize a fragile marriage).

3. **Biologic.** Some patients may have pain disorder, rather than another mental disorder, because of sensory and limbic structural or chemical abnormalities that predispose them to pain.

4. **Psychodynamics.** Patients may be symbolically expressing an intrapsychic conflict through the body. Persons may unconsciously regard emotional pain as weak and displace it to the body. Pain can be a method to obtain love or can be used as a punishment. Defense mechanisms involved in the disorder include displacement, substitution, and repression.

C. **Diagnosis.** The disorder must have a psychological factor judged to be significantly involved in the pain symptoms and their ramifications (emotional distress and social or occupational impairment).

   Major depressive disorder is present in about 25% to 50% of patients with pain disorder, and dysthymic disorder or depressive disorder symptoms are reported in 60% to 100% of the patients.

D. **Differential diagnosis.** Physical pain can be difficult to distinguish from psychogenic pain, as the two are not mutually exclusive.

1. **Physical pain due to a medical condition.** Difficult to distinguish since physical pain is also sensitive to emotional and situational factors. Pain that does not vary, wax, or wane or is not relieved by analgesics is more often psychogenic. Absence of a medical or surgical condition to account for pain is an important factor.

2. **Hypochondriasis.** Tend to have more symptoms than patients with pain disorder.

3. **Conversion disorder.** Usually have more motor and sensory disturbances than pain disorder.

4. **Course and prognosis.** Variable course but tends to be chronic. Patients with comorbid depression have poor prognosis as do patients with secondary gain (e.g., litigation).

E. **Treatment**

1. **Pharmacotherapy.** Antidepressants, particularly selective serotonin reuptake inhibitors (SSRIs) and serotonin norepinephrine reuptake inhibitors (SNRIs), are useful. Tricyclics are also used but have more side effects.

   Augmentation with small doses of amphetamine may benefit some patients, but dosages must be monitored carefully. Avoid opioids for analgesia because of risk of abuse.

2. **Psychotherapy.** Psychodynamic therapy is of use in motivated patients. Cognitive therapy has proved beneficial in altering negative life attitudes. Other approaches include hypnosis, biofeedback acupuncture, and massage.

 CLINICAL HINT:
Do not confront patients with comments such as "This is all in your head." For the patient, the pain is real. An entry point is to examine how the pain affects the patient's life, not whether the pain is imaginary.

VI. Other Specified or Unspecified Somatic Symptom Disorder

This DSM-5 category is used to describe conditions characterized by one or more unexplained physical symptoms of at least 6 months' duration, which are below the threshold for a diagnosis of somatic symptom disorder. The symptoms are not caused, or fully explained, by another medical, psychiatric, or substance abuse disorder, and they cause clinical significant distress or impairment.

Two types of symptom patterns may be seen: those involving the autonomic nervous system and those involving sensations of fatigue or weakness. In *autonomic arousal disorder,* symptoms are limited to bodily functions innervated by the autonomic nervous system and include cardiovascular, respiratory, gastrointestinal, urogenital, and dermatologic systems. Other patients complain of mental and physical fatigue, physical weakness, exhaustion, and inability to perform everyday activities. Other conditions included in this unspecified category of somatic symptom disorder are pseudocyesis and conditions that may not have met the 6-month criterion of the other somatic symptom disorders.

For more detailed discussion of this topic, see Chapter 18, Somatic Symptom and Related Disorders, p. 1827, and Chapter 19, Factitious Disorder, p. 1846 in CTP/X.

17

Personality Disorders

I. General Introduction

A. Definition. Personality disorder is an enduring pattern of behavior and inner experiences that deviates significantly from the individual's cultural standards; is rigidly pervasive; has an onset in adolescence or early adulthood; is stable through time; leads to unhappiness and impairment; and manifests in at least two of the following four areas: cognition, affectivity, interpersonal function, or impulse control. When personality traits are rigid and maladaptive and produce functional impairment or subjective distress, a personality disorder may be diagnosed. See Table 17-1.

B. Classification. *DSM-5* groups the personality disorders into three clusters.

1. **Cluster A.** The *odd and eccentric cluster* consists of the paranoid, schizoid, and schizotypal personality disorder. These disorders involve the use of fantasy and projection and are associated with a tendency toward psychotic thinking. Patients may have a biologic vulnerability toward cognitive disorganization when stressed.

2. **Cluster B.** The *dramatic, emotional, and erratic cluster* includes the histrionic, narcissistic, antisocial, and borderline personality disorders. These disorders involve the use of dissociation, denial, splitting, and acting out. Mood disorders may be common.

3. **Cluster C.** The *anxious or fearful cluster* includes the avoidant, dependent, and obsessive-compulsive personality disorders. These disorders involve the use of isolation, passive aggression, and hypochondriasis.

4. Personality disorder traits; individuals frequently exhibit traits that are not limited to a single personality disorder. When a patient meets the criteria for more than one personality disorder, clinicians should diagnose each; this circumstance is not uncommon.

II. Odd and Eccentric Cluster

A. Paranoid personality disorder

1. **Definition.** Characterized by their intense distrust and suspiciousness of others, patients with paranoid personality disorder are often hostile, irritable, hypersensitive, envious, or angry, and will not take responsibly for their own actions, often projecting such responsibility onto others. They may be bigots, injustice collectors, pathologically jealous spouses, or litigious cranks.

2. **Epidemiology**

   a. The prevalence is 0.5% to 2.5% in the general population; 10% to 30% for inpatients; and 2% to 10% for outpatients.

   b. The prevalence is higher among minorities, immigrants, and the deaf.

Table 17-1
General Personality Disorder

- A fixed behavioral pattern at odds with cultural norms that affects at least 2 of:
  - Cognitive perceptions of the world and oneself
  - Emotional/affective response
  - Social interaction
  - Impulse control
- This pattern must have been detectable before adulthood
  (In children and adolescents, features must have been present for at least 1 year)
  (Antisocial personality disorder cannot be diagnosed before age 18)

    c. The incidence is increased in relatives of patients with schizophrenia and delusional disorders.

    d. The disorder is more common in men than in women.

3. Etiology

    a. A genetic component is established.

    b. Nonspecific early family difficulties are often present. Histories of childhood abuse are common.

4. Psychodynamics

    a. The classic defenses are projection, denial, and rationalization.

    b. Shame is a prominent feature.

    c. The superego is projected onto authority.

    d. Unresolved separation and autonomy issues are a factor.

5. Diagnosis. The critical feature of such patients is a pervasive and unwarranted tendency to perceive the actions of others as deliberately demeaning or threatening. This tendency begins by early adulthood. Patients expect to be exploited or harmed by others and frequently dispute the loyalty and trustworthiness of family, friends, or associates without justification. These patients tend to be reluctant to confide. They have a formal manner, can exhibit considerable muscle tension, and may scan the environment. They are often humorless and serious. Although the premises of their arguments may be false at times, their speech is goal directed and logical. Projection is employed, and they can be quite prejudiced. Some are involved in extremist groups. In marriage and sexual relationships, they are often pathologically jealous and question the fidelity of their partners. They tend to internalize their own emotions and use the defense of projection. They attribute to others the impulses and thoughts that they are unable to accept themselves. Ideas of reference and logically defended beliefs are common. See Table 17-2.

6. Differential diagnosis

    a. Delusional disorder. The patient has fixed delusions.

    b. Paranoid schizophrenia. The patient has hallucinations and a formal thought disorder.

    c. Schizoid, borderline, and antisocial personality disorders. The patient does not show similar active involvement with others and is less stable.

    d. Substance abuse (e.g., stimulants) can produce paranoid features.

Table 17-2
Paranoid Personality Disorder

- A pattern of skepticism toward others and paranoid suspicion of their motives, as evidenced by ≥4 of:
  - Suspicion that others are out to trick or take advantage of oneself
  - Obsession with friends' infidelity
  - Refusal to trust others because of fear that they will switch loyalties
  - Constant detection of covert and damaging interpretations of innocuous matters
  - Inability to set aside grievances and snubs
  - Eagerness to detect (imagined) character assaults
  - Constant mistrust of partner's sexual fidelity
- Can occur alongside schizophrenia, but must suffuse the personality even during nonpsychotic episodes

7. **Course and prognosis.** In some patients the disorder is lifelong, while in others it is a harbinger of schizophrenia. In general, patients with paranoid personality disorder have problems working and living with others. Occupational and marital problems are common.

8. **Treatment**

   a. **Psychotherapy.** Psychotherapy is the treatment of choice. Therapists should be straightforward and remember that trust and toleration of intimacy are difficult areas for such patients. Group therapy is not a method of choice with these patients, although it can be useful in improving social skills and diminishing suspiciousness.

   b. **Pharmacotherapy.** Pharmacotherapy is useful in dealing with agitation and anxiety. In most cases, an antianxiety agent such as diazepam (Valium) or clonazepam (Klonopin) is sufficient. It may sometimes be necessary to use an antipsychotic, such as olanzapine (Zyprexa) or haloperidol (Haldol), in small dosages and for brief periods to manage agitation and quasi-delusional thinking. The antipsychotic drug pimozide (Orap) has been successfully used to reduce paranoid ideation in some patients.

B. **Schizoid personality disorder**

1. **Definition.** Often perceived as eccentric and introverted, patients with schizoid personality disorder are characterized by their isolated lifestyles and their lack of interest in social interaction.

2. **Epidemiology**

   a. This disorder may affect 7.5% of the general population.

   b. The incidence is increased among family members of schizophrenic and schizotypal personality disorder probands.

   c. The incidence is greater among men than among women, with a possible ratio of 2:1.

3. **Etiology**

   a. Genetic factors are likely.

   b. A history of disturbed early family relationships often is elicited.

4. **Psychodynamics**

   a. Social inhibition is pervasive.

   b. Social needs are repressed to ward off aggression.

Table 17-3
Schizoid Personality Disorder

- A temperament characterized by social disengagement as well as constricted affect, demonstrated more fully by ≥4 of:
  - Distaste for close relations, including family
  - Habitual preference to be alone
  - Asexuality
  - Lack of hobbies
  - Absence of friends or close relations with nonrelatives
  - Inattention to the reactions of others
  - Emotional apathy
- Can occur alongside schizophrenia, but must suffuse the personality even during nonpsychotic episodes

5. **Diagnosis.** These patients are ill at ease with others and may show poor eye contact. Their affect is often constricted, aloof, or inappropriately serious. Humor may be adolescent or off the mark. They may give short answers, avoid spontaneous speech, and use occasional odd metaphors. They may be fascinated with inanimate objects or metaphysical constructs, or interested in mathematics, astronomy, or philosophical movements. Their sensorium is intact, their memory functions well, and their proverb interpretations are appropriately abstract. See Table 17-3.

6. **Differential diagnosis**
   a. **Paranoid personality disorder.** The patient is involved with others, has a history of aggressive behavior, and projects his or her feelings onto others.
   b. **Schizotypal personality disorder.** The patient exhibits oddities and eccentricities of manners, has schizophrenic relatives, and may not have a successful work history.
   c. **Avoidant personality disorder.** The patient is isolated but wants to be involved with others.
   d. **Schizophrenia.** The patient exhibits thought disorder and delusional thinking.

7. **Course and prognosis.** Onset of this disorder usually occurs in early childhood. Course is long lasting, but not necessarily lifelong. Complications of delusional disorder, schizophrenia, other psychoses, or depression may develop.

8. **Treatment**
   a. **Psychotherapy.** Unlike paranoid personality disorder, schizoid patients are often introspective, and they may become devoted, if distant, psychotherapy patients. As trust builds, the patient may reveal a plethora of fantasies, imaginary friends, and fears of unbearable dependence—even of merging with the therapist. In group therapy, schizoid patients may be silent for long periods of time, but they do not completely lack involvement. The other group members become important to the patient as time goes by and may become the patient's only social contacts.

     b. Pharmacotherapy. Small dosages of antipsychotics, antidepressants, and psychostimulants have been effective in some patients. Serotonergic agents may make patients less sensitive to rejection. Benzodiazepines may be of use to diminish interpersonal anxiety.

C. Schizotypal personality disorder

  1. Definition. Persons with schizotypal personality disorder are characterized by magical thinking, peculiar notations, ideas of reference, illusions, and derealization. Such individuals are perceived as strikingly odd or strange, even to laypersons.

  2. Epidemiology

    a. The prevalence of this disorder is 3%.

    b. The prevalence is increased in families of schizophrenic probands. A higher concordance in monozygotic twins has been shown.

    c. The sex ratio is unknown; however, it is frequently diagnosed in women with fragile X syndrome.

  3. Etiology. Etiologic models of schizophrenia may apply. See Chapter 8.

  4. Psychodynamics. Dynamics of magical thinking, splitting, isolation of affect.

  5. Diagnosis. Schizotypal personality disorder is diagnosed on the basis of the patient's oddities of thinking, behavior, and appearance. Taking the history of such patients may be difficult due to their bizarre way of communicating. These patients may be superstitious or claim powers of clairvoyance and may believe that they have other special powers of thought and insight. They may be isolated and have few friends due to their inability to maintain interpersonal relationships and their inappropriate actions. While under stress, patients may decompensate and show psychotic symptoms. See Table 17-4.

  6. Differential diagnosis

    a. Paranoid personality disorder. The patient is suspicious and guarded, but lacks odd behavior.

Table 17-4
Schizotypal Personality Disorder

- A temperament characterized by social deficits stemming from odd behavior and thinking, ultimately hampering close friendships and demonstrated by ≥5 of:
  - Ideas but not delusions of reference (suspicions that real world events revolve around or are targeting oneself)
  - Strange ideas that clash even with cultural superstitions
  - Extraordinary or extrasensory perceptions
  - Abnormal logic or language
  - Paranoia
  - Odd affect
  - Outlandish or otherwise bizarre behavior and appearance
  - Social isolation
  - Social anxiety that is irremediable because of paranoia
- Can occur alongside schizophrenia, but must suffuse the personality even during nonpsychotic episodes

   b. **Schizoid personality disorder.** The patient has no particular eccentricities.
   c. **Borderline personality disorder.** The patient shows emotional instability, intensity, and impulsiveness.
   d. **Schizophrenia.** The patient's reality testing is lost.
7. **Course and prognosis.** Up to 10% of patients commit suicide. Schizophrenia can develop in some patients. Prognosis is guarded.
8. **Treatment**
   a. **Psychotherapy.** Treatment of patients with schizotypal personality disorder is similar to that of schizoid patients. Patients have eccentric patterns of thinking and some may be involved in cults, strange religious practices, and the occult. Clinicians must not appear skeptical nor ridicule or judge schizotypal patients for these beliefs.
   b. **Pharmacotherapy.** In dealing with ideas of reference, illusions, and other symptoms, antipsychotic agents may be useful and can be combined with psychotherapy. Antidepressants may be used when depression is present.

III. Dramatic, Impulsive, and Erratic Cluster
A. Antisocial personality disorder
1. **Definition.** Persons with antisocial personality disorder are characterized by their inability to conform to the social norms which govern individual behavior. Such persons are impulsive, egocentric, irresponsible, and cannot tolerate frustration. Patients with antisocial personality disorder reject discipline and authority and have an underdeveloped conscience. It should be noted that though this disorder is associated with criminality; it is not synonyms with it.
2. **Epidemiology**
   a. The prevalence is 3% in men (it may be as high as 7%) and 1% in women in the general population. In prison populations, it may be as high as 75%.
   b. Antisocial personality disorder, somatization disorder, and alcoholism cluster in some families. The disorder is five times more common among first-degree relatives of men than among controls.
   c. The disorder is more common in lower socioeconomic groups.
   d. Predisposing conditions include attention-deficit/hyperactivity disorder (ADHD) and conduct disorder.
3. **Etiology**
   a. Adoptive studies demonstrate that genetic factors are involved in this disorder.
   b. Brain damage or dysfunction is a feature of this disorder, which can be secondary to such conditions as perinatal brain injury, head trauma, and encephalitis.
   c. Histories of parental abandonment or abuse are very common. Repeated, arbitrary, or harsh punishment by parents is thought to be a factor.

4. Psychodynamics

  a. Patients with this disorder are impulse-ridden, with associated ego deficits in planning and judgment.

  b. Superego deficits or lacunae are present; conscience is primitive or poorly developed.

  c. Object relational difficulties are significant, with a failure in empathy, love, and basic trust.

  d. Aggressive features are prominent.

  e. Associated features are sadomasochism, narcissism, and depression.

5. Diagnosis. Patients with antisocial personality disorder can fool the most experienced clinician. They may appear composed and credible, but beneath the façade lies tension, hostility, irritability, and rage. A stress interview, one where patients are vigorously confronted with inconsistencies in their histories, may be needed to reveal the pathology. A diagnostic workup should include a thorough neurologic examination. Patients often show abnormal electroencephalogram (EEG) results and soft neurologic signs suggestive of minimal brain damage in childhood. Typical experiences beginning in childhood include lying, truancy, running away from home, thefts, fights, substance abuse, and illegal activities. Promiscuity, spouse abuse, child abuse, and drunk driving are common. Patients lack remorse for their actions and appear to lack a conscience. See Table 17-5.

6. Differential diagnosis

  a. Adult antisocial behavior. The patient does not meet all the criteria of antisocial personality disorder.

  b. Substance use disorders. The patient may exhibit antisocial behavior as a consequence of substance abuse and dependence.

  c. Mental retardation. The patient may demonstrate antisocial behavior as a consequence of impaired intellect and judgment.

  d. Psychoses. The patient may engage in antisocial behavior as a consequence of psychotic delusions.

  e. Borderline personality disorder. The patient often attempts suicide and exhibits self-loathing and intense, ambivalent attachments.

  f. Narcissistic personality disorder. The patient is law-abiding.

Table 17-5
Antisocial Personality Disorder

- A neglect of and indifference to others' concerns that pervades all personal relations and is demonstrated by ≥3 of:
  - Disregard for social customs and rules culminating in lawbreaking
  - Mendacity
  - Carelessness and lack of premeditated behavior
  - Combativeness and a pattern of brawls
  - Inattentiveness to safety
  - Inability to uphold one's obligations
  - Merciless and unrepentant conduct
- Must be in a person at least 18 years old who displayed behavior consistent with conduct disorder before the age of 15

g. **Personality change secondary to a general medical condition.** The patient has had a different premorbid personality or shows features of an organic disorder.

h. **ADHD.** Cognitive difficulties and impulse dyscontrol are present.

7. **Course and prognosis.** The prognosis of antisocial personality disorder varies. The condition often significantly improves after early or middle adulthood. Complications include death by violence, substance abuse, suicide, physical injury, legal and financial difficulties, and depressive disorders.

8. **Treatment**

a. **Psychotherapy.** Psychotherapy is often difficult if not impossible. It improves if the patient is institutionalized so that they cannot act out. Self-help groups, especially with other antisocial personalities, are often useful. Firm limits are crucial before treatment can begin. Clinicians must deal with patients' self-destructive behavior. They must frustrate the patient's desire to run from honest human encounters and overcome the patient's fear of intimacy. In doing so, therapists face the challenge of separating control from punishment and of separating the need to be confrontational from the patient's unconscious fear of rejection.

b. **Pharmacotherapy.** Pharmacotherapy is used to deal with symptoms such as anxiety, anger, and depression, but drugs must be used judiciously due to the risk of substance abuse. If the patient exhibits evidence of ADHD, psychostimulants such as methylphenidate (Ritalin) may be useful. There have been attempts to alter catecholamine metabolism with drugs and to control impulsive behavior with antiepileptic drugs such as carbamazepine (Tegretol) or valproate (Depakote), especially in cases of abnormal wave forms on an EEG. β-Adrenergics have been used to reduce aggression.

B. **Borderline personality disorder**

1. **Definition.** Patients with borderline personality disorder are literally on the border between neurosis and psychosis. They exhibit extraordinarily unstable mood, affect, behavior, object relations, and self-image. Suicide attempts and acts of self-mutilation are common occurrences among borderline patients. These individuals are very impulsive, and suffer from identity problems as well as feelings of emptiness and boredom. Borderline personality disorder has also been called *ambulatory schizophrenia, as-if personality, pseudoneurotic schizophrenia,* and *psychotic character disorder.*

2. **Epidemiology**

a. The prevalence of borderline personality disorder is about 2% of the general population, 10% of outpatients, 20% of inpatients, and 30% to 60% of patients with personality disorders.

b. It is more common in women than in men.

c. Of these patients, 90% have one other psychiatric diagnosis, and 40% have two.

    d. The prevalence of mood and substance-related disorders and antisocial personality disorder in families is increased.

    e. The disorder is five times more common among relatives of probands with the disorder. The prevalence of borderline personality disorder is increased in the mothers of borderline patients.

3. Etiology

    a. Brain damage may be present and represent perinatal brain injury, encephalitis, head injury, and other brain disorders.

    b. Histories of physical and sexual abuse, abandonment, or overinvolvement are the rule.

4. Psychodynamics

    a. Splitting. The patient divides persons into those who like and those who hate the patient, and into those who are all "good" and all "bad." These feelings are changeable and can become a problem for a treatment team managing a patient.

    b. Primitive idealization. The patient views others just as in splitting but with continuing idealization and instead blames himself.

    c. Projective identification. The patient attributes idealized positive or negative features to another, then seeks to engage the other in various interactions that confirm the patient's belief. The patient tries, unconsciously, to induce the therapist to play the projected role.

    d. The patient has both intense aggressive needs and intense object hunger, often alternating.

    e. The patient has a marked fear of abandonment.

    f. The rapprochement subphase of separation–Individuation (theory of M. Mahler) is unresolved; object constancy is impaired. This results in a failure of internal structuralization and control.

    g. Turning against the self. self-hate, self-loathing—is prominent.

    h. Generalized ego dysfunction results in identity disturbance.

5. Diagnosis. Patients with borderline personality disorder are marked by their pervasive and excessive instability of affects, self-image, and interpersonal relationships and their distinct impulsivity. They tend to have micropsychotic episodes, often with paranoia or transient dissociative symptoms. Self-destructive, self-mutilating, or suicidal gestures, threats, or acts occur frequently. They are impulsive in regard to money and sex and engage in substance abuse, reckless driving, or binge eating. They may show shortened rapid eye movement (REM) latency and sleep continuity disturbances, abnormal dexamethasone suppression test (DST) results, and abnormal thyrotropin-releasing hormone (TRH) test results. Pananxiety and chaotic sexuality are also common features. Patients with borderline personality disorder always appear to be in a state of crisis. Mood swings are common. See Table 17-6.

6. Differential diagnosis

    a. Psychotic disorder. Impaired reality testing persists.

    b. Mood disorders. The mood disturbance is usually nonreactive. Major depressive disorder with atypical features is often a difficult differential

Table 17-6
Borderline Personality Disorder

- Temperamental instability of relationships and self-concept marked by ≥5 of:
  - Desperate attempts to avoid desertion or abandonment
  - Propensity to form relationships that whipsaw between positive and negative extremes
  - Unsteady and negative self-image
  - Impetuosity to a self-damaging extent
  - Habitual suicidal behavior or expressed gestures
  - Emotional lability
  - Emotional vacuity
  - Uncontrollable temper
  - Dissociation or paranoia

diagnosis. At times, only a treatment trial will tell. Atypical patients often have sustained episodes of depression, however.

   c. Personality change secondary to a general medical condition. Results of testing for medical illness are positive.

   d. Schizotypal personality disorder. The affective features are less severe.

   e. Antisocial personality disorder. The defects in conscience and attachment ability are more severe.

   f. Histrionic personality disorder. Suicide and self-mutilation are less common. The patient tends to have more stable interpersonal relationships.

   g. Narcissistic personality disorder. Identity formation is more stable.

   h. Dependent personality disorder. Attachments are stable.

   i. Paranoid personality disorder. Suspiciousness is more extreme and consistent.

7. Course and prognosis. Prognosis is variable; some improvement may occur in later years. Suicide, self-injury, mood disorders, somatoform disorders, psychoses, substance abuse, and sexual disorders are possible complications.

8. Treatment. Patients with borderline personality disorder can be problematic. The patient may have "affect storms" and require considerable attention.

   a. Psychotherapy. Psychotherapy is the treatment of choice, although it is difficult for both the therapist and the patient. Patients easily regress, act out their impulses, and show labile or fixed negative or positive transferences, which are difficult to analyze. Projective identification and splitting may also make treatment problematic; therefore, a reality-oriented approach is preferred to exploration of the unconscious. Behavior therapy may be useful to control impulses and angry outbursts and to reduce sensitivity to criticism and rejection. Social skills training is useful to improve their interpersonal behavior. Dialectical behavior therapy may be used in cases of parasuicidal behavior such as frequent cutting. Intensive psychotherapy in the hospital setting is useful on both an individual basis and a group basis.

    b. Pharmacotherapy. Antipsychotics are useful in controlling anger, hostility, and brief psychotic episodes. Antidepressants are useful in improving depressed mood. Monoamine oxidase inhibitors (MAOIs) may be effective in modulating impulse behavior. Benzodiazepines, particularly alprazolam (Xanax), can be helpful with anxiety and depression, but some patients show a disinhibition with these drugs. Anticonvulsants such as carbamazepine (Tegretol) may improve global functioning. Serotonergic agents such as fluoxetine (Prozac) have proved to be useful.

C. Histrionic personality disorder

  1. Definition. Characterized by the flamboyant, dramatic, excitable and overreactive behavior, persons with histrionic person personality disorder are intent on gaining attention. They tend to be immature, dependent, and are often seductive. These individuals have difficulty maintaining long lasting relationships.

  2. Epidemiology

    a. The prevalence of histrionic personality disorder is 2% to 3%. Of the patients in treatment, 10% to 15% are reported to have this disorder.

    b. The prevalence is greater in women than in men, but the disorder is probably underdiagnosed in men.

    c. This disorder may be associated with somatization disorder, mood disorders, and alcohol use.

  3. Etiology

    a. Early interpersonal difficulties may have been resolved by dramatic behavior.

    b. Distant or stern father with a seductive mother may be a pattern.

  4. Psychodynamics

    a. Fantasy in "playing a role," with emotionality and a dramatic style, is typical.

    b. Common defenses include repression, regression, identification, somatization, conversion, dissociation, denial, and externalization.

    c. A faulty identification with the same-sex parent and an ambivalent and seductive relationship with the opposite-sex parent are often noted.

    d. Fixation at the early genital level.

    e. Prominent oral traits.

    f. Fear of sexuality, despite overt seductiveness.

  5. Diagnosis. Patients with histrionic personality disorder are often cooperative and eager to be helped. Gestures and dramatic punctuation in their conversation are common and their language is colorful. Cognitive test results are usually normal; however, a lack of perseverance may be shown on arithmetic or concentration tasks. Emotionality may also be shallow or insincere and patients may be forgetful of affect-laden material. They tend to exaggerate thoughts and feelings to get attention, and display temper tantrums, tears, and accusations when they do not get the attention they crave. They constantly need reassurance and their relationships tend to be superficial. See Table 17-7.

Table 17-7
Histrionic Personality Disorder

- A thoroughgoing pattern of unrestrained sentimentality and desire for the spotlight as manifest by ≥5 of:
  - Unease when not in the spotlight
  - Tendency to fraternize in a sexually suggestive manner
  - Fickle and superficial emotionality
  - Use or enhancement of physical features to attract others' notice
  - Hazy, sketchy speech
  - Melodramatic emotional expression
  - Impressionability
  - Skewed perception of the intimacy of ordinary relationships

   6. **Differential diagnosis**

      a. Borderline personality disorder. More overt despair and suicidal and self-mutilating features; the disorders can coexist.

      b. Somatization disorder. Physical complaints predominate.

      c. Conversion disorder. Physical symptoms are prominent.

      d. Dependent personality disorder. The emotional flamboyance is lacking.

   7. **Course and prognosis.** The course is variable. Patients often show fewer symptoms with age; however, because they lack the energy of earlier years, the decrease in symptoms may be more apparent than real. Possible complications are somatization disorders, conversion disorders, dissociative disorders, sexual disorders, mood disorders, and substance abuse.

   8. **Treatment**

      a. Psychotherapy. Histrionic patients are often unaware of their real feelings, so clarification of their feelings is essential to the therapeutic process. Treatment is usually individual psychotherapy, insight oriented or supportive, depending on ego strength. The focus is on the patient's deeper feelings and use of superficial drama as a defense against them.

      b. Pharmacotherapy. Pharmacotherapy can be adjunctive when symptoms are targeted. Antidepressants can be used for depression and somatic complaints. Antianxiety agents are useful for anxiety. Antipsychotics can be used for derealization and illusions.

  D. Narcissistic personality disorder

   1. **Definition.** Persistent pattern of grandiosity, a heightened sense of self-importance, preoccupation with fantasies of ultimate success, exaggerated responses to criticism, an overconcern with self-esteem and self-image, and disturbance in interpersonal relationships.

   2. **Epidemiology**

      a. The established prevalence is less than 1% in the general population.

      b. The prevalence is 2% to 16% in the clinical population.

      c. More common in men than in women.

      d. A familial transmission is suspected.

   3. **Etiology.** A commonly cited factor is a failure in maternal empathy, with early rejection or loss.

Table 17-8
Narcissistic Personality Disorder

- A temperament defined by heightened sense of self, the seeking of reverence from others, and callousness marked by ≥5 of:
  - Exaggerated sense of self-worth
  - Imagined possession of extreme power, intelligence, glamour, or other typically beneficial qualities
  - Abiding sense of exclusivity
  - A need for adulation or adoration
  - A sense of privilege
  - Selfish use of others
  - Callousness and ignorance of others
  - Jealousness of others
  - Hubris

4. **Psychodynamics.** Grandiosity and empathic failure defend against primitive aggression. The grandiosity is commonly viewed as a compensation for a sense of inferiority.

5. **Diagnosis.** Patients with narcissistic personality disorder have a grandiose sense of self-importance, whether in fantasy or in behavior. They have a great need for admiration, lack empathy, and often have chronic, intense envy. They handle criticism or defeat poorly; they either become enraged or depressed. Fragile self-esteem and interpersonal relationships are evident. Common stresses produced by their behavior are interpersonal difficulties, occupational problems, rejection, and loss. See Table 17-8.

6. **Differential diagnosis**
   a. **Antisocial personality disorder.** The patient overtly disregards the law and the rights of others.
   b. **Paranoid schizophrenia.** The patient has overt delusions.
   c. **Borderline personality disorder.** The patient shows greater emotionality, greater instability.
   d. **Histrionic personality disorder.** The patient displays more emotion.

7. **Course and prognosis.** The disorder can be chronic and difficult to treat. Aging is handled poorly because it is a narcissistic injury; therefore, they are more vulnerable to midlife crises. Possible complications include mood disorders, transient psychoses, somatoform disorders, and substance use disorders. The overall prognosis is guarded.

8. **Treatment**
   a. **Psychotherapy.** Patients must renounce narcissism to make progress, making treatment rather difficult. Some clinicians suggest psychoanalytic approaches to effect change, but more research is needed. Group therapy has proved useful in helping patients share with others and develop an empathic response to others.
   b. **Pharmacotherapy.** Lithium (Eskalith) is useful in patients with mood swings while antidepressants, especially serotonergic agents, are useful in depression.

IV. Anxious or Fearful Cluster

A. Obsessive-compulsive personality disorder

1. Definition. Characterized by perfectionism, orderliness, inflexibility, stubbornness, emotional constriction, and indecisiveness. Also called *anancastic personality disorder*.

2. Epidemiology

a. The prevalence is 1% in the general population and 3% to 10% in outpatients.

b. The prevalence is greater in men than in women.

c. Familial transmission is likely.

d. The concordance is increased in monozygotic twins.

e. The disorder is diagnosed most often in oldest children.

3. Etiology. Patients may have backgrounds characterized by harsh discipline.

4. Psychodynamics

a. Isolation, reaction formation, undoing, intellectualization, and rationalization are the classic defenses.

b. Emotions are distrusted.

c. Issues of defiance and submission are psychologically important.

d. Fixation at the anal period.

5. Diagnosis. Patients with obsessive-compulsive personality disorder have a stiff, formal, and rigid demeanor. They lack spontaneity and their mood is usually serious. In an interview, patients may be anxious about not being in control and their answers to questions are unusually detailed. Patients with obsessive-compulsive personality disorder are preoccupied with rules, regulations, orderliness, neatness, and details. Patients lack interpersonal skills; they often lack a sense of humor, alienate people, and are unable to compromise. However, they are eager to please powerful figures and carry out these people's wishes in an authoritarian manner. See Table 17-9.

6. Differential diagnosis. The patient with obsessive-compulsive disorder has true obsessions or compulsions, whereas the patient with obsessive-compulsive personality disorder does not.

7. Course and prognosis. The course of this disorder is variable and unpredictable. The patient may flourish in arrangements in which methodical or detailed work is required. The patient's personal life is likely to remain

Table 17-9
Obsessive-Compulsive Personality Disorder

- An enduring focus on neatness and control (≥4 of the following):
  - Excessive concern with regulations, timing, organization, or specific detail
  - Perfectionistic performance standards that prevent accomplishment
  - Prioritization of productivity and labor at the expense of leisure or rest
  - Overly rigid adherence to rules and moral standards
  - Hoarding possessions
  - Unwillingness to cede control
  - Parsimonious spending habits
  - Hardheaded temperament

barren. Complications of anxiety disorders, depressive disorders, and somatoform disorders may develop.

8. Treatment

a. Psychotherapy. Patients with obsessive-compulsive personality disorder are aware of their suffering and often seek treatment on their own. Treatment is often long and complex, and counter transference problems are common. Patients value free association and nondirective therapy.

b. Pharmacotherapy. Clonazepam (Klonopin) is useful in reducing symptoms. Clomipramine (Anafranil) and serotonergic agents such as fluoxetine, with dosages of 60 to 80 mg/day, may be useful if obsessive-compulsive signs and symptoms break through. Atypical antipsychotics such as quetiapine (Seroquel) may be of use in severe cases.

B. Avoidant personality disorder

1. Definition. Patients have a shy or timid personality and show an intense sensitivity to rejection. They are not asocial and show a great desire for companionship; however, they have a strong need for reassurance and a guarantee of uncritical acceptance. They are sometimes described as having an inferiority complex.

2. Epidemiology

a. The prevalence is 0.05% to 1% of the general population and 10% of outpatients.

b. Possible predisposing factors include avoidant disorder of childhood or adolescence or a deforming physical illness.

3. Etiology. Overt parental deprecation, overprotection, or phobic features in the parents themselves are possible etiologic factors.

4. Psychodynamics

a. The avoidance and inhibition are defensive.

b. The overt fears of rejection cover underlying aggression, either oedipal or preoedipal.

5. Diagnosis. In clinical interviews, patients are often anxious about talking to the interviewer. Their nervous and tense manner appears to wax and wane with their perception of whether the interviewer likes them. Patients may be vulnerable to the interviewer's comments and suggestions and may perceive a clarification or an interpretation as criticism. See Table 17-10.

Table 17-10
Avoidant Personality Disorder

- A temperament characterized by social withdrawal because of increased sensitivity to others' criticism demonstrated by ≥4 of:
  - Avoidance of social situations because of a desire to minimize criticism
  - Disengagement from relationships because of fear of others' disapproval
  - Unwillingness to become intimate due to a sense of embarrassment
  - Excessive concern about social rejection
  - Withdrawal from new social situations
  - Negative self-concept
  - Avoidance of risk and novelty because of fear of shame and ridicule

6. **Differential diagnosis**
   a. **Schizoid personality disorder.** The patient has no overt desire for involvement with others.
   b. **Social phobia.** Specific social situations, rather than personal relationships, are avoided. The disorders may coexist.
   c. **Dependent personality disorder.** The patient does not avoid attachments and has a greater fear of abandonment. Disorders may coexist.
   d. **Borderline and histrionic personality disorders.** The patient is demanding, irritable, and unpredictable.
7. **Course and prognosis.** Patients function best in a protected environment. Possible complications are social phobia and mood disorders.
8. **Treatment**
   a. **Psychotherapy.** Psychotherapeutic treatment depends on solidifying an alliance with patients. As trust develops, it is crucial that a clinician conveys an accepting attitude toward the patient's fears, especially that of rejection. Clinicians should be cautious about giving assignments to exercise the patient's new social skills outside of therapy, because failure may reinforce patients' poor self-esteem. Group therapy is helpful in gaining an understanding of the effects that sensitivity to rejection has on themselves and others. Assertive training in behavior therapy may help teach patients to openly express their needs and to enhance their self-esteem.
   b. **Pharmacotherapy.** Pharmacotherapy is useful in managing anxiety and depression. β-Adrenergic receptor antagonists, such as atenolol (Tenormin), is helpful in managing hyperactivity in the autonomic nervous system, which is especially high when approaching feared situations. Serotonergic agents are helpful with rejection sensitivity. Dopaminergic agents may cause more novelty-seeking behavior in these patients, but the patient needs to be psychologically prepared for any new experiences that may occur as a result.

C. **Dependent personality disorder**
   1. **Definition.** Patients are predominantly dependent and submissive. They lack self-confidence and get others to assume responsibility for major areas of their lives.
   2. **Epidemiology**
      a. The disorder is more prevalent in women than in men; however, it may be underdiagnosed in men.
      b. The disorder is common, possibly accounting for 2.5% of all personality disorders.
      c. More common in young children than in older ones.
   3. **Etiology.** Chronic physical illness, separation anxiety, or parental loss in childhood may predispose.
   4. **Psychodynamics**
      a. Unresolved separation issues are present.
      b. The dependent stance is a defense against aggression.

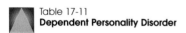

Table 17-11
Dependent Personality Disorder

- A recurrent state of subordination to the care of others manifest by ≥5 of:
  - Indecisiveness and reliance on other parties when making everyday choices
  - Deferral of responsibility for most aspects of life to others
  - Reluctance to voice opposition
  - Diffidence precluding taking actions on one's initiative
  - Willingness to debase oneself for approval
  - Feelings of isolation or desolation when alone because of fears of incompetence
  - Recurrent need to seek replacement support figures
  - Excessive anxiety about having to take care of oneself

---

5. **Diagnosis.** Persons with dependent personality disorder have an intense need to be taken care of, which leads to clinging behavior, submissiveness, fear of separation, and interpersonal dependency. In interviews, they appear rather compliant; they try to cooperate, welcome specific questions, and look for guidance. They are passive and have difficulty expressing disagreement. Patients are pessimistic, passive, indecisive, and fear expressing sexual or aggressive feelings. In *folie à deux* (shared psychotic disorder), one member of the pair usually suffers from this disorder; the submissive partner takes on the delusional system of the more aggressive, assertive partner on whom he or she is dependent. See Table 17-11.

6. **Differential diagnosis**
   a. **Agoraphobia.** The patient is afraid of leaving or being away from home.
   b. **Histrionic and borderline personality disorders.** The patient has a series of dependent relationships and is overly manipulative.

7. **Course and prognosis.** The course of dependent personality disorder is variable. Depressive complications are possible if a relationship is lost. The prognosis can be favorable with treatment. The patient may not be able to tolerate the "healthy" step of leaving an abusive relationship.

8. **Treatment**
   a. **Psychotherapy.** Insight-oriented therapies are helpful in enabling patients to understand the antecedents of their behavior, thereby enabling them to become more independent, assertive, and self-reliant. Behavior therapy, assertiveness training, family therapy, and group therapy have also been successful. Clinicians must respect patients' feelings of attachment in pathologic relationships.
   b. **Pharmacotherapy.** Pharmacotherapy has been used in managing specific symptoms such as anxiety or depression. Alprazolam (Xanax) has been useful in patients who experience panic attacks. If a patient's depression or withdrawal symptoms respond to psychostimulants, they may be used. Benzodiazepines and serotonergic agents have also been used successfully.

V. Other Specified Personality Disorders

In DSM-5, the category other specified personality disorder is reserved for disorders that do not fit into any of the personality disorder categories described above. Passive-aggressive personality and depressive personality are examples. A narrow spectrum of behavior or a particular trait—such as oppositionalism, sadism, or masochism—can also be classified in this category. A patient with features of more than one personality disorder but without the complete criteria of any one disorder can be assigned this classification.

A. Passive-aggressive personality

Passive-aggressive personality was once considered a psychiatric diagnosis but is no longer classified as such. It is included here because persons with this personality type are not uncommon.

1. **Definition.** Patients with this disorder show aggression in passive ways characterized by obstructionism, procrastination, stubbornness, and inefficiency. It is also called *negativistic personality disorder*.

2. **Epidemiology.** Unknown.

3. **Etiology**

   a. May involve learned behavior and parental modeling.

   b. Early difficulties with authority common.

4. **Psychodynamics**

   a. Conflicts regarding authority, autonomy, and dependence.

   b. Uses passive modes to express defiance and aggression.

5. **Diagnosis.** Patients with passive-aggressive personality disorder are passive, sullen, and argumentative. They resist demands for adequate performance in social and occupational tasks and unreasonably criticize and scorn authority. They complain of being misunderstood and unappreciated and exaggerate personal misfortune. They are both envious and resentful of those whom they deem more fortunate. They tend to alternate between hostile defiance and guilt.

6. **Differential diagnosis**

   a. **Histrionic and borderline personality disorders.** The patient's behavior is more flamboyant, dramatic, and openly aggressive.

   b. **Antisocial personality disorder.** The patient's defiance is overt.

   c. **Obsessive-compulsive personality disorder.** The patient is overtly perfectionistic and submissive.

7. **Course and prognosis.** Association with depressive disorders and alcohol abuse in approximately 50% of patients. Prognosis is guarded without treatment.

8. **Treatment**

   a. **Psychotherapy.** Psychotherapy can be successful with these patients but requires that clinicians point out the consequences of passive-aggressive behaviors as they occur. Such confrontations may be more helpful than a correct interpretation in changing patients' behavior. Clinicians must treat suicide gestures as a covert expression of anger rather than as object loss in major depressive disorder.

  b. Pharmacotherapy. Antidepressants are used when clinical indications of depression and suicidal ideation exist. Some patients respond to benzodiazepines and psychostimulants, depending on the clinical features.

B. Depressive personality

  1. Definition. Patients are characterized by depressive traits that last that have been prevalent throughout their lives, such as pessimism, self-doubt, and chronic unhappiness. They are introverted passive and duty bound.

  2. Epidemiology

    a. The disorder is thought to be common, but no data are available.

    b. Probably occurs equally in men and women.

    c. Probably occurs in families with depression.

  3. Etiology. Chronic physical illness, separation anxiety, or parental loss in childhood may predispose.

  4. Psychodynamics

    a. Unresolved separation issues are present.

    b. The dependent stance is a defense against aggression.

  5. Diagnosis. Patients with depressive personality disorder often complain of chronic feelings of unhappiness. They admit to low self-esteem and have difficulty finding anything joyful, hopeful, or optimistic in their lives. They are self-critical and derogatory and are likely to denigrate their work, themselves, and their relationships with others. Their physiognomy often reflects their mood—poor posture, depressed facies, soft voice, and psychomotor retardation.

  6. Differential diagnosis

    a. Dysthymic disorder. Fluctuations in mood are greater than in depressive personality disorder.

    b. Avoidant personality disorder. The patient tends to be more anxious than depressed.

  7. Course and prognosis. A risk for dysthymic disorder, major depressive disorder, and current or lifetime mood disorder is thought to be likely.

  8. Treatment

    a. Psychotherapy. Insight-oriented psychotherapy enables patients to gain insight into the psychodynamics of their illness and to appreciate the effect it has on their interpersonal relationships. Cognitive therapy corrects the cognitive manifestation of their low self-esteem and pessimism. Group therapy, interpersonal therapy, and self-help measures are also useful.

    b. Pharmacotherapy. Pharmacotherapy for depressive personality disorder patients includes the use of antidepressant medications. Serotonergic agents are especially useful. Small dosages of psychostimulants, such as amphetamine at 5 to 15 mg/day, have been helpful for some patients. These approaches should be combined with psychotherapy for best results.

C. Sadomasochistic personality. Not an official diagnostic but is of major interest to physicians clinically and historically. It is characterized by elements of sadism, the desire to cause others pain sexually, physically, or psychologically, and masochism, inflicting pain on oneself either sexually or morally. Treatment with insight-oriented psychotherapy, including psychoanalysis, can be effective.

D. Sadistic personality. Patients show a pervasive pattern of cruel, demeaning, and aggressive behavior toward others. Physical cruelty and violence are used to inflict pain on others with no actual goal. Such patients are usually fascinated with weapons, violence, injury, and torture. It is often related to parental abuse.

E. Personality change due to a general medical condition
Personality change due to a general medical condition is a significant occurrence. These include brain disease, damage, and dysfunction, which includes organic personality disorder, postencephalitic syndrome, and postconcussional syndrome. It is characterized by a marked change in personality style and traits from a previous level of functioning.

   1. Diagnosis and clinical features. A change in personality from previous patterns of behavior with impaired impulse control and expression of emotions. Euphoria or apathy may be prominent as well as excitement and facile jocularity with injury to the frontal lobes. Frontal lobe syndrome consists of indifference and apathy, lack of concerns and temper outbursts that can result in violent behavior. Persons with temporal lobe epilepsy characteristically show humorlessness, hypergraphia, hyperreligiosity, and marked aggressiveness during seizures. See Table 17-12.

   2. Etiology. Structural damage to the brain is usually the cause of the personality change, and head trauma is probably the most common cause.

Table 17-12
Personality Change Due to Another Medical Condition

- An enduring change in personality attributable to a medical condition
  (In children, this must last more than a year)
  (Delirium is a red flag)
- Subtypes include:
  - Labile: marked by heightened emotional variability
  - Disinhibited: marked by indomitable impulses or appetites
  - Aggressive: marked by violent or enraged behavior
  - Apathetic: marked by detachment
  - Paranoid: marked by distrust
  - Combined: marked by a mixture of any of the subtypes
  - Other: adhering to none of the outlined subtypes
  - Unspecified

Table 17-13
Medical Conditions Associated with Personality Change

Head trauma
Cerebrovascular diseases
Cerebral tumors
Epilepsy (particularly, complex partial epilepsy)
Huntington's disease
Multiple sclerosis
Endocrine disorders
Heavy metal poisoning (manganese, mercury)
Neurosyphilis
Acquired immune deficiency syndrome (AIDS)

The conditions most often associated with personality change are listed in Table 17-13.

F. Anabolic steroids

Large number of high school and college athletes and bodybuilders are using anabolic steroids for physical development. These include oxymetholone (Anadrol), somatropin (Humatrope), stanozolol (Winstrol), and testosterone. Anabolic steroids can cause persistent alterations of personality and behavior.

1. **Differential diagnosis.** In differentiating the specific syndrome from other disorders in which personality change may occur—such as schizophrenia, delusional disorder, mood disorders, and impulse control disorders—physicians must consider the presence in personality change disorder of a specific organic causative factor.

2. **Course and prognosis.** In structural damage to the brain, the disorder tends to persist. In head trauma or vascular accident damage and may be permanent. The personality change can evolve into dementia in cases of brain tumor, multiple sclerosis, and Huntington's disease.

3. **Treatment.** Management of personality change disorder involves treatment of the underlying organic condition when possible. Psychopharmacological treatment of specific symptoms may be indicated in some cases, such as imipramine or fluoxetine for depression.

   Patients with severe cognitive impairment need counseling and patients' families may require emotional support.

VI. Psychobiological Model of Treatment

The psychobiological model of treatment combines psychotherapy and pharmacotherapy and can be systematically matched to the personality structure and stage of character development. The newest development is treating personality disorders pharmacologically. Table 17-14 summarizes drug choices for various target symptoms of personality disorders.

A. Temperament

Temperament refers to the body's biases in the modulation of conditioned behavioral responses to prescriptive physical stimuli. It is conceptualized as the stylistic component ("how") of behavior, as differentiated from the motivation ("why") and the content ("what") of behavior. Four major

Table 17-14
Pharmacotherapy of Target Symptom Domains of Personality Disorders

Target Symptom	Drug of Choice	Contraindication[a]
I. Behavior dyscontrol		
Aggression or impulsivity		
Affective aggression (hot temper with normal EEG)	Lithium[a]	? Benzodiazepines
	Serotonergic drugs[a]	Stimulants
	Anticonvulsants[a]	
	Low-dosage antipsychotics	
Predatory aggression (hostility or cruelty)	Antipsychotics[a]	Benzodiazepines
	Lithium	Stimulants
	β-Adrenergic receptor antagonists	
Organic-like aggression	Imipramine[a]	
	Cholinergic agonists (donepezil)	
Ictal aggression (abnormal EEG)	Carbamazepine[a]	Antipsychotics
	Diphenylhydantoin[a]	Stimulants
	Benzodiazepines	
II. Mood dysregulation		
Emotional lability	Lithium[a]	? Tricyclic drugs
	Antipsychotics	
Depression		
Atypical depression, dysphoria	MAOIs[a]	
	Serotonergic drugs[a]	
	Antipsychotics	
Emotional detachment	Serotonin-dopamine antagonists[a]	? Tricyclic drugs
	Atypical antipsychotics	
III. Anxiety		
Chronic cognitive	Serotonergic drugs[a]	Stimulants
	MAOIs[a]	
	Benzodiazepines	
Chronic somatic	MAOIs[a]	
	β-Adrenergic receptor antagonists	
Severe anxiety	Low-dose antipsychotics	
	MAOIs	
IV. Psychotic symptoms		
Acute and psychosis	Antipsychotics[a]	Stimulants
Chronic and low-level psychotic-like symptoms	Low-dose antipsychotics[a]	

[a]Drug of choice or major contraindication. EEG, electroencephalogram; MAOI, monoamine oxidase inhibitor.

temperament traits have been identified and include: harm avoidance, novelty seeking, reward dependence, and persistence.

B. Biologic character traits

Four character traits have been described and mentioned in Table 17-15. It summarizes contrasting sets of behaviors that distinguish extreme scorers on the four dimensions of temperament.

1. Harm avoidance

High harm avoidance is observed as fear of uncertainty, social inhibition, shyness with strangers, rapid fatigability, and pessimistic worry in anticipation of problems even in situations that do not worry other persons. Persons low in harm avoidance are carefree, courageous, energetic, outgoing, and optimistic even in situations that worry most persons.

Table 17-15
Descriptors of Individuals Who Score High or Low on the Four Temperament Dimensions

	Descriptors of Extreme Variants	
Temperament Dimension	High	Low
Harm avoidance	Pessimistic	Optimistic
	Fearful	Daring
	Shy	Outgoing
	Fatigable	Energetic
Novelty seeking	Exploratory	Reserved
	Impulsive	Deliberate
	Extravagant	Thrifty
	Irritable	Stoical
Reward dependence	Sentimental	Detached
	Open	Aloof
	Warm	Cold
	Affectionate	Independent
Persistence	Industrious	Lazy
	Determined	Spoiled
	Enthusiastic	Underachiever
	Perfectionist	Pragmatist

2. Novelty seeking

Novelty seeking is observed as exploratory activity in response to novelty, impulsiveness, extravagance in approach to cues of reward, and active avoidance of frustration. Individuals high in novelty seeking are quick tempered, curious, easily bored, impulsive, extravagant, and disorderly. Persons low in novelty seeking are slow tempered, uninquiring, stoical, reflective, frugal, reserved, tolerant of monotony, and orderly.

3. Reward dependence

Individuals high in reward dependence are tender hearted, sensitive, socially dependent, and sociable. Individuals low in reward dependence are practical, tough minded, cold, socially insensitive, irresolute, and indifferent if alone.

4. Persistence

Highly persistent persons are hard-working, perseverant, and ambitious overachievers who tend to intensify their effort in response to anticipated rewards and view frustration and fatigue as personal challenges. Individuals low in persistence are indolent, inactive, unstable, and erratic; they tend to give up easily when faced with frustration, rarely strive for higher accomplishments, and manifest little perseverance even in response to intermittent reward.

C. Psychobiology of temperament

Temperament traits of harm avoidance, novelty seeking, reward dependence, and persistence are defined as heritable differences underlying automatic responses to danger, novelty, social approval, and intermittent reward, respectively. The neurobiologic model of learning in animals is summarized in Table 17-16. This model distinguishes four dissociable brain systems for behavioral inhibition (harm avoidance), behavioral activation (novelty

Table 17-16
Four Dissociable Brain Systems Influencing Stimulus–Response Patterns Underlying Temperament

Brain System (Related Personality Dimension)	Principal Neuromodulators	Relevant Stimuli	Behavioral Response
Behavioral inhibition (harm avoidance)	GABA Serotonin (dorsal raphe)	Aversive conditioning (pairing CS and UCS) Conditioned signals for punishment and frustrative nonreward	Formation of aversive CS Passive avoidance Extinction
Behavioral activation (novelty seeking)	Dopamine	Novelty CS of reward CS or UCS of relief of monotony or punishment	Exploratory pursuit Appetitive approach Active avoidance Escape
Social attachment (reward dependence)	Norepinephrine Serotonin (median raphe)	Reward conditioning (pairing CS and UCS)	Formation of appetitive CS
Partial reinforcement (persistence)	Glutamate Serotonin (dorsal raphe)	Intermittent (partial) reinforcement	Resistance to extinction

CS, conditioned stimulus; GABA, γ-aminobutyric acid; UCS, unconditioned stimulus.
Adapted from Cloninger CR. A systematic method for clinical description and classification of personality variables. *Arch Gen Psychiatry.* 1987;44:573.

seeking), social attachment (reward dependence), and partial reinforcement (persistence).

They have been shown to be universal across different cultures, ethnic groups, and political systems. In summary, these aspects of personality are called temperament because they are heritable, manifest early in life, are developmentally stable, and are consistent in different cultures.

For more detailed discussion of this topic, see Chapter 57, Personality Disorders, Section 57.3i, p. 4103, in CTP/X.

18
Sexual Dysfunction and Gender Dysphoria

Sexual dysfunctions are an inability to respond to sexual stimulation, or the experience of pain during the sexual act. It is defined by disturbance in the subjective sense of pleasure or desire associated with sex, or by the objective performance. In the *Diagnostic and Statistical Manual of Mental Disorders, fifth edition* (DSM-5), the sexual dysfunctions include male hypoactive sexual desire disorder, female sexual interest/arousal disorder, erectile disorder, female orgasmic disorder, delayed ejaculation, premature (early) ejaculation, genito-pelvic pain/penetration disorder, substance/medication-induced sexual dysfunction, other specified sexual dysfunction, and unspecified sexual dysfunction. If more than one dysfunction exists, they should all be diagnosed. Sexual dysfunctions can be **lifelong or acquired, generalized or situational,** and result from **psychological factors, physiologic factors,** or **combined factors.** As per DSM-5 dysfunction due to a general medical condition, substance use, or adverse effects of medication should be noted. Sexual dysfunction may be diagnosed in conjunction with another psychiatric disorder (depressive disorders, anxiety disorders, personality disorders, and schizophrenia).

I. **Desire, Interest, and Arousal Disorders**
   A. **Male hypoactive sexual desire disorder.** Characterized by a lack or absence of sexual fantasies and desire for minimum duration of 6 months. Men may have never experienced erotic/sexual thoughts and the dysfunction can be lifelong. The prevalence is greatest in the younger (6% of men ages 18 to 24) and older (40% of men ages 66 to 74) with only 2% aged 16 to 44 affected by this disorder.

   Patients with desire problems often use inhibition of desire defensively, to protect against unconscious fears about sex. Lack of desire can also result from chronic stress, anxiety, or depression or the use of various psychotropic drugs and other drugs that depress the central nervous system (CNS). In sex therapy clinic populations, lack of desire is one of the most common complaints among married couples, with women more affected than men.

   The diagnosis should not be made unless the lack of desire is a source of distress to a patient. See Table 18-1.
   B. **Female sexual interest/arousal disorder.** The combination of interest (or desire) and arousal reflects that women do not necessarily move stepwise from desire to arousal, but experience desire synchronously with, or even following feelings of arousal. Consequently, women may experience either/

Table 18-1
Male Hypoactive Sexual Desire Disorder

Reduced or no sexual appetite or libido for ≥6 months
Many factors such as age and culture should inform whether the patient fits within the bounds for normal sexual desire

---

or both inability to feel interest or arousal, difficulty achieving orgasm or experience pain. Usual complaints include decrease or paucity of erotic feelings, thoughts and fantasies; a decreased impulse to initiate sex; a decreased or absent receptivity to partner overtures and an inability to respond to partner stimulation.

Subjective sense of arousal is poorly correlated with genital lubrication in both normal and dysfunctional women. A woman complaining of lack of arousal may lubricate vaginally, but may not experience a subjective sense of excitement. The prevalence is generally underestimated. In one study of subjectively happily married couples, 33% of women described arousal problems. Difficulty in maintaining excitement can reflect psychological conflicts (e.g., anxiety, guilt, and fear) or physiologic changes. Alterations in testosterone, estrogen, prolactin, and thyroxin levels have been implicated in female sexual arousal disorder. In addition, medications with antihistaminic or anticholinergic properties cause a decrease in vaginal lubrication. Relationship problems are particularly relevant to acquired interest/arousal disorder. In one study of couples with markedly decreased sexual interaction, the most prevalent etiology was marital discord. See Table 18-2.

C. **Male erectile disorder.** In lifelong male erectile disorder one has never been able to obtain an erection while in acquired type one has successfully achieved penetration at some time in his sexual life.

Erectile disorder is reported in 10% to 20% of all men and is the chief complaint of more than 50% of all men treated for sexual disorders. Lifelong male erectile disorder is rare; it occurs in about 1% of men younger than age 35. The incidence increases with age and has been reported around 2% to 8% of the young adult population. The rate increases to 40% to 50% in men between ages of 60 and 70.

Male erectile disorder can be organic or psychological, or a combination but in young and middle-aged men the cause is usually psychological. A

Table 18-2
Female Sexual Interest/Arousal Disorder

Reduced or no sexual appetite or libido for ≥6 months ≥3 of:
- Decreased interest in sex
- Decrease in thoughts about sex or imaginative scenarios
- Decreased receptivity to and engagement in sex
- Decreased enjoyment of sexual situations
- Decreased responsiveness to sexual cues
- Decrease in genital and nongenital reactions to sex
Cannot be a sequela of severe relationship distress or significant stressors

---

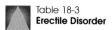

Table 18-3
Erectile Disorder

Difficulty achieving or maintaining an erection, or in attaining erectile stiffness throughout almost all sexual efforts for ≥6 months
Cannot be a sequela of severe relationship distress or significant stressors

history of spontaneous erections, morning erections, or good erections with masturbation or with partners other than the usual one indicates functional impotence. Psychological causes of erectile dysfunction include a punitive conscience or superego, an inability to trust, or feelings of inadequacy. Erectile dysfunction also may reflect relationship difficulties between partners. See Table 18-3.

II. Orgasm Disorders

A. Female orgasmic disorder. Female orgasmic disorder (anorgasmia or *inhibited female orgasm*) is a recurrent or persistent delay in or absence of orgasm following a normal sexual excitement phase. In lifelong female orgasmic disorder, one has never experienced an orgasm by any kind of stimulation while in acquired orgasmic disorder one has previously experienced at least one orgasm. The disorder is more common among unmarried women. The estimated proportion of married women over age 35 who never have achieved orgasm is 5%. The proportion is higher in unmarried women and younger women. The overall prevalence of inhibited female orgasm is 30%. Psychological factors associated with inhibited orgasm include fears of impregnation or rejection by the sex partner, hostility toward men, feelings of guilt about sexual impulses, or marital conflicts. See Table 18-4.

B. Delayed ejaculation. In male delayed ejaculation (*retarded ejaculation)*, a man achieves ejaculation during coitus with great difficulty, if at all. The problem occurs mostly during coital activity. Lifelong inhibited male orgasm usually indicates more severe psychopathology. Acquired ejaculatory inhibition frequently reflects interpersonal difficulties. The incidence is low compared to premature ejaculation and in one group of men was only 3.8%. A general prevalence of 5% has been reported but more recently increased rates have been seen. This has been attributed to the increasing use of antidepressants like selective serotonin reuptake inhibitors (SSRIs), which cause delayed orgasm. See Table 18-5.

C. Premature (early) ejaculation. In premature ejaculation, men persistently or recurrently achieve orgasm and ejaculation before they wish to. The diagnosis is made when a man regularly ejaculates before or

Table 18-4
Female Orgasmic Disorder

Reduction in frequency, immediacy, or intensity of orgasm
Cannot be a sequela of severe relationship distress or significant stressors

Table 18-5
Delayed Ejaculation

Increase in latency or decrease in regularity of ejaculation during almost all sexual efforts for ≥6 months
Cannot be a sequela of severe relationship distress or significant stressors

within approximately 1 minute after penetration. It is more prevalent among young men, men with a new partner, and college-educated men than among men with less education; the problem with the latter group is thought to be related to concern for partner satisfaction. Premature ejaculation is the chief complaint of 35% to 40% of men treated for sexual disorders.

Difficulty in ejaculatory control may be associated with anxiety regarding the sex act and with unconscious fears about the vagina. It may also be the result of conditioning if the man's early sexual experiences occurred in situations in which discovery would have been embarrassing. A stressful marriage exacerbates the disorder.

Behavioral techniques are used in treatment. However, a subgroup of premature ejaculators may be biologically predisposed; they are more vulnerable to sympathetic stimulation or they have a shorter bulbocavernosus reflex nerve latency time, and they should be treated pharmacologically with SSRIs or other antidepressants. A side effect of these drugs is the inhibition of ejaculation.

The developmental background and the psychodynamics found in premature ejaculation and in erectile disorder are similar. See Table 18-6.

III. Sexual Pain Disorders
   A. Genito-pelvic pain/penetration disorder. In DSM-5, this disorder refers to one or more of the following complaints, of which any two or more may occur together: difficulty having intercourse; genito-pelvic pain; fear of pain or penetration; and tension of the pelvic floor muscles. Previously, these were diagnosed as *dyspareunia* or *vaginismus* and could coexist and lead to fear of pain with sex. These diagnoses are categorized into one diagnostic category but for the purposes of clinical discussion the distinct categories of dyspareunia and vaginismus remain clinically useful. See Table 18-7.
      1. Dyspareunia. Dyspareunia is recurrent or persistent genital pain occurring before, during, or after intercourse. Dyspareunia is related to vaginismus and repeated episodes of vaginismus can lead to dyspareunia.

Table 18-6
Premature (Early) Ejaculation

Undesired ejaculation during the first minute after (vaginal) penetration
Ejaculation occurs prematurely during almost all sexual encounters
(Duration criteria do not exist for other penetration sites.)

Table 18-7
Genito-Pelvic Pain/Penetration Disorder

Problems with at least one of:
- Vaginal penetration
- Extreme pelvic/vaginal pain during penetration attempts
- Anxiety about such pain
- Pelvic muscle clenching during penetration

Though GPP should cause distress, it cannot be a sequela of severe relationship distress or significant stressors

DSM-5 cites that 15% of women in North America report recurrent pain during intercourse.

Chronic pelvic pain is a common complaint in women with a history of rape or childhood sexual abuse. Painful coitus can result from tension and anxiety and makes intercourse unpleasant or unbearable. Dyspareunia is uncommon in men and is usually associated with a medical condition (e.g., Peyronie's disease). Dyspareunia may present as any of the four complaints listed under genito-pelvic pain/penetration disorder and should be diagnosed as genito-pelvic pain/penetration disorder.

2. **Vaginismus.** Defined as a constriction of the outer third of the vagina due to involuntary pelvic floor muscle tightening or spasm, vaginismus interferes with penile insertion and intercourse.

Vaginismus may be complete, that is no penetration of the vagina is possible. In a less severe form, pain makes penetration difficult, but not impossible.

It mostly afflicts highly educated women and of high socioeconomic groups. A sexual trauma, such as rape, or unpleasant first coital experience may cause vaginismus. A strict religious upbringing in which sex is associated with sin is frequent in these patients.

IV. **Sexual Dysfunction Due to a General Medical Condition**
   A. **Male erectile disorder due to a general medical condition.** Statistics indicate that 20% to 50% of men with erectile disorder have an organic basis for the disorder. A physiologic etiology is likely in men older than 50 and the most likely cause in men older than age 60. The organic causes of male erectile disorder are listed in Table 18-8.

Following procedures may help differentiate organically caused erectile disorder from functional erectile disorder.

1. Monitoring nocturnal penile tumescence (erections during rapid eye movement sleep)
2. Monitoring tumescence with a strain gauge
3. Measuring blood pressure in the penis with a penile plethysmograph

Other diagnostic include glucose tolerance tests, plasma hormone assays, liver and thyroid function tests, prolactin and follicle-stimulating hormone (FHS) determinations, and cystometric examinations.

Table 18-8
Diseases and Other Medical Conditions Implicated in Male Erectile Disorder

Infectious and parasitic diseases	Neurologic disorders
Elephantiasis	Multiple sclerosis
Mumps	Transverse myelitis
Cardiovascular disease[a]	Parkinson's disease
Atherosclerotic disease	Temporal lobe epilepsy
Aortic aneurysm	Traumatic and neoplastic spinal cord diseases[a]
Leriche's syndrome	Central nervous system tumor
Cardiac failure	Amyotrophic lateral sclerosis
Renal and urologic disorders	Peripheral neuropathy
Peyronie's disease	General paresis
Chronic renal failure	Tabes dorsalis
Hydrocele and varicocele	Pharmacologic factors
Hepatic disorders	Alcohol and other dependence-inducing substances
Cirrhosis (usually associated with	(heroin, methadone, morphine, cocaine, amphetamines,
alcohol dependence)	and barbiturates)
Pulmonary disorders	Prescribed drugs (psychotropic drugs, antihypertensive
Respiratory failure	drugs, estrogens, and antiandrogens)
Genetics	Poisoning
Klinefelter's syndrome	Lead (plumbism)
Congenital penile vascular and	Herbicides
structural abnormalities	Surgical procedures[a]
Nutritional disorders	Perineal prostatectomy
Malnutrition	Abdominal-perineal colon resection
Vitamin deficiencies	Sympathectomy (frequently interferes with ejaculation)
Obesity	Aortoiliac surgery
Endocrine disorders[a]	Radical cystectomy
Diabetes mellitus	Retroperitoneal lymphadenectomy
Acromegaly	Miscellaneous
Addison's disease	Radiation therapy
Chromophobe adenoma	Pelvic fracture
Adrenal neoplasia	Any severe systemic disease or debilitating condition
Myxedema	
Hyperthyroidism	

[a]In the United States an estimated 2 million men are impotent because they have diabetes mellitus; an additional 300,000 are impotent because of other endocrine diseases; 1.5 million are impotent as a result of vascular disease; 180,000 because of multiple sclerosis; 400,000 because of traumas and fractures leading to pelvic fractures or spinal cord injuries; and another 650,000 are impotent as a result of radical surgery, including prostatectomies, colostomies, and cystectomies.

B. Dyspareunia due to a general medical condition. An estimated 30% of all surgical procedures on the female genital area result in temporary dyspareunia. In addition, 30% to 40% of women with the complaint who are seen in sex therapy clinics have pelvic pathology. Organic abnormalities leading to dyspareunia and vaginismus include irritated or infected hymenal remnants, episiotomy scars, Bartholin's gland infection, various forms of vaginitis and cervicitis, endometriosis, and adenomyosis. Postcoital pain has been reported by women with myomata, endometriosis, and adenomyosis, and is attributed to the uterine contractions during orgasm. Postmenopausal women may have dyspareunia resulting from thinning of the vaginal mucosa and reduced lubrication.

    Two conditions not readily apparent on physical examination that produce dyspareunia are vulvar vestibulitis and interstitial cystitis.

Table 18-9
Neurophysiology of Sexual Dysfunction

	DA	5-HT	NE	ACh	Clinical Correlation
Erection	↑		α, β ↓ ↑	M	Antipsychotics may lead to erectile dysfunction (DA block); DA agonists may lead to enhanced erection and libido; priapism with trazodone (α_1, block); β-blockers may lead to impotence
Ejaculation and orgasm	± ↓		α_1 ↑	M	α-Blockers (tricyclic drugs, MAOIs, thioridazine) may lead to impaired ejaculation; 5-HT agents may inhibit orgasm

↑, facilities; ↓, inhibits or decreases; ±, some; ACh, acetylcholine; DA, dopamine; 5-HT, serotonin; M, modulates; NE, norepinephrine; minimal.
Reprinted with permission from Segraves R. *Psychiatric Times.* 1990.

C. **Male hypoactive sexual desire disorder and female interest/arousal disorder due to a general medical condition.** Sexual desire commonly decreases after major illness or surgery, particularly when the body image is affected after such procedures as mastectomy, ileostomy, hysterectomy, and prostatectomy. In some cases, biochemical correlates are associated with hypoactive sexual desire disorder (Table 18-9). Drugs that depress the CNS or decrease testosterone production can decrease desire.

D. **Other male sexual dysfunction due to a general medical condition.** Delayed ejaculation can have physiologic causes and can occur after surgery on the genitourinary tract, such as prostatectomy. It may also be associated with Parkinson's disease and other neurologic disorders involving the lumbar or sacral sections of the spinal cord. The antihypertensive drug guanethidine monosulfate (Ismelin), methyldopa (Aldomet), the phenothiazines, the tricyclic drugs, and the SSRIs, among others, have been implicated in retarded ejaculation (Table 18-10).

E. **Other female sexual dysfunction due to a general medical condition.** Some medical conditions—specifically, endocrine diseases such as hypothyroidism, diabetes mellitus, and primary hyperprolactinemia—can affect a woman's ability to have orgasms.

F. **Substance/medication-induced sexual dysfunction.** The diagnosis of substance-induced sexual dysfunction is used when evidence of substance intoxication or withdrawal is apparent from the history, physical examination, or laboratory findings. The disturbance in sexual function must be predominant in the clinical picture. See Table 18-11. In general, sexual function is negatively affected by serotonergic agents, dopamine antagonists, drugs that increase prolactin, and drugs that affect the autonomic nervous system. With commonly abused substances, dysfunction occurs within a month of significant substance intoxication or withdrawal. In small doses, some substances (e.g., amphetamine) may enhance sexual performance, but abuse impairs erectile, orgasmic, and ejaculatory capacities.

Oral contraceptives are reported to decrease libido in some women, and some drugs with anticholinergic side effects may impair arousal as well as orgasm. Benzodiazepines have been reported to decrease libido,

Table 18-10
Pharmacologic Agents Implicated in Male Sexual Dysfunctions

Drug	Impairs Erection	Impairs Ejaculation
Psychiatric drugs		
Selective serotonin reuptake inhibitors[a]		
Citalopram (Celexa)	–	+
Fluoxetine (Prozac)	–	+
Paroxetine (Paxil)	–	+
Sertraline (Zoloft)	–	+
Cyclic drugs		
Imipramine (Tofranil)	+	+
Protriptyline (Vivactil)	+	+
Desipramine (Pertofrane)	+	+
Clomipramine (Anafranil)	+	+
Amitriptyline (Elavil)	+	+
Monoamine oxidase inhibitors		
Tranylcypromine (Parnate)	+	
Phenelzine (Nardil)	+	+
Pargyline (Eutonyl)	–	+
Isocarboxazid (Marplan)	–	+
Other mood-active drugs		
Lithium (Eskalith)	+	
Amphetamines	+	+
Trazodone (Desyrel)[b]	–	–
Venlafaxine (Effexor)	–	+
Antipsychotics[c]		
Fluphenazine (Prolixin)	+	
Thioridazine (Mellaril)	+	+
Chlorprothixene (Taractan)	–	+
Mesoridazine (Serentil)	–	+
Perphenazine (Trilafon)	–	+
Trifluoperazine (Stelazine)	–	+
Reserpine (Serpasil)	+	+
Haloperidol (Haldol)	–	+
Antianxiety agent[d]		
Chlordiazepoxide (Librium)	–	+
Antihypertensive drugs		
Clonidine (Catapres)	+	
Methyldopa (Aldomet)	+	+
Spironolactone (Aldactone)	+	–
Hydrochlorothiazide (Hydrodiuril)	+	–
Guanethidine (Ismelin)	+	+
Commonly abused substances		
Alcohol	+	+
Barbiturates	+	+
Cannabis	+	–
Cocaine	+	+
Heroin	+	+
Methadone	+	–
Morphine	+	+
Miscellaneous drugs		
Antiparkinsonian agents	+	+
Clofibrate (Atromid-S)	+	–
Digoxin (Lanoxin)	+	–
Glutethimide (Doriden)	+	+
Indomethacin (Indocin)	+	–
Phentolamine (Regitine)	–	+
Propranolol (Inderal)	+	–

[a]SSRIs also impair desire.
[b]Trazodone has been causative in some cases of priapism.
[c]Impairment of sexual function is less likely with atypical antipsychotics. Priapism has occasionally occurred in association with the use of antipsychotics.
[d]Benzodiazepines have been reported to decrease libido, but in some patients the diminution of anxiety caused by those drugs enhances sexual function.

Table 18-11
Substance/Medication-Induced Sexual Dysfunction

A distressing change in sexual function during or soon after intoxication of or withdrawal from a substance/medication that is known to produce such symptoms.
(Red flags include delirium and symptoms of the sexual dysfunction outside of the influence of the substance/medication.)

but in some patients the diminution of anxiety caused by those drugs enhances sexual function. Both increase and decrease in libido have been reported with psychoactive agents. Alcohol may foster the initiation of sexual activity by removing inhibition, but it also impairs performance. Sexual dysfunction associated with the use of a drug disappears when the drug is discontinued. Table 18-12 lists psychiatric medications that may inhibit female orgasm.

G. Pharmacologic agents implicated in sexual dysfunction. Almost every pharmacologic agent, particularly those used in psychiatry, has been associated with an effect on sexuality. The effects of psychoactive drugs are detailed later in this section. For a detailed list of medication that impact sexual functioning, see Table 18-13.

    1. Antipsychotic drugs. Most antipsychotic drugs are dopamine receptor antagonists that also block adrenergic and cholinergic receptors, thus accounting for the adverse sexual effects.

    2. Antidepressant drugs. The tricyclic and tetracyclic antidepressants have anticholinergic effects that interfere with erection and delay ejaculation. Clomipramine (Anafranil) has been reported to increase sex drive in some persons. Selegiline (Deprenyl), a selective MAO type B (MAO_B) inhibitor, and bupropion (Wellbutrin) also increase sex drive.

Table 18-12
Some Psychiatric Drugs Implemented in Inhibited Female Orgasm[a]

Tricyclic antidepressants	Dopamine receptor antagonists
Imipramine (Tofranil)	Thioridazine (Mellaril)
Clomipramine (Anafranil)	Trifluoperazine (Stelazine)
Nortriptyline (Aventyl)	
	Selective serotonin reuptake inhibitors
Monoamine oxidase inhibitors	Fluoxetine (Prozac)
Tranylcypromine (Parnate)	Paroxetine (Paxil)
Phenelzine (Nardil)	Sertraline (Zoloft)
Isocarboxazid (Marplan)	Fluvoxamine (Luvox)
	Citalopram (Celexa)

[a]The interrelation between female sexual dysfunction and pharmacologic agents has been less extensively evaluated than male reactions. Oral contraceptives are reported to decrease libido in some women, and some drugs with anticholinergic side effects may impair arousal as well as orgasm. Prolonged use of oral contraceptives may also cause physiologic menopausal-like changes resulting in genito-pelvic pain/penetration disorder. Benzodiazepines have been reported to decrease libido, but in some patients the diminution of anxiety caused by those drugs enhances sexual function. Both increase and decrease in libido have been reported with psychoactive agents. It is difficult to separate those effects from the underlying condition or from improvement of the condition. Sexual dysfunction associated with the use of a drug disappears when use of the drug is discontinued.

Table 18-13
Some Pharmacologic Agents Implicated in Sexual Dysfunctions

Drug	Impairs Erection	Impairs Ejaculation
Psychiatric drugs		
Cyclic drugs[a]		
Imipramine (Tofranil)	+	+
Protriptyline (Vivactil)	+	+
Desipramine (Pertofrane)	+	+
Clomipramine (Anafranil)	+	+
Amitriptyline (Elavil)	+	+
Trazodone (Desyrel)[b]	−	−
Monoamine oxidase inhibitors		
Tranylcypromine (Parnate)	+	
Phenelzine (Nardil)	+	+
Pargyline (Eutonyl)	−	+
Isocarboxazid (Marplan)	−	+
Other mood-active drugs		
Lithium (Eskalith)	+	
Amphetamines	+	+
Fluoxetine (Prozac)[e]	−	+
Antipsychotics[c]		
Fluphenazine (Prolixin)	+	
Thioridazine (Mellaril)	+	+
Chlorprothixene (Taractan)	−	+
Mesoridazine (Serentil)	−	+
Perphenazine (Trilafon)	−	+
Trifluoperazine (Stelazine)	−	+
Reserpine (Serpasil)	+	+
Haloperidol (Haldol)	−	+
Antianxiety agent[d]		
Chlordiazepoxide (Librium)	−	+
Antihypertensive drugs		
Clonidine (Catapres)	+	
Methyldopa (Aldomet)	+	+
Spironolactone (Aldactone)	+	−
Hydrochlorothiazide	+	−
Guanethidine (Ismelin)	+	+
Commonly abused substances		
Alcohol	+	+
Barbiturates	+	+
Cannabis	+	−
Cocaine	+	+
Heroin	+	+
Methadone	+	−
Morphine	+	+
Miscellaneous drugs		
Antiparkinsonian agents	+	+
Clofibrate (Atromid-S)	+	−
Digoxin (Lanoxin)	+	−
Glutethimide (Doriden)	+	+
Indomethacin (Indocin)	+	−
Phentolamine (Regitine)	−	+
Propranolol (Inderal)	+	−

[a]The incidence of male erectile disorder associated with the use of tricyclic drugs is low.
[b]Trazodone has been causative in some cases of priapism.
[c]Impairment of sexual function is not a common complication of the use of antipsychotics. Priapism has occasionally occurred in association with the use of antipsychotics.
[d]Benzodiazepines have been reported to decrease libido, but in some patients the diminution of anxiety caused by those drugs enhances sexual function.
[e]All SSRIs can produce sexual dysfunction, more commonly, in men.

SSRIs and SNRIs lower the sex drive and difficulty reaching orgasm occur in both sexes.

  a. Lithium. Lithium (Eskalith) regulates mood and, in the manic state, may reduce hypersexuality, possibly by a dopamine antagonist activity. In some patients, impaired erection has been reported.

  b. Sympathomimetics. Psychostimulants raise the plasma levels of norepinephrine and dopamine. Libido is increased; however, with prolonged use, men may experience a loss of desire and erections.

  c. α-Adrenergic and β-adrenergic receptor antagonists. α-Adrenergic and β-adrenergic receptor antagonists diminish tonic sympathetic nerve outflow from vasomotor centers in the brain and that can cause impotence, decrease the volume of ejaculate, and produce retrograde ejaculation.

  3. Anticholinergics. The anticholinergics block cholinergic receptors and cause dryness of the mucous membranes (including those of the vagina) and erectile disorder. However, amantadine may reverse SSRI-induced orgasmic dysfunction through its dopaminergic effect.

  4. Antihistamines. Drugs such as diphenhydramine (Benadryl) may inhibit sexual function. Cyproheptadine, although an antihistamine, is a serotonin antagonist and reverses sexual adverse effects produced by SSRIs.

  5. Antianxiety agents. Benzodiazepines diminish anxiety, and as a result they improve sexual function in persons inhibited by anxiety.

  6. Alcohol. Alcohol can produce erectile disorders in men but paradoxically increase testosterone levels in women. This may account for women to have increased libido after drinking small amounts of alcohol.

  7. Opioids. Opioids, such as heroin, have adverse sexual effects, such as erectile failure and decreased libido. The alteration of consciousness may enhance the sexual experience in occasional users.

V. Treatment

Treatment focuses on the exploration of unconscious conflicts, motivation, fantasy, and various interpersonal difficulties. Methods that have proved effective singly or in combination include (1) training in behavioral–sexual skills, (2) systematic desensitization, (3) directive marital therapy, (4) psychodynamic approaches, (5) group therapy, (6) pharmacotherapy, (7) surgery, and (8) hypnotherapy. Evaluation and treatment must address the possibility of accompanying personality disorders and physical conditions. The addition of behavioral techniques is often necessary to cure the sexual problem.

  A. Dual-sex therapy. The theoretical basis of dual-sex therapy is the concept of the marital unit or dyad as the object of therapy. In dual-sex therapy, treatment is based on a concept that the couple must be treated when a dysfunctional person is in a relationship. There is a roundtable session in which a male and female therapy team clarifies, discusses, and works through problems with the couple and open communication between the partners is urged.

B. Specific techniques and exercises

Various techniques are used to treat the various sexual disorders.

1. **Vaginismus.** The woman is advised to dilate her vaginal opening with her fingers or with dilators.

2. **Premature ejaculation.** The squeeze technique is used to raise the threshold of penile excitability. The patient or his partner forcibly squeezes the coronal ridge of the glans at the first sensation of impending ejaculation. The erection is diminished and ejaculation inhibited. A variation is the stop–start technique. Stimulation is stopped as excitement increases, but no squeeze is used.

3. **Male erectile disorder.** The man is sometimes told to masturbate to demonstrate that full erection and ejaculation are possible.

4. **Female orgasmic disorder (primary anorgasmia).** The woman is instructed to masturbate, sometimes with the use of a vibrator. The use of fantasy is encouraged.

5. **Retarded ejaculation.** It is managed by extravaginal ejaculation initially and gradual vaginal entry after stimulation to the point of near ejaculation.

C. Hypnotherapy. Hypnotherapists focus specifically on the anxiety-producing situation—that is, the sexual interaction that results in dysfunction. The successful use of hypnosis enables patients to gain control over the symptom that has been lowering self-esteem and disrupting psychological homeostasis. The focus of treatment is on symptom removal and attitude alteration. Hypnosis may be added to a basic individual psychotherapy program to accelerate the effects of psychotherapeutic intervention.

D. Behavior therapy. The behavior therapist enables the patient to master the anxiety through a standard program of systematic desensitization, which is designed to inhibit the learned anxious response by encouraging behaviors antithetical to anxiety. The patient first deals with the least anxiety-producing situation in fantasy and progresses by steps to the most anxiety-producing situation. Medication, hypnosis, and special training in deep muscle relaxation are sometimes used to help with the initial mastery of anxiety. Sexual exercises may be prescribed starting with those activities that have proved most pleasurable and successful in the past.

E. Mindfulness. Mindfulness is a cognitive technique that has been helpful in the treatment of sexual dysfunction. The patient is directed to focus on the moment and maintain an awareness of sensations—visual, tactile, auditory, and olfactory—that he or she experiences in the moment.

F. Group therapy. A therapy group provides a strong support system for a patient who feels ashamed, anxious, or guilty about a particular sexual problem. It is a useful forum in which to counteract sexual myths, correct misconceptions, and provide accurate information about sexual anatomy, physiology, and varieties of behavior. Group therapy can be an adjunct to other forms of therapy or the prime mode of treatment. Techniques, such as role playing and psychodrama, may be used in treatment.

Table 18-14
Pharmacokinetics of the PDE-5 Inhibitors

	Sildenafil 100 mg	Vardenafil 20 mg	Tadalafil 20 mg
Maximum concentration	450 ng/mL	20.9 ng/mL	378 ng/mL
Time to maximum concentration	1.0 hours	0.7 hours	2.0 hours
Half-life	4 hours	3.9 hours	17.5 hours

From Arnold LM. Vardenafil & Tadalafil: Options for erectile dysfunction. *Curr Psychiatr.* 2004;3(2):46.

G. Analytically oriented sex therapy. One of the most effective treatment modalities is the integration of sex therapy (training in behavioral–sexual skills) with psychodynamic and psychoanalytically oriented psychotherapy. Psychodynamic conceptualizations are added to behavioral techniques for the treatment of patients.

H. Biologic treatments. Biologic treatments, including pharmacotherapy, surgery, and mechanical devices, are used to treat specific cases of sexual disorder. Most of the recent advances involve male sexual dysfunction. Current studies are under way to test biologic treatment of sexual dysfunction in women.

I. Pharmacotherapy. Most pharmacologic treatments involve male sexual dysfunctions. Studies are being conducted to test the use of drugs to treat women. Pharmacotherapy may be used to treat sexual disorders of physiologic, psychological, or mixed causes. In the latter two cases, pharmacologic treatment is usually used in addition to a form of psychotherapy.

J. Treatment of erectile disorder and premature ejaculation. The major new medications to treat sexual dysfunction are sildenafil (Viagra) and its congeners (Table 18-14); oral phentolamine (Vasomax); alprostadil (Caverject), and injectable medications; papaverine, prostaglandin E1, phentolamine, or some combination of these (Edex); and a transurethral alprostadil (MUSE), all used to treat erectile disorder.

 CLINICAL HINT:
When prescribing any of these drugs, be sure to explain to the patient that the pill does not produce an erection spontaneously. Sexual stimulation is necessary if an erection is to occur.

Sildenafil (Viagra), a nitric oxide enhancer, facilitates the inflow of blood to the penis necessary for an erection for about 4 hours. The medication does not work in the absence of sexual stimulation. Its use is contraindicated for people taking organic nitrates. New nitric oxide enhancers are vardenafil (Levitra) and tadalafil (Cialis). Tadalafil is effective for up to 36 hours.

Other medications act as vasodilators in the penis. They include oral prostaglandin (Vasomax); alprostadil (Caverject), an injectable phentolamine; and a transurethral alprostadil suppository (MUSE). α-Adrenergic agents such as methylphenidate (Ritalin), dextroamphetamine (Dexedrine), and yohimbine (Yocon) are also used to treat erectile disorder. SSRIs and heterocyclic antidepressants alleviate premature ejaculation because of their side effect of inhibiting orgasm.

Flibanserin, a drug to increase desire in women was approved for use in 2015. Sold under the trade name **Addyi,** is used for the treatment of premenopausal women with hypoactive sexual desire disorder. Adverse events include dizziness, nausea, fatigue, day-time sleepiness, and interrupted night-time sleep. Drinking alcohol will cause severe drop in blood pressure. Because of limited post marketing data, clinicians should be cautious about prescribing the drug.

K. Treatment of sexual aversion disorder. Cyclic antidepressants and SSRIs are used if people with this dysfunction are considered phobic of the genitalia.

L. Hormone therapy. Androgens increase the sex drive in women and in men with low testosterone concentrations. Women may experience virilizing effects, some of which are irreversible (e.g., deepening of the voice). In men, prolonged use of androgens produces hypertension and prostatic enlargement.

Estrogens use may cause decreased libido; in such cases, a combined preparation of estrogen and testosterone has been used effectively.

M. Antiandrogens and antiestrogens. Estrogens and progesterone are antiandrogens that have been used to treat compulsive sexual behavior in men, usually in sex offenders.

VI. Other Specified Sexual Dysfunctions
Many sexual disorders are not classifiable as sexual dysfunctions or as paraphilias. These unclassified disorders are rare, poorly documented, not easily classified, or not specifically described in DSM-5. Never-the-less they are syndromes that therapists have seen clinically. See Table 18-15.

A. Postcoital dysphoria. Occurs during the resolution phase of sexual activity, when persons normally experience a sense of general well-being and muscular and psychological relaxation. Some persons become depressed, tense, anxious, and irritable, and show psychomotor agitation. They often want to get away from their partners and may become verbally or even physically abusive and is more common in men.

B. Couple problems. At times, a complaint arises from the spousal unit or the couple, rather than from an individual dysfunction. For example, one

Table 18-15
Other Specified Sexual Dysfunction

Sexual dysfunction not meeting full criteria (e.g., sexual aversion)

Table 18-16
Signs of Sexual Addiction

1. Out-of-control behavior
2. Severe adverse consequences (medical, legal, interpersonal) due to sexual behavior
3. Persistent pursuit of self-destructive or high-risk sexual behavior
4. Repeated attempts to limit or stop sexual behavior
5. Sexual obsession and fantasy as a primary coping mechanism
6. The need for increasing amounts of sexual activity
7. Severe mood changes related to sexual activity (e.g., depression, euphoria)
8. Inordinate amount of time spent in obtaining sex, being sexual, or recovering from sexual experience
9. Interference of sexual behavior in social, occupational, or recreational activities

Data from Carnes P. *Don't Call It Love*. New York: Bantam Books; 1991.

partner may prefer morning sex, but the other functions more readily at night, or the partners have unequal frequencies of desire.

C. Body image problems. Some persons are ashamed of their bodies and insist on sex only during total darkness, not allow certain body parts to be seen or touched, or seek unnecessary operative procedures to deal with their imagined inadequacies. Body dysmorphic disorder should be ruled out.

D. Sex addiction and compulsivity. The concept of sex addiction developed over the last two decades to refer to persons who compulsively seek out sexual experiences and whose behavior becomes impaired if they are unable to gratify their sexual impulses.

In DSM-5, the terms *sex addiction* or *compulsive sexuality* are not used, nor is it a disorder that is universally recognized or accepted. Such persons show repeated and increasingly frequent attempts to have a sexual experience, deprivation of which gives rise to symptoms of distress.

The signs of sexual addiction are listed in Table 18-16.

E. Types of behavioral patterns. The paraphilias constitute the behavioral patterns most often found in the sex addict. The essential features of a paraphilia are recurrent, intense sexual urges or behaviors, including exhibitionism, fetishism, frotteurism, sadomasochism, cross-dressing, voyeurism, and pedophilia. Paraphilias are associated with clinically significant distress and almost invariably interfere with interpersonal relationships, and they often lead to legal complications.

   1. Distress about sexual orientation. Distress about sexual orientation is characterized by dissatisfaction with sexual arousal patterns, and it is usually applied to dissatisfaction with homosexual arousal patterns, a desire to increase heterosexual arousal, and strong negative feelings about being homosexual.

   Treatment of sexual orientation distress also known as conversion or reparative therapy is controversial.

   Another and more prevalent style of intervention is directed at enabling persons with persistent and marked distress about sexual orientation to live comfortably with homosexuality without shame, guilt, anxiety, or depression. Gay counseling centers are engaged with patients in such treatment programs. The American Psychiatric Association opposes conversion therapy on two grounds: it is based on the assumption that homosexuality is a disease and that it has not been proved to work. Opponents of conversion therapy consider it to be not only unethical but illegal and some groups advocate laws that prohibit therapists from engaging in or advocating such approaches. Overall, conversion therapy has been discredited.

2. **Persistent genital arousal disorder.** Persistent genital arousal disorder (PGAD) has previously been called persistent sexual arousal syndrome. It has been diagnosed in women who complain of a continual feeling of sexual arousal, which is uncomfortable, demands release, and interferes with life pleasures and activities. These women masturbate frequently, sometimes incessantly, because climax provides relief. However, the relief is temporary and the sense of arousal returns rapidly and remains. The sense of arousal in these cases is neither pleasurable nor exciting. One case of attempted suicide has been reported with this syndrome. There is some speculation that this disorder is due to nerve damage or anomaly, but the etiology is unknown.

3. **Female premature orgasm.** A case of multiple spontaneous orgasms without sexual stimulation was seen in a woman; the cause was an epileptogenic focus in the temporal lobe. Instances have been reported of women taking antidepressants (e.g., fluoxetine and clomipramine) who experience spontaneous orgasm associated with yawning.

4. **Postcoital headache.** Postcoital headache, characterized by headache immediately after coitus, may last for several hours. It is usually described as throbbing and is localized in the occipital or frontal area. The cause is unknown.

5. **Orgasmic anhedonia.** Orgasmic anhedonia is a condition in which a person has no physical sensation of orgasm, even though the physiologic component (e.g., ejaculation) remains intact.

6. **Masturbatory pain.** Persons may experience pain during masturbation. Organic causes should always be ruled out; a small vaginal tear or early Peyronie's disease can produce a painful sensation. The condition should be differentiated from compulsive masturbation.

VII. Gender Dysphoria

A. **Introduction.** The term *gender dysphoria* refers to those persons with a marked incongruence between their experienced or expressed gender and the one they were assigned at birth.

The term *gender identity* refers to the sense one has of being male or female, which corresponds most often to the person's anatomical sex. Persons with gender dysphoria express their discontent with their assigned sex as a desire to have the body of the other sex or to be regarded socially as a person of the other sex.

The term *transgender* is a general term used to refer to those who identify with a gender different from the one they were born with (sometimes referred to as their assigned gender).

B. Gender identity disorders. A group of disorders that have as their main symptom a persistent preference for the role of the opposite sex and the feeling that one was born into the wrong sex.

People with disordered gender identity try to live as or pass as members of the opposite sex. *Transsexuals* want biologic treatment (surgery, hormones) to change their biologic sex and acquire the anatomic characteristics of the opposite sex. The disorders may coexist with other pathology or be circumscribed, with patients functioning ably in many areas of their lives.

C. Diagnosis, signs, and symptoms

1. Children. Gender dysphoria in children is incongruence between expressed and assigned gender, with the most important criterion being a desire to be another gender or insistence that one is another gender. Many children with gender dysphoria prefer clothing typical of another gender, preferentially choose playmates of another gender, enjoy games and toys associated with another gender, and take on the roles of another gender during play. Children may express a desire to have different genitals, state that their genitals are going to change, or urinate in the position (standing or sitting) typical of another gender.

2. Adolescents and adults. Adolescents and adults diagnosed with gender dysphoria must also show an incongruence between expressed and assigned gender. In addition, they must meet at least two of six criteria, half of which are related to their current (or in the cases of early adolescents, future) secondary sex characteristics or desired secondary sex characteristics. Other criteria include a strong desire to be another gender, be treated as another gender, or the belief that one has the typical feelings and reactions of another gender.

D. Epidemiology

1. Unknown, but rare.

2. Male-to-female ratio is 4:1.

3. Almost all gender-disordered females have a homosexual orientation.

4. Fifty percent of gender-disordered males have a homosexual orientation, and 50% have a heterosexual, bisexual, or asexual orientation.

5. The prevalence rate for transsexualism is 1 per 10,000 males and 1 per 30,000 females.

E. Etiology

Biologic. Testosterone affects brain neurons that contribute to masculinization of the brain in such areas as the hypothalamus. Whether testosterone contributes to so-called masculine or feminine behavioral patterns in gender identity disorders remains controversial. Sex steroids influence the expression of sexual behavior in mature men and women (i.e., testosterone can increase libido and aggressiveness in men and women, while estrogen or progesterone can decrease libido and aggressiveness in men).

Table 18-17
Classification of Intersexual Disorders[a]

Syndrome	Description
Virilizing adrenal hyperplasia (andrenogenital syndrome)	Results from excess androgens in fetus with XX genotype; most common female intersex disorder; associated with enlarged clitoris, fused labia, hirsutism in adolescence.
Turner's syndrome	Results from absence of second female sex chromosome (XO); associated with web neck, dwarfism, cubitus valgus; no sex hormones produced; infertile; usually assigned as females because of female-looking genitals.
Klinefelter's syndrome	Genotype is XXY; male habitus present with small penis and rudimentary testes because of low androgen production; weak libido; usually assigned as male.
Androgen insensitivity syndrome (testicular-feminizing syndrome)	Congenital X-linked recessive disorder that results in inability of tissues to respond to androgens; external genitals look female and cryptorchid testes present; assigned as females, even though they have XY genotype; in extreme form patient has breasts, normal external genitals, short blind vagina, and absence of pubic and axillary hair.
Enzymatic defects in XY genotype (e.g., 5-α reductase deficiency, 17-hydroxysteroid deficiency)	Congenital interruption in production of testosterone that produces ambiguous genitals and female habitus; usually assigned as female because of female-looking genitalia.
Hermaphroditism	True hermaphrodite is rare and characterized by both testes and ovaries in same person (may be 46 XX or 46 XY).
Pseudohermaphroditism	Usually the result of endocrine or enzymatic defect (e.g., adrenal hyperplasia) in persons with normal chromosomes; female pseudohermaphrodites have masculine-looking genitals but are XX; male pseudohermaphrodites have rudimentary testes and external genitals and are XY; assigned as males or females, depending on morphology of genitals.

[a]Intersexual disorders include a variety of syndromes that produce persons with gross anatomic or physiologic aspects of the opposite sex.

Psychosocial. The absence of same-sex role models and explicit or implicit encouragement from caregivers to behave like the other sex contributes to gender identity disorder in childhood. Mothers may be depressed or withdrawn. Inborn temperamental traits sometimes result in sensitive, delicate boys and energetic, aggressive girls. Physical and sexual abuse may predispose.

F. Differential diagnosis

Transvestic fetishism. Cross-dressing for purpose of sexual excitement; can coexist (dual diagnosis).

Intersex conditions. See Table 18-17.

Schizophrenia. Rarely, true delusions of being other sex.

G. Course and prognosis

Children. Course varies. Symptoms may diminish spontaneously or with treatment. Prognosis depends on age of onset and intensity of symptoms. The disorder begins in boys before the age of 4 years, and peer conflict develops at about the age of 7 or 8 years. Tomboyism is generally better tolerated. The age of onset is also early for girls, but most give up masculine behavior by adolescence. Fewer than 10% of children go on to transsexualism.

Adults. Course tends to be chronic.

Transsexualism—after puberty, distress with one's biologic sex and a desire to eliminate one's primary and secondary sex characteristics and acquire those of the other sex. Most transsexuals have had gender identity disorder in childhood; cross-dressing is common; associated mental disorder is common, especially borderline personality disorder or depressive disorder; suicide is a risk, but persons may mutilate their sex organs to coerce surgeons to perform sex reassignment surgery.

H. Treatment

Children. Improve existing role models or, in their absence, provide one from the family or elsewhere (e.g., big brother or sister). Caregivers are helped to encourage sex-appropriate behavior and attitudes. Any associated mental disorder is addressed.

Adolescents. Difficult to treat because of the coexistence of normal identity crises and gender identity confusion. Acting out is common, and adolescents rarely have a strong motivation to alter their stereotypic cross-gender roles.

Adults.

1. **Psychotherapy.** Set the goal of helping patients become comfortable with the gender identity they desire; the goal is not to create a person with a conventional sexual identity. Therapy also explores sex-reassignment surgery and the indications and contraindications for such procedures, which severely distressed and anxious patients often decide to undergo impulsively.

2. **Sex-reassignment surgery.** Definitive and irreversible. Patients must go through a 3- to 12-month trial of cross-dressing and receive hormone treatment. Seventy percent to 80% of patients are satisfied by the results. Dissatisfaction correlates with severity of pre-existing psychopathology. A reported 2% commit suicide.

3. **Hormonal treatments.** Many patients are treated with hormones in lieu of surgery.

VIII. Paraphilias

Paraphilias or perversions are sexual stimuli or acts that are deviations from normal sexual behaviors, but are necessary for some persons to experience arousal and orgasm. Individuals with paraphilic interests can experience sexual pleasure, but they are inhibited from responding to stimuli that are normally considered erotic. DSM-5 lists pedophilia, frotteurism, voyeurism, exhibitionism, sexual sadism, sexual masochism, fetishism, and transvestism with explicit diagnostic criteria because of their threat to others and/or because they are relatively common paraphilias. They are more common in men than in women. Cause is unknown. A biologic predisposition (abnormal electroencephalogram, hormone levels) may be reinforced by psychologic factors, such as childhood abuse. Psychoanalytic theory holds that paraphilia

Table 18-18
Paraphilias

Disorder	Definition	General Considerations	Treatment
Exhibitionism	Exposing genitals in public; rare in females.	Person wants to shock female—her reaction is affirmation to patient that penis is intact.	Insight-oriented psychotherapy, aversive conditioning. Female should try to ignore exhibitionistic male, who is offensive but not dangerous, or call police.
Fetishism	Sexual arousal with inanimate objects (e.g., shoes, hair, clothing).	Almost always in men. Behavior often followed by guilt.	Insight-oriented psychotherapy; aversive conditioning; implosion, i.e., patient masturbates with fetish until it loses its arousal effect (masturbatory satiation).
Frotteurism	Rubbing genitals against female to achieve arousal and orgasm.	Occurs in crowded places, such as subways usually by passive, nonassertive men.	Insight-oriented psychotherapy; aversive conditioning; group therapy; antiandrogenic medication.
Pedophilia	Sexual activity with children under age 13; most common paraphilia.	95% heterosexual, 5% homosexual. High risk of repeated behavior. Fear of adult sexuality in patient; low self-esteem. 10–20% of children have been molested by age 18.	Place patient in treatment unit; group therapy; insight-oriented psychotherapy; antiandrogen medication to diminish sexual urge.
Sexual masochism	Sexual pleasure derived from being abused physically or mentally or from being humiliated (moral masochism).	Defense against guilt feelings related to sex—punishment turned inwards.	Insight-oriented psychotherapy; group therapy.
Sexual sadism	Sexual arousal resulting from causing mental or physical suffering to another person.	Mostly seen in men. Named after Marquis de Sade. Can progress to rape in some cases.	Insight-oriented psychotherapy; aversive conditioning.
Transvestic fetishism	Cross-dressing.	Most often used in heterosexual arousal. Most common is male-to-female cross-dressing. Do not confuse with transsexualism-wanting to be opposite sex.	Insight-oriented psychotherapy.
Voyeurism	Sexual arousal by watching sexual acts (e.g., coitus or naked person). Can occur in women but more common in men. Variant is listening to erotic conversations (e.g., telephone sex).	Masturbation usually occurs during voyeuristic activity. Usually arrested for loitering or peeping-tomism.	Insight-oriented psychotherapy; aversive conditioning.
Other paraphilias Excretory paraphilias	Defecating (coprophilia) or urinating (urophilia) on a partner or vice versa.	Fixation at anal stage of development; klismaphilia (enemas).	Insight-oriented psychotherapy.
Zoophilia	Sex with animals.	More common in rural areas; may be opportunistic.	Behavior modification, insight-oriented psychotherapy.

results from fixation at one of the psychosexual phases of development or is an effort to ward off castration anxiety. Learning theory holds that association of the act with sexual arousal during childhood leads to conditioned learning.

Paraphiliac activity often is compulsive. Patients repeatedly engage in deviant behavior and are unable to control the impulse. When stressed, anxious, or depressed, the patient is more likely to engage in the deviant behavior. The patient may make numerous resolutions to stop the behavior but is generally unable to abstain for long, and acting out is followed by strong feelings of guilt. Treatment techniques, which result in only moderate success rates, include insight-oriented psychotherapy, behavior therapy, and pharmacotherapy alone or in combination. Table 18-18 lists the common paraphilias.

For more detailed discussion of this topic, see Chapter 21, Normal Sexuality and Sexual Disorders, p. 1953, in CTP/X.

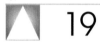 **19**

Feeding and Eating Disorders

I. Anorexia Nervosa

The term *anorexia nervosa* is derived from the Greek term for "loss of appetite" and a Latin word implying nervous origin. Anorexia nervosa is a syndrome characterized by three essential criteria: (1) a self-induced starvation to a significant degree, (2) a relentless drive for thinness or a morbid fear of fatness, and (3) the presence of medical signs and symptoms resulting from starvation. It is often associated with disturbances of body image—the perception that one is distressingly large despite obvious thinness.

A. Epidemiology. The most common age of onset is between 14 and 18 years. Anorexia nervosa is estimated to occur in about 0.5% to 1% of adolescent girls. It occurs 10 to 20 times more often in females than in males. The prevalence of young women with some symptoms of anorexia nervosa who do not meet the diagnostic criteria is estimated to be close to 5%. It seems to be most frequent in developed countries, and it may be seen with greatest frequency among young women in professions that require thinness, such as modeling and ballet. It is associated with depression, social phobia, and obsessive-compulsive disorder. See Table 19-1 lists comorbid psychiatric conditions associated with anorexia nervosa.

B. Etiology. Biologic, social, and psychological factors are implicated in the causes of anorexia nervosa. Some evidence points to higher concordance rates in monozygotic twins than in dizygotic twins. Major mood disorders are more common in family members than in the general population.

1. Biologic factors. Starvation results in many biochemical changes, some of which are also present in depression, such as hypercortisolemia and nonsuppression by dexamethasone. An increase in familial depression, alcohol dependence, or eating disorders has been noted. Some evidence of increased anorexia nervosa in sisters has also been noted. Neurobiologically, a reduction in 3-methoxy-4-hydroxyphenylglycol (MHPG) in urine and cerebrospinal fluid (CSF) suggests lessened norepinephrine turnover and activity. Endogenous opioid activity appears lessened as a consequence of starvation. Table 19-2 lists the neuroendocrine changes associated with anorexia nervosa. In one positron emission tomography (PET) study, caudate nucleus metabolism was higher during the anorectic state than after weight gain. Magnetic resonance imaging (MRI) may show volume deficits of gray matter during illness, which may persist during recovery. A genetic predisposition may be a factor.

2. Social factors. Patients with anorexia nervosa find support for their practices in society's emphasis on thinness and exercise. Families of children who present with eating disorders, especially binge-eating or purging

Table 19-1
Comorbid Psychiatric Conditions Associated with Anorexia Nervosa

Diagnosis	Restricting-Type Anorexia Nervosa (%)	Binge-Eating and Purging Type Anorexia Nervosa (%)
Any affective disorder	57	100
Intermittent depressive disorder	29	44
Major depression	57	66
Minor depression	0	11
Mania/hypomania	0	33
Any anxiety disorder	57	67
Phobic disorder	43	11
Panic disorder	29	22
Generalized anxiety disorder	14	11
Obsessive-compulsive disorder	14	56
Any substance abuse/dependence	14	33
Drug	14	22
Alcohol	0	33
Schizophrenia	0	0
Any codiagnoses	71	100
3 or more codiagnoses	71	100
Female	100	89
Single	71	89
Age ($x \pm$ SD)	23.6 ± 10.8	25.0 ± 6.4
No. of codiagnoses ($x \pm$ SD)	2.3 ± 2.5	3.8 ± 1.4

SD, standard deviation.

Table 19-2
Neuroendocrine Changes in Anorexia Nervosa and Experimental Starvation

Hormone	Anorexia Nervosa	Weight Loss
Corticotropin-releasing hormone (CRH)	Increased	Increased
Plasma cortisol levels	Mildly increased	Mildly increased
Diurnal cortisol difference	Blunted	Blunted
Luteinizing hormone (LH)	Decreased, prepubertal pattern	Decreased
Follicle-stimulating hormone (FSH)	Decreased, prepubertal pattern	Decreased
Growth hormone (GH)	Impaired regulation	Same
	Increased basal levels and limited response to pharmacologic probes	
Somatomedin C	Decreased	Decreased
Thyroxine (T_4)	Normal or slightly decreased	Normal or slightly decreased
Triiodothyronine (T_3)	Mildly decreased	Mildly decreased
Reverse T_3	Mildly increased	Mildly increased
Thyrotropin-stimulating hormone (TSH)	Normal	Normal
TSH response to thyrotropin-releasing hormone (TRH)	Delayed or blunted	Delayed or blunted
Insulin	Delayed release	–
C-peptide	Decreased	–
Vasopressin	Secretion uncoupled from osmotic challenge	–
Serotonin	Increased function with weight restoration	
Norepinephrine	Reduced turnover	Reduced turnover
Dopamine	Blunted response to pharmacologic probes	–

subtypes, may exhibit high levels of hostility, chaos, and isolation and low levels of nurturance and empathy. Vocational and avocational interests interact with other vulnerability factors to increase the probability of developing eating disorders (i.e., ballet in young women and wrestling in high school boys).

3. **Psychological and psychodynamic factors.** Patients with the disorder substitute their preoccupations, which are similar to obsessions, with eating and weight gain for other, normal adolescent pursuits. These patients typically lack a sense of autonomy and selfhood.

C. **Diagnosis and clinical features.** The onset of anorexia nervosa usually occurs between the ages of 10 and 30 years. It is present when (1) an individual voluntarily reduces and maintains an unhealthy degree of weight loss or fails to gain weight proportional to growth; (2) an individual experiences an intense fear of becoming fat, has a relentless drive for thinness despite obvious medical starvation, or both; (3) an individual experiences significant starvation-related medical symptomatology, often, but not exclusively, abnormal reproductive hormone functioning, but also hypothermia, bradycardia, orthostasis, and severely reduced body fat stores; and (4) the behaviors and psychopathology are present for at least 3 months. In addition, patients have a significantly less than minimally normal weight and a marked fear of gaining weight. Obsessive-compulsive behavior, depression, and anxiety are other psychiatric symptoms of anorexia nervosa most frequently noted in the literature. Poor sexual adjustment is frequently described in patients with the disorder.

D. **Subtypes**

1. **Restricting type.** Present in approximately 50% of cases. Food intake is highly restricted (usually with attempts to consume fewer than 300 to 500 calories per day and no fat grams), and the patient may be relentlessly and compulsively overactive, with overuse athletic injuries. Persons with restricting anorexia nervosa often have obsessive-compulsive traits with respect to food and other matters.

2. **Binge-eating/purging type.** Patients alternate attempts at rigorous dieting with intermittent binge or purge episodes, with the binges, if present, being either subjective (more than the patient intended, or because of social pressure, but not enormous) or objective. Purging represents a secondary compensation for the unwanted calories, most often accomplished by self-induced vomiting, frequently by laxative abuse, less frequently by diuretics, and occasionally with emetics. The suicide rate is higher than in those with the restricting type.

E. **Pathology and laboratory examination.** A complete blood count often reveals leukopenia with a relative lymphocytosis in emaciated patients with anorexia nervosa. If binge eating and purging are present, serum electrolyte determination reveals hypokalemic alkalosis. Fasting serum glucose concentrations are often low during the emaciated phase, and serum salivary amylase concentrations are often elevated if the patient is vomiting. The ECG may show ST-segment and T-wave changes, which are usually secondary to

Table 19-3
Medical Complications of Eating Disorders

Disorder and System Affected	Consequence
Anorexia nervosa	
Vital signs	Bradycardia, hypotension with marked orthostatic changes, hypothermia, poikilothermia
General	Muscle atrophy, loss of body fat
Central nervous system	Generalized brain atrophy with enlarged ventricles, decreased cortical mass, seizures, abnormal electroencephalogram
Cardiovascular	Peripheral (starvation) edema, decreased cardiac diameter, narrowed left ventricular wall, decreased response to exercise demand, superior mesenteric artery syndrome
Renal	Prerenal azotemia
Hematologic	Anemia of starvation, leukopenia, hypocellular bone marrow
Gastrointestinal	Delayed gastric emptying, gastric dilatation, decreased intestinal lipase and lactase
Metabolic	Hypercholesterolemia, nonsymptomatic hypoglycemia, elevated liver enzymes, decreased bone mineral density
Endocrine	Low luteinizing hormone, low follicle-stimulating hormone, low estrogen or testosterone, low/normal thyroxine, low triiodothyronine, increased reverse triiodothyronine, elevated cortisol, elevated growth hormone, partial diabetes insipidus, increased prolactin
Bulimia nervosa and binge-eating and purging type anorexia nervosa	
Metabolic	Hypokalemic alkalosis or acidosis, hypochloremia, dehydration
Renal	Prerenal azotemia, acute and chronic renal failure
Cardiovascular	Arrhythmias, myocardial toxicity from emetine (ipecac)
Dental	Lingual surface enamel loss, multiple caries
Gastrointestinal	Swollen parotid glands, elevated serum amylase levels, gastric distention, irritable bowel syndrome, melanosis coli from laxative abuse
Musculoskeletal	Cramps, tetany

electrolyte disturbances; emaciated patients have hypotension and bradycardia. Other medical complications are listed in Table 19-3.

F. Differential diagnosis

1. **Medical conditions and substance use disorders.** Medical illness (e.g., cancer, brain tumor, gastrointestinal disorders, drug abuse) that can account for weight loss.

2. **Depressive disorder.** Depressive disorders and anorexia nervosa have several features in common, such as depressed feelings, crying spells, sleep disturbance, obsessive ruminations, and occasional suicidal thoughts. However, generally a patient with a depressive disorder has decreased appetite, whereas a patient with anorexia nervosa claims to have normal appetite and to feel hungry; only in the severe stages of anorexia nervosa do patients actually have decreased appetite. Also, in contrast to depressive agitation, the hyperactivity seen in anorexia nervosa is planned and ritualistic. The preoccupation with recipes, the caloric content of foods, and the preparation of gourmet feasts is typical with anorexia nervosa not with depressive disorder. In depressive disorders, patients have no intense fear of obesity or disturbance of body image. Comorbid major depression or dysthymia has been found in 50% of patients with anorexia.

3. **Somatization disorder.** Weight loss not as severe; no morbid fear of becoming overweight; amenorrhea unusual.
4. **Schizophrenia.** Delusions about food (e.g., patients believe the food to be poisoned). Patients rarely fear becoming obese and are not as hyperactive.
5. **Bulimia nervosa.** Patient's weight loss is seldom more than 15%. Bulimia nervosa develops in 30% to 50% of patients with anorexia nervosa within 2 years of the onset of anorexia.

 CLINICAL HINT:
Anorexia nervosa patients often give a history of few or no sexual
experiences and generally have low libido; Bulimia patients are often
sexually active with a normal or high libido.

G. **Course and prognosis.** The course of anorexia nervosa varies greatly—spontaneous recovery without treatment, recovery after a variety of treatments, a fluctuating course of weight gains followed by relapses, and a gradually deteriorating course resulting in death caused by complications of starvation. The short-term response of patients to almost all hospital treatment programs is good. Those who have regained sufficient weight, however, often continue their preoccupation with food and body weight, have poor social relationships, and exhibit depression. In general, the prognosis is not good. Studies have shown a range of mortality rates from 5% to 18%. About half of patients with anorexia nervosa eventually have the symptoms of bulimia, usually within the first year after the onset of anorexia nervosa.

H. **Treatment**
   1. **Hospitalization.** The first consideration in the treatment of anorexia nervosa is to restore patients' nutritional state. Patients with anorexia nervosa who are 20% below the expected weight for their height are recommended for inpatient programs, and patients who are 30% below their expected weight require psychiatric hospitalization for 2 to 6 months. Inpatient psychiatric programs for patients with anorexia nervosa generally use a combination of a behavioral management approach, individual psychotherapy, family education and therapy, and, in some cases, psychotropic medications. Patients must become willing participants for treatment to succeed in the long run. After patients are discharged from the hospital, clinicians usually find it necessary to continue outpatient supervision of the problems identified in the patients and their families.
   2. **Psychotherapy**
      a. **Cognitive-behavioral therapy (CBT).** Cognitive and behavioral therapy principles can be applied in both inpatient and outpatient settings. Behavior therapy has been found effective for inducing weight gain; no large, controlled studies of cognitive therapy with behavior

therapy in patients with anorexia nervosa have been reported. Patients are taught to monitor their food intake, their feelings and emotions, their binging and purging behaviors, and their problems in interpersonal relationships. Patients are taught cognitive restructuring to identify automatic thoughts and to challenge their core beliefs. Problem solving is a specific method whereby patients learn how to think through and devise strategies to cope with their food-related and interpersonal problems. Patients' vulnerability to rely on anorectic behavior as a means of coping can be addressed if they can learn to use these techniques effectively.

b. **Dynamic psychotherapy.** Patients' resistance may make the process difficult and painstaking. Because patients view their symptoms as constituting the core of their specialness, therapists must avoid excessive investment in trying to change their eating behavior. The opening phase of the psychotherapy process must be geared to building a therapeutic alliance. Patients may experience early interpretations as though someone else were telling them what they really feel and thereby minimizing and invalidating their own experiences. Therapists who empathize with patients' points of view and take an active interest in what their patients think and feel, however, convey to patients that their autonomy is respected. Above all, psychotherapists must be flexible, persistent, and durable in the face of patients' tendencies to defeat any efforts to help them.

c. **Family therapy.** A family analysis should be done for all patients with anorexia nervosa who are living with their families, as a basis for a clinical judgment on what type of family therapy or counseling is advisable. In some cases, family therapy is not possible; however, issues of family relationships can then be addressed in individual therapy. Sometimes, brief counseling sessions with immediate family members is the extent of family therapy required.

3. **Pharmacotherapy.** Some reports support the use of cyproheptadine (Periactin), a drug with antihistaminic and antiserotonergic properties, for patients with the restricting type of anorexia nervosa. Amitriptyline (Elavil) has also been reported to have some benefit. Concern exists about the use of tricyclic drugs in low-weight, depressed patients with anorexia nervosa, who may be vulnerable to hypotension, cardiac arrhythmia, and dehydration. Once an adequate nutritional status has been attained, the risk of serious adverse effects from the tricyclic drugs may decrease; in some patients, the depression improves with weight gain and normalized nutritional status. Other medications that have been tried by patients with anorexia nervosa with variable results include clomipramine (Anafranil), pimozide (Orap), and chlorpromazine (Thorazine). Trials of fluoxetine (Prozac) have resulted in some reports of weight gain, and serotonergic agents may yield positive responses. In patients with anorexia nervosa and coexisting depressive disorders, the depressive condition should be treated.

II. Bulimia Nervosa

Bulimia nervosa is defined as binge eating combined with inappropriate ways of stopping weight gain. Social interruption or physical discomfort—that is, abdominal pain or nausea—terminates the binge eating, which is often followed by feelings of guilt, depression, or self-disgust. Unlike patients with anorexia nervosa, those with bulimia nervosa may maintain a normal body weight.

A. **Epidemiology.** Bulimia nervosa is more prevalent than anorexia nervosa. Estimates of bulimia nervosa range from 1% to 4% of young women. As with anorexia nervosa, bulimia nervosa is significantly more common in women than in men, but its onset is often later in adolescence than that of anorexia nervosa. The onset may even occur in early adulthood. Approximately 20% of college women experience transient bulimic symptoms at some point during their college years. Although bulimia nervosa is often present in normal-weight young women, they sometimes have a history of obesity. In industrialized countries, the prevalence is about 1% of the general population.

B. **Etiology**

1. **Biologic factors.** Serotonin and norepinephrine have been implicated. Because plasma endorphin levels are raised in some bulimia nervosa patients who vomit, the feeling of well-being after vomiting that some of these patients experience may be mediated by raised endorphin levels. Increased frequency of bulimia nervosa is found in first-degree relatives of persons with the disorder.

2. **Social factors.** Patients with bulimia nervosa, as with those with anorexia nervosa, tend to be high achievers and to respond to societal pressures to be slender. As with anorexia nervosa patients, many patients with bulimia nervosa are depressed and have increased familial depression, but the families of patients with bulimia nervosa are generally less close and more conflictual than the families of those with anorexia nervosa. Patients with bulimia nervosa describe their parents as neglectful and rejecting.

3. **Psychological factors.** Patients with bulimia nervosa have difficulties with adolescent demands, but are more outgoing, angry, and impulsive than patients with anorexia nervosa. Alcohol dependence, shoplifting, and emotional lability (including suicide attempts) are associated with bulimia nervosa. These patients generally experience their uncontrolled eating as more ego-dystonic and seek help more readily.

C. **Diagnosis and clinical features.** Bulimia nervosa is present when (1) episodes of binge eating occur relatively frequently (twice a week or more) for at least 3 months; (2) compensatory behaviors are practiced after binge eating to prevent weight gain—primarily self-induced vomiting, laxative abuse, diuretics, or abuse of emetics (80% of cases), and, less commonly, severe dieting and strenuous exercise (20% of cases); (3) weight is not severely lowered as in anorexia nervosa; and (4) the patient has a morbid fear of fatness, a relentless drive for thinness, or both and a disproportionate amount of self-evaluation depends on body weight and shape. When making a diagnosis of bulimia nervosa, clinicians should explore the possibility that the patient has experienced a brief or prolonged prior bout of anorexia nervosa, which is present in approximately half of those with bulimia nervosa. Binging usually precedes vomiting by about 1 year. Depression, sometimes called *postbinge anguish*, often follows the episode. During binges, patients eat food that is sweet, high in calories, and generally soft or smooth textured, such as cakes and pastry. The food is eaten secretly and rapidly and is sometimes not even chewed. Most patients are sexually active. Pica and struggles during meals are sometimes revealed in the histories of patients with bulimia nervosa.

D. Subtypes
1. **Purging type.** Patients regularly engage in self-induced vomiting or the use of laxatives or diuretics. May be at risk for certain medical complications, such as hypokalemia from vomiting or laxative abuse and hypochloremic alkalosis. Those who vomit repeatedly are at risk for gastric and esophageal tears, although these complications are rare.
2. **Nonpurging type.** Patients use strict dieting, fasting, or vigorous exercise but do not regularly engage in purging. Patients tend to be obese.

E. Pathology and laboratory examinations. Bulimia nervosa can result in electrolyte abnormalities and various degrees of starvation. In general, thyroid function remains intact in bulimia nervosa, but patients may show nonsuppression on the dexamethasone-suppression test. Dehydration and electrolyte disturbances are likely to occur in patients with bulimia nervosa who purge regularly. These patients commonly exhibit hypomagnesemia and hyperamylasemia. Although not a core diagnostic feature, many patients with bulimia nervosa have menstrual disturbances. Hypotension and bradycardia occur in some patients.

F. Differential diagnosis
1. **Anorexia nervosa.** The diagnosis of bulimia nervosa cannot be made if the binge-eating and purging behaviors occur exclusively during episodes of anorexia nervosa. In such cases, the diagnosis is anorexia nervosa, binge eating–purging type.
2. **Neurologic disease.** Clinicians must ascertain that patients have no neurologic disease, such as epileptic-equivalent seizures, central nervous system tumors, Klüver–Bucy syndrome, or Kleine–Levin syndrome.
3. **Seasonal affective disorder.** Patients with bulimia nervosa who have concurrent seasonal affective disorder and patterns of atypical depression (with overeating and oversleeping in low-light months) may manifest seasonal worsening of both bulimia nervosa and depressive features. In these cases, binges are typically much more severe during winter months.
4. **Borderline personality disorder.** Patients sometimes binge eat, but the eating is associated with other signs of the disorder.
5. **Major depressive disorder.** Patients rarely have peculiar attitudes or idiosyncratic practices regarding food.

G. Course and prognosis. Bulimia nervosa is characterized by higher rates of partial and full recovery compared with anorexia nervosa. Those treated fare much better than those untreated. Untreated patients tend to remain chronic or may show small but generally unimpressive degrees of improvement with time. A history of substance use problems and a longer duration of the disorder at presentation predicted worse outcome.

H. Treatment

1. **Hospitalization.** Most patients with uncomplicated bulimia nervosa do not require hospitalization. In some cases—when eating binges are out of control, outpatient treatment does not work, or a patient exhibits such additional psychiatric symptoms as suicidality and substance abuse—hospitalization may become necessary. In addition, electrolyte and metabolic disturbances resulting from severe purging may necessitate hospitalization.

 CLINICAL HINT:
Bulimia patients should have careful dental checkups since the acid content of vomit often erodes tooth enamel.

---

2. **Psychotherapy**

   a. **Cognitive-behavioral therapy.** CBT should be considered the benchmark, first-line treatment for bulimia nervosa. CBT implements a number of cognitive and behavioral procedures to (1) interrupt the self-maintaining behavioral cycle of bingeing and dieting and (2) alter the individual's dysfunctional cognitions; beliefs about food, weight, body image; and overall self-concept.

   b. **Dynamic psychotherapy.** Psychodynamic treatment of patients with bulimia nervosa has revealed a tendency to concretize introjective and projective defense mechanisms. In a manner analogous to splitting, patients divide food into two categories: items that are nutritious and those that are unhealthy. Food that is designated nutritious may be ingested and retained because it unconsciously symbolizes good introjects. But junk food is unconsciously associated with bad introjects and, therefore, is expelled by vomiting, with the unconscious fantasy that all destructiveness, hate, and badness are being evacuated. Patients can temporarily feel good after vomiting because of the fantasized evacuation, but the associated feeling of "being all good" is short lived because it is based on an unstable combination of splitting and projection.

3. **Pharmacotherapy.** Antidepressant medications have been shown to be helpful in treating bulimia. This includes the selective serotonin reuptake inhibitors (SSRIs), such as fluoxetine but in high dosages (60 to 80 mg a day). Imipramine (Tofranil), desipramine (Norpramin), trazodone (Desyrel), and monoamine oxidase inhibitors (MAOIs) have been helpful. In general, most of the antidepressants have been effective at

doses usually given in the treatment of depressive disorders. Carbamaze-pine (Tegretol) and lithium (Eskalith) have not shown impressive results as treatments for binge eating, but they have been used in the treatment of patients with bulimia nervosa with comorbid mood disorders, such as bipolar I disorder.

III. Binge-Eating Disorder and Other Eating Disorders

A. **Binge-eating disorder.** Defined as recurrent binge eating during which one eats an abnormally large amount of food over a short time. It is the most common of eating disorders and more prevalent in females. Associated with impulsive personality styles and the cause is unknown. It is characterized by four features: (1) eating more rapidly than normal and to the point of being uncomfortably full, (2) eating large amounts of food even when not hungry, (3) eating alone, and (4) feeling guilty or otherwise upset about the episode. Binges must occur at least once a week for at least 3 months. Treatment modalities include cognitive-behavioral therapy (CBT) and pharmacother-apy with SSRIs.

B. **Other specified feeding or eating disorder.** Includes eating conditions that may cause significant distress but do not meet the full criteria for a clas-sified eating disorder. Conditions included in this category include night eating syndrome, purging disorder, and subthreshold forms of anorexia ner-vosa, bulimia nervosa, and binge-eating disorder.

For more detailed discussion of this topic, see Chapter 22, Feeding and Eating Disorders, p. 2065, in CTP/X.

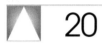

20
Obesity and Metabolic Syndrome

I. Introduction
The global epidemic of obesity has resulted in an alarming increase in associated morbidity and mortality and is the leading cause of preventable death in the United States.

II. Definition
Obesity refers to an excess of body fat.
- **A.** In healthy individuals, body fat accounts for approximately 25% of body weight in women and 18% in men.
- **B.** Overweight refers to weight above some reference norm, typically standards derived from actuarial or epidemiologic data. In most cases, increasing weight reflects increasing obesity.
- **C.** Body mass index (BMI) is calculated by dividing weight in kilograms by height in meters squared. Although there is debate about the ideal BMI, it is generally thought that a BMI of 20 to 25 kg/m^2 represents healthy weight, a BMI of 25 to 27 kg/m^2 is associated with somewhat elevated risk, a BMI above 27 kg/m^2 represents clearly increased risk, and a BMI above 30 kg/m^2 carries greatly increased risk.
- **D.** There is a higher prevalence of morbid psychiatric illness by 40% to 60% in obese patients. These include binge eating disorder, substance use disorders, psychotic disorders (schizophrenia), mood disorders, anxiety disorders, personality disorders, attention-deficit/ hyperactivity disorder (ADHD), and posttraumatic stress disorder (PTSD).

III. Epidemiology
- **A.** In the United States, over 50% of the population is overweight (defined as a BMI of 25.0 to 29.9 kg/m^2, whereas 36% are obese (defined as a BMI >30 kg/m^2). Extreme obesity (BMI ≥40 kg/m^2) is found in about 3% of men and 7% of women.
- **B.** The prevalence of obesity is highest in minority populations, particularly among non-Hispanic black women.
- **C.** More than one-half of these individuals 40 years of age or older are obese and more than 80% are overweight.
- **D.** The prevalence of overweight and obesity in children and adolescents in the United States has also increased substantially. About 18% of adolescents and about 10% of 2- to 5-year olds are overweight.

IV. Etiology

Persons accumulate fat by eating more calories than are expended as energy; thus, intake of energy exceeds its dissipation. If fat is to be removed from the body, fewer calories must be put in or more calories must be taken out than are put in. An error of no more than 10% in either intake or output would lead to a 30-pound change in body weight in 1 year.

A. Satiety is the feeling that results when hunger is satisfied. A metabolic signal derived from food receptor cells, probably in the hypothalamus, to produce satiety. Studies have shown evidence for dysfunction in serotonin, dopamine, and norepinephrine involvement in regulating eating behavior through the hypothalamus. Other hormonal factors that may be involved include corticotrophin releasing factor, neuropeptide Y, gonadotropin-releasing hormone, and thyroid-stimulating hormone. A new substance, obestatin, made in the stomach, is a hormone that in animal experiments produces satiety and may have potential use as a weight loss agent in humans.

Eating is also affected by cannabinoid receptors, which, when stimulated, increases appetite. Marijuana acts on that receptor, which accounts for the "munchies" associated with marijuana use. The drug rimonabant is an inverse agonist to the cannabidiol receptor, meaning that it blocks appetite. It may have clinical use.

The olfactory system may play a role in satiety. Experiments have shown that strong stimulation of the olfactory bulbs in the nose with food odors by use of an inhaler saturated with a particular smell produces satiety for that food. This may have implications for therapy of obesity.

V. Genetic Factors

About 80% of patients who are obese have a family history of obesity, although no specific genetic marker of obesity has been found. Studies show that identical twins raised apart can both be obese, an observation that suggests a hereditary role. Table 20-1 lists the genetic factors affecting body weight.

VI. Developmental Factors

A. Obesity that begins early in life is characterized by adipose tissue with an increased number of adipocytes (fat cells) of increased size. Obesity that begins in adult life, on the other hand, results solely from an increase in the size of the adipocytes. In both instances, weight reduction produces a decrease in cell size.

B. The distribution and amount of fat vary in individuals, and fat in different body areas has different characteristics. Fat cells around the waist, flanks, and abdomen (the so-called potbelly) are more active metabolically than those in the thighs and buttocks.

C. A hormone called leptin, made by fat cells, acts as a fat thermostat. When the blood level of leptin is low, more fat is consumed; when high, less fat is consumed.

Table 20-1
Genetic Factors Affecting Body Weight

	Genetic Factor Description
Leptin	Highly expressed in areas of the hypothalamus that control feeding behavior, hunger, body temperature, and energy expenditure. The mechanisms by which leptin suppresses feeding and exerts its effects on metabolism are largely unknown.
Neuropeptide Y	Synthesized in many areas of the brain; it is a potent stimulator of feeding. Leptin appears to suppress feeding in part by inhibiting expression of neuropeptide Y.
Ghrelin	An acylated, 28–amino acid peptide secreted primarily by the stomach. Ghrelin circulates in the blood and activates neuropeptide Y neurons in the hypothalamic arcuate nucleus, thereby stimulating food intake.
Melanocortin	Acts on certain hypothalamic neurons that inhibit feeding. Targeted disruptions of the melanocortin-4 receptor in mice are associated with development of obesity.
Carboxypeptidase E	The enzyme necessary for processing proinsulin and perhaps other hormones, such as neuropeptide Y. Mice with mutations in this gene gradually become obese as they age and develop hyperglycemia that can be suppressed by treatment with insulin.
Mitochondrial uncoupling proteins	First discovered in brown fat and subsequently identified in white fat and muscle cells. May play an important role in energy expenditure and body weight regulation.
Tubby protein	Highly expressed in the paraventricular nucleus of the hypothalamus and other regions of the brain. Mice with naturally occurring or engineered mutations in the tubby gene show adult onset of obesity, but the mechanisms involved are not known.

Adapted from Comuzzie AG, Williams JT, Martin LJ, Blanger J. Searching for genes underlying normal variation in human adiposity. *J Mol Med.* 2001;79:57.

VII. Physical Activity Factors

The marked decrease in physical activity in affluent societies seems to be the major factor in the rise of obesity as a public health problem. Physical inactivity restricts energy expenditure and may contribute to increased food intake. Although food intake increases with increasing energy expenditure over a wide range of energy demands, intake does not decrease proportionately when physical activity falls below a certain minimum level.

VIII. Brain-Damage Factors

Destruction of the ventromedial hypothalamus can produce obesity in animals, but this is probably a very rare cause of obesity in humans. There is evidence that the central nervous system, particularly in the lateral and ventromedial hypothalamic areas, adjusts to food intake in response to changing energy requirements so as to maintain fat stores at a baseline determined by a specific set point. This set point varies from one person to another and depends on height and body build.

IX. Health Factors

In only a small number of cases is obesity the consequence of identifiable illness. Such cases include a variety of rare genetic disorders, such as Prader–Willi syndrome, as well as neuroendocrine abnormalities (Table 20-2).

Table 20-2
Illnesses that Can Explain Some Cases of Obesity

Genetic (dysmorphic) obesities
Autosomal recessive
X-linked
Chromosomal (e.g., Prader–Willi syndrome)
Neuroendocrine obesities
Hypothalamic syndromes
Cushing's syndrome
Hypothyroidism
Polycystic ovarian syndrome (Stein–Leventhal syndrome)
Pseudohypoparathyroidism
Hypogonadism
Growth hormone deficiency
Insulinoma and hyperinsulinism
Iatrogenic obesities
Drugs (psychiatric)
Hypothalamic surgery (neuroendocrine)

Adapted from Bray GA. An approach to the classification and evaluation of obesity. In: Bjorntorp P, Brodoff BN, eds. *Obesity*. Philadelphia, PA: Lippincott Williams & Wilkins; 1992.

Hypothalamic obesity results from damage to the ventromedial region of the hypothalamus (VMH), which has been studied extensively in laboratory animals and is a known center of appetite and weight regulation. In humans, damage to the VMH may result from trauma, surgery, malignancy, or inflammatory disease.

Some forms of depression, particularly seasonal affective disorder, are associated with weight gain. Most persons who live in seasonal climates report increases in appetite and weight during the fall and winter months, with decreases in the spring and summer. Depressed patients usually lose weight, but some gain weight, e.g., atypical depression.

X. Other Clinical Factors

A variety of clinical disorders are associated with obesity. Cushing's disease is associated with a characteristic fat distribution and moon-like face. Myxedema is associated with weight gain, although not invariably. Other neuroendocrine disorders include adiposogenital dystrophy (Fröhlich's syndrome), which is characterized by obesity and sexual and skeletal abnormalities.

XI. Psychotropic Drugs

Long-term use of steroid medications is associated with significant weight gain, as is the use of several psychotropic agents. Patients treated for major depression, psychotic disturbances, and bipolar disorder typically gain 3 to 10 kg, with even larger gains with chronic use. This can produce the so-called metabolic syndrome discussed later.

XII. Psychological Factors

Although psychological factors are evidently crucial to the development of obesity, how such psychological factors result in obesity is not known. The food-regulating mechanism is susceptible to environmental influence, and cultural, family, and psychodynamic factors have all been shown to contribute to the development of obesity. Although many investigators have proposed that specific family histories, precipitating factors, personality structures, or unconscious conflicts cause obesity, overweight persons may suffer from any conceivable psychiatric disorder and come from a variety of disturbed backgrounds. Many obese patients are emotionally disturbed persons who, because of the availability of the overeating mechanism in their environments, have learned to use hyperphagia as a means of coping with psychological problems. Some patients may show signs of serious mental disorder when they attain normal weight because they no longer have that coping mechanism.

XIII. Diagnosis and Clinical Features

The diagnosis of obesity, if done in a sophisticated way, involves the assessment of body fat. Because this is rarely practical, the use of height and weight to calculate BMI is recommended.

In most cases of obesity, it is not possible to identify the precise etiology, given the multitude of possible causes and their interactions. Instances of secondary obesity (described in Table 20-3) are rare but should not be overlooked.

Table 20-3
Psychiatric Medications and Changes in Body Weight

Tendency to Increase Appetite and Body Weight		
Greatest	**Intermediate**	**Least**
Antidepressant drugs		
Amitriptyline (Elavil)	Doxepin (Adapin, Sinequan)	Amoxapine (Asendin)
	Imipramine (Tofranil)	Desipramine (Norpramin)
	Mirtazapine (Remeron)	Trazodone (Desyrel)
	Nortriptyline (Pamelor)	Tranylcypromine (Parnate)
		Fluoxetine (Prozac)[a]
	Phenelzine (Nardil)	Sertraline (Zoloft)[a]
		Bupropion (Wellbutrin)[a]
	Trimipramine (Surmontil)	Venlafaxine (Effexor)[a]
Mood stabilizers		
Lithium (Eskalith)	Carbamazepine (Tegretol)	Topiramate (Topamax)
Valproic acid (Depakene)		
Antipsychotic drugs		
Chlorpromazine (Thorazine)	Haloperidol (Haldol)	Ziprasidone (Geodon)
		Aripiprazole (Abilify)
Clozapine (Clozaril)	Trifluoperazine (Stelazine)	Molindone (Moban)[a]
Thioridazine (Mellaril)	Perphenazine (Trilafon)	Asenapine (Saphris)
Mesoridazine (Serentil)	Thiothixene (Navane)	
Olanzapine (Zyprexa)	Fluphenazine (Permitil, Prolixin)	
Quetiapine (Seroquel)		
Risperidone (Risperdal)		

[a]May decrease appetite and facilitate weight loss.
Adapted from Allison DB, Mentore JL, Heo M, Chandler LP, Capeller JC, Infante MC, Weiden PJ. Antipsychotic-induced weight gain: A comprehensive research synthesis. *Am J Psychiatry.* 1999;156:1686; Bernstein JG. Management of psychotropic drug-induced obesity. In: Bjorntorp P, Brodoff BN, eds. *Obesity.* Philadelphia, PA: Lippincott Williams & Wilkins; 1992.

The habitual eating patterns of many obese persons often seem similar to patterns found in experimental obesity. Impaired satiety is a particularly important problem. Obese persons seem inordinately susceptible to food cues in their environment, to the palatability of foods, and to the inability to stop eating if food is available. Obese persons are usually susceptible to all kinds of external stimuli to eating, but they remain relatively unresponsive to the usual internal signals of hunger. Some are unable to distinguish between hunger and other kinds of dysphoria.

XIV. Differential Diagnosis

A. **The night-eating syndrome**, in which persons eat excessively after they have had their evening meal, seems to be precipitated by stressful life circumstances and, once present, tends to recur daily until the stress is alleviated. Night-eating may also occur as a result of using sedatives to sleep that may produce sleep-walking and eating. This has been reported with the use of Zolpidem (Ambien) in patients.

B. **The binge-eating disorder** is characterized by sudden, compulsive ingestion of very large amounts of food in a short time, usually with great subsequent agitation and self-condemnment. Binge eating also appears to represent a reaction to stress. In contrast to the night-eating syndrome, however, these bouts of overeating are not periodic, and they are far more often linked to specific precipitating circumstances. (See Chapter 19 for a complete discussion of bulimia.) The Pickwickian syndrome is said to exist when a person is 100% over desirable weight and has associated respiratory and cardiovascular pathology.

C. **Body dysmorphic disorder (dysmorphophobia).** Some obese persons feel that their bodies are grotesque and loathsome and that others view them with hostility and contempt. This feeling is closely associated with self-consciousness and impaired social functioning. Emotionally healthy obese persons have no body image disturbances, and only a minority of neurotic obese people have such disturbances. The disorder is confined mainly to persons who have been obese since childhood; even among them, less than half suffer from it. (Body dysmorphic disorder is discussed further in Chapter 13 on Obsessive-Compulsive and Related Disorders.)

XV. Metabolic Syndrome

The metabolic syndrome consists of a cluster of metabolic abnormalities associated with obesity and that contribute to an increased risk of cardiovascular disease and type II diabetes. The syndrome is diagnosed when a patient has three or more of the following five risk factors: (1) abdominal obesity, (2) high triglyceride level, (3) low high-density lipoprotein (HDL) cholesterol level, (4) hypertension, and (5) an elevated fasting blood glucose level (see Table 20-4). The syndrome is believed to occur in about 30% of the US population, but it is also well known in other industrialized countries around the world.

Table 20-4
World Health Organization Clinical Criteria for Metabolic Syndrome

Insulin resistance, identified by one of the following:
- Type 2 diabetes
- Impaired fasting glucose
- Impaired glucose tolerance
- Or for those with normal fasting glucose levels (<100 mg/dL), glucose uptake below the lowest quartile for background population under investigation under hyperinsulinemic, euglycemic conditions

Plus any two of the following:
- Antihypertensive medication and/or high blood pressure (≥140 mm Hg systolic or ≥90 mm Hg diastolic)
- Plasma triglycerides ≥150 mg/dL (≥1.7 mmol/L)
- BMI >30 kg/m^2 and/or waist:hip ratio >0.9 in men, >0.85 in women
- Urinary albumin excretion rate ≥20 µg/min or albumin:creatinine ratio ≥30 mg/g

The cause of the syndrome is unknown, but obesity, insulin resistance, and a genetic vulnerability are involved. Treatment involves weight loss, exercise, and the use of statins and antihypertensives as needed to lower lipid levels and blood pressure. Because of the increased risk of mortality, it is important that the syndrome be recognized early and treated.

Second-generation (atypical) antipsychotic medication has been implicated as a cause of metabolic syndrome. In patients with schizophrenia, treatment with these medications can cause a rapid increase in body weight in the first few months of therapy that may continue for more than 1 year. In addition, insulin resistance leading to type II diabetes has been associated with an artherogenic lipid profile.

Clozapine and olanzapine (Zyprexa) are the two drugs most implicated, but other atypical antipsychotics may also be involved. Patients prescribed second-generation antipsychotic medication should be monitored periodically with fasting blood glucose levels at the beginning of treatment and during its course. Lipid profiles should also be obtained (see Table 20-5).

Table 20-5
Screen Patients Before Prescribing Antipsychotics

- Personal history of obesity
- Family history of obesity
- Diabetes
- Dyslipidemias
- Hypertension
- Cardiovascular disease
- Body mass index
- Waist circumference at level of umbilicus
- Blood pressure
- Fasting plasma glucose
- Fasting lipid profile

Data from American Diabetes Association; 2004.

Psychological reactions to the metabolic syndrome depend on the signs and symptoms experienced by the patient. Those who suffer primarily from obesity must deal with self-esteem issues from being overweight as well as the stress of participating in weight loss programs. In many cases of obesity, eating is a way of satisfying deep-seated dependency needs. As weight is lost, some patients become depressed or anxious. Cases of psychosis have been reported in a few markedly obese patients during or after the process of losing a vast amount of weight. Other metabolic discrepancies, particularly variations in blood sugar, may be accompanied by irritability or other mood changes. Finally, fatigue is a common occurrence in patients with this syndrome. As the condition improves, especially if exercise is part of the regimen, fatigue eventually diminishes, but patients may be misdiagnosed as having a dysthymic disorder or chronic fatigue syndrome if metabolic causes of fatigue are not considered.

XVI. Course And Prognosis

A. **Effects on health.** Obesity has adverse effects on health and is associated with a broad range of illnesses (Table 20-6). There is a strong correlation between obesity and cardiovascular disorders. Hypertension (blood pressure >160/95 mm Hg) is three times higher for persons who are overweight, and hypercholesterolemia (blood cholesterol >250 mg/dL) is twice as common. Studies show that blood pressure and cholesterol levels can be reduced by weight reduction. Diabetes, which has clear genetic determinations, can often be reversed with weight reduction, especially type II diabetes (mature-onset or noninsulin-dependent diabetes mellitus).

Obese men, regardless of smoking habits, have a higher mortality from colon, rectal, and prostate cancer than men of normal weight. Obese women have a higher mortality from cancer of the gallbladder, biliary passages, breast (postmenopause), uterus (including cervix and endometrium), and ovaries than women of normal weight.

B. **Longevity.** The more overweight a person is, the higher is that person's risk for death. A person who reduces weight to acceptable levels has a mortality decline to normal rates. Weight reduction may be lifesaving for patients with extreme obesity, defined as weight that is twice the desirable weight. Such patients may have cardiorespiratory failure, especially when asleep (sleep apnea).

A number of studies have demonstrated that decreasing caloric intake by 30% or more in young or middle-aged laboratory animals prevents or retards age-related chronic diseases and significantly prolongs maximal life span. The mechanisms through which this effect is mediated are not known, but they may include reductions in metabolic rate, oxidative stress and inflammation, improved insulin sensitivity, and changes in neuroendocrine and sympathetic nervous system function. Whether long-term calorie restriction with adequate nutrition slows aging in humans is not yet known.

Table 20-6
Health Disorders Thought to Be Caused or Exacerbated by Obesity

Heart
Premature coronary heart disease
Left ventricular hypertrophy
Angina pectoris
Sudden death (ventricular arrhythmia)
Congestive heart failure
Vascular system
Hypertension
Cerebrovascular disorder (cerebral infarction or hemorrhage)
Venous stasis (with lower-extremity edema, varicose veins)
Respiratory system
Obstructive sleep apnea
Pickwickian syndrome (alveolar hypoventilation)
Secondary polycythemia
Right ventricular hypertrophy (sometimes leading to failure)
Hepatobiliary system
Cholelithiasis and cholecystitis
Hepatic steatosis
Hormonal and metabolic functions
Diabetes mellitus (insulin independent)
Gout (hyperuricemia)
Hyperlipidemias (hypertriglyceridemia and hypercholesterolemia)
Kidney
Proteinuria and, in very severe obesity, nephrosis
Renal vein thrombosis
Joints, muscles, and connective tissue
Osteoarthritis of knees
Bone spurs of the heel
Osteoarthrosis of spine (in women)
Aggravation of preexisting postural faults
Neoplasia
In women: increased risk of cancer of endometrium, breast, cervix, ovary, gallbladder, and biliary
    passages
In men: increased risk of cancer of colon, rectum, and prostate

Reprinted from Vanitallie TB. Obesity: Adverse effects on health and longevity. *Am J Clin Nutr.* 1979; 32:2723, with permission.

XVII. Prognosis

The prognosis for weight reduction is poor, and the course of obesity tends toward inexorable progression. Of patients who lose significant amounts of weight, 90% regain it eventually. The prognosis is particularly poor for those who become obese in childhood. Juvenile-onset obesity tends to be more severe, more resistant to treatment, and more likely to be associated with emotional disturbance than is adult obesity.

XVIII. Discrimination Toward the Obese

Overweight and obese individuals are subject to significant prejudice and discrimination in the United States and other industrialized nations. In a culture in which beauty ideals include highly unrealistic thinness, overweight people are blamed for their condition and are the subject of teasing, bias, and discrimination (sometimes called "fatism"). Income and earning power are reduced in overweight people, and untoward social conditions, such as absence of romantic relationships, are more common. Furthermore, obese individuals face limited access to health care and may receive biased diagnoses and treatment from medical and mental health providers.

XIX. Treatment

Many patients routinely treated for obesity may develop anxiety or depression. A high incidence of emotional disturbances has been reported among obese persons undergoing long-term, in-hospital treatment by fasting or severe calorie restriction. Obese persons with extensive psychopathology, those with a history of emotional disturbance during dieting, and those in the midst of a life crisis should attempt weight reduction, if at all, cautiously and under careful supervision.

A. **Diet.** The basis of weight reduction is simple—establish a caloric deficit by bringing intake below output. The simplest way to reduce caloric intake is by means of a low-calorie diet. The best long-term effects are achieved with a balanced diet that contains readily available foods. For most persons, the most satisfactory reducing diet consists of their usual foods in amounts determined with the aid of tables of food values that are available in standard books on dieting. Such a diet gives the best chance of long-term maintenance of weight loss. Total unmodified fasts are used for short-term weight loss, but they have associated morbidity including orthostatic hypotension, sodium diuresis, and impaired nitrogen balance.

Ketogenic diets are high-protein, high-fat diets used to promote weight loss. They have high cholesterol content and produce ketosis, which is associated with nausea, hypotension, and lethargy. Many obese persons find it tempting to use a novel or even bizarre diet. Whatever effectiveness these diets may have in large part results from their monotony. When a dieter stops the diet and returns to the usual fare, the incentives to overeat are multiplied.

In general, the best method of weight loss is a balanced diet of 1,100 to 1,200 calories. Such a diet can be followed for long periods but should be supplemented with vitamins, particularly iron, folic acid, zinc, and vitamin B_6. Table 20-7 contains details and comparisons of various types of diets.

B. **Exercise.** Increased physical activity is an important part of a weight-reduction regimen. Because caloric expenditure in most forms of physical activity is directly proportional to body weight, obese persons expend more calories than persons of normal weight with the same amount of activity. Furthermore, increased physical activity may actually decrease food intake by formerly sedentary persons. This combination of increased caloric expenditure and decreased food intake makes an increase in physical activity a highly desirable feature of any weight-reduction program. Exercise also helps maintain weight loss. It is essential in the treatment of the metabolic syndrome.

1. **Lifestyle change.** A lifestyle change empowers the patient to set goals of weight management. Simple lifestyle modification strategies that patients should be encouraged to follow include:

Table 20-7
Types of Diets

Type of Diet	Calorie Deficit	Weight Loss	Important Supplementary Measures	Content
Low-calorie diet (LCD)	−500 to −1,000 cal/day	0.5–1 kg/wk	Diet record very important for success	Carbs 55% Protein 15% Fat <30%
Very low-calorie diet (VLCD)	800 cals/day	15–25% in 8–12 wks	Support and electrolyte monitoring	Protein 70–100 g/day full replacement of vitamin/mineral/electrolytes
Fasting	<200 cals/day	50% of weight loss is water weight	Dangerous and not done anymore	Liquids
Popular diets				
1. South Beach diet/ New Diet Revolution/ Zone diet	<30 g of carb/day	20 lbs in 6 mos	Difficult to follow over a long period. Cardiac or renal effects need to be evaluated	High fat, low carb
2. Weight Watchers/ Jenny Craig/ Nutrisystem	Goal is to provide great range of food choice while maintaining a negative energy balance	1–2 lbs/wk	Has been shown to reduce cholesterol and blood pressure	Mod fat, balanced nutrient reduction, 20–30% fat, 15–20% protein, 55–60% carbs
3. Ornish program/ Pritikin program	Mostly vegetarian diet, no caffeine, no caloric restriction, just one type of food	—	Combines meditation, stress reduction, and smoking cessation	Very low fat, <10–19% cals from fat/20% protein, and 70% complex carbs like fruit and grain

a. Personal behavior during a meal:
 1. Eat slowly and savor each mouthful
 2. Chew each bite 30 times before swallowing
 3. Put the fork down between bites
 4. Delay eating for 2 to 3 minutes and converse
 5. Postpone a snack for 10 minutes
 6. Serve food on a smaller plate
 7. Divide portions in half so another portion may be permitted
b. Reduce eating cues:
 1. Eat only at one designated place
 2. Leave the table as soon as eating is done
 3. Do not combine eating with other activities (e.g., reading or watching television)
 4. Do not put bowls of food on the table
 5. Stock home with healthier food choices
 6. Shop for groceries from a list after a full meal
 7. Plan meals
 8. Keep a food diary to link eating with hunger and nonhunger episodes
 9. Substitute other activities for snacking

Table 20-8
Common Drugs for the Treatment of Obesity

Generic Name	Trade Name(s)	Usual Dosage Range (mg/day)
Amphetamine and dextroamphetamine	Adderall	5–20
Methamphetamine	Desoxyn	10–15
Benzphetamine	Didrex	75–150
Phendimetrazine	Bontril, Plegine, Prelu-2, X-Trozine	105
Phentermine hydrochloride	Adipex-P, Fastin, Oby-trim	18.75–37.5
Resin	Ionamin	15–30
Diethylpropion hydrochloride	Tenuate	75
Mazindol	Snorex, Mazanor	3–9
Orlistat	Xenical	360
Naltrexone/Bupropion	Contrave	32/360
Lorcaserin	Belviq	10 twice a day
Phentermine-topiramate	Qsymia	3.75–15 phentermine 23–92 topiramate

C. **Pharmacotherapy.** In recent times, FDA has approved medications for the treatment of obesity, some more effective than others. Drug treatment is effective because it suppresses appetite, but tolerance to this effect may develop after several weeks of use. An initial trial period of 4 weeks with a specific drug can be used; then, if the patient responds with weight loss, the drug can be continued to see whether tolerance develops. If a drug remains effective, it can be dispensed for a longer time until the desired weight is achieved. For a list of medications, see Table 20-8.

1. **Orlistat.** One weight-loss medication approved by the Food and Drug Administration (FDA) for long-term use (in 1999) is orlistat (Xenical), which is a selective gastric and pancreatic lipase inhibitor that reduces the absorption of dietary fat (which is then excreted in stool). In clinical trials, orlistat (120 mg, three times a day), in combination with a low-calorie diet, induced losses of approximately 10% of initial weight in the first 6 months, which were generally well maintained for periods up to 24 months. Side effects include oily stool, flatulence, and fecal urgency.

2. **Lorcaserin.** Lorcaserin (Belviq) is approved for the treatment of obesity in adults. It is a selective serotonin agonist and suppresses appetite. Dosage is 10 mg twice a day. Side effects include headaches, dizziness, fatigue, nausea, dry mouth, and constipation. Rarely it may cause suicidal thoughts as well as memory and comprehension problems.

3. **Phentermine-topiramate.** Phentermine-topiramate (Qsymia) has been approved by the FDA for weight loss in conjunction with diet and exercise. Start at low dose (3.75 mg phentermine/23 mg topiramate extended release) to recommended dose (7.5 mg/46 mg). High doses (15 mg/92 mg) can be used in some patients. Side effects include paraesthesia, dry mouth, altered taste, increased heart rate, possible birth defects, and psychiatric problems (depression, suicidal thoughts, impaired memory, and concentration).

4. **Naltrexone HCl/Bupropion HCl.** Naltrexone/Bupropion (Contrave) is indicated for chronic weight management in adults with BMI of

more than 30 or 27 with at least one comorbid condition (hypertension, hyperlipidemia, and type II DM). It includes bupropion and antidepressant that decreases appetite and naltrexone that control hunger and food cravings. Target dose of 32mg/360 mg is reached by week 4. Common side effects include elevated blood pressure, constipation, dizziness, tremor, and depression.

5. **Rimonabant.** An alternative to psychostimulants, Rimonabant has a unique mechanism of action: It is a selective cannabinoid-1 receptor blocker. Rimonabant has been shown to reduce body weight and improve cardiovascular risk factors in obese patients. It appears to help suppress metabolic abnormalities that lead to type II diabetes, obesity, and atherosclerosis. The use of Rimonabant to mitigate psychopharmacologic metabolic disturbances may be justified in some patients.

D. **Surgery.** Surgical methods that cause malabsorption of food or reduce gastric volume have been used in persons who are markedly obese. *Gastric bypass* is a procedure in which the stomach is made smaller by transecting or stapling one of the stomach curvatures. In *gastroplasty*, the size of the stomach stoma is reduced so that the passage of food slows. Results are successful, although vomiting, electrolyte imbalance, and obstruction may occur. A syndrome called dumping, which consists of palpitations, weakness, and sweating, may follow surgical procedures in some patients if they ingest large amounts of carbohydrates in a single meal. The surgical removal of fat (lipectomy) has no effect on weight loss in the long run nor does liposuction, which has value only for cosmetic reasons. Bariatric surgery is now recommended in individuals who have serious obesity-related health complications and a BMI of greater than 35 kg/m^2 (or a BMI >40 kg/m^2 in the absence of major health complications). Before surgery, candidates should have tried to lose weight using the safer, more traditional options of diet, exercise, and weight loss medication.

E. **Psychotherapy.** Some patients may respond to insight-oriented psychodynamic therapy with weight loss, but this treatment has not had much success. Uncovering the unconscious causes of overeating may not alter the behavior of persons who overeat in response to stress, although it may serve to augment other treatment methods. Years after successful psychotherapy, many persons who overeat under stress continue to do so. Obese persons seem particularly vulnerable to overdependency on a therapist, and the inordinate regression that may occur during the uncovering psychotherapies should be carefully monitored.

Behavior modification has been the most successful of the therapeutic approaches for obesity and is considered the method of choice. Patients are taught to recognize external cues that are associated with eating and to keep diaries of foods consumed in particular circumstances, such as at the movies or while watching television, or during certain emotional states, such as anxiety or depression. Patients are also taught to develop new eating patterns, such as eating slowly, chewing food well, not reading while eating, and not eating between meals or when not seated. Operant

Table 20-9
Key Recommendations for Healthy Weight

- Weight loss to lower elevated blood pressure in overweight and obese persons with high blood pressure.
- Weight loss to lower elevated levels of total cholesterol, low-density lipoprotein (LDL) cholesterol, and triglycerides, and to raise low levels of high-density lipoprotein (HDL) cholesterol in overweight and obese persons with dyslipidemia.
- Weight loss to lower elevated blood glucose levels in overweight and obese persons with type 2 diabetes.
- Use the body mass index (BMI) to classify overweight and obesity and to estimate relative risk of disease compared with normal weight.
- The waist circumference should be used to assess abdominal fat content.
- The initial goal of weight loss therapy should be to reduce body weight by about 10% from baseline. With success, and if warranted, further weight loss can be attempted.
- Weight loss should be about 1–2 lbs/wk for a period of 6 mos, with the subsequent strategy based on the amount of weight lost.
- Low-calorie diets (LCD) for weight loss in overweight and obese persons. Reducing fat as part of an LCD is a practical way to reduce calories.
- Reducing dietary fat alone without reducing calories is not sufficient for weight loss. However, reducing dietary fat, along with reducing dietary carbohydrates, can help reduce calories.
- A diet that is individually planned to help create a deficit of 500–1,000 kcal/day should be an integral part of any program aimed at achieving a weight loss of 1–2 lbs/wk.
- Physical activity should be part of a comprehensive weight loss therapy and weight control program because it (1) modestly contributes to weight loss in overweight and obese adults, (2) may decrease abdominal fat, (3) increases cardiorespiratory fitness, and (4) may help with maintenance of weight loss.
- Physical activity should be an integral part of weight loss therapy and weight maintenance. Initially, moderate levels of physical activity for 30–45 min, 3–5 days a week, should be encouraged. All adults should set a long-term goal to accumulate at least 30 min or more of moderate-intensity physical activity on most, and preferably all, days of the week.
- The combination of a reduced calorie diet and increased physical activity is recommended because it produces weight loss that may also result in decreases in abdominal fat and increases in cardiorespiratory fitness.
- Behavior therapy is a useful adjunct when incorporated into treatment for weight loss and weight maintenance.
- Weight loss and weight maintenance therapy should employ the combination of LCDs, increased physical activity, and behavior therapy.
- After successful weight loss, the likelihood of weight loss maintenance is enhanced by a program consisting of dietary therapy, physical activity, and behavior therapy, which should be continued indefinitely. Drug therapy can also be used. However, drug safety and efficacy beyond 1 yr of total treatment have not been established.
- A weight maintenance program should be a priority after the initial 6 months of weight loss therapy.

Formulated from the Obesity Education Institute, National Institute of Health.

conditioning therapies that use rewards such as praise or new clothes to reinforce weight loss have also been successful. Group therapy helps to maintain motivation, to promote identification among members who have lost weight, and to provide education about nutrition.

F. **Comprehensive approach.** The National Heart, Lung, and Blood Institute formulated key recommendations for patients and the public regarding weight loss. These are listed in Table 20-9.

For more detailed discussion of this topic, see Chapter 27, Psychosomatic Medicine: Obesity, Section 27.4, p. 2210, in CTP/X.

21

Normal Sleep and Sleep–Wake Disorders

I. General Introduction

Sleep is an essential process for proper brain functioning and serves a restorative, homeostatic function, and appears to be crucial for normal thermoregulation and energy conservation. It is one of the most significant of human behaviors, occupying roughly one-third of human life. Approximately 30% of adults in the United States experience a sleep disorder during their lifetime, and over half do not seek treatment. Lack of sleep can lead to the inability to concentrate, memory complaints, deficits in neuropsychological testing, and decreased libido. Additionally, sleep disorders can have serious consequences, including fatal accidents related to sleepiness. Disturbed sleep can be a primary diagnosis itself or a component of another medical or psychiatric disorder. Careful diagnosis and specific treatment are essential. Female sex, advanced age, medical and mental disorders, and substance abuse are associated with an increased prevalence of sleep disorders.

II. Sleep Deprivation

May lead to ego disorganization, hallucinations, and delusions. REM-deprived patients may exhibit irritability and lethargy.

III. Sleep Requirements

Short sleepers require fewer than 6 hours of sleep while long sleepers need more than 9 hours each night to function adequately. Short sleepers are generally efficient, ambitious, socially adept, and content. Long sleepers tend to be mildly depressed, anxious, and socially withdrawn.

IV. Sleep–Wake Rhythm

Sleep is also influenced by biologic rhythms as well as external factors—such as the light–dark cycle, daily routines, meal periods, and other external synchronizers. It develops over first 2 years of life. Sleep patterns are not physiologically the same when persons sleep in the daytime or during the time when they are accustomed to being awake; the psychological and behavioral effects of sleep differ as well.

A. Sleep stages. Sleep is comprised of two physiologic states: rapid eye movement (REM) sleep and non-rapid eye movement (NREM) sleep. NREM sleep consists of four sleep stages, named stage I through stage IV. Dreaming occurs mostly in REM sleep, but additionally, some dreaming occurs in stages III and IV sleep. Sleep is measured with a polysomnograph, which simultaneously measures brain activity (electroencephalogram [EEG]), eye

Table 21-1
Sleep Stages

Awake:	Low voltage, random, very fast
Drowsy:	Alpha waves (8–12 CPS), random and fast
Stage I:	Theta waves (3–7 CPS), slight slowing
Stage II:	Further slowing, K complex (triphasic complexes), sleep spindles, true sleep onset
Stage III:	Delta waves (0.5–2 CPS), high amplitude slow waves.
Stage IV:	At least 50% delta waves. Stages III and IV comprise delta sleep.
REM:	Sawtooth waves, similar to drowsy sleep on EEG

CPS, cycles per second.

movement (electro-oculogram), and muscle tone (electromyogram). Other physiologic tests can be applied during sleep and measured along with the above. EEG findings are used to describe sleep stages (Table 21-1).

It takes the average person 15 to 20 minutes to fall asleep; this is the sleep latency. During the next 45 minutes, one descends from stages I and II of sleep to stages III and IV. Stages III and IV comprise the deepest sleep; that is, the largest stimulus is needed to arouse one in these stages of sleep. Approximately 45 minutes after stage IV begins, the first REM period is reached. Therefore, the average REM latency (the time from sleep onset to REM onset) is 90 minutes. Throughout the night, one cycles through the four stages of sleep followed by REM sleep. As the night progresses, each REM period becomes longer, and stages III and IV disappear. Hence, further into the night, persons sleep more lightly and dream (mostly REM sleep) more. The sleep stages in an adult are approximately 25% REM sleep and 75% NREM sleep, consisting of 5% in stage I, 45% in stage II, 12% in stage III, and 13% in stage IV. This distribution remains relatively constant into old age, although a reduction occurs in both slow-wave sleep and REM sleep in older persons.

B. Characteristics of REM sleep (also called paradoxical sleep)
  1. Autonomic instability
     a. Increased heart rate (HR), blood pressure (BP), and respiratory rate (RR).
     b. Increased variability in HR, BP, and RR from minute to minute.
     c. Appears similar to an awake person on EEG.
  2. Tonic inhibition of skeletal muscle tone leading to paralysis.
  3. Rapid eye movements.
  4. Dreaming.
  5. Reduced hypercapnic respiratory drive, no increase in tidal volume as partial pressure of carbon dioxide decreases.
  6. Relative poikilothermia (cold-bloodedness).
  7. Penile tumescence or vaginal lubrication.
  8. Deafness.

V. Sleep Disorder Classification
The DSM-5 classifies sleep disorders on the basis of clinical diagnostic criteria and presumed etiology. The 10 sleep–wake disorders described in DSM-5 are only a fraction of the known sleep disorders; they provide a framework for clinical assessment. The current classification includes the following sleep disorders each of which is described in detail below.

A. **Insomnia disorder.** DSM-5 defines insomnia disorder as dissatisfaction with sleep quantity or quality associated with one or more of the following symptoms: difficulty in initiating sleep, difficulty in maintaining sleep with frequent awakenings or problems returning to sleep, and early morning awakening with inability to return to sleep.

Insomnia can be categorized in terms of how it affects sleep (e.g., sleep-onset insomnia, sleep-maintenance insomnia, or early-morning awakening). Insomnia can also be classified according to its duration (e.g., transient, short term, and long term).

Primary insomnia is diagnosed by nonrestorative sleep or difficulty in initiating or maintaining sleep, and the complaint continues for at least a month (according to ICD-10, the disturbance must occur at least three times a week for a month).

1. Insomnia is the most common type of sleep disorder.
2. Causes are listed in Table 21-2.
3. Treatment includes deconditioning techniques, transcendental meditation, relaxation tapes, sedative-hypnotic drugs, and nonspecific measures such as sleep hygiene, described in Table 21-3.

B. **Hypersomnolence disorder.** Diagnosed when there is no other cause found for greater than 1 month of excessive somnolence (daytime sleepiness) or excessive amounts of daytime sleep. Usually begins in childhood. Can be a consequence of (1) insufficient sleep, (2) basic neurologic dysfunction in brain systems regulating sleep, (3) disrupted sleep, or (4) the phase of an individual's circadian rhythm. Treatment consists of stimulant drugs.

Table 21-2
Common Causes of Insomnia

Symptom	Insomnia Secondary to Medical Conditions	Insomnia Secondary to Psychiatric or Environmental Conditions
Difficulty in falling asleep	Any painful or uncomfortable condition	Anxiety
	CNS lesions	Tension anxiety, muscular
	Conditions listed below, at times	Environmental changes
Difficulty in remaining asleep	Sleep apnea syndromes	Circadian rhythm sleep disorder
	Nocturnal myoclonus and restless legs syndrome	Depression, especially primary depression
	Dietary factors (probably)	Environmental changes
	Episodic events (parasomnias)	Circadian rhythm sleep disorder
	Direct substance effects (including alcohol)	Posttraumatic stress disorder
	Substance withdrawal effects (including alcohol)	Schizophrenia
	Substance interactions	
	Endocrine or metabolic diseases	
	Infectious, neoplastic, or other diseases	
	Painful or uncomfortable conditions	
	Brainstem or hypothalamic lesions or diseases	
	Aging	

Courtesy of Ernest L. Hartmann, M.D.

Table 21-3
Nonspecific Measures to Induce Sleep (Sleep Hygiene)

1. Arise at the same time daily.
2. Limit daily in-bed time to the usual amount before the sleep disturbance.
3. Discontinue CNS-acting drugs (caffeine, nicotine, alcohol, stimulants).
4. Avoid daytime naps (except when sleep chart shows they induce better night sleep).
5. Establish physical fitness by means of a graded program of vigorous exercise early in the day.
6. Avoid evening stimulation; substitute radio or relaxed reading for television.
7. Try very hot, 20-min, body temperature-raising bath soaks near bedtime.
8. Eat at regular times daily; avoid large meals near bedtime.
9. Practice evening relaxation routines, such as progressive muscle relaxation or meditation.
10. Maintain comfortable sleeping conditions.

From Regestein QR. Sleep disorders. In: Stoudemire A, ed. *Clinical Psychiatry for Medical Students.* Philadelphia, PA: Lippincott, 1990:578, with permission.

1. **Types of hypersomnia**
    a. **Kleine–Levin syndrome.** Rare condition consisting of recurrent periods of prolonged sleep (from which patients may be aroused) with intervening periods of normal sleep and alert waking.
        (1) Periodic disorder of episodic hypersomnolence.
        (2) Usually affects young men, ages 10 to 21.
        (3) May sleep excessively for several weeks and awaken only to eat (voraciously).
        (4) Associated with hypersexuality, extreme hostility, irritability, and occasionally hallucinations during episode.
        (5) Amnesia follows attacks.
        (6) May resolve spontaneously after several years.
        (7) Patients are normal between episodes.
        (8) Treatment consists of stimulants (amphetamines, methylphenidate [Ritalin], and pemoline [Cylert]) for hypersomnia and preventive measures for other symptoms. Lithium also has been used successfully.
    b. **Menstrual-related hypersomnia.** Recurrent episodes of hypersomnia related to the menstrual cycle, experiencing intermittent episodes of marked hypersomnia at, or shortly before, the onset of their menses.
    c. **Idiopathic hypersomnia.** Disorder of excessive sleepiness in which patients do not have the ancillary symptoms associated with narcolepsy. It is associated with long nonrefreshing naps, difficulty awakening, sleep drunkenness, and automatic behaviors with amnesia. Other symptoms include migraine-like headaches, fainting spells, syncope, orthostatic hypotension, and Raynaud-type phenomena with cold hands and feet.
    d. **Other types include**
        Behaviorally induced insufficient sleep syndrome
        Hypersomnia due to a medical condition
        Hypersomnia due to drug or substance abuse

2. Treatment

Regularizing sleep periods

Wake promoting drugs like modafinil (Provigil)

Traditional psychostimulants

C. Narcolepsy

1. Narcolepsy consists of the following characteristics:

  a. Excessive daytime somnolence (sleep attacks) is the primary symptom of narcolepsy.

   (1) Distinguished from fatigue by irresistible sleep attacks of short duration (less than 15 minutes).

   (2) Sleep attacks may be precipitated by monotonous or sedentary activity.

   (3) Naps are highly refreshing and effects usually last 30 to 120 minutes.

  b. Cataplexy

   (1) Reported by over 50% of narcoleptic patients.

   (2) Brief (seconds to minutes) episodes of muscle weakness or paralysis.

   (3) No loss of consciousness if episode is brief.

   (4) When attack is over, the patient is completely normal.

   (5) May manifest as partial loss of muscle tone (weakness, slurred speech, buckled knees, dropped jaw).

   (6) Often triggered by laughter (common), anger (common), athletic activity, excitement or elation, sexual intercourse, fear, or embarrassment.

   (7) Flat affect or lack of expressiveness develops in some patients as an attempt to control emotions.

   (8) A diagnosis of cataplexy automatically results in a diagnosis of narcolepsy. If cataplexy does not occur, multiple other characteristics are necessary for the diagnosis of narcolepsy.

  c. Sleep paralysis

   (1) Temporary partial or complete paralysis in sleep–wake transitions.

   (2) Conscious but unable to move or open eyes.

   (3) Most commonly occurs on awakening.

   (4) Generally described as an anxiety-provoking, "scary" event.

   (5) Generally lasts less than 1 minute.

   (6) Reported by 25% to 50% of the general population though for a much shorter duration.

  d. Hypnagogic and hypnopompic hallucinations

   (1) Dreamlike experience during transition from wakefulness to sleep and vice versa.

   (2) Vivid auditory or visual hallucinations or illusions.

  e. Sleep-onset REM periods (SOREMPs)

   (1) Defined as appearance of REM within 15 minutes of sleep onset (normally approximately 90 minutes).

(2) Narcolepsy can be distinguished from other disorders of excessive daytime sleepiness by SOREMPs seen on polysomnographic recording.

(3) A multiple sleep latency test (MSLT) measures excessive sleepiness. An MSLT consists of at least four recorded naps at 2-hour intervals. More than two SOREMPs are considered diagnostic of narcolepsy (seen in 70% of patients with narcolepsy, in fewer than 10% of patients with other hypersomnias).

f. Increased incidence of other clinical findings in narcolepsy

(1) Periodic leg movement.

(2) Sleep apnea—predominantly central.

(3) Short sleep latency.

(4) Frequent nighttime arousals; from REM sleep to stage I or wakefulness, the patient usually is unaware of the awakenings.

(5) Memory problems.

(6) Ocular symptoms—blurring, diplopia, flickering.

(7) Depression.

(8) Automatic behaviors can occur for which people have no memory.

2. Onset and clinical course

a. Typically, full syndrome emerges in late adolescence or early 20s.

b. Once established, condition is chronic without major remissions.

c. A long delay may occur between the earliest symptoms (excessive somnolence) and the late appearance of cataplexy.

3. Causes

a. Plausibly caused by an abnormality of REM-inhibiting mechanisms.

b. Human leukocyte antigen (HLA)-DR2 and narcolepsy.

(1) Strong (>70%) association between narcolepsy and HLA-DR2, a type of human lymphocyte antigen.

(2) HLA-DR2 is also found in up to 30% of unaffected persons.

(3) Recent research involving hypocretin, a neurotransmitter, suggests that hypocretin is significantly reduced in narcolepsy patients.

4. Treatment

a. Regular bedtime.

b. Daytime naps scheduled at a regular time of day.

c. Safety considerations, such as caution while driving and avoiding furniture with sharp edges.

d. Stimulants (e.g., modafinil [Provigil]) for daytime sleepiness. High-dose propranolol (Inderal) may be effective.

e. Tricyclics and selective serotonin reuptake inhibitors (SSRIs) for REM-related symptoms, especially cataplexy. Other treatments are listed in Table 21-4.

D. Breathing-related sleep disorder. Characterized by sleep disruption that is caused by a sleep-related breathing disturbance, leading to excessive

Table 21-4
Narcolepsy Drugs Currently Available

Drug	Maximal Daily Dosage (mg) (All Drugs Administered Orally)
Treatment of excessive daytime somnolence (EDS)	
Stimulants	
Methylphenidate	≤60
Pernoline	≤150
Modafinil	≤400
Amphetamine–dextroamphetamine	≤60
Dextroamphetamine	≤60
Adjunct-effect drugs (i.e., improve EDS if associated with stimulant)	
Protriptyline	≤10
Treatment of cataplexy, sleep paralysis, and hypnogogic hallucinations	
Tricyclic antidepressants (with atropinelike side effects)	
Protriptyline	≤20
Imipramine	≤200
Clomipramine	≤200
Desipramine	≤200
Antidepressants (without major atropinelike side effects)	
Bupropion	≤300
SSRIs	
Sertraline	≤200 mg
Citalopram	≤40 mg

Adapted from Guilleminault C. Narcolepsy syndrome. In: Kryger MH, Roth T, Dement WC, eds. *Principles and Practice of Sleep Medicine.* Philadelphia, PA: Saunders, 1989:344.

sleepiness, insomnia, or hypersomnia. Breathing disturbances include apneas, hypoapneas, and oxygen desaturations.

1. **Apnea.** The two types of sleep apnea are (1) obstructive and (2) central sleep apnea (CSA), which have numerous subtypes. Greater than 40% of patients evaluated for somnolence using polysomnography are found to have sleep apnea. Sleep apnea may account for a number of unexplained deaths.

   a. **Obstructive sleep apnea (OSA)**

      (1) Caused by cessation of air flow through the nose or mouth in the presence of continuing thoracic breathing movements, resulting in decreases in arterial oxygen saturation and a transient arousal, after which respiration resumes normally.

      (2) Typically occurs in middle-aged, overweight men (Pickwickian syndrome).

      (3) Also occurs more frequently in patients with smaller jaws or micrognathia, acromegaly, and hypothyroidism.

      (4) Main symptoms are loud snoring with intervals of apnea.

      (5) Additional symptoms include extreme daytime sleepiness with long and unrefreshing daytime sleep attacks.

      (6) Other symptoms include severe morning headaches, morning confusion, depression, and anxiety.

(7) Medical consequences include cardiac arrhythmias, systemic and pulmonary hypertension, and decreased sexual drive or function with progressive worsening without treatment.

(8) Apnic events occur in both REM (more severe) and NREM (more frequent) sleep.

(9) Each event lasts 10 to 20 seconds. There are usually 5 to 10 events per hour of sleep.

(10) In severe cases, patients may have more than 300 episodes of apnea per night.

(11) Patients are unaware of episodes of apnea.

(12) Treatment consists of nasal continuous positive airway pressure (CPAP), uvulopharyngopalatoplasty, weight loss, buspirone (Buspar), and SSRIs and tricyclic drugs (to reduce REM periods, the stage during which obstructive apnea is usually more frequent). If a specific abnormality of the upper airway is found, surgical intervention is indicated.

(13) Sedatives and alcohol should be avoided because they can considerably exacerbate the condition, which may then become life threatening.

b. Central sleep apnea (CSA). Defined as the absence of breathing due to lack of respiratory effort. Disorder of ventilatory control with repeated episodes of apneas and hypopneas occur in a periodic or intermittent pattern during sleep caused by variability in respiratory effort.

(1) Rare, usually in elderly.

(2) Treatment consists of mechanical ventilation or nasal CPAP.

(3) There are three subtypes of CSA:

Idiopathic CSA: They present with daytime sleepiness, insomnia, or awakening with shortness of breath.

Cheyne–Stokes breathing: Prolonged hyperpneas alternate with apnea and hypopnea episodes that are associated with reduced ventilatory effort.

CSA comorbid with opioid use: Chronic use of long-acting opioid medications and impairment of neuromuscular respiratory control.

(4) Other types of CSA:

CSA due to medical condition that is not Cheyne–Stokes

CSA due to drug or substance abuse

Primary sleep apnea of infancy

2. Sleep-related hypoventilation. Central apnea followed by an obstructive phase.

a. Impaired ventilation that appears or greatly worsens only during sleep and in which significant apneic episodes are absent.

b. The ventilatory dysfunction is characterized by inadequate tidal volume or respiratory rate during sleep.

c. Death may occur during sleep (Ondine's curse).

d. Central alveolar hypoventilation is treated with mechanical ventilation (e.g., nasal ventilation).

e. Types of sleep-related hypoventilation

Idiopathic hypoventilation. Shallow breathing longer than 10 seconds in duration associated with arterial oxygen desaturation and frequent arousals from sleep associated with the breathing disturbances or bradytachycardia.

Congenital central alveolar hypoventilation. Called Ondine's curse, results from a failure in automatic control of breathing.

Comorbid sleep-related hypoventilation. Consequence of a medical condition, for example, pulmonary parenchymal or vascular pathology, lower airway obstruction, or neuromuscular or chest wall disorders.

E. Circadian rhythm sleep disorders.

1. Includes a wide range of conditions involving a misalignment between desired and actual sleep periods.

2. The six types are (1) delayed sleep phase, (2) advanced sleep phase type, (3) irregular sleep–wake type, (4) non–24-hour sleep–wake type, (5) shift work type, and (6) Jet lag type.

3. Quality of sleep is basically normal.

4. Self-limited. Resolves as body readjusts to new sleep–wake schedule.

5. Adjusting to an advance of sleep time is more difficult than adjusting to a delay.

6. Most effective treatment of sleep–wake schedule disorders is a regular schedule of bright light therapy to entrain the sleep cycle and is more useful for transient than for persistent disturbances. Melatonin, a natural hormone that induces sleep, which is produced by the pineal gland, has been used orally to alter sleep–wake cycles, but its effect is uncertain.

F. Parasomnias. Characterized by physiologic or behavioral phenomena that occur during or are potentiated by sleep. Wakefulness, NREM sleep, and REM sleep can be characterized as three basic states that differ in their neurologic organization.

1. NREM sleep arousal disorders

a. Sleepwalking disorder (*somnambulism*)

(1) Complex activity—with brief episodes of leaving bed and walking about without full consciousness.

(2) Usually begins between the ages of 4 and 8, with peak prevalence at about 12 years old; generally disappears spontaneously with age.

(3) About 15% of children have an occasional episode and is more common in boys.

(4) Patients often have familial history of other parasomnias.

(5) Amnesia for the event—patient does not remember the episode.

(6) Occurs during deep NREM sleep (stages III and IV sleep).

(7) Initiated during first third of the night.

(8) Can usually be guided back to bed.

(9) Can sometimes be initiated by placing a child who is in stage IV sleep in the standing position.

(10) In adults and elderly persons, may reflect psychopathology—rule out central nervous system (CNS) pathology.

(11) Drugs that suppress stage IV sleep, such as benzodiazepines, can be used to treat somnambulism.

(12) Potentially dangerous. Precautions include window guards and other measures to prevent injury.

(13) Treatment includes education and reassurance.

Specialized forms of sleepwalking include sleep-related eating behavior and sexsomnia.

a. Sleep-related eating

Episodes of ingesting food during sleep with amnesia.

b. Sexsomnia

Person engages in sexual activities (e.g., masturbation, fondling, sexual intercourse) during sleep without conscious awareness.

b. Sleep terror disorder

(1) Sudden awakening, usually sitting up, with intense anxiety.

(2) Autonomic overstimulation, movement, crying out, increased heart rate, and diaphoresis.

(3) Especially common in children (about 1% to 6%), more common in boys, and tends to run in families.

(4) Patient does not remember the event in the morning.

(5) Occurs during deep, non-REM sleep, usually stage III or IV sleep.

(6) Often occurs within the first few hours' sleep.

(7) Occurrence starting in adolescence or later may be the first symptom of temporal lobe epilepsy.

(8) Treatment rarely needed in childhood.

(9) Awakening child before night terror for several days may eliminate terrors for extended periods.

(10) In rare cases, when medication is required, diazepam in small doses at bedtime may be beneficial.

2. Parasomnias usually associated with REM sleep

a. REM sleep behavior disorder (including parasomnia overlap disorder and status dissociatus)

(1) Loss of atonia during REM sleep, with emergence of complex, often violent behaviors (acting out dreams).

(2) Chronic and progressive, chiefly in elderly men.

(3) Potential for serious injury.

(4) Neurologic cause in many cases such as small stroke or early Parkinson's disease.

(5) May occur as rebound to sleep deprivation.

(6) May develop in patients treated with stimulants and SSRIs.

(7) Treat with 0.5 to 2.0 mg of clonazepam daily, or 100 mg of carbamazepine (Tegretol) three times daily.

b. Recurrent isolated sleep paralysis
  (1) Isolated symptom.
  (2) Hypnagogic hallucinations
  (3) Last one to several; minutes
  (4) Episode terminates with touch, noise (some external stimulus), or voluntary repetitive eye movements.

3. Nightmare disorder
  a. Nightmares are vivid dreams in which one awakens frightened.
  b. About 50% of the adult population may report occasional nightmares.
  c. Almost always occur during REM sleep.
  d. Can occur at any time of night, but usually after a long REM period late in the night.
  e. Good recall (quite detailed).
  f. Less anxiety, vocalization, motility, and autonomic discharge than in sleep terrors.
  g. No harm results from awakening a person who is having a nightmare.
  h. No specific treatment; benzodiazepines, tricyclics, and SSRIs may be of help.

4. Other parasomnias
  a. Sleep enuresis
    (1) Primary
      (a) One urinates during sleep while in bed
      (b) Continuance of bed-wetting since infancy
      (c) Parental primary enuresis increases the likelihood in children.
    (2) Secondary
      (a) Relapse after toilet training is complete and there was a period during which the child remained dry.
      (b) Associated with nocturnal seizures, sleep deprivation, and urologic anomalies.
          Treatment modalities include medicines (imipramine, oxybutynin chloride, and synthetic vasopressin), behavioral treatments (bladder training, using conditioning devices (bell and pad), and fluid restriction).
  b. Sleep-related groaning (Catathrenia)
    (1) Prolonged, frequently loud groans during any stage of sleep.
    (2) There is no known treatment.
  c. Sleep-related hallucinations
    (1) At sleep onset (hypnagogic) or on awakening (hypnopompic).
    (2) Common in narcolepsy.
    (3) Vivid and frightening images.
  d. Sleep-related eating disorder
    (1) Inability to get back to sleep after awakening unless the individual eats or drinks.
    (2) Mostly in infants and children.

5. **Parasomnias due to drug or substance use and parasomnia due to medical condition.** Many drugs trigger parasomnias including alcohol that can lead to sleepwalking. Other drugs include biperiden (Akineton), tricyclic antidepressants, monoamine oxidase inhibitors (MAOIs), caffeine, venlafaxine (Effexor), selegiline (Eldepryl), and serotonin agonist. Sleep-related breathing disorders trigger sleepwalking, enuresis, sleep terror, confusional arousal, and nightmares. Neurologic conditions include Parkinson's disease, dementia, progressive supranuclear palsy, among others.

G. **Sleep-related movement disorders**

1. **Restless legs syndrome (Ekbom syndrome)**

   a. Uncomfortable sensations in legs at rest.

   b. Peaks in middle age; occurs in 5% of the population.

   c. Can interfere with falling asleep, though symptoms not limited to sleep.

   d. Relieved by movement.

   e. Patient may have associated sleep-related myoclonus.

   f. Associated with pregnancy, renal disease, iron deficiency, and vitamin B_{12} deficiency.

   g. Treatment includes benzodiazepines, levodopa, quinine, opioids, propranolol, valproate, carbamazepine, and carbidopa. A new drug, ropinirole (Requip), has been reported to be effective.

2. **Periodic leg movement disorder (formerly called *nocturnal myoclonus*).**

   a. Stereotypic, periodic leg movements (every 20 to 60 seconds) during NREM sleep (at least five leg movements per hour).

   b. No seizure activity.

   c. Most prevalent in patients over age 55.

   d. Frequent awakenings.

   e. Unrefreshing sleep.

   f. Daytime sleepiness a major symptom.

   g. Patient unaware of the myoclonic events.

   h. Associated with renal disease, iron deficiency, and vitamin B_{12} deficiency. May also be associated with attention-deficit/hyperactivity disorder (ADHD).

   i. Various drugs have been reported to help. These include clonazepam (Klonopin), opioids, quinine, and levodopa (Larodopa).

   j. Other treatments include stress management and anxiety-relieving programs.

3. **Sleep-related leg cramps**

   a. Occur during wakefulness

   b. Painful and affect calf muscles.

   c. Precipitated by metabolic disorders, mineral deficiencies, diabetes and pregnancy.

4. **Sleep bruxism (tooth grinding)**

   a. Occurs throughout the night, though primarily occurs in stages I and II sleep or during partial arousals or transitions.

    b. Occurs in greater than 5% of the population.

    c. Treatment consists of bite plates to prevent dental damage.

  5. Sleep rhythmic movement disorder (*jactatio capitis nocturna*)

    a. Rhythmic head or body rocking just before or during sleep; may extend into light sleep.

    b. Usually limited to childhood.

    c. No treatment required in most infants and young children. Crib padding or helmets may be used. Behavior modification, benzodiazepines, and tricyclic drugs may be effective.

H. Sleep-related movement disorder due to drug or substance use and sleep-related movement disorder due to medical condition. A variety of drugs, substances, and comorbid conditions can produce or exacerbate sleep-related movement disorders. Stimulants can produce rhythmic movement disorders and bruxism. Antidepressants (including most tricyclics and SSRIs), antiemetics, lithium (Eskalith), calcium-channel blockers, antihistamines, and neuroleptics can provoke restless legs symptoms and periodic limb movement disorder. Neurologic diseases that are associated with daytime movement disorders can also be associated with sleep-related movement disorders. Stress, anxiety, and sleep deprivation may contribute to bruxism.

  1. Isolated symptoms, apparently normal variants, and unresolved issues

    a. Sleep talking (somniloquy)

      (1) Common in children and adults

      (2) Sometimes accompanies night terrors and sleepwalking.

      (3) Found in all stages of sleep.

      (4) Requires no treatment.

    b. Long sleeper

    c. Short sleeper

    d. Snoring

    e. Sleep starts (hypnic jerk)

    f. Benign sleep myoclonus of infancy

    g. Hypnagogic foot tremor and alternating leg muscle activation during sleep

    h. Propriospinal myoclonus at sleep onset

    i. Excessive fragmentary myoclonus

VI. Sleep Disorders of Clinical Significance

  A. Insufficient sleep. Characterized by complaints of daytime sleepiness, irritability, inability to concentrate, and impaired judgment by a person who persistently fails to sleep enough to support alert wakefulness.

  B. Sleep drunkenness

    1. Inability to become fully alert for sustained period after awakening.

    2. Most commonly seen in persons with sleep apnea or after sustained sleep deprivation.

    3. Can occur as an isolated disorder.

    4. No specific treatment. Stimulants may be of limited value.

C. **Altitude insomnia**
1. Insomnia secondary to change in sleep onset ventilatory set point and resulting breathing problems.
2. More severe at higher altitudes as oxygen level declines.
3. Patients may awaken with apnea.
4. Acetazolamide (Diamox) can increase ventilatory drive and decrease hypoxemia.

VII. **Significance of Sleep Disorders in Clinical Practice**
One who complains of insomnia for greater than 1 year is 40 times more likely than the general population to have a diagnosable psychiatric disorder. In 35% of patients who present to sleep disorder centers with a complaint of insomnia, the underlying cause is a psychiatric disorder. Half of these patients have major depression. Roughly 80% of patients with major depression complain of insomnia. In patients with major depression, sleep involves relatively normal onset, but repeated awakenings in the second half of the night, premature morning awakening, decreased stages III and IV sleep, a short REM latency, and a long first REM period. Treatment for insomnia in a depressed patient may include use of a sedating antidepressant, for example, treating with amitriptyline (Elavil). Post-traumatic stress disorder patients typically describe insomnia and nightmares.

Hypersomnia related to a mental disorder is usually found in a variety of conditions such as the early stages of mild depressive disorder, grief, personality disorders, dissociative disorders, and somatoform disorders. Treatment of the primary disorder should resolve the hypersomnia.

VIII. **Sleep Disorder Resulting from a General Medical Condition**
Though not listed as a category in DSM-5, clinicians should be aware of the following medical disorders associated with sleep disorders.
A. Insomnia, hypersomnia, parasomnia, or a combination can be caused by a general medical condition, such as:
1. **Sleep-related epileptic seizures.** Seizures occur almost exclusively during sleep (sleep epilepsy).
2. **Sleep-related cluster headaches.** Sleep-related cluster headaches are severe and unilateral, appear often during sleep, and are marked by an on–off pattern of attacks.
3. **Chronic paroxysmal hemicrania.** Chronic paroxysmal hemicrania is a unilateral headache that occurs frequently and has a sudden onset (only occurs during REM).
4. **Sleep-related abnormal swallowing syndrome.** A condition during sleep in which inadequate swallowing results in aspiration of saliva, coughing, and choking. It is intermittently associated with brief arousals or awakenings.
5. **Sleep-related asthma**. Asthma that is exacerbated by sleep. In some people may result in significant sleep disturbances.
6. **Sleep-related cardiovascular symptoms.** Associated with disorders of cardiac rhythm, congestive heart failure, valvular disease, and blood

pressure variability that may be induced or exacerbated by alterations in cardiovascular physiology during sleep.

7. **Sleep-related gastroesophageal reflux.** Patient awakes from sleep with burning substernal pain, a feeling of tightness or pain in the chest, or a sour taste in the mouth. Often associated with hiatal hernia. Gastroesophageal reflux disorder (GERD) can also lead to sleep-related asthma due to reflux into the lungs.

8. **Sleep-related hemolysis (paroxysmal nocturnal hemoglobinuria).** Rare, acquired, chronic hemolytic anemia. The hemolysis and consequent hemoglobinuria are accelerated during sleep so that the morning urine appears brownish red.

9. Painful conditions, such as arthritis, may lead to insomnia.

B. Treatment, whenever possible, should be of the underlying medical condition.

IX. Sleep and Aging

A. Subjective reports by elderly.

1. Time in bed increases.
2. Number of nocturnal awakenings increases.
3. Total sleep time at night decreases.
4. Sleep latency increases.
5. Dissatisfaction with sleep.
6. Tired and sleepy in the daytime.
7. More frequent napping.

B. Objective evidence of age-related changes in sleep cycle.

1. Reduced total REM sleep.
2. Reduced stages III and IV.
3. Frequent awakenings.
4. Reduced duration of nocturnal sleep.
5. Need for daytime naps.
6. Propensity for phase advance.

C. Certain sleep disorders are more common in the elderly.

1. Nocturnal myoclonus.
2. Restless legs syndrome.
3. REM sleep behavior disturbance.
4. Sleep apnea.
5. Sundowning (confusion from sedation).

D. Medications and medical disorders also contribute to the problem.

For more detailed discussion of this topic, see Chapter 23, Sleep Disorders, p. 2083, in CTP/X.

22

Disruptive, Impulse-Control, and Conduct Disorders

I. Impulse-Control Disorders

A. Introduction. Psychodynamic, psychosocial, and biologic factors all play an important role in impulse-control disorders. Persons with impulse-control disorders are unable to resist an intense, drive, or temptation to perform a particular act that is obviously harmful to themselves, others, or both. Before the event, the individual usually experiences mounting tension and arousal, sometimes—but not consistently—mingled with conscious anticipatory pleasure. Completing the action brings gratification and relief. Within a variable time afterward, the individual experiences a conflation of remorse, guilt, self-reproach, and dread. These feelings may stem from obscure unconscious conflicts or awareness of the deed's impact on others (including the possibility of serious legal consequences in syndromes such as kleptomania). Shameful secretiveness about the repeated impulsive activity frequently expands to pervade the individual's entire life, often significantly delaying treatment. Five conditions comprise the category of *disruptive*, *impulse-control*, and *conduct disorders.* They include two that are associated with childhood: (1) oppositional defiant disorder and (2) conduct disorder, both of which are discussed in the child psychiatry section in Chapter 25.

1. **Intermittent explosive disorder**—episodes of aggression resulting in harm to others.

2. **Kleptomania**—repeated shoplifting or stealing.

3. **Pyromania**—deliberately setting fires.

4. **Other specified or unspecified disorders**—a residual category for disorders that do not meet the criteria for the disorders described earlier. These include:

   a. **Internet compulsion (addiction).** Persons spend almost all their waking hours at the computer, are repetitive and constant, and they are unable to resist strong urges to use the computer or to "surf the Web."

   b. **Mobile or cell phone compulsion.** Persons compulsively use mobile phones to call others—friends, acquaintances, or business associates. Factors include fear of being alone, the need to satisfy unconscious dependency needs, or undoing a hostile wish toward a loved one.

   c. **Repetitive self-mutilation.** Persons cut themselves or damage their bodies in a compulsive manner. DSM-5 has a category called "non-suicidal self-injury" to refer to persons who repeatedly damage their bodies, who, however, do not wish to die. Cutting or inflicting bodily pain may release endorphins or raise dopamine levels, which contribute to a euthymic or elated mood.

    d. Compulsive sexual behavior (sex addiction). Persons repeatedly seek out sexual gratification, often in perverse ways (e.g., exhibitionism). They are unable to control their behavior and may not experience feelings of guilt after an episode of acting-out behavior.

B. Epidemiology

    1. Intermittent explosive disorder, pathologic gambling, pyromania—men affected more than women.

    2. Kleptomania, trichotillomania—women affected more than men. The female-to-male ratio is 3:1 in clinical samples.

    3. Pathologic gambling—affects up to 3% of adult population in the United States. The disorder is more common in men than in women, and the rate is higher in locations where gambling is legal.

C. Etiology. It is unknown. Some disorders (e.g., intermittent explosive disorder) may be associated with abnormal electroencephalogram (EEG) results, mixed cerebral dominance, or soft neurologic signs. Alcohol or drugs (e.g., marijuana) reduce the patient's ability to control impulses (disinhibition).

D. Psychodynamics. Acting out of impulses relates to the need to express sexual or aggressive drive. Gambling is often associated with underlying depression and represents an unconscious need to lose and experience punishment.

E. Differential diagnosis (see Table 22-1).

    1. Temporal lobe epilepsy. Characteristic foci of EEG abnormalities in the temporal lobe account for aggressive outbursts, kleptomania, and pyromania.

Table 22-1
Differential Diagnosis, Course, and Prognosis for Impulse-Control Disorders

Disorder	Differential Diagnosis	Course and Prognosis
Intermittent explosive disorder	Delirium, dementia Personality change due to a general medical condition, aggressive type Substance intoxication or withdrawal Oppositional defiant disorder, conduct disorder, antisocial disorder, manic episode, schizophrenia Purposeful behavior, malingering Temporal lobe epilepsy	May increase in severity with time
Kleptomania	Ordinary theft Malingering Antisocial personality disorder, conduct disorder Manic episode Delusions, hallucinations (e.g., schizophrenia) Dementia Temporal lobe epilepsy	Frequently arrested for shoplifting
Pyromania	Arson: profit, sabotage, revenge, political statement Childhood experimentation Conduct disorder Manic episode Antisocial personality disorder Delusions, hallucinations (e.g., schizophrenia) Dementia Mental retardation Substance intoxication Temporal lobe epilepsy	Often produces increasingly larger fires over time

2. **Head trauma.** Brain imaging techniques may show residual signs of trauma.

3. **Bipolar I disorder.** Gambling may be an associated feature of manic episodes.

4. **Substance-related disorder**. History of drug or alcohol use or a positive test result on drug screen may suggest that the behavior is drug- or alcohol-related.

5. **Medical condition.** Rule out brain tumor, degenerative brain disease, and endocrine disorder (e.g., hyperthyroidism) on the basis of characteristic findings for each.

6. **Schizophrenia.** Delusions or hallucinations account for impulsive behavior.

F. **Course and prognosis.** Course usually is chronic for all impulse-control disorders (see Table 22-1).

G. **Treatment**

1. **Intermittent explosive disorder.** Combined pharmacotherapy and psychotherapy are most effective. May have to try different medications (e.g., β-adrenergic receptor antagonists, anticonvulsants [carbamazepine (Tegretol), lithium (Eskalith)]) before result is achieved. Serotonergic drugs such as buspirone (BuSpar), trazodone (Desyrel), and selective serotonin reuptake inhibitors (SSRIs) (e.g., fluoxetine [Prozac]) may be helpful. Benzodiazepines can aggravate the condition through disinhibition. Other measures include supportive psychotherapy, behavior therapy with limit setting, and family therapy. Group therapy must be used cautiously if the patient is liable to be aggressive toward other group members.

 CLINICAL HINT:
The successful use of SDAs (quetiapine [Seroquel]) to control acting out of impulses has been reported.

2. **Kleptomania.** Insight-oriented psychotherapy is helpful in understanding motivation (e.g., guilt, need for punishment) and to control poor impulse. Behavior therapy is used for learning new patterns of behavior. SSRIs, tricyclics, trazodone, lithium, and valproate (Depakote) may be effective in some patients.

3. **Pyromania.** Insight-oriented therapy, behavior therapy. Patients require close supervision because of repeated fire-setting behavior and consequent danger to others. May require inpatient facility, night hospital, or other structured setting. Fire setting by children must be treated in a timely manner. Treatment should include family therapy and close supervision.

4. **Other specified or unspecified disorders**
   a. **Internet compulsion (addiction).** A subset of Web pages offer a chance to evaluate one's Internet use as possibly pathologic and offer both education and online counseling.
   b. **Mobile phone compulsion.** Understanding of psychodynamic fear of being alone, excessive dependency and needs, and phobic tendencies

may be of help in changing behavior. Cognitive therapy and behavioral modification techniques are useful.

c. Repetitive self-mutilation. Cognitive and behavioral techniques may be helpful. Studies have shown naltrexone to be helpful.

d. Compulsive sexual behavior. Abstinence is goal achieved through self-help groups such as sex-addicts anonymous. In severe cases, anti-androgen medication maybe used in men. Underlying psychiatric conditions, most commonly depression, should be treated.

For more detailed discussion of this topic, see Chapter 24, Impulse-Control Disorders, p. 2110, in CTP/X.

Psychosomatic Medicine

I. Psychosomatic Disorders

A. Definition. Psychosomatic (psychophysiologic) medicine has been a specific area of study within the field of psychiatry for more than 75 years. It is informed by two basic assumptions: There is a unity of mind and body (reflected in term mind–body medicine); and psychological factors must be taken into account when considering all disease states. Although most physical disorders are influenced by stress, conflict, or generalized anxiety, some disorders are more affected than others. A number of physical disorders meet these criteria and are listed in Table 23-1.

B. Theories

1. **Stress factors.** This etiologic theory states that any prolonged stress can cause physiologic changes that result in a physical disorder. Each person has a shock organ that is genetically vulnerable to stress: Some patients are cardiac reactors, others are gastric reactors, and others are skin reactors. Persons who are chronically anxious or depressed are more vulnerable to physical or psychosomatic disease. Table 23-2 lists life stressors that may herald a psychosomatic disorder.

2. **Neurotransmitter response.** Stress activates noradrenergic system that releases catecholamines and serotonin which are increased. Dopamine is increased via mesoprefrontal pathways.

3. **Endocrine response.** Corticotropin-releasing factor (CRF) is secreted from hypothalamus which releases cortisol. Glucocorticoids promote energy use in the short term. Increased thyroid hormone turnover also occurs during stress states.

4. **Immune response.** Release of humoral immune factors (called cytokines) such as interleukin-1 and -2 occurs. Cytokines can increase glucocorticoids. Some persons develop severe organ damage from overload of cytokine release under stress.

5. **Physiological factors**

   a. Hans Selye described the *general adaption syndrome*, which is the sum of all the nonspecific systemic reactions of the body that follow prolonged stress. The hypothalamic–pituitary–adrenal axis is affected, with excess secretion of cortisol producing structural damage to various organ systems.

   b. George Engel postulated that in the stressed state, all neuroregulatory mechanisms undergo functional changes that depress the body's homeostatic mechanisms, so that the body is left vulnerable to infection and other disorders. Neurophysiologic pathways thought to mediate stress reactions include the cerebral cortex, limbic system,

Table 23-1
Physical Conditions Affected by Psychological Factors

Disorder	Observations/Comments/Theory/Approach
Angina, arrhythmias, coronary spasms	Type A person is aggressive, irritable, easily frustrated, and prone to coronary artery disease. Arrhythmias common in anxiety states. Sudden death from ventricular arrhythmia in some patients who experience massive psychological shock or catastrophe. Lifestyle changes: cease smoking, curb alcohol intake, lose weight, lower cholesterol to limit risk factors. Propranolol (Inderal) prescribed for patients who develop tachycardia as part of social phobia—protects against arrhythmia and decreased coronary blood flow.
Asthma	Attacks precipitated by stress, respiratory infection, allergy. Examine family dynamics, especially when child is the patient. Look for overprotectiveness and try to encourage appropriate independent activities. Propranolol and beta blockers contraindicated in asthma patients for anxiety. Psychological theories: strong dependency and separation anxiety; asthma wheeze is suppressed cry for love and protection.
Connective tissue diseases: systemic lupus erythematosus, rheumatoid arthritis	Disease can be heralded by major life stress, especially death of loved one. Worsens with chronic stress, anger, or depression. Important to keep patient as active as possible to minimize joint deformities. Treat depression with antidepressant medications or psychostimulants, and treat muscle spasm and tension with benzodiazepines.
Headaches	Tension headache results from contraction of strap muscles in neck, constricting blood flow. Associated with anxiety, situational stress. Relaxation therapy, antianxiety medication useful. Migraine headaches are unilateral and can be triggered by stress, exercise, foods high in tyramine. Manage with ergotamine (Cafergat). Propranolol prophylaxis can produce associated depression. Sumatriptan (Imitrex) can be used to treat nonhemiplegic and nonbasilar migraine attacks.
Hypertension	Acute stress produces catecholamines (epinephrine), which raise systolic blood pressure. Chronic stress associated with essential hypertension. Look at lifestyle. Prescribe exercise, relaxation therapy, biofeedback. Benzodiazepines of use in acute stress if blood pressure rises as shock organ. Psychological theories: inhibited rage, guilt over hostile impulses, need to gain approval from authority.
Hyperventilation syndrome	Accompanies panic disorder, generalized anxiety disorder with associated hyperventilation, tachycardia, vasoconstriction. May be hazardous in patients with coronary insufficiency. Antianxiety agents of use: Some patients respond to monoamine oxidase inhibitors, tricyclic antidepressants, or serotonergic agents.
Inflammatory bowel diseases: Crohn's disease, irritable bowel syndrome, ulcerative colitis	Depressed mood associated with illness; stress exacerbates symptoms. Onset after major life stress. Patients respond to stable doctor-patient relationship and supportive psychotherapy in addition to bowel medication. Psychological theories: passive personality, childhood intimidation, obsessive traits, fear of punishment, masked hostility.
Metabolic and endocrine disorders	Thyrotoxicosis following sudden severe stress. Glycosuria in chronic fear and anxiety. Depression alters hormone metabolism, especially adrenocorticotropic hormone (ACTH).
Neurodermatitis	Eczema in patients with multiple psychosocial stressors—especially death of loved one, conflicts over sexuality, repressed anger. Some respond to hypnosis in symptom management.
Obesity	Hyperphagia reduces anxiety. Night-eating syndrome associated with insomnia. Failure to perceive appetite, hunger, and satiation. Psychological theories: conflicts about orality and pathologic dependency. Behavioral techniques, support groups, nutritional counseling, and supportive psychotherapy useful. Treat underlying depression.

(continued)

Table 23-1
Physical Conditions Affected by Psychological Factors *(Continued)*

Disorder	Observations/Comments/Theory/Approach
Osteoarthritis	Lifestyle management includes weight reduction, isometric exercises to strengthen joint musculature, maintenance of physical activity, pain control. Treat associated anxiety or depression with supportive psychotherapy.
Peptic ulcer disease	Idiopathic type not related to specific bacterium or physical stimulus. Increased gastric acid and pepsin relative to mucosal resistance: both sensitive to anxiety, stress, coffee, alcohol. Lifestyle changes. Relaxation therapy. Psychological theories: strong frustrated dependency needs, cannot express anger, superficial self-sufficiency.
Raynaud's disease	Peripheral vasoconstriction associated with smoking, stress, Lifestyle changes: cessation of smoking, moderate exercise. Biofeedback can raise hand temperature by increased vasodilation.
Syncope, hypotension	Vasovagal reflex with acute anxiety or fear produces hypotension and fainting. More common in patients with hyperreactive autonomic nervous system. Aggravated by anemia, antidepressant medications (produce hypotension as side effect).
Urticaria, angioedema	Idiopathic type not related to specific allergens or physical stimulus. May be associated with stress, chronic anxiety, depression. Pruritus worse with anxiety; self-excoriation associated with repressed hostility. Some phenothiazines have antipruritic effect. Psychological theories: conflict between dependence–independence, unconscious guilt feelings, itching as sexual displacement.

hypothalamus, adrenal medulla, and sympathetic and parasympathetic nervous systems. Neuromessengers include such hormones as cortisol and thyroxine (Table 23-3).

    c. Walter Cannon demonstrated that under stress the autonomic nervous system is activated to ready the organism to the "fight or flight" response. When there is no option for either, psychosomatic disorders may result.

C. Causes. A host of medical and neurologic disorders (see Table 23-4) may present with psychiatric symptoms, which must be differentiated from psychiatric disorders. Some psychiatric disorders have associated physical symptoms. In most cases, there is no demonstrable organic pathologic lesion to account for the symptoms (e.g., aphonia in conversion disorder). See Table 23-5.

Table 23-2
Ranking of 10 Life-Change Stressors

1. Death of spouse
2. Divorce
3. Death of close family member
4. Marital separation
5. Serious personal injury or illness
6. Fired from work
7. Jail term
8. Death of a close friend
9. Pregnancy
10. Business readjustment

Adapted from Richard H. Rahe, M.D., and Thomas Holmes.

Table 23-3
Functional Responses to Stress

Neurotransmitter response
  Increased synthesis of brain norepinephrine.
  Increased serotonin turnover may result in eventual depletion of serotonin.
  Increased dopaminergic transmission.
Endocrine response
  Increased adrenocortotropic hormone (ACTH) stimulates adrenal cortisol.
  Testosterone decrease with prolonged stress.
  Decrease in thyroid hormone.
Immune response
  Immune activation occurs with release of hormonal immune factors (cytokines) in acute stress.
  Number and activity of natural killer cells decreased in chronic stress.

D. Treatment

1. **Collaborative approach.** Collaborate with internist or surgeon who manages the physical disorder and with psychiatrist attending to psychiatric aspects.

2. **Psychotherapy**

   a. **Supportive psychotherapy.** When patients have a therapeutic alliance, they are able to ventilate fears of illness, especially death fantasies, with the psychiatrist. Many patients have strong dependency needs, which are partially gratified in treatment.

   b. **Dynamic insight-oriented psychotherapy.** Explore unconscious conflicts regarding sex and aggression. Anxiety associated with life stresses is examined and mature defenses are established. More patients will benefit from supportive psychotherapy than insight-oriented therapy when they have psychosomatic disorders.

   c. **Group therapy.** Group therapy is of use for patients who have similar physical conditions (e.g., patients with colitis, those undergoing hemodialysis). They share experiences and learn from one another.

   d. **Family therapy.** Family relationships and processes are explored, with emphasis placed on how the patient's illness affects other family members.

   e. **Cognitive–behavioral therapy**

      1. **Cognitive.** Patients learn how stress and conflict translate into somatic illness. Negative thoughts about disease are examined and altered.

      2. **Behavioral.** Relaxation and biofeedback techniques affect the autonomic nervous system positively. Of use in asthma, allergies, hypertension, and headache.

   f. **Hypnosis.** Effective in smoking cessation and dietary change augmentation.

   g. **Biofeedback.** Control of certain autonomic nervous system functions by training. Used for tension, migraine headaches, and hypertension.

   h. **Acupressure and acupuncture.** Alternative therapy used with variable results in almost all psychosomatic disorders.

Text continues on page 353.

Table 23-4
Medical Problems that Present with Psychiatric Symptoms

Disease	Sex and Age Prevalence	Common Medical Symptoms	Psychiatric Symptoms and Complaints	Impaired Performance and Behavior	Diagnostic Problems
AIDS	Males > females; IV drug abusers, homosexuals, female sex partners of bisexual men	Lymphadenopathy, fatigue, opportunistic infections, Kaposi's sarcoma	Depression, anxiety, disorientation	Dementia with global impairment	Seropositive HIV virus is diagnostic when clinical signs present
Hyperthyroidism (thyrotoxicosis)	Females 3:1; 20–50 yrs	Tremor, sweating, loss of weight and strength, heat intolerance	Anxiety, depression	Occasional hyperactive or grandiose behavior	Long lead time; rapid onset resembles anxiety attack
Hypothyroidism (myxedema)	Females 5:1; 30–50 yrs	Puffy face, dry skin, cold intolerance	Lethargy, anxiety with irritability, thought disorder, somatic delusions, hallucinations	Myxedema madness; delusional, paranoid, belligerent behavior	Madness may mimic schizophrenia; mental status is clear, even during most disturbed behavior
Hyperparathyroidism	Females 3:1, 40–60 yrs	Weakness, anorexia, fractures, colculi, peptic ulcers		Anorexia and fatigue of slow-growing adenoma resembles involutional depression
Hypoparathyroidism	Females, 40–60 yrs	Hyperreflexia, spasms, tetany	Either state may cause anxiety, hyperactivity, and irritability or depression, apathy, and withdrawal	Either state may proceed to a toxic psychosis: confusion, disorientation, and clouded sensorium	None; rare condition except after surgery
Hyperadrenalism (Cushing's disease)	Adults, both sexes	Weight gain, fat alteration, easy fatigability	Varied; depression, anxiety, thought disorder with somatic delusions	Rarely produces aberrant behavior	Bizarre somatic delusions caused by bodily changes; resemble those of schizophrenia
Adrenal cortical insufficiency (Addison's disease)	Adults, both sexes	Weight loss, hypotension, skin pigmentation	Depression—negativism, apathy; thought disorder—suspiciousness	Toxic psychosis with confusion and agitation	Long lead time; weight loss, apathy, despondency resemble involutional depression
Porphyria—acute intermittent type	Females, 20–40 yrs	Abdominal crises, paresthesias, weakness	Anxiety—sudden onset, severe; mood swings	Extremes of excitement or withdrawal; emotional or angry outbursts	Patients often have truly neurotic lifestyles; crises resemble conversion reactions or anxiety attacks

(continued)

Table 23-4
Medical Problems that Present with Psychiatric Symptoms (Continued)

Disease	Sex and Age Prevalence	Common Medical Symptoms	Psychiatric Symptoms and Complaints	Impaired Performance and Behavior	Diagnostic Problems
Pernicious anemia	Females, 40–60 yrs	Weight loss, weakness, glossitis, extremity neuritis	Depression—feelings of guilt and worthlessness	Eventual brain damage with confusion and memory loss	Long lead time, sometimes many months; easily mistaken for involutional depression; normal early blood studies may give false reassurance
Hepatolenticular degeneration (Wilson's disease)	Males 2:1; adolescence	Liver and extrapyramidal symptoms	Mood swings—sudden and changeable; anger—explosive	Eventual brain damage with memory and IQ loss; combativeness	In late teens, may resemble adolescent storm, incorrigibility, or schizophrenia
Hypoglycemia (islet cell adenoma)	Adults, both sexes	Tremor, sweating, hunger, fatigue, dizziness	Anxiety—fear and dread; depression with fatigue	Agitation, confusion; eventual brain damage	Can mimic anxiety attack or acute alcoholism; bizarre behavior may draw attention away from somatic symptoms
Intracranial tumors	Adults, both sexes	None early; headache, vomiting, papilledema later	Varied: depression, anxiety, personality changes	Loss of memory, judgment; self-criticism; clouding of consciousness	Tumor location may not determine early symptoms
Pancreatic carcinoma	Males 3:1, 50–70 yrs	Weight loss, abdominal pain, weakness, jaundice	Depression, sense of imminent doom but without severe guilt	Loss of drive and motivation	Long lead time; exact age and symptoms of involutional depression
Pheochromocytoma	Adults, both sexes	Headache, sweating during elevated blood pressure	Anxiety, panic, fear, apprehension, trembling	Inability to function during an attack	Classic symptoms of anxiety attack; intermittently normal blood pressures may discourage further studies
Multiple sclerosis	Females, 20–40 yrs	Motor and sensory losses, scanning speech, nystagmus	Varied; personality changes, mood swings, depression; bland euphoria uncommon	Inappropriate behavior resulting from personality changes	Long lead time; early neurologic symptoms mimic hysteria or conversion disorders
Systemic lupus erythematosus	Females 8:1; 20–40 yrs	Multiple symptoms of cardiovascular, genitourinary, gastrointestinal, other systems	Varied; thought disorder, depression, confusion	Toxic psychosis unrelated to steroid treatment	Long lead time, perhaps many years; psychiatric picture variable over time; thought disorder resembles schizophrenia, steroid psychosis

Adapted from Maurice J. Martin, M.D.

Table 23-5
Conditions Mimicking Psychosomatic Disorders

Diagnosis	Definition and Example
Conversion disorder	There is an alteration of physical function that suggests a physical disorder but is an expression of psychological conflict (e.g., psychogenic aphonia). The symptoms are falsely neuroanatomic in distribution, are symbolic in nature, and allow much secondary gain.
Body dysmorphic disorder	Preoccupation with an imagined physical defect in appearance in a normal-appearing person (e.g., preoccupation with facial hair).
Hypochondriasis	Imaged overconcern about physical disease when objective examination reveals none to exist (e.g., angina pectoris with normal heart functioning).
Somatization disorder	Recurrent somatic and physical complaints with no demonstrable physical disorder despite repeated physical examinations and no organic basis.
Pain disorder	Preoccupation with pain with no physical disease to account for intensity. It does not follow a neuroanatomic distribution. There may be a close correlation between stress and conflict and the initiation or exacerbation of pain.
Physical complaints associated with classic psychological disorders	Somatic accompaniment of depression (e.g., weakness, asthenia).
Physical complaints with substance abuse disorder	Bronchitis and cough associated with nicotine and tobacco dependence.

   i. Relaxation exercises
      1. Muscle relaxation. Patients are taught to relax muscle groups, such
         as those involved in "tension headaches." When they encountered,
         and were aware of, situations that caused tension in their muscles, the
         patients were trained to focus on the muscles involved.
   j. Time management. Time-management methods are designed to
      help individuals restore a sense of balance to their lives. To accom-
      plish this goal, individuals might be asked to keep a record of how
      they spend their time each day, noting the amount of time spent
      in important categories, such as work, family, exercise, or leisure
      activities. With awareness comes increased motivation to make
      changes.
3. Pharmacotherapy
   a. Always take nonpsychiatric symptoms seriously and use appropri-
      ate medication (e.g., laxatives for simple constipation). Consult with
      referring physician.
   b. Use antipsychotic drugs when associated psychosis is present. Be
      aware of side effects and their impact on the disorder.
   c. Antianxiety drugs diminish harmful anxiety during period of acute
      stress. Limit use so as to avoid dependency, but do not hesitate to
      prescribe in a timely manner.
   d. Antidepressants can be used with depression resulting from a
      medical condition. Selective serotonin reuptake inhibitors (SSRIs)
      can help when the patient obsesses or ruminates about his or her
      illness.

II. Consultation–Liaison Psychiatry

Psychiatrists serve as consultants to medical colleagues (either another psychiatrist or, more commonly, a nonpsychiatric physician) or to other mental health professionals (psychologist, social worker, or psychiatric nurse). In addition, consultation–liaison psychiatrists provide consultation regarding patients in medical or surgical settings and provide follow-up psychiatric treatment as needed. Consultation–liaison psychiatry is associated with all the diagnostic, therapeutic, research, and teaching services that psychiatrists perform in the general hospital and serves as a bridge between psychiatry and other specialties.

Because more than 50% of medical inpatients have psychiatric problems that may require treatment, the consultation–liaison psychiatrist is important in the hospital setting. Table 23-6 lists the most common consultation–liaison problems encountered in general hospitals.

Table 23-6
Common Consultation-Liaison Problems

Reason for Consultation	Comments
Suicide attempt or threat	High-risk factors are men over 45, no social support, alcohol dependence, previous attempt, incapacitating medical illness with pain, and suicidal ideation. If risk is present, transfer to psychiatric unit or start 24-hr nursing care.
Depression	Suicidal risks must be assessed in every depressed patient (see above); presence of cognitive defects in depression may cause diagnostic dilemma with dementia; check for history of substance abuse or depressant drugs (e.g., reserpine, propranolol); use antidepressants cautiously in cardiac patients because of conduction side effects, orthostatic hypotension.
Agitation	Often related to cognitive disorder, withdrawal from drugs (e.g., opioids, alcohol, sedative-hypnotics); haloperidol most useful drug for excessive agitation; use physical restraints with great caution; examine for command hallucinations or paranoid ideation to which patient is responding in agitated manner; rule out toxic reaction to medication.
Hallucinations	Most common cause in hospital is delirium tremens; onset 3–4 days after hospitalization. In intensive care units, check for sensory isolation; rule out brief psychotic disorder, schizophrenia, cognitive disorder. Treat with antipsychotic medication.
Sleep disorder	Common cause is pain; early morning awakening associated with depression; difficulty in falling asleep associated with anxiety. Use antianxiety or antidepressant agent, depending on cause. Those drugs have no analgesic effect, so prescribe adequate painkillers. Rule out early substance withdrawal.
No organic basis for symptoms	Rule out conversion disorder, somatization disorder, factitious disorder, and malingering; glove and stocking anesthesia with autonomic nervous system symptoms seen in conversion disorder; multiple body complaints seen in somatization disorder; wish to be hospitalized seen in factitious disorder; obvious secondary gain in malingering (e.g., compensation case).
Disorientation	Delirium versus dementia; review metabolic status, neurologic findings, substance history. Prescribe small dose of antipsychotics for major agitation; benzodiazepines may worsen condition and cause sundown syndrome (ataxia, confusion); modify environment so patient does not experience sensory deprivation.
Noncompliance or refusal to consent to procedure	Explore relationship of patient and treating doctor; negative transference is most common cause of noncompliance; fears of medication or of procedure require education and reassurance. Refusal to give consent is issue of judgment; if impaired, patient can be declared incompetent, but only by a judge; cognitive disorder is main cause of impaired judgment in hospitalized patients.

Table 23-7
Transplantation and Surgical Problems

Organ	Biologic Factors	Psychological Factors
Kidney	50–90% success rate; may not be done if patient is over age 55; increasing use of cadaver kidneys rather than those from living donors	Living donors must be emotionally stable; parents are best donors, siblings may be ambivalent; donors are subject to depression. Patients who panic before surgery may have poor prognoses; altered body image with fear of organ rejection is common. Group therapy for patients is helpful.
Bone marrow	Used in aplastic anemias and immune system disease	Patients are usually ill and must deal with death and dying; compliance is important. The procedure is commonly done in children who present problems of prolonged dependence; siblings are often donors and may be angry or ambivalent about procedure.
Heart	End-stage coronary artery disease and cardiomyopathy	Donor is legally dead; relatives of the deceased may refuse permission or be ambivalent. No fallback is available if the organ is rejected; kidney rejection patient can go on hemodialysis. Some patients seek transplantation hoping to die. Postcardiotomy delirium is seen in 25% of patients.
Breast	Radical mastectomy versus lumpectomy	Reconstruction of breast at time of surgery leads to postoperative adaptation; veteran patients are used to counsel new patients; lumpectomy patients are more open about surgery and sex than are mastectomy patients; group support is helpful.
Uterus	Hysterectomy performed on 10% of women over 20	Fear of loss of sexual attractiveness with sexual dysfunction may occur in a small percentage of women; loss of childbearing capacity is upsetting.
Brain	Anatomic location of lesion determines behavioral change	Environmental dependence syndrome in frontal lobe tumors is characterized by inability to show initiative; memory disturbances are involved in periventricular surgery; hallucinations are involved in parieto-occipital area.
Prostate	Cancer surgery has more negative psychobiologic effects and is more technically difficult than surgery for benign hypertrophy	Sexual dysfunction is common except in trans-urethral prostatectomy. Perineal prostatectomy produces the absence of emission, ejaculation, and erection; penile implant may be of use.
Colon and rectum	Colostomy and ostomy are common outcomes, especially for cancer	One-third of patients with colostomies feel worse about themselves than before bowel surgery; shame and self-consciousness about the stoma can be alleviated by self-help groups that deal with those issues.
Limbs	Amputation performed for massive injury, diabetes, or cancer	Phantom-limb phenomenon occurs in 98% of cases; the experience may last for years; sometimes the sensation is painful, and neuroma at the stump should be ruled out; the condition has no known cause or treatment; it may stop spontaneously.

III. Special Medical Settings

Besides the usual medical wards in a hospital, special settings produce uncommon, distinctive forms of stress.

A. ICU. ICUs contain seriously ill patients who have life-threatening illnesses (e.g., coronary care units). Among the defensive reactions encountered

Text continues on page 358.

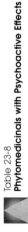

Table 23-8
Phytomedicinals with Psychoactive Effects

Name	Ingredients	Use	Adverse Effects	Interactions	Dosage[a]	Comments
Echinacea L. *Echinacea purpurea*	Flavonoids,[b] polysaccharides, caffeic acid derivatives, alkamides	Stimulates immune system; for lethargy, malaise, respiratory and lower urinary tract infections	Allergic reaction, fever, nausea, vomiting	Undetermined.	1–3 g/day	Use in HIV and AIDS patients is controversial.
Ephedra, ma-huang L. *Ephedra sinica*	Ephedrine, pseudoephedrine	Stimulant: for lethargy, malaise, diseases of respiratory tract	Sympathomimetic overload: arrythmias, increased blood pressure, headache, irritability, nausea, vomiting	Synergistic with sympathomimetics, serotoninergic agents. Avoid with MAOIs.	1–2 g/day	Administer for short periods as tachyphylaxis and dependence can occur.
Ginkgo L. *Ginkgo biloba*	Flavonoids,[b] ginkgolide, A, B	Symptomatic relief of delirium, dementia; improves concentration and memory deficits; possible antidote to SSRI induced sexual dysfunction	Allergic skin reactions, gastrointestinal upset, muscle spasms, headache	Anticoagulant: Use with caution because of its inhibitory effect on platelet-activating factor; increased bleeding possible.	120–240 mg/day	Studies indicate improved cognition in Alzheimer's patients after 4 to 5 weeks of use, possibly because of increased blood flow.
Ginseng L. *Panax ginseng*	Triterpenes, ginsenosides	Stimulant: for fatigue, elevation of mood immune system	Insomnia, hypertonia, and edema (called *ginseng abuse syndrome*)	Not to be used with sedatives, hypnotic agents, MAOIs, antidiabetic agents, or steroids.	1–2 g/day	Several varieties exist: Korean (most highly valued), Chinese, Japanese, American (*Panax quinquefolius*).

Herb	Constituents	Action	Adverse effects	Interactions	Dosage	Comments
Kava kava L. *Piperis methysticum rhizoma*	Kava lactones, kava pyrone	Sedative-hypnotic, antispasmodic	Lethargy, impaired cognition, dermatitis with long-term unreported use	Synergistic with anxiolytics, alcohol; avoid with levodopa and dopaminergic agents.	600-800 mg/day	May be GABAergic. Contraindicated in patients with endogenous depression; may increase the danger of suicide.
St. John's wort *L. Hypericum Perforatum*	Hypericin, flavonoids, xanthones	Antidepressant, sedative, anxiolytic	Headaches, photosensitivity (may be severe), constipation	Report of manic reaction when used with sertraline (Zoloff). Do not combine with SSRIs or MAOIs; possible serotonin syndrome. Do not use with alcohol, opioids.	100-950 mg/day	Under investigation by National Institutes of Health. May act as MAOI or SSRI. Allow 4- to 6-wk trial for mild depressive moods; if no apparent improvement, another therapy should be tried. May be chemically unstable.
Valerian L. *Valeriana officinalis*	Valepotriates, valerenic acid, caffeic acid	Sedative, muscle relaxant, hypnotic	Cognitive and motor impairment, gastrointestinal upset, hepatotoxicity; with long-term use: contact allergy, headache, restlessness, insomnia, mydriasis, cardiac dysfunction	Avoid concomitant use with alcohol or CNS depressants.	1-2 g/day	

ªNo reliable, consistent, or valid data on dosages or adverse effects are available for most phytomedicinals.

ᵇFlavonoids are common to many herbs. They are plant by-products that act as antioxidants (i.e., agents that prevent the deterioration of material such as DNA via oxidation).

MAOI, monoamine oxidase inhibitor; GABA, γ-aminobutyric acid; SSRI, selective serotonin reuptake inhibitor.

are fear, anxiety, acting out, signing out against medical advice, hostility, dependency, depression, grief, and delirium.

B. Hemodialysis. Patients on hemodialysis have a lifelong dependency on machines and health care providers. They have problems with prolonged dependency, regression to childhood states, hostility, and negativism in following doctors' directions. It is advisable that all patients for whom dialysis is being considered undergo a psychological evaluation.

Dialysis dementia is a disorder characterized by a loss of cognitive functions, dystonias, and seizures. It usually ends in death. It tends to occur in patients who have been on dialysis for long periods of time.

C. Surgery. Patients who have undergone severe surgical procedures have a variety of psychological reactions, depending on their premorbid personality and the nature of the surgery. These reactions are summarized in Table 23-7.

IV. Alternative (or Complementary) Medicine

Increasing the use at present. One in three persons uses such therapies at some point for such common ailments as depression, anxiety, chronic pain, low back pain, headaches, and digestive problems. Some commonly taken herbal preparations with psychoactive properties are listed in Table 23-8.

For more detailed discussion of this topic, see Chapter 27, Psychosomatic Medicine, p. 2177 and Chapter 31, Complementary, Alternative, and Integrative Approaches in Mental Health Care, p. 2542, in CTP/X.

24
Suicide, Violence, and Emergency Psychiatric Medicine

I. Suicide
A. Definition

1. The word *suicide* is derived from Latin, meaning "self-murder." If successful, it is a fatal act that fulfills the person's wish to die. Various terms used to describe para-suicidal thoughts or behaviors—that is, suicidality, ideation—should be used with clear meaning and purpose. See Table 24-1 for definitions of terms related to suicide.

2. Identification of the potentially suicidal patient is among the most critical tasks in psychiatry.

B. Incidence and prevalence

1. About 40,000 persons commit suicide per year in the United States.

2. The rate is 12.5 persons per 100,000.

3. About 250,000 persons attempt suicide per year.

4. The United States is at the midpoint worldwide in numbers of suicides (e.g., 25 persons per 100,000 in Scandinavian countries). The rate is the lowest in Spain and Italy.

C. Associated risk factors. Table 24-2 lists high- and low-risk factors in the evaluation of suicide risk.

1. **Gender.** Men commit suicide three times more often than women. Women attempt suicide four times more often than men.

2. **Method.** Men's higher rate of successful suicide is related to the methods they use (e.g., firearms, hanging), while women more commonly take an overdose of psychoactive substances or a poison.

3. **Age.** Rates increase with age.

   a. Among men, the suicide rate peaks after age 45; among women, it peaks after age 65.

   b. Older persons attempt suicide less often but are more successful.

   c. After age 75, the rate rises in both sexes.

   d. Currently, the most rapid rise is among male 15- to 24-year olds.

4. **Race.** In the United States, two of every three suicides are committed by male white persons. The risk is lower in non-whites. The suicide rates are higher than average in Native Americans and Inuits.

5. **Religion.** Rate is the highest in Protestants; the lowest in Catholics, Jews, and Muslims.

6. **Marital status.** Rate is twice as high in single persons than in married persons. Divorced, separated, or widowed persons have rates four to five times higher than married persons. Divorced men register 69 suicides

Table 24-1
Terms Comprising Suicidal Ideation and Behavior

Aborted suicide attempt: Potentially self-injurious behavior with explicit or implicit evidence that the person intended to die but stopped the attempt before physical damage occurred.
Deliberate self-harm: Willful self-inflicting of painful, destructive, or injurious acts without intent to die.
Lethality of suicidal behavior: Objective danger to life associated with a suicide method or action. Note that lethality is distinct from and may not always coincide with an individual's expectation of what is medically dangerous.
Suicidal ideation: Thought of serving as the agent of one's own death; seriousness may vary depending on the specificity of suicidal plans and the degree of suicidal intent.
Suicidal intent: Subjective expectation and desire for a self-destructive act to end in death.
Suicide attempt: Self-injurious behavior with a nonfatal outcome accompanied by explicit or implicit evidence that the person intended to die.
Suicide: Self-inflicted death with explicit or implicit evidence that the person intended to die.

Table 24-2
Evaluation of Suicide Risk

Variable	High Risk	Low Risk
Demographic and social profile		
Age	Over 45 yrs	Below 45 yrs
Sex	Male	Female
Marital status	Divorced or widowed	Married
Employment	Unemployed	Employed
Interpersonal relationship	Conflictual	Stable
Family background	Chaotic or conflictual	Stable
Health		
Physical	Chronic illness	Good health
	Hypochondriac	Feels healthy
	Excessive substance intake	Low substance use
Mental	Severe depression	Mild depression
	Psychosis	Neurosis
	Severe personality disorder	Normal personality
	Substance abuse	Social drinker
	Hopelessness	Optimism
Suicidal activity		
Suicidal ideation	Frequent, intense, prolonged	Infrequent, low intensity, transient
Suicide attempt	Multiple attempts	First attempt
	Planned	Impulsive
	Rescue unlikely	Rescue inevitable
	Unambiguous wish to die	Primary wish for change
	Communication internalized (self-blame)	Communication externalized (anger)
	Method lethal and available	Method of low lethality or not readily available
Resources		
Personal	Poor achievement	Good achievement
	Poor insight	Insightful
	Affect unavailable or poorly controlled	Affect available and appropriately controlled
Social	Poor rapport	Good rapport
	Socially isolated	Socially integrated
	Unresponsive family	Concerned family

From Adam K. Attempted suicide. *Psychiatric Clin North Am.* 1985;8:183, with permission.

Table 24-3
Medical and Mental Disorders Associated with Increased Suicide Risk

- AIDS
- Amnesia
- Attention-deficit/hyperactivity disorder (ADHD)
- Bipolar disorder
- Borderline personality disorder
- Delirium
- Dementia
- Dysthymic disorder
- Eating disorders
- Impulse-control disorders
- Learning disability
- Major depression
- Panic disorder
- Posttraumatic stress disorder
- Schizoaffective disorder
- Schizophrenia
- Substance-use disorders

per 100,000, compared with 18 per 100,000 for divorced women. Death of spouse increases risk. For women, having young children at home is protective against suicide. Homosexual persons are at higher risk than heterosexuals.

7. **Physical health.** Medical or surgical illness is a high-risk factor, especially if associated with pain or chronic or terminal illness (Table 24-3).

8. **Mental illness**

   a. **Depressive disorders.** Mood disorders are the diagnoses most commonly associated with suicide. Fifty percent of all persons who commit suicide are depressed. Fifteen percent of depressed patients kill themselves. Patients with mood disorder accompanied by panic or anxiety attacks are at the highest risk.

   b. **Schizophrenia.** The onset of schizophrenia is typically in adolescence or early childhood, and most of these patients who commit suicide do so during the first few years of their illness. In the United States, an estimated 4,000 schizophrenic patients commit suicide each year. Ten percent of persons who commit suicide are schizophrenic with prominent delusions. Patients who have command hallucinations telling them to harm themselves are at increased risk.

   c. **Alcohol and other substance dependence.** Alcohol dependence increases the risk of suicide, especially if the person is also depressed. Studies show that many alcohol-dependent patients who eventually commit suicide are rated depressed during hospitalization and that up to two-thirds are assessed as having mood disorder symptoms during the period in which they commit suicide. The suicide rate for persons who are heroin dependent or dependent on other drugs is approximately 20 times the rate for the general population.

   d. **Personality disorders**. Borderline personality disorder is associated with a high rate of para-suicidal behavior. An estimated 5% of patients with antisocial personality disorder commit suicide, especially those in prisons. Prisoners have the highest suicide rate of any group.

e. **Dementia and delirium.** Increased risk in patients with dementia and delirium, especially secondary to alcohol abuse or with psychotic symptoms.

f. **Anxiety disorder.** Unsuccessful suicide attempts are made by almost 20% of patients with a panic disorder and social phobia. If depression is an associated feature, the risk of suicide rises. Panic disorder has been diagnosed in 1% of persons who successfully kill themselves.

9. **Other risk factors**
   a. Unambiguous wish to die.
   b. Unemployment.
   c. Sense of hopelessness.
   d. Rescue unlikely.
   e. Hoarding pills.
   f. Access to lethal agents or to firearms.
   g. Family history of suicide or depression.
   h. Fantasies of reunion with deceased loved ones.
   i. Occupation: dentist, physician, nurse, scientist, police officer, farmer.
   j. Previous suicide attempt.
   k. History of childhood physical or sexual abuse.
   l. History of impulsive or aggressive behavior.
   m. Social context—Key features of the epidemiology of suicide, however, can vary among different countries or ethnic groups. For example, in China, women commit suicide more than men. Rates vary from some South American countries reporting rates of 3/100,000 to rates in the Russian Federation of 60/100,00. See Table 24-4 for questions about suicidal feelings and behaviors.

D. **Management of the suicidal patient.** A general strategy for evaluating and managing suicidal patients is presented in Table 24-5.

1. Do not leave a suicidal patient alone; remove any potentially dangerous objects from the room.

2. Assess whether the attempt was planned or impulsive. Determine the lethality of the method, the chances of discovery (whether the patient was alone or notified someone), and the reaction to being saved (whether the patient is disappointed or relieved). Also, determine whether the factors that led to the attempt have changed.

3. Patients with severe depression may be treated on an outpatient basis if their families can supervise them closely and if treatment can be initiated rapidly. Otherwise, hospitalization is necessary.

4. The suicidal ideation of alcoholic patients generally remits with abstinence in a few days. If depression persists after the physiologic signs of alcohol withdrawal have resolved, a high suspicion of major depression is warranted. All suicidal patients who are intoxicated by alcohol or drugs must be reassessed when they are sober.

Text continues on page 365.

Table 24-4
Questions About Suicidal Feelings and Behaviors

Begin with questions that address the patient's feeling about living
Have you ever felt that life was not worth living?
Did you ever wish you could go to sleep and just not wake up?

Follow on with specific questions that ask about thoughts of death, self-harm, or suicide
Is death something you have thought about recently?
Have things ever reached the point that you have thought of harming yourself?

For individuals who have thoughts of self-harm or suicide
When did you first notice such thoughts?
What led up to the thoughts (e.g., interpersonal and psychosocial precipitants, including real or imagined losses; specific symptoms such as mood changes, anhedonia, hopelessness, anxiety, agitation, psychosis)?
How often have those thoughts occurred, including frequency, obsessional quality, controllability?
How close have you come to acting on those thoughts?
How likely do you think it is that you will act on them in the future?
Have you ever started to harm (or kill) yourself but stopped before doing something (e.g., holding knife or gun to your body but stopping before acting, going to edge of bridge but not jumping)?
What do you envision happening if you actually killed yourself (e.g., escape, reunion with significant other, rebirth, reactions of others)?
Have you made a specific plan to harm or kill yourself? (If so, what does the plan include?)
Do you have guns or other weapons available to you?
Have you made any particular preparations (e.g., purchasing specific items, writing a note or a will, making financial arrangements, taking steps to avoid discovery, rehearsing the plan)?
Have you spoken to anyone about your plans?
How does the future look to you?
What things would lead you to feel more (or less) hopeful about the future (e.g., treatment, reconciliation of relationship, resolution of stressors)?
What things would make it more (or less) likely that you would try to kill yourself?
What things in your life would lead you to want to escape from life or be dead?
What things in your life make you want to go on living?
If you began to have thoughts of harming or killing yourself again, what would you do?

For individuals who have attempted suicide or engaged in self-damaging action(s), parallel questions to those in the previous section can address the prior attempt(s). Additional questions can be asked in general terms or can refer to the specific method used and may include:
Can you describe what happened (e.g., circumstances, precipitants, view of future, use of alcohol or other substances, method, intent, seriousness of injury)?
What thoughts were you having beforehand that led up to the attempt?
What did you think would happen (e.g., going to sleep versus injury versus dying, getting a reaction out of a particular person)?
Were other people present at the time?
Did you seek help afterward yourself, or did someone get help for you?
Had you planned to be discovered, or were you found accidentally?
How did you feel afterward (e.g., relief versus regret at being alive)?
Did you receive treatment afterward (e.g., medical versus psychiatric, emergency department versus inpatient versus outpatient)?
Has your view of things changed, or is anything different for you since the attempt?
Are there other times in the past when you have tried to harm (or kill) yourself?

For individuals with repeated suicidal thoughts or attempts
About how often have you tried to harm (or kill) yourself?
When was the most recent time?
Can you describe your thoughts at the time that you were thinking most seriously about suicide?
When was your most serious attempt at harming or killing yourself?
What led up to it, and what happened afterward?

(continued)

Table 24-4
Questions About Suicidal Feelings and Behaviors *(Continued)*

For individuals with psychosis, ask specifically about hallucinations and delusions

Can you describe the voices (e.g., single versus multiple, male versus female, internal versus external, recognizable versus nonrecognizable)?

What do the voices say (e.g., positive remarks versus negative remarks versus threats)? (If the remarks are commands, determine if they are for harmless versus harmful acts; ask for examples.)

How do you cope with (or respond to) the voices?

Have you ever done what the voices ask you to do? (What led you to obey the voices? If you tried to resist them, what made it difficult?)

Have there been times when the voices told you to hurt or kill yourself? (How often? What happened?)

Are you worried about having a serious illness or that your body is rotting?

Are you concerned about your financial situation even when others tell you there's nothing to worry about?

Are there things that you've been feeling guilty about or blaming yourself for?

Consider assessing the patient's potential to harm others in addition to himself or herself

Are there others who you think may be responsible for what you are experiencing (e.g., persecutory ideas, passivity experiences)?

Are you having any thoughts of harming them?

Are there other people you would want to die with you?

Are there others who you think would be unable to go on without you?

Direct and specific questions about suicide are essential in suicide assessment. The psychiatrist should ask about suicidal thoughts, plans, and behaviors. Accepting a negative response to an initial question about suicidal ideation may not be enough to determine actual suicide risk. A denial of suicidal ideation that is inconsistent with the patient's presentation or current depressive symptomatology may indicate a need for additional questioning or collateral sources of information. These questions may be helpful when asking about specific aspects of a patient's suicidal thoughts, plans, and behaviors.

From the *Practice Guidelines for Assessment and Treatment of the Suicidal Patient.* 2nd ed. American Psychiatric Association Practice Guidelines for the Treatment of Psychiatric Disorders Compendium (Copyright 2004), with permission.

Table 24-5
General Strategy in Evaluating Patients

I. Protect yourself
- A. Know as much as possible about the patients before meeting them.
- B. Leave physical restraint procedures to those who are trained to handle them.
- C. Be alert to risks for impending violence.
- D. Attend to the safety of the physical surroundings (e.g., door access, room objects).
- E. Have others present during the assessment if needed.
- F. Have others in the vicinity.
- G. Attend to developing on alliance with the patient (e.g., do not confront or threaten patients with paranoid psychoses).

II. Prevent harm
- A. Prevent self-injury and suicide. Use whatever methods are necessary to prevent patients from hurting themselves during the evaluation.
- B. Prevent violence toward others. During the evaluation, briefly assess the patient for the risk of violence. If the risk is deemed significant, consider the following options:
  1. Inform the patient that violence is not acceptable.
  2. Approach the patient in a nonthreatening manner.
  3. Reassure and calm the patient or assist in reality testing.
  4. Offer medication.
  5. Inform the patient that restraint or seclusion will be used if necessary.
  6. Have teams ready to restrain the patient.
  7. When patients are restrained, always closely observe them and frequently check their vital signs. Isolate restrained patients from agitating stimuli. Immediately plan a further approach—medication, reassurance, medical evaluation.

III. Rule out cognitive disorders

IV. Rule out impending psychosis

5. Suicidal ideas in schizophrenic patients must be taken seriously, because they tend to use violent, highly lethal, and sometimes bizarre methods.

6. Patients with personality disorders benefit mostly from empathic confrontation and assistance in solving the problem that precipitated the suicide attempt and to which they have usually contributed.

7. Long-term hospitalization is recommended for conditions that contribute to self-mutilation; brief hospitalization does not usually affect such habitual behavior. Para-suicidal patients may benefit from long-term rehabilitation, and brief hospitalization may be necessary from time to time, but short-term treatment cannot be expected to alter their course significantly.

 CLINICAL HINTS: SUICIDE

- *Ask about suicidal ideas, especially plans to harm oneself. Asking about suicide does not plant the idea.*
- *Do not hesitate to ask patients if they "want to die." A straightforward approach is the most effective.*
- *Understand what and how suicide solves a problem, feel in control of such thoughts, and the degree they can see and pursue other solutions.*
- *Conduct the interview in a safe place. Patients have been known to throw themselves out of a window.*
- *Do not offer false reassurance (e.g., "Most people think about killing themselves at some time").*
- *Always ask about past suicide attempts, which can be related to future attempts.*
- *Always ask about access to firearms; access to weapons increases the risk in a suicidal patient.*
- *Explore how people understand their ability, strategies, and desire to alert others of impending self-harm.*
- *Do not release patients from the emergency department if you are not certain that they will not harm themselves.*
- *Never assume that family or friends will be able to watch a patient 24 hours a day. If that is required, admit the patient to the hospital.*
- *Never worry alone—If you are unsure about the level of risk or course of action involve others.*

E. **Legal issues**

1. Successful suicide is a major cause of lawsuits against psychiatrists.

2. Courts recognize that not all suicides can be prevented, but they do require thorough evaluation of suicide risk and careful treatment plan.

3. Careful documentation of suicidal patients is necessary, including record of decision-making process (e.g., discharge of patient from hospital to home, provision for follow-up care).

4. Take care especially with patients for whom suicidality is a concern to document formulation of risk—shorthand phrases such as "contracts for safety" do not substitute for more specific description of the features of mental status or ideation that suggest an adequate treatment alliance and behavior of the patient to alert the clinician of heightened risk.

II. Violence
A. Definition
1. Intentional act of doing bodily harm to another person.
2. Includes assault, rape, robbery, and homicide.
3. Physical and sexual abuse of adults, children, and the elderly are included in violent acts.

B. Incidence and prevalence
1. About 8 million violent acts are committed each year in the United States.
2. Lifetime risk of becoming a homicide victim is about 1 in 85 for men and 1 in 280 for women. Men are the victims of violence more often than women.

C. Disorders associated with violence.
The psychiatric conditions most commonly associated with violence include such psychotic disorders as schizophrenia and mania (particularly if the patient is paranoid or is experiencing command hallucinations), intoxication with alcohol and drugs, withdrawal from alcohol and sedative–hypnotics, catatonic excitement, agitated depression, personality disorders characterized by rage and poor impulse control (e.g., borderline and antisocial personality disorders), and cognitive disorders (especially those associated with frontal and temporal lobe involvement).

D. Predicting violent behavior.
See Table 24-6. Best predictors are past acts of violence. Predictors, however, are often very nonspecific among psychiatric populations. Some evidence suggests that a fluctuating course or altered pattern of symptoms in a psychiatric illness, rather than the cumulative specific symptoms per se, might be predictive of greater violence risk.
1. Several symptom scales such as the MOAS or the Broset have been studied with respect to the prediction of violence, although mostly in terms of immediate risk in inpatient treatment settings. One key value of such scales may be to fix more concerted attention and management of staff to patients as well as track clinical course.

E. Evaluation and management
1. Protect yourself. Assume that violence is always a possibility, and be on guard for a sudden violent act. Never interview an armed patient. The patient should always surrender a weapon or potential weapon to secure personnel. Know as much as possible about the patient before the interview. Never interview a potentially violent patient alone or in an office with the door closed. Consider removing neckties, necklaces, and other articles of clothing or jewelry you are wearing that the patient can grab or pull. Stay within sight of other staff members. Leave physical restraint

Table 24-6
Assessing and Predicting Violent Behavior

Signs of impending violence

Recent acts of violence, including property violence.

Verbal or physical threats (menacing).

Carrying weapons or other objects that may be used as weapons (e.g., forks, ashtrays).

Progressive psychomotor agitation.

Alcohol or other substance intoxication.

Paranoid features in a psychotic patient.

Command violent auditory hallucinations—some but not all patients are at high risk.

Brain diseases, global or with frontal lobe findings; less commonly with temporal lobe findings (controversial).

Catatonic excitement.

Certain manic episodes.

Certain agitated depressive episodes.

Personality disorders (rage, violence, or impulse dyscontrol).

Assess the risk for violence

Consider violent ideation, wish, intention, plan, availability of means, implementation of plan, wish for help.

Consider demographics—sex (male), age (15–24), socioeconomic status (low), social supports (few).

Consider the patient's history: violence, nonviolent antisocial acts, impulse dyscontrol (e.g., gambling, substance abuse, suicide or self-injury, psychosis).

Consider overt stressors (e.g., marital conflict, real or symbolic loss).

to staff members who are trained in that. Do not give the patient access to areas where weapons may be available (e.g., a crash cart or a treatment room). Do not sit close to a paranoid patient, who may feel threatened. Keep yourself at least an arm's length away from any potentially violent patient. Do not challenge or confront a psychotic patient. Be alert to the signs of impending violence. Always leave yourself a route of rapid escape in case the patient attacks you. Never turn your back on the patient.

2. Signs of impending violence include recent violent acts against people or property, clenched teeth and fists, verbal threats (menacing), possession of weapons or objects potentially usable as weapons, psychomotor agitation (considered to be an important indicator), alcohol or drug intoxication, paranoid delusions, and command hallucinations.

3. Physical restraint should be applied only by persons with appropriate training. Patients with suspected phencyclidine intoxication should not be physically restrained (limb restraints especially should be avoided) because they may injure themselves. Usually, a benzodiazepine or an antipsychotic is given immediately after physical restraints have been applied to provide a chemical restraint, but the choice of drug depends on the diagnosis. Provide a nonstimulating environment.

4. Perform a definitive diagnostic evaluation. The patient's vital signs should be assessed, a physical examination performed, and a psychiatric history obtained. Evaluate the patient's risk for suicide and create a treatment plan that provides for the management of potential subsequent violence. Elevated vital signs may suggest withdrawal from alcohol or sedative–hypnotics.

5. Explore possible psychosocial interventions to reduce the risk for violence. If violence is related to a specific situation or person, try to separate the patient from that situation or person. Try family interventions and other modifications of the environment. Would the patient still be potentially violent while living with other relatives?

6. Hospitalization may be necessary to detain the patient and prevent violence. Constant observation may be necessary, even on a locked inpatient psychiatric ward.

7. If psychiatric treatment is not appropriate, you may involve the police and the legal system.

8. Intended victims must be warned of the continued possibility of danger (e.g., if the patient is not hospitalized).

 CLINICAL HINTS: VIOLENT PATIENTS

- *If the patient is brought to the emergency department by police with restraining devices (e.g., handcuffs), do not immediately remove them.*
- *Conduct the interview in a safe environment with attendants on call should the patient become agitated.*
- *Position yourself so that you cannot be blocked by the patient from exiting the examination room.*
- *Do not interview a patient if sharp or potentially dangerous objects are in the interview room (e.g., a letter opener on a desk).*
- *Trust your feelings. If you feel apprehensive or fearful, terminate the interview.*
- *Ask about past attempts at violence (including cruelty to animals). They are predictors for future violent events.*
- *Admit a patient for observation if there is any question of his or her being a danger to others.*
- *Never worry alone—If you are unsure about the level of risk or course of action involve others.*

F. **History and diagnosis.** Risk factors for violence include a statement of intent, formulation of a specific plan, available means, male sex, young age (15 to 24 years), low socioeconomic status, poor social support system, past history of violence, other antisocial acts, poor impulse control, history of suicide attempts, and recent stressors. A history of violence is the best predictor of violence. Additional important factors include a history of childhood victimization; a childhood history of the triad of bed-wetting, fire setting, and cruelty to animals; a criminal record; military or police service; reckless driving; and a family history of violence. Again, see Table 24-7 for commonly attributed risk factors.

G. **Drug treatment**

1. Drug treatment depends on the specific diagnosis.

Table 24-7
Risk Factors for Violence

Current mental status findings
Hostile, irritable, menacing, threatening
Agitation
Victim(s) apparently picked out
Weapons available
Acute Intoxication
Paranoia
Delusions or hallucinations, especially command-type or that are used by patients to explain or justify their behavior
Impaired empathy

Disorders
Mania (when characterized by prominent irritability), as in bipolar disorder or schizoaffective disorder, bipolar type
Paranoid schizophrenia
Anabolic steroid abuse
Personality change (with disinhibition, e.g., frontal lobe syndrome)
Dementia
Delirium
Mental retardation
Paranoid personality disorder
Antisocial personality disorder
Borderline personality disorder
Alcohol intoxication
Stimulant intoxication (cocaine, amphetamines)
Intermittent explosive disorder
Delusional disorder

Personal history
History of violent behavior, impulsivity, in similar circumstances
Recent act(s) of violence/destruction of property
History of being physically abused in childhood
Growing up in a family where parents were violent toward each other
Childhood history of enuresis, cruelty to animals, and fire setting (the "triad")

Demographic
Male > female
Young (late teens or early 20s) > older

2. Benzodiazepines and antipsychotics are used most often to tranquilize a patient. Haloperidol (Haldol) given at a dose of 5 mg by mouth or intramuscularly; 2 mg of risperidone (Risperdal) by mouth; or 2 mg of lorazepam (Ativan) by mouth or intramuscularly may be tried initially. An intramuscular of olanzapine is also commonly used.

3. If the patient is already taking an antipsychotic, give more of the same drug. If the patient's agitation has not decreased in 20 to 30 minutes, repeat the dose.

4. Avoid antipsychotics in patients who are at risk for seizures.

5. Benzodiazepines may be ineffective in patients who are tolerant, and they may cause disinhibition, which can potentially exacerbate violence.

6. For patients with epilepsy, first try an anticonvulsant (e.g., carbamazepine [Tegretol] or gabapentin [Neurontin]) and then a benzodiazepine (e.g., clonazepam [Klonopin]). Chronically violent patients sometimes respond to beta-blockers (e.g., propranolol [Inderal]).

Text continues on page 376.

Table 24-8
Common Psychiatric Emergencies

Syndrome or Presenting Symptom	Emergency Problem	Emergency Treatment Issues
Abuse of child or adults	Is there another explanation? Protect from further injury.	Management of medical problems: psychiatric evaluation; notification of protective services.
AIDS	Unrealistic or obsessive concern about having contracted the illness; changes in behavior secondary to organic effects; symptoms of depression or anxiety in someone who has the illness; grief over the loss of a friend or lover from AIDS.	Explore the patient's primary concern; if there is a realistic possibility of the patient's having contracted the virus, arrange for counseling and HIV titer; rule out an organic component in the HIV-positive patient, facilitate grieving for the patient who has suffered a loss by identifying the depression and referring for brief psychotherapy treatment or AIDS-support group.
Adjustment disorder	Agitation, sleep disorder, or depression; substance abuse; anxiety.	Explore briefly the meaning of the loss that has precipitated the adjustment reaction; refer for brief focused therapy; do not prescribe medications for the symptoms of adjustment disorder in the emergency department, because many of the symptoms abate once the patient is aware of their origins and has a chance to deal with the associated feelings.
Adolescent crisis	Suicidal ideation or attempts, running-away behaviors, drug use, pregnancy, psychosis, assaultive behavior toward family members, eating disorders.	Family crisis intervention is ideal if that can be accomplished; for the adolescent who is completely estranged from the family, inquire about an interested adult relative or friend who can be involved; evaluate for sexual or other physical abuse; evaluate for suicidal ideation; refer to adolescent crisis services if those are available; consider hospitalization if necessary.
Agoraphobia	Determination of the reason for the patient's emergency department visit.	Agoraphobia is a long-standing problem; refer the patient for psychiatric treatment; do not prescribe medications in the emergency department unless there will be continuity of care in follow-up.
Akathisia	Is this a new onset? Is the patient on maintenance antipsychotics?	Determine the causative agent; diphenhydramine (Benadryl) orally or intravenously, or benztropine (Cogentin) orally or intramuscularly. Explain to patient and family the cause of the symptom.
Alcohol-related emergencies	Confusion; psychosis; assaultive behavior, suicidal ideation or behavior; hallucinations.	Determine blood alcohol concentration; concentrations above 300 mg/dL suggest fairly long-standing alcohol abuse; assess the need for emergency intervention; antipsychotic agents as needed for psychotic symptoms; confront the patient about the degree of alcohol abuse and hold in emergency department until level decreases sufficiently for an appropriate assessment of suicidality and judgment; refer to an alcohol treatment program.

Alcohol idiosyncratic intoxication	Marked aggressive or assaultive behavior; "the patient just isn't himself (or herself)."	Rule out organic cause; benzodiazepines as needed to calm the patient; decrease external stimulation and restrain the patient, if necessary; after a determination is made that the patient can be safely discharged, warn the patient about the likelihood that the idiosyncratic reaction will recur with further drinking.
Alcohol withdrawal	Irritability, shakiness: confusion and disorientation; abnormal vital signs, including tachycardia, hyperthermia, and hypertension.	Benzodiazepines as needed to reduce symptoms; observe patient closely and monitor vital signs over several hours to detect onset of delirium tremens; when the patient is ready for discharge, inform the patient firmly about the diagnosis of alcohol dependence and refer for treatment.
Korsakoff's syndrome, Wernicke's encephalopathy	Confusion, amnesia; multiple organic symptoms, including ataxia, confusion, and disturbances of eye muscles.	Determine onset if possible; institute treatment with thiamine; determine capacity for patient to care for self; hospitalize, if necessary; inform the patient firmly about the diagnosis of alcoholism.
Amnesia	Identification; differential diagnosis, particularly of an organic component.	Explore circumstances in which patient came to the emergency department; consider an amobarbital (Amytal) interview; evaluate patient to rule out organic cause.
Amphetamine, cocaine, or amphetamine-like intoxication	Psychosis; agitation or assaultive behavior; paranoia.	Decrease stimulation, consider restraints and antipsychotics to control behavior, consider hospitalization as amphetamine-induced psychotic disorder may persist for weeks to months; cocaine withdrawal may produce suicidal feelings.
Anxiety, acute	Differential diagnosis, particularly of medical or substance-induced cause; management of the acute symptomatology.	Explore patient's capacity for insight regarding the precipitant; refer for outpatient psychiatric treatment; avoid prescribing medications from the emergency department because the principal agents that are effective are also commonly abused.
Borderline personality disorder	Determination of the immediate need for the emergency department visit; determination of the patient's agenda.	Evaluate for acute suicidal ideation; consider hospitalization if clinician is uncomfortable; state limits as clearly as able to enforce; state clear follow-up plan.
Catatonia	Differential diagnosis of an organic cause; management of the acute symptoms.	Rule out organic causes; consider rapid tranquilization if the emergency department has the capacity to monitor the patient over several hours.
Delirium, dementia	Fluctuating sensorium; determine acuity; differential diagnosis; need for physical restraint while the patient is evaluated.	Evaluate patient for organic cause; remember that prescribed medications are very common causes for acute cognitive disorders.
Delusions	Degree to which delusional beliefs interfere with the patient's ability to negotiate activities of daily living; degree to which the patient's response to these delusional beliefs is likely to cause problems for the patient.	Explore the time of onset, the pervasiveness of the delusions, and the degree to which the delusional beliefs interfere with the patient's daily functioning, particularly if there is anything to suggest that the patient might try to harm self or others because of these delusions; rule out organic causes; refer for ongoing treatment, or hospitalize if there is an immediate life threat or need for further organic evaluation.

(continued)

Table 24-8
Common Psychiatric Emergencies *(Continued)*

Syndrome or Presenting Symptom	Emergency Problem	Emergency Treatment Issues
Depression	Recognition of the diagnosis; onset; risk of suicide; assessment of the need to protect the patient.	Explore onset of symptoms; evaluate for suicidal ideation; evaluate nonpsychiatric causes; drug-related depression; consider hospitalization if the patient does not respond to the interpersonal interaction of the emergency evaluation or seems hopeless or helpless even after the evaluation; tell the patient the presumptive diagnosis and refer for treatment; initiation of pharmacologic treatment for depression should not take place from an emergency department unless there will be continuity of care for the patient in the some system.
Dystonia, acute	Patient's psychological and physical discomfort; identification of causative agent.	Determine the causative agent; treat with diphenhydramine or benztropine and contact the agency or therapist that prescribed the medication for follow-up care; refer the patient back to treating agency after explaining the cause of the symptoms.
Family crises, marital cases	Determination of danger to members of the family; resolution of the crisis sufficiently to get the couple or family out of the emergency department.	Offer an opportunity for the family unit to meet briefly to explore the issue that brought them to the emergency department; do not make any recommendations that seem self-evident, because there is always more than meets the eye when a crisis propels a family to use an emergency department as an intervention; rule out issues of domestic violence, child abuse, or substance abuse; refer as appropriate.
Geriatric crises	Identification of contributory medical or pharmacologic problems; identification of family agenda.	Determine acuity; try to uncover the family agenda; rule out organicity, especially as it relates to the reason for the emergency department visit now; rule out elder abuse; refer as appropriate.
Grief and bereavement	Identification of an excessive or pathologic reaction, determination of the need for professional referral; facilitation of the grieving process in the emergency department.	Explore any extreme or pathologic reactions to the loss, especially undue use of medications, drugs, or alcohol; rule out major depressive disorder; acknowledge the validity of the feelings, and refer for appropriate treatment or to support groups as necessary; avoid prescribing any medications from the emergency department unless there is the capacity for continuity of care and follow-up.
Hallucinations	Onset; differential diagnosis, particularly for a medical or substance-related cause.	Evaluate for possible organic cause, especially for visual, tactile, or olfactory hallucinations; assess for suicidal or homicidal content and consider hospitalization or referral for immediate care, if indicated.
High fever	Potential life threat; determine cause; potential offenders include lithium, anticholinergics, agranulocytosis induced by clozapine (Clozaril) or phenothiazines; neuroleptic malignant syndrome.	Emergency treatment for high fever; stop offending medication and treat underlying cause.

Homicidal and assaultive behavior	Danger to staff and other patients; determination of risk for suicide; cause of the behavior.	Determine whether there is an acute psychiatric condition determining the homicidal or assaultive behavior; use sufficient personnel and restraints to ensure the safety of staff and other patients; rule out medical or substance-related components.
Hyperventilation	Physical symptoms; patient's anxiety with respect to the symptoms.	Explain briefly to the patient how the symptoms are caused by hyperventilation; instruct the patient to breathe into a paper bag for several minutes; it may be useful to encourage the patient to hyperventilate again in the clinician's presence to confirm the cause of the symptoms.
Insomnia	Determination of an acute precipitant; identification of the patient's primary concern.	Determine the cause of the symptoms, rule out depression or incipient psychosis; refer as appropriate, do not prescribe medications from the emergency department for the condition.
Lithium (Eskalith) toxicity	Medical instability; contributing medical conditions.	Monitor for significant medical instability and consider hospitalization; stop lithium immediately; institute supportive measures as indicated.
Mania	Danger to self or others; need for restraints before behavior escalates out of control in the emergency department.	Reduce stimulation and consider the use of restraints; rule out organic cause if there is no history of a bipolar disorder or if the symptoms are significantly worse; consider hospitalization, especially if patient is unable to appreciate need for treatment.
Neuroleptic malignant syndrome	Medical instability; correct identification of the problem; need for rapid response.	Institute life support measures as indicated; the illness can progress rapidly; hospitalize; make clear to the receiving physicians the presumptive diagnosis.
Opioid intoxication or withdrawal	Correct identification of the problem.	Administer naloxone (Norcan) for overdose; opiate withdrawal is not life threatening, and patient may be treated symptomatically for relief of discomfort; refer to proper treatment program.
Panic reactions	Identification of an acute precipitant; response to the patient's need for immediate relief.	Talk the patient down; look for an organic cause, especially for a first episode; attempt to identify the acute precipitant, but it is a chronic problem that must be referred for adequate management; there is some evidence that encouraging the patient to face the precipitating stimulus again as soon as possible minimizes the long-term disability associated with panic reactions.
Paranoia	Underlying psychosis; possible organic cause.	Consider an underlying psychosis; stimulant abuse is the most common organic cause for paranoid symptoms; refer the patient as appropriate, or consider hospitalization if the paranoia poses a threat to the patient's life or to others'; suicidal behavior is not uncommon in acute paranoia.
Parkinsonism	Identification of the cause (i.e., idiopathic vs. side effects of medication).	Prescribe an anti-parkinsonian agent and refer the patient to the original prescribing physician or to a neurologist or psychiatrist as indicated.

(continued)

Table 24-8
Common Psychiatric Emergencies *(Continued)*

Syndrome or Presenting Symptom	Emergency Problem	Emergency Treatment Issues
Phencyclidine intoxication	Identification of causative agent; danger to self or others.	Reduce stimulation; observe for significant physiologic disturbances, such as temperature elevation; avoid antipsychotics; hospitalize, if necessary to protect the patient during intoxication, which may last for several days.
Phobias	Reason for current emergency department visit.	Assess onset of symptoms and the degree to which they are interfering with the patient immediately; refer for long-term management, probably to a behavioral treatment program.
Photosensitivity or rash	Confirm cause (phenothiazines).	Advise patient of necessary precautions (sunscreen, hat, avoidance of strong sunlight).
Posttraumatic stress disorder	Identification of the precipitant; identification of symptoms that are particularly disruptive to normal functioning, such as substance abuse, sleep disturbances, isolation.	Assess onset of symptoms; try to identify the precipitant for the current visit; refer to a brief treatment program if a specific precipitant can be identified.
Priapism	Discomfort, anxiety; determine whether patient is on trazodone (Desyrel).	Discontinue trazodone; consult urologist if symptom persists.
Psychosis	Acuity; differential diagnosis; danger to self or others from suicidal ideation or psychotic ideation.	Evaluate for organic cause; explore possible precipitants; take whatever measures are indicated to protect the patient and others; consider rapid neuroleptization if medical or substance-related cause can be clearly ruled out.
Rape	Identification of any extreme features of the assault; need for support; medical components.	Be sure that all medical and forensic issues have been addressed, such as chain of evidence, prevention of pregnancy, and sexually transmitted disease; facilitate the patient's exploration of feelings about the assault; facilitate access to rape crisis counseling.
Repeaters	Reason for the return visit; emergency issues; danger to self or others; reason for failure of prior management or referral.	Once genuine reasons for a return visit have been ruled out, review how the emergency department may be encouraging the patient to use such a method of receiving care and attention rather than more traditional channels; consider substance abuse or medical condition as possible overlooked conditions.
Schizophrenia	Onset; reason for current emergency department visit; question whether there is a breakdown of long-term case management.	Determine reason for use of the emergency department rather than the patient's identified treatment program; contact program before making any decisions about treatment or hospitalization; consider suicide potential.

Sedative intoxication	Medical management; exploration of motivation (was it a suicidal act?) for intoxication.	Initiate treatment as indicated; consider suicidal intent even if patient denies it.
Seizures	Patient safety; determination of cause.	Observe for postictal confusion; discontinue or lower seizure-inducing medication; refer or hospitalize for comprehensive evaluation.
Substance abuse	Onset; reason for use of the emergency department; identification of agent; level of need for treatment (intoxication, withdrawal, or desire for abstinence).	Institute treatment as indicated for medically unstable patients; refer all others to formal treatment programs and do not institute treatment in the emergency department.
Suicidal behavior	Seriousness of intent; seriousness of attempt; need for medical intervention; need for hospitalization.	Consider hospitalization, particularly if patient has made prior attempts; has a family history of suicide; has had a significant recent loss, particularly by suicide; and does not seem to respond to the interpersonal interaction with the physician; hospitalize if uneasy.
Suicide thoughts or threats	Seriousness of intent; ability of patient to control thoughts; determination of usefulness of prior or current psychiatric treatment.	As above.
Tardive dyskinesia	Patient's discomfort; reason for emergency department visit; question whether there has been a breakdown of outpatient management.	This is a long-term problem, not an acute one; reduction of antipsychotic often increases the symptoms of tardive dyskinesia; refer the patient for appropriate psychiatric treatment.
Tremor	New onset? Determine cause, such as lithium toxicity, tardive dyskinesia, substance withdrawal, anxiety.	Treat according to cause.
Violence	Danger to others; determination of underlying psychiatric basis for behavior.	Use sufficient strength, in terms of numbers and competence of staff, and restraints to control the behavior quickly; delay or hesitation may escalate the violence; assess, and treat the patient as indicated according to the underlying cause; file charges if there has been any damage or injury because of the patient's behavior.

Table by Beverly J. Fauman, M.D.

III. Other Psychiatric Emergencies

A psychiatric emergency is a disturbance in thoughts, feelings, or actions that requires immediate treatment. It may be caused or accompanied by a medical or surgical condition that requires timely evaluation and treatment. Emergencies can occur in any location—home, office, street, and medical, surgical, and psychiatric units. Under ideal conditions, the patient will be brought to the psychiatric emergency unit, where physicians and psychiatrists who specialize in emergency medicine can evaluate the situation and institute treatment. Table 24-8 lists a broad range of conditions that fall into the category of psychiatric emergencies.

For more detailed discussion of this topic, see Chapter 32, Psychiatric Emergencies, p. 2610 and Chapter 28, Section 28.2, Adult Antisocial Behavior, Criminality, and Violence, p. 2413, in CTP/X.

25
Child Psychiatry

I. Child Development

The transactional nature of development in childhood consists of a continuous interplay between biologic predisposition and environmental experiences. It is widely accepted that adverse childhood experiences are likely to alter the trajectory of development in a given individual, and that during early development the brain is especially vulnerable to injury. Changes in both white matter and gray matter in the brains of children are linked to increase in acquisition of subtle social skills and on their potential to adapt to new and challenging demands.

Development results from interplay of maturation of the central nervous system (CNS), neuromuscular apparatus, and endocrine system and various environmental influences (e.g., parents and teachers, who can either facilitate or thwart a child's attainment of his or her developmental potential). This potential is specific to each person's given genetic predisposition to (1) intellectual level and (2) mental disorders, temperament, and certain personality traits.

A. Phases of development. The phases of development are divided into four areas: (1) the fetus, from 8 weeks to birth; (2) infancy, from birth to 15 months; (3) the preschool period from 2½ to 6 years; and (4) and the middle years from 6 to 12 years followed by adolescence which by convention ends at age 18.

The tables that follow list the developmental milestones at various stages of which the clinician should be aware.

Table 25-1 describes the landmarks of normal behavioral development from birth to 6 years.

Table 25-2 describes the development of language from 0 to 6 months until age 55 months. In the first age range, vocalizations begin and in the second age range, true communication such as telling of stories is present.

Table 25-3 describes emotional development in which feelings and reactions to others are described. This table is important in the diagnosis of a new disorder first described in DSM-5 called social (pragmatic) communication disorder described later in this section.

B. Psychological theories of development. A variety of theories have been developed to explain the psychological development of children. The most cited are those of Sigmund Freud, Margaret Mahler, Erik Erickson, and Jean Piaget. Their work is outlined in Table 25-4.

C. Attachment theory. John Bowlby studied the attachment of infants to mothers and concluded that early separations of infants from their mothers had severe negative effects on children's emotional and intellectual development. He described attachment behavior which develops during the

Text continues on page 387.

Table 25-1
Landmarks of Normal Behavioral Development

Age	Motor and Sensory Behavior	Adaptive Behavior	Personal and Social Behavior
Birth to 4 wks	Hand to mouth reflex, grasping reflex Rooting reflex (puckering lips in response to perioral stimulation); Moro reflex (digital extension when startled); sucking reflex; Babinski reflex (toes spread when sole of foot touched) Differentiates sounds (orients to human voice) and sweet and sour tastes Visual tracking Fixed focal distance of 8 in Makes alternating crawling movements Moves head laterally when placed in prone position	Anticipatory feeding-approach behavior at 4 days Responds to sound of rattle and bell Regards moving objects momentarily	Responsiveness to mother's face, eyes, and voice within first few hours of life Endogenous smile Independent play (until 2 yrs) Quiets when picked up Impassive face
4 wks	Tonic neck reflex positions predominate Hands fisted Head sags but can hold head erect for a few seconds Visual fixation, stereoscopic vision (12 wks)	Follows moving objects to the midline Shows no interest and drops objects immediately	Regards face and diminishes activity Responds to speech Smiles preferentially to mother
16 wks	Symmetrical postures predominate Holds head balanced Head lifted 90 degrees when prone on forearm Visual accommodation	Follows a slowly moving object well Arms activate on sight of dangling object	Spontaneous social smile (exogenous) Aware of strange situations
28 wks	Sits steadily, leaning forward on hands Bounces actively when placed in standing position	One-hand approach and grasp of toy Bangs and shakes rattle Transfers toys	Takes feet to mouth Pats mirror image Starts to imitate mother's sounds and actions
40 wks	Sits alone with good coordination Creeps Pulls self to standing position Points with index finger	Matches two objects at midline Attempt to imitate scribble	Separation anxiety manifest when taken away from mother Responds to social play, such as pat-a-cake and peekaboo Feeds self cracker and holds own bottle
52 wks	Walks with one hand held Stands alone briefly	Seeks novelty	Cooperates in dressing

Age	Gross Motor	Fine Motor/Adaptive	Personal-Social
15 mos	Toddles Creeps up stairs		Points or vocalizes wants Throws objects in play or refusal
18 mos	Coordinated walking, seldom falls Hurls ball Walks up stairs with one hand held	Builds a tower of three or four cubes Scribbles spontaneously and imitates a writing stroke	Feeds self in part, spills Pulls toy on string Carries or hugs a special toy, such as a doll Imitates some behavioral patterns with slight delay
2 yrs	Runs well, no falling Kicks large ball Goes up and down stairs alone Fine motor skills increase	Builds a tower of six or seven cubes Aligns cubes, imitating train Imitates vertical and circular strokes Develops original behaviors	Pulls on simple garment Domestic mimicry Refers to self by name Says "no" to mother Separation anxiety begins to diminish Organized demonstrations of love and protest Parallel play (plays side by side but does not interact with other children)
3 yrs	Rides tricycle Jumps from bottom steps Alternates feet going up stairs	Builds tower of nine or ten cubes Imitates a three-cube bridge Copies a circle and a cross	Puts on shoes Unbuttons buttons Feeds self well Understands taking turns
4 yrs	Walks down stairs one step to a tread Stands on one foot for 5-8 sec	Copies a cross Repeats four digits Counts three objects with correct pointing	Washes and dries own face Brushes teeth Associative or joint play (plays cooperatively with other children)
5 yrs	Skips, using feet alternately Usually has complete sphincter control Fine coordination improves	Copies a square Draws a recognizable human with a head, a body, limbs Counts 10 objects accurately	Dresses and undresses self Prints a few letters Plays competitive exercise games
6 yrs	Rides two-wheel bicycle	Prints name Copies triangle	Ties shoelaces

Adapted from Arnold Gessell, M.D., and Stella Chess, M.D.

Table 25-2
Language Development

Age and Stage of Development	Mastery of Comprehension	Mastery of Expression
0–6 mos	Shows startle response to loud or sudden sounds; attempts to localize sounds, turning eyes or head; appears to listen to speakers, may respond with smile; Recognizes warning, angry, and friendly voices; responds to hearing own name	Has vocalizations other than crying; has differential cries for hunger, pain; makes vocalizations to show pleasure; plays at making sounds Babbles (a repeated series of sounds)
7–11 mos Attending-to-Language	Shows listening selectivity (voluntary control over responses to sounds); listens to music or singing with interest; recognizes "no," "hot," own name; looks at pictures being named for up to 1 min; listens to speech without being distracted by other sounds	Responds to own name with vocalizations; imitates the melody of utterances; uses jargon (own language); has gestures (shakes head for no); has exclamation ("oh-oh"); plays language games (pat-a-cake, peekaboo)
12–18 mos Single-Word	Shows gross discriminations between dissimilar sounds (bells vs. dog vs. horn vs. mother's or father's voice); understands basic body parts, names of common objects; Acquires understanding of some new words each week; can identify simple objects (baby, ball, etc.) from a group of objects or pictures; understands up to 150 words by age 18 mos	Uses single words (mean age of first word is 11 mos; by age 18 mos, child is using up to 20 words); "Talks" to toys, self, or others using long patterns of jargon and occasional words; approximately 25% of utterances are intelligible; all vowels articulated correctly; initial and final consonants often omitted
12–24 mos Two-Word Messages	Responds to simple directions ("Give me the ball") Responds to action commands ("Come here," "Sit down") Understands pronouns (me, him, her, and you) Begins to understand complex sentences ("When we go to the store, I'll buy you some candy")	Uses two-word utterances ("Mommy sock," "all gone," "ball here"); imitates environmental sounds in play ("moo," "mmm, mmm," etc.); refers to self by name, begins to use pronouns; echoes two or more last words of sentences; begins to use three-word telegraphic utterances ("all gone ball," "me go now"); utterances 26–50% intelligible; uses language to ask for needs
24–36 mos Grammar Formation	Understands small body parts (elbow, chin, eyebrow); understands family name categories (grandma, baby) Understands size (little one, big one) Understands most adjectives Understands functions (why do we eat, why do we sleep)	Uses real sentences with grammatical function words (can, will, the, and a); usually announces intentions before acting "conversations" with other children, usually just monologues jargon and echolalia gradually drop from speech; increased vocabulary (up to 270 words at 2 yrs, 895 words at 3 yrs); speech 50–80% intelligible P, b, m articulated correctly; speech may show rhythmic disturbances
36–54 mos Grammar Development	Understands prepositions (under, behind, and between) Understands many words (up to 3,500 at 3 yrs, 5,500 at 4 yrs) Understands cause and effect (What do you do when you're hungry? cold?) Understands analogies (Food is to eat, milk is to ____)	Correct articulation of n, w, ng, h, t, d, k, and g; uses language to relate incidents from the past; uses wide range of grammatical forms: plurals, past tense, negatives, questions; plays with language: rhymes, exaggerates; Speech 90% intelligible, occasional errors in the ordering of sounds within words; able to define words; egocentric use of language rare; can repeat a 12-syllable sentence correctly; some grammatical errors still occur

(continued)

Table 25-2
Language Development (Continued)

Age and Stage of Development	Mastery of Comprehension	Mastery of Expression
55 mos on True Communication	Understands concepts of number, speed, time, space; understands left and right; understands abstract terms; is able to categorize items into semantic classes	Uses language to tell stories, share ideas, and discuss alternatives; increasing use of varied grammar; spontaneous self-correction of grammatical errors; stabilizing of articulation f, v, s, z, l, r, th, and consonant clusters; speech 100% intelligible

Reprinted from Sadock BJ, Sadock VA, Ruiz P, Sadock BJ. *Kaplan & Sadock's Concise Textbook of Clinical Psychiatry*. Philadelphia: Wolters Kluwer; 2017; and Rutter M, Hersov L, eds. *Child and Adolescent Psychiatry*. London: Blackwell; 1985, with permission.

Table 25-3
Emotional Development

Stages First Seen	Emotional Skills	Emotional Behavior
Gestational–Infancy: 0–2 yrs		
0–2 mos onward	Love, evoked by touching Fear, evoked by loud noise Rage, evoked by body restrictions Brain pathways for emotion forming	Social smile and joy shown Responds to emotions of others All emotions there
3–4 mos onward	Self-regulation of emotions starts; brain pathways of emotion growing	Laughter possible and more control over smiles; anger shown
7–12 mos	Self-regulation of emotion grows	Able to elicit more responsiveness
	Increased intensity of basic three	Denies to cope with stress
1–2 yrs	Shame and pride appear; envy, embarrassment appear Displaces onto other children	Some indications of empathy starting; expressions of feeling: "I like you, Daddy" "I'm sorry" Likes attention and approval; enjoys play alone or next to peers
Early Childhood: 2–5 yrs		
3–6 yrs	Can understand causes of many emotions Can begin to find ways for regulating emotions and for expressing them Identifies with adult to cope	Empathy increases with understanding More response and less reaction; self-regulation: "Use your words to say that you are angry with him" Aggression becomes competition By age 5, shows sensitivity to criticism and cares about feelings of others
Middle Childhood:		Ego rules until age 6
5–11 yrs	Can react to the feelings of others	Empathy becomes altruism: "I feel so bad about their fire, I'm going to give them some of my things"
7–11 yrs	More aware of other's feelings	Superego dominates

Reprinted from Sadock BJ, Sadock VA, Ruiz P, Sadock BJ. *Kaplan & Sadock's Concise Textbook of Clinical Psychiatry*. Philadelphia: Wolters Kluwer; 2017; and adapted from Magda Campbell, M.D. and Wayne Green, M.D.

Table 25-4
A Synthesis of Developmental Theorists

Age (yrs)	Margaret Mahler	Sigmund Freud	Erik Erikson	Jean Piaget	Comments
0–1	Normal autistic phase (birth to 4 wks) • State of half-sleep, half-wake • Major task of phase is to achieve homeostatic equilibrium with the environmentNormal symbiotic phase (3-4 wks to 4-5 mos) • Dim awareness of caretaker, but infant still functions as if he or she and caretaker are in state of undifferentiation or fusion • Social smile characteristic (2-4 mos) The subphases of separation–individuation proper First subphase: differentiation (5-10 mos) • Process of hatching from autistic shell (i.e., developing more alert sensorium that reflects cognitive and neurologic maturation) • Beginning of comparative scanning (i.e., comparing what is and what is not mother) • Characteristic anxiety: stronger anxiety, which involves curiosity and fear (most prevalent around 8 mos)	Oral phase (birth to 1 yr) • Major site of tension and gratification is the mouth, lips, tongue—includes biting and sucking activities	Basic trust vs. basic mistrust (oral sensory) (birth to 1 yr) • Social mistrust demonstrated via ease of feeding, depth of sleep, bowel relaxation • Depends on consistency and sameness of experience provided by caretaker • Second 6 mos teething and biting move infant "from getting to taking" • Weaning leads to "nostalgia for lost paradise" • If basic trust is strong, child maintains hopeful attitude	Sensorimotor phase (birth to 2 yrs) • Intelligence rests mainly on actions and movements coordinated under schemata: (*Schemata* are a pattern of behavior in response to a particular environmental stimulus.) • Environment is mastered through *assimilation and accommodation* (*Assimilation* is the incorporation of new environmental stimuli; *accommodation* is the modification of behavior to adapt to new stimuli.) • *Object permanence* is achieved by age 2 yrs. Object still exists in mind if disappears from view; search for hidden object • Reversibility in action begins	In contrast to Mahler, other observers of mother–infant pairs are impressed with a mutuality and complementarity (not autism or fusion), which provides a groundwork for relatedness and language development, as if there were a prewiring for these abilities. Piaget and others emphasize the infant's active striving to manipulate the inanimate environment. This supplements Freud's work because the infant and young child's motivation for behavior is not simply to relieve drive tension and attain oral, anal, and phallic gratification.

1-2					
	Second subphase: practicing (10–16 mos) • Beginning of this phase marked by upright locomotion—child has new perspective and also mood of elation • Mother used as home base • Characteristic anxiety: separation anxiety Third subphase: rapprochement (16–24 mos) • Infant now a toddler—more aware of physical separateness, which dampens mood of elation • Child tries to bridge gap between self and mother—concretely seen as bringing objects to mother • Mother's efforts to help toddler often not perceived as helpful, temper tantrums typical • Characteristic event: rapprochement crisis, wanting to be soothed by mother and yet not able to accept her help • Symbol of rapprochement: child standing on threshold of door not knowing which way to turn, helpless frustration • Resolution of crisis occurs as child's skills improve and child able to get gratification from doing things on own	Anal phase (1–3 yrs) • Anus and surrounding area major source of interest • Acquisition of voluntary sphincter control (toilet training)	Autonomy vs. shame and doubt (muscular-anal) (1–3 yrs) • Biologically includes learning to walk, feed self, talk • Muscular maturation sets stage for "holding on and letting go" • Need for outer control, firmness of caretaker before development of autonomy • *Shame* occurs when child is overtly self-conscious via negative exposure • *Self-doubt* can evolve if parents overtly shame child (e.g. about elimination)	Preoperational phase (2–7 yrs) • Appearance of symbolic functions, associated with language acquisition • *Egocentrism:* child understands everything exclusively from own perspective • Thinking is illogical and magical • Nonreversible thinking with absence of conversation— *Animism:* belief that inanimate objects are alive (i.e., have feelings and intentions) —"*Imminent justice*," belief that punishment for bad deeds is inevitable	Supplementing the work of Freud and Mahler, theorists have postulated that severe problems in mother-infant/toddler interactions contribute to the formation of pathologic character traits, gender identity disorder, or personality disorders. Angry, frustrating, narcissistic caretakers often produce angry, needy children and adults who cannot tolerate the normal frustrations and disappointments in relationships and whose character formation is grossly distorted.

(continued)

Table 25-4

A Synthesis of Developmental Theorists (Continued)

Age (yrs)	Margaret Mahler	Sigmund Freud	Erik Erikson	Jean Piaget	Comments
2–3	Fourth subphase: consolidation and object constancy (24–36 mos) • Child better able to cope with mother's absence and engage substitutes • Child can begin to feel comfortable with mother's absences by knowing she will return • Gradual internalization of image of mother as reliable and stable and better sense of time, child can tolerate delay and endure separations				
3–4 4–5		Phallic-oedipal phase (3–5 yrs) • Genital focus of interest, stimulation, and excitement • Penis is organ of interest for both sexes • Genital masturbation common • Intense preoccupation with *castration anxiety* (fear of genital loss or injury) • *Penis envy* (discontent with one's own genitals and wish to possess genitals of male) seen in girls in this phase • *Oedipus complex* universal: child wishes to have sex with and marry parent of opposite sex and simultaneously be rid of parent of same sex	Initiative vs. guilt (locomotor genital) (3–5 yrs) • *Initiative* arises in relation to tasks for the sake of activity, both motor and intellectual • Guilt may arise over goals contemplated (especially aggressive) • Desire to mimic adult world; involvement in oedipal struggle leads to resolution via social role identification • Sibling rivalry frequent		Researchers have amended Freud's work. Children of both sexes explore and are aware of their own genitals during the second year of life and, with proper parental reinforcement, begin to correctly identify themselves as girls or boys. Penis envy is neither universal nor normative. Freud emphasized problems with oedipal resolution in psychopathogenesis. His theory accounts for only a part of psychopathology.

5–6	• Latency phase (from 5–6 yrs to 11–12 yrs) • State of relative quiescence of sexual drive with resolution of oedipal complex • Sexual drives channeled into more socially appropriate aims (i.e., schoolwork and sports)			Contrary to Freud, the onset of latency (school age or middle childhood) is now considered primarily a consequence of changes in the CNS and less dependent on the nondemonstrable quiescence and sublimation of sexual drive. During the years 6–8, changes in the CNS are reflected in
6–11	• Formation for *superego*, one of three psychic structures in mind responsible for moral and ethical development, including conscience • Other two psychic structures are *ego*, a group of functions mediating between drives and the external environment, and *id*, repository of sexual and aggressive drives • The id is present at birth, and the ego develops gradually from rudimentary structure present at birth	• Industry vs. inferiority (latency) (6–11 yrs) • Child is busy building, creating, and accomplishing • Receives systematic instruction as well as fundamentals of technology • Danger of sense of inadequacy and inferiority if child despairs of his or her tools/skills and status among peers • Socially decisive age	• Concrete (operational) phase (7–11 yrs) • Emergence of logical (cause–effect) thinking, including reversibility and ability to sequence and serialize • Understanding of part–whole relationships and classifications • Child able to take others' point of view • Conservation of number, length, weight, and volume	Developmental progress of perceptual-sensory-motor functioning and thought processes. In Piaget's framework, it is the transition from the preoperational to the concrete (operational) phase. Compared with preschoolers, latency children are capable of greater learning, independent functioning, and socialization. Friendships develop with less dependence on parents (and less preoccupation with intrafamilial oedipal rivalries). Today, superego development is considered more prolonged gradual and less related to oedipal resolution.

(continued)

Table 25-4
A Synthesis of Developmental Theorists (Continued)

Age (yrs)	Margaret Mahler	Sigmund Freud	Erik Erikson	Jean Piaget	Comments
11+		Genital phase (from 11–12 yrs and beyond) • Final stage of psychosexual development—begins with puberty and the biologic capacity for orgasm but involves the capacity for true intimacy	Identity vs. role diffusion (11 yrs through end of adolescence) • Struggle to develop ego *identity* (sense of inner sameness and continuity) • Preoccupation with appearance, hero worship, ideology • *Group identity* (peers) develops • Danger of *role confusion*, doubts about sexual and vocational identity • *Psychosocial moratorium*, stage between morality learned by the child and the ethics to be developed by the adult	Formal (abstract) phase (11 yrs through end of adolescence) • Hypothetical-deductive reasoning, not only on basis of objects but also on basis of hypotheses or propositions • Capable of thinking about one's thoughts • Combinative structures emerge, permitting flexible grouping of elements in a system • Ability to use two systems of reference simultaneously • Ability to grasp concept of probabilities	The interplay of child and caretaker is emphasized in the attachment theory of John Bowlby. Mary Ainsworth developed the "strange situation" protocol for examining infant–caretaker separations. "Goodness of fit" between child and caretaker is also stressed in the work on temperament by Chess and Thomas. Infants have inborn differences in certain behavioral dimensions, such as activity level, approach, or withdrawal, intensity of reaction. How parents respond to these behaviors influences development. Lawrence Kohlberg, who was influenced by Piaget, described three levels of moral development: pre-conventional, in which moral decisions are made to avoid punishment; conventional role conformity, with decisions made to maintain friend-ships; and in adolescence self-accepted moral princi-ples, (i.e., voluntary compli-ance with ethical principles).

Adapted from Sylvia Karasu, M.D., and Richard Oberfield, M.D.

Table 25-5
Types of Attachment

Secure Attachment	Children show fewer adjustment problems; however, these children have typically received more consistent and developmentally appropriate parenting for most of their life. The parents of securely attached children are likely better able to maintain these aspects of parenting through a divorce. Given that the family factors that lead to divorce also impact the children, there could be fewer securely attached children in divorcing families.
Insecure/ Avoidant Attachment	Children become anxious, clinging, and angry with the parent. These children typically come from families with adults who were also insecurely attached to their families and, thus, were unable to provide the kind of consistency, emotional responsiveness, and care that securely attached parents could offer. Such parents have a more difficult time with divorce, and are more likely to become rejecting.
Insecure/ Ambivalent Attachment	Children generally are raised with disorganized, neglecting, and inattentive parenting. The parents are even less able to provide stability and psychological strength for them after a divorce and, as a result, the children are even more likely to become clinging but inconsolable in their distress, as well as to act out, suffer mood swings, and become oversensitive to stress.

Reprinted from Sadock BJ, Sadock VA, Ruiz P, Sadock BJ. *Kaplan & Sadock's Concise Textbook of Clinical Psychiatry.* Philadelphia: Wolters Kluwer; 2017.

first year of life, as maintenance of physical contact between the mother and child when the child is hungry, frightened, or in distress. Table 25-5 describes the types of attachments that occur between the child and mother or caregiver.

II. Psychiatric Examination of the Child

A comprehensive evaluation of a child includes interviews with the parents, the child, and the family; gathering of information regarding the child's current school functioning; and often, a standardized assessment of the child's intellectual level and academic achievement. In some cases, standardized measures of developmental level and neuropsychological assessments are useful. Psychiatric evaluations of children are rarely initiated by the child, so clinicians must obtain information from the family and the school to understand the reasons for evaluations. In some cases, the court or a child protective service agency may initiate a psychiatric evaluation. Children often have difficulty with chronology of symptoms and are sometimes reticent to report behaviors that got them into trouble. Very young children often cannot articulate their experiences verbally and are better at showing their feelings and preoccupations in a play situation.

Table 25-6 outlines the topics to be covered in the examinations of the child.

III. Classification of Childhood Mental Disorders

Children with some exceptions are subject to the same disorders that occur in adults, for example, depression and anxiety. DSM-5 no longer has a classification of disorders that occur only in childhood or adolescence. Nevertheless, there are some disorders that have their onset during this period that

Table 25-6
Child Psychiatric Evaluation

Identifying data
Identified patient and family members
Source of referral
Informants
History
Chief complaint
History of present illness
Developmental history and milestones
Psychiatric history
Medical history, including immunizations
Family social history and parents' marital status
Educational history and current school functioning
Peer relationship history
Current family functioning
Family psychiatric and medical histories
Current physical examination
Mental status examination
Neuropsychiatric examination (when applicable)
Developmental, psychological, and educational testing
Formulation and summary
DSM-5 diagnosis
Recommendations and treatment plan

Reprinted from Sadock BJ, Sadock VA, Ruiz P. Sadock BJ. *Kaplan & Sadock's Concise Textbook of Clinical Psychiatry.* Philadelphia: Wolters Kluwer; 2017.

are classified under the heading of neurodevelopmental disorders. They are described in this section.

A. Specific learning disorder. Specific learning disorder is diagnosed when reading, writing, and mathematical skills are significantly lower than expected.

  1. Reading disorder. Formally known as dyslexia, reading disorder is characterized by an impaired ability to recognize words, poor comprehension, and slow and inaccurate reading.

    a. Diagnosis. Reading ability is significantly below that expected of a child of the same age, education, and measured intelligence. It is usually identified by the age of 7 years (second grade); however, in some cases, particularly when the disorder is associated with high intelligence it may not be apparent until the age of 9 years (fourth grade). Associated problems include language difficulties and difficulties in properly sequencing words. Younger children tend to feel shame and humiliation, while older children tend to be angry and depressed and exhibit low self-esteem.

    b. Epidemiology
    Occurs in 4% to 8% of school-aged children.
    Occurs in somewhat more frequently in boys compared to girls.

    c. Etiology
    Possible link to chromosome 6 and chromosome 15.
    Occipital lobe lesions and hemispheric abnormality have been linked.
    Occurs in 35% to 40% of first-degree relatives.

d. Differential diagnosis

Intellectual disability: Reading, along with other skills, is below the achievement expected for a child's chronologic age.

Hearing and visual impairments should be ruled out with screening tests.

e. Course and prognosis. Most school-aged children do not need remediation past grade school, with only severe disorders requiring help into middle and high school level.

f. Treatment

Remediation: Effective remediation programs begin with teaching the child to make accurate associations between letters and sounds. Once these skills have been mastered, remediation can target larger components of reading, such as syllables and words. Positive coping strategies include small, structured reading groups that offer individual attention.

Psychotherapy: Coexisting emotional and behavioral problems are treated by appropriate psychotherapeutic means. Parental counseling may be helpful. Social skills improvement is an important component of psychotherapy.

Pharmacology: Use only for an associated psychiatric disorder, such as ADHD.

2. **Mathematics disorder.** Also known as dyscalculia. Child has difficulty with learning and remembering numerals, remembering and applying basic facts about numbers, and is slow and inaccurate in computation.

   a. Diagnosis. Mathematical ability is significantly below what is expected when considering the child's age, education, and measured intelligence. Children have difficulty learning the names for numbers and signs for addition and subtraction, memorizing multiplication tables, applying computations to word problems, and doing calculations at a reasonable pace.

   b. Epidemiology

   Occurs in approximately 3% to 6% of school-aged children.

   May occur more often in females.

   c. Etiology

   In part genetic factors.

   Possible right hemisphere deficit, principally in occipital lobe areas.

   d. Differential diagnosis

   Intellectual disability: Arithmetic difficulties are accompanied by a generalized impairment in overall intellectual functioning.

   ADHD or conduct disorder should not be overlooked during diagnosis.

   e. Course and prognosis. This disorder is usually identified by the age of 8 years (third grade); however, it can be seen as early as 6 years (first grade) or as late as 10 years (fifth grade). Children with moderate mathematics disorder who do not receive intervention may have complications such as continuing academic difficulties, shame, poor self-concept, frustration, and depression. Such complications can lead to reluctance to attend school, truancy, and hopelessness about academic success.

f. Treatment

Remediation: Combines effective teaching of mathematical concepts along with continuous practice. Computerized learning programs have been developed (Project-MATH)

Psychoeducation: Provides positive feedback for good performance in social areas.

3. Written expression. Characterized by frequent grammatical and punctuation errors and poor spelling and handwriting skills.

a. Diagnosis. Child underperforms in composing written text when compared to similar-aged children and intellectual ability. The child has poor spelling, poor punctuation, poor handwriting, and poor organization of written stories. Features manifest in grade school. The child often becomes angry and frustrated because of feelings inadequacy and failure in academic performance. In severe cases, depressive disorders may be present.

b. Epidemiology

Occurs in approximately 5% to 15% of school-aged children.

Three times more likely in males.

c. Etiology

Causes believed to be similar to those of reading disorder.

Strong concordance between children and first-degree relatives with disorder of written expression.

d. Differential diagnosis. The confounding effects of ADHD and depressive disorder may interfere with the ability to concentrate. Therefore, treatment of the above disorders may improve the child's writing performance. Disorder of written expression may occur with other language and learning disorders such as reading disorder, receptive language disorder, expressive language disorder, mathematics disorder, developmental coordination disorder, and disruptive behavior and attention-deficit disorders (ADDs).

e. Course and prognosis. In severe cases, symptoms appear by age 7 (second grade); in less severe cases, the disorder may appear by age 10 (fifth grade) or later. Patients with mild to moderate cases usually do well if they receive remedial education early in grade school. Severe cases require continual, extensive remedial treatment through high school and college. Prognosis relies on the severity of the disorder, the age or grade in which intervention is received, the length and continuity of treatment, and the presence or absence of associated or secondary emotional or behavioral problems.

f. Treatment

Remediation: Treatment includes continuous practice of spelling and sentence writing and review of grammar. Intensive and individually tailored creative writing therapy may provide additional benefit.

Psychotherapy: Psychological therapy including individual, group, or family therapy may be useful in cases of secondary behavioral and emotional problems.

B. Motor skills disorder: There are three major types: developmental coordination disorder; tic disorders (includes Tourette's disorder); and stereotypic movement disorder.

1. Developmental coordination disorder. Is characterized by poor performance in daily activities requiring coordination. This may present with delays in achieving such motor milestones as sitting, crawling, and walking. The disorder may also manifest by clumsy gross and fine motor skills, resulting in poor athletic performance and poor handwriting.

a. Diagnosis. Disorder may manifest as early as infancy. Diagnosis is based on a history of delay in achieving early motor milestones. The diagnosis may be associated with below-normal scores on performance subtests of standardized intelligence tests and by normal or above-normal scores on verbal subtests. Testing can be done by asking child to hop, skip, jump, stand on one leg, and so on.

b. Epidemiology

Prevalence is approximately 5% of school-aged children.

Male-to-female ratio may range from 2:1 to 4:1; however, bias may exist.

c. Etiology

Unknown but probably multifactorial.

Risk factors may include prematurity, hypoxia, perinatal malnutrition, and low birth weight.

Frequently found in children with hyperactivity and learning disorders.

d. Differential diagnosis

Neuromuscular disorders, for example, cerebral palsy: Patients exhibit more global muscle and neurologic impairment.

Attention-deficit/hyperactivity disorder (ADHD): Rule out physical carelessness seen in individuals with ADHD.

Intellectual disability: Coordination usually does not stand out as a significant deficit compared with other skills.

e. Course and prognosis.

Few data available on outcome. Although clumsiness may continue, some children are able to compensate by developing interest in other skills. Clumsiness generally persists into adolescence and adult life.

f. Treatment. Usually includes versions of sensory integration programs and modified forms of physical education. Sensory integration programs consist of physical activities that increase awareness of motor and sensory function. Adaptive physical education programs incorporate certain sports actions, such as kicking or throwing a ball. Patients may benefit from social skills groups and other prosocial interventions. Secondary academic and emotional problems and coexisting communication disorders should be considered for individual treatments. Parental counseling may be beneficial in reducing parents' anxiety and guilt, increasing their awareness, and facilitating their confidence.

2. **Stereotypic movement disorder.** A repetitive, nonfunctional motor behavior that seems to be compulsive.

   a. **Diagnosis.** Diagnostically, repetitive, seemingly nonfunctional behaviors that last for at least 4 weeks and interfere with normal activities or cause physical injury. Common behaviors include hand shaking, head banging, nail biting, nose picking, and hair pulling. In extreme cases, severe mutilation and life-threatening injuries may result, and secondary infection and septicemia may follow self-inflicted trauma.

   b. **Epidemiology.** Ten percent to 20% of intellectually disabled children are affected by symptoms. More prevalent in males than females. Often seen in blindness.

   c. **Etiology**

   Associated with an increase in dopamine activity.

   d. **Differential diagnosis**

   Tic disorders: Tics are often associated with distress.

   Obsessive–compulsive disorder (OCD): The compulsions must be ego-dystonic.

   e. **Course and prognosis.** The duration and course are variable, as the symptoms may wax and wane. When present later in childhood or in noncomforting manner, symptoms range from brief episodes occurring under stress to an ongoing pattern in the context of a chronic condition (i.e., intellectual disability or pervasive development disorder).

   f. **Treatment**

   Behavioral: Techniques including reinforcement and behavioral shaping are successful in some cases.

   Pharmacotherapy: Dopamine antagonists and opiate antagonists have reduced self-injurious behaviors. Fenfluramine (Pondimin) can diminish stereotypic behaviors in autistic children. Clomipramine (Anafranil) and fluoxetine can decrease self-injurious and other stereotypical movements.

3. **Persistent (chronic) motor or vocal tic disorder.** A group of neuropsychiatric disorders that behind in childhood or adolescence and may be constant or wax and wane over time. DSM-5 includes Tourette's disorder and chronic motor or vocal tic disorder under this category.

   a. **Tourette's disorder.**

   Multiple motor tics and one or more vocal tics that occur several times a day for more than 1 year.

   (1) **Diagnosis.** Multiple motor tics and one or more vocal tics; these can be simple or complex. Simple motor tics appear first in the face and neck and include eye blinking, head jerking, and facial grimacing. These progress downwardly. Complex motor tics include hitting oneself and jumping. Simple vocal tics include coughing, grunting, or sniffing. Complex vocal tics include coprolalia (use

of vulgar words), palilalia (repeating own words), and echolalia (repeating another's words). ADHD, learning problems, and obsessive–compulsive symptoms are associated with the disorder and are increased in first-degree relatives.

(2) Epidemiology

Four to five cases per 10,000.

Motor component generally occurs by 7 years; vocal tics emerge by 11 years, on average.

Male-to-female ratio is 3:1.

(3) Etiology. Genetic contribution strongly supported by increased prevalence in first-degree relatives and higher concordance rates in monozygotic than dizygotic twins. There is evidence of neurobiologic substrate–nonspecific electroencephalogram (EEG) abnormalities as well as abnormal computed tomography (CT) findings. Abnormal dopamine levels may be implicated as dopamine antagonists generally diminish tics and stimulants worsen or precipitate tics. Additionally, abnormal levels of homovanillic acid in the CSF have been demonstrated.

(4) Differential diagnosis. Stereotypic movement disorders; tics seem to be voluntary and often produce a sense of comfort.

(5) Course and prognosis. Untreated, the disorder is usually chronic with waxing and waning symptoms. Severely affected persons may have serious emotional problems, including major depressive disorder.

(6) Treatment

Psychotherapy: Includes family and patient education and learning behavioral techniques. Behavioral techniques and pharmacotherapy may have a synergistic effect.

Pharmacotherapy: High-potency antipsychotics, such as haloperidol (Haldol), lead to improvement in 85% of patients but are associated with acute dystonic reactions and parkinsonian symptoms. Pimozide is also effective, but it prolongs the QT interval and thus requires electrocardiographic (ECG) monitoring. These drugs are being replaced with atypicals such as risperidone and olanzapine with similar success. Clonidine, a noradrenergic antagonist, has shown benefit in 40% to 70% of patients, although it is not presently approved for use in Tourette's disorder. Another α-adrenergic agonist, guanfacine (Tenex), is also used.

b. Chronic motor or vocal tic disorder. Rapid and repetitive involuntary muscle contractions resulting in movements or vocalizations. The disorder must have onset before the age of 18 years.

(1) Diagnosis. Same as Tourette's disorder except that the patient has either single or multiple motor tics or vocal tics, but not both. Chronic vocal tics are less conspicuous than in Tourette's disorder and much rarer than chronic motor tics. Vocal tics are not loud or intense and are primarily produced by the vocal cords. Onset is usually in early childhood.

(2) Epidemiology

It is 100 to 1,000 times more frequent than Tourette's disorder; estimate is 1% to 2%.

School-aged males are at higher risk.

(3) Etiology

Chronic motor or vocal tic disorder and Tourette's disorder aggregate in some families.

High concordance in monozygotic twins.

(4) Differential diagnosis. Chronic motor tics must be differentiated from other motor movements such as choreiform movements, myoclonus, restless legs syndrome, akathisia, and dystonias. Involuntary vocal utterances can occur in neurologic disorders, such as Huntington's disease and Parkinson's disease.

(5) Course and prognosis. Children whose tics begin between ages of 8 and 8 years have the best outcomes. Symptoms usually last for 4 to 6 years and stop in early adolescence. Children whose tics involve the limbs or trunk tend to do less well than those with facial tics.

(6) Treatment

Psychotherapy: Treatment depends on the severity and the frequency of the tics; the patient's subjective distress; the effects of the tics on school, work or job performance and socialization; and the presence of any other concomitant mental disorder. Psychotherapy may be used to minimize the secondary emotional problems caused by the tics. Behavioral techniques, particularly habit reversal treatment, are effective.

Pharmacotherapy: Antipsychotic medication has been helpful in some cases, but the risk must be weighed against the possible clinical benefits because of adverse effects, including development of tardive dyskinesia.

C. Communication disorders. Communication disorders are characterized by impairment in understanding and expressing language and the production of speech. There are four major communication disorders including a new communication disorder described in DSM-5 called Social (pragmatic) Communication Disorder.

1. Language disorder. Characterized by deficits in vocabulary, tenses, production of complex sentences, and recall of words. There are two types: expressive in which language can be understood but not expressed and receptive in which language cannot be understood.

a. Diagnosis. Patient presents selective deficits in expressed or received language skills. Diagnosis should be confirmed by standardized tests of expressive language and nonverbal intelligence. Severity of the disorder can be determined by the child's verbal and sign language in various places (i.e., the schoolyard, classroom, home, and playroom) and interaction with other children. In severe cases, the disorder presents by approximately 18 months.

b. Epidemiology

Occurs in 3% to 5% of school-aged children.

Two to three times more common in males.

History of relatives with other communication disorders.

c. Etiology

Subtle cerebral damage and maturational lags in cerebral development may be a cause.

Associated with left-handedness and ambilaterality.

Concordance for monozygotic twins.

Genetic, environmental, and educational factors appear to play a role.

d. Differential diagnosis

Intellectual disability: Child has an overall impairment in intellectual functioning, and nonverbal intellectual capacity is not within normal limits.

Autism spectrum disorder: Child has no inner language or appropriate use of gestures and shows characteristic symptoms of autism.

Aphasia or dysphasia: Child has a history of early normal language development; onset of the disordered language is after a head trauma or other neurologic disorder (i.e., seizure disorder).

Selective mutism: Child has a history of normal language development.

e. Course and prognosis. The rapidity and degree of recovery depends on the severity of the disorder, the child's motivation to participate in therapies, and the timely institution of speech and other therapeutic interventions. As many as 50% of children with mild cases recover spontaneously, while severe cases continue to display some features of language impairment. Prognosis in receptive type is not as good as in expressive types.

f. Treatment

Remedial: Language therapy is aimed at using words to improve communication strategies and social interactions. Benefit from individual learning experiences.

Psychotherapy: Can be used as a positive model for more effective communication and broadening social skills in patients where language impairment has affected self-esteem. Supportive parental counseling may be useful in some cases.

Family therapy: Beneficial in patients with associated emotional and behavioral problems. Family counseling in which parents and children can develop more effective, less frustrating means of communicating is beneficial.

2. Speech sound disorder. The child presents impairment in sound production by substituting one sound for another or omitting sounds that are part of words.

a. Diagnosis. Delay or failure to produce developmentally expected speech sounds accompanied by normal language development. The child is unable to articulate certain phonemes correctly and may omit, substitute, or distort the affected phonemes. Most children usually outgrow the disorder by third grade; however, spontaneous recovery is unlikely after fourth grade.

b. Epidemiology

Variable prevalence of 0.5% by mid- to late adolescence.

Two to three times more common in males.

Common among first-degree relatives.

c. Etiology

Likely to include perinatal problems, genetics, auditory processing problems, hearing impairment, and structural abnormalities related to speech.

Genetic studies indicate a high concordance among monozygotic twins.

d. Differential diagnosis

Physical abnormalities causing articulation errors must be ruled out. Dysarthria is less likely to spontaneously remit.

Hearing impairment, intellectual disability, and pervasive developmental disorders (PDDs) should be ruled out.

e. Course and prognosis. Spontaneous remission of symptoms is common in children whose misarticulations involve only a few phonemes. Articulation problems that persist after the age of 5 years may be comorbid with other speech and language impairments. Auditory perceptual problems are more likely in children with articulation problems after the age of 5 years. Spontaneous remission is rare after the age of 8 years (fourth grade).

f. Treatment. Speech therapy is the most successful form of treatment. It is indicated when the child's intelligibility is poor; the child is over the age of 8 years; the speech problem interferes with peer relations, learning, and self-image; the disorder is so severe that many consonants are misarticulated; and errors involve omissions and substitution of phonemes rather than distortions. Parental counseling and monitoring of child–peer relations and school behavior may be beneficial.

3. **Stuttering (childhood-onset fluency disorder).** A condition characterized by involuntary disruptions in the flow of speech.

   a. Diagnosis. Disturbance in normal fluency and time patterning of speech. Stuttering appears between the ages of 18 months and 9 years, with peaks at 2 to 3.5 years and 5 to 7 years. Symptoms gradually develop over weeks or months with a repetition of initial consonants.

   b. Epidemiology

   Prevalence is 3% to 4%.

   Affects three to four times more males.

   Typical onset is 2 to 7 years of age with a peak at 5 years of age.

   Spontaneous remission in about 80% of young children.

   c. Etiology. Unknown; organic deficits and learning models have been proposed.

d. Differential diagnosis

Normal speech dysfluency: Patients are nonfluent with their speech but seem to be at ease.

Spastic dysphonia: Patients have an abnormal breathing pattern.

Cluttering: Rapid spurts of words or phrases.

e. Course and prognosis. Course is usually long term with periods of remissions and exacerbations. Fifty percent to 80% of patients recover spontaneously, mostly with mild cases.

f. Treatment

Remediation: Speech therapy, relaxation techniques, and breathing exercises have been employed. Other approaches using distraction include teaching the patient to talk in time to rhythmic movements of the arm, hand, or finger, but this only removes stuttering temporarily. Relaxation techniques are based on the premise that the relaxed state and stuttering are incompatible.

Psychotherapy: Classic psychoanalysis, insight-oriented psychotherapy, group therapy, and other psychotherapeutic techniques have not been successful in treating stuttering, but individual psychotherapy can be helpful in cases that include associated poor self-image, anxiety, or depression. Family therapy should be considered if there is evidence of family dysfunction, a family contribution to symptoms, or family stress caused by trying to cope with, or help, the stutter.

Pharmacotherapy: Treatments such as haloperidol (Haldol) have been used in an attempt to increase relaxation; however, there are no data to assess its efficacy. Recent studies have suggested the use of serotonin–dopamine antagonists (SDA) including olanzapine (Zyprexa) and risperidone (Risperdal) but data is inconclusive.

4. **Social (pragmatic) communication disorder.** A disorder characterized by persistent deficits in using verbal and nonverbal communication for social purposes.

a. Diagnosis

The child has limited communication skills in social situations.

Not able to infer meaning in interactions with others and is unable to pick up social cues from others. Does not engage in give and take conversation.

b. Epidemiology. This is a new diagnosis with limited data. Prevalence to be determined.

c. Differential diagnosis

Autism spectrum disorder (ASD): ASD patients have repetitive behaviors and interests.

Attention-deficit/hyperactivity disorder: Core features of impulsivity and reduced attention span with hyperactivity are absent. May be co-morbid however.

Social anxiety disorder: Communication skills not impaired.

Intellectual disability: No signs of diminished intelligence. IQ testing within normal range.

    d. Course and prognosis. Limited data but course is variable. Improves with time.

    e. Treatment. Limited data but specific training in social skills using role-playing techniques may be of use.

D. Autism spectrum disorder (ASD). ASD is characterized by qualitative deficits in reciprocal social interaction and communication skills and restricted patterns of behavior.

    1. Diagnosis. Among the principle criteria for diagnosing autism are deficits in language development and difficulty using language to communicate. At first glance, patients do not show physical signs of the disorder; however, they do have minor physical abnormalities such as ear malformations. Autistic children do not demonstrate special attention to important people in their lives and have impaired eye contact and attachment behavior to family members and notable deficits in interacting with peers. They are unable to make attributions about the motivation or intentions of others; therefore, they cannot develop empathy. Activities and play are often rigid, repetitive, and monotonous. Common behavior problems include hyperkinesis, hypokinesis, aggression, head banging, biting, scratching, hair pulling, and resistance to change in routine. Prodigious cognitive or visuomotor capabilities may occur in a small subgroup (known as autistic savants).

        There are 3 levels: Level 1 has social interaction and speech; Level 2 minimal speech and interaction; Level 3 no speech or social interaction.

    2. Epidemiology

    Occurs in 1 in 68 children.

    Four to five times more common in males; females with the disorder are more likely to have more severe mental retardation.

    Onset before age of 3 years.

    3. Etiology

    Higher concordance rate in monozygotic than dizygotic twins; at least 2% to 4% of siblings are affected.

    Biologic factors implicated due to high rates of seizure disorder and mental retardation.

    Immunologic incompatibility and prenatal and perinatal insults might be contributory factors.

    Magnetic resonance imaging (MRI) studies have demonstrated increased brain volume in occipital, parietal, and temporal lobes.

    Subgroups have abnormal levels of dopamine and serotonin metabolites in cerebrospinal fluid (CSF). Psychosocial and family stressors are associated with exacerbation of symptoms.

    4. Differential diagnosis

    Schizophrenia with childhood onset: Is rare in children under the age of 5 and is accompanied by hallucinations or delusions, with a lower incidence of seizures and mental retardation and a more even IQ.

    Intellectual disorder with behavioral symptoms: Children usually relate to adults and other children in accordance with their mental age; they use the language they do have to communicate with others; and they have a relatively even profile of impairments without splinter functions.

Acquired aphasia with convulsion: Child is normal for several years before losing both receptive and expressive language. Most have a few seizures and generalized EEG abnormalities at onset that do not persist. A profound language comprehension disorder then follows, characterized by deviant speech pattern and speech impairment.

Congenital deafness or severe hearing impairment: Infants have a history of relatively normal babbling that tapers off gradually and may stop from 6 months to 1 year of age. Children respond only to loud sounds. Auditory or auditory-evoked potentials indicate significant hearing loss. Children usually relate to their parents, seek their affection, and enjoy being held as infants.

Psychosocial deprivation: Children improve rapidly when placed in a favorable and enriched psychosocial environment.

5. **Course and prognosis.** Autism spectrum disorder is generally a lifelong disorder with a guarded prognosis. Two-thirds remain severely handicapped and dependent. Improved prognosis if IQ > 70 and communication skills are seen by ages 5 to 7 years.

6. **Treatment**

Remediation: Structured classroom training in combination with behavioral methods is the most effective treatment method. Language and academic remediation are often required.

Psychotherapy: Parents are often distraught and need support and counseling.

Pharmacotherapy: The administration of antipsychotic medication reduces aggressive or self-injurious behavior. SDAs such as risperidone (Risperdal), olanzapine (Zyprexa), quetiapine (Seroquel), clozapine (Clozaril), and ziprasidone (Geodon) have been used. Selective serotonin reuptake inhibitors (SSRIs), including fluoxetine (Prozac), and citalopram (Celexa) have been studied in autism spectrum disorder, because of the association between the compulsive behaviors in OCD and stereotypic behaviors seen in autism. Atomoxetine (Strattera) has also shown improvement in children with PDD.

E. **Attention-deficit/hyperactivity disorder**

Disorders with a persistent and marked pattern of inattention and/or hyperactive and impulsive behavior. Includes 3 types: hypoactive-impulsive, inattentive and combined type.

1. **Diagnosis.** Consists of a persistent pattern of inattention and/or hyperactivity and impulsive behavior that is more severe than expected of children of similar age and level of development. Symptoms must be present before the age of 12 years, must be present in at least two settings, and must interfere with the appropriate social, academic, and extracurricular functioning. Principle signs are based on history of child's developmental patterns and direct observation in situations requiring attention.

Typical signs include talking excessively, persevering, fidgeting, frequent interruptions, impatience, difficulty organizing and finishing tasks, distractibility, and forgetfulness.

2. Epidemiology

Occurs in 3% to 7% of grade-schoolers.

Male-to-female ratio is 3:1 to 5:1.

Symptoms often present by 3 years.

3. Etiology

Possible causes include perinatal trauma and genetic and psychosocial factors.

Evidence of noradrenergic and dopaminergic dysfunction in neurotransmitter systems.

Frontal lobe hypoperfusion and lower frontal lobe metabolic rates have also been noted.

Soft neurologic signs are found in higher rates among children with ADHD.

4. Differential diagnosis

Bipolar disorder and childhood-onset schizophrenia: There is more waxing and waning of symptoms in bipolar disorder and hallucinations or delusions in childhood schizophrenia.

Learning disorders: Inability to do math or read is not because of inattention.

Depressive disorder: Distinguished by hypoactivity and withdrawal.

Anxiety disorder: May be manifested by overactivity and easy distractibility.

5. Course and prognosis

Course is variable. Most patients undergo partial remission. Inattention is frequently the last remitting symptom. Patients are vulnerable to antisocial behavior, substance use disorders, and mood disorders. Learning problems often continue throughout life.

Table 25-7 describes the differential diagnosis of autism and childhood-onset schizophrenia and Table 25-8 of language disorder.

6. Treatment

Psychotherapy: Multimodality treatment is often necessary for child and family. These include social skills groups, behavioral intervention, individual psychotherapy, family therapy, and special education when indicated.

Pharmacotherapy: Pharmacologic agents shown to have significant efficacy and excellent safety records are CNS stimulants such as methylphenidate (Ritalin, Ritalin SR, Concerta, Metadate CD, Metadate ER) and dextroamphetamine and amphetamine salt combinations (Adderall, Adderall XR). A prodrug of amphetamine, lisdexamfetamine (Vynase) was approved for once-daily dosing. The Daytrana patch (active ingredient methylphenidate) has been approved by the FDA in the treatment of ADHD in children age 6 to 12 years. Daytrana comes in patches that can deliver 15, 20, and 30 mg when worn for

Table 25-7
Autism Spectrum Disorder versus Childhood-Onset Schizophrenia

Criteria	Autism Spectrum Disorder	Schizophrenia (with Onset Before Puberty)
Age of onset	Early developmental period	Rarely under 5 yrs of age
Incidence	1%	<1 in 10,000
Sex ratio (M:F)	4:1	1.67:1 (slight preponderance of males)
Family history of schizophrenia	Not increased	Likely increased
Prenatal and perinatal complications	Increased	Not increased
Behavioral characteristics	Poor social relatedness; may have aberrant language, speech or echolalia; stereotyped phrases; may have stereotypies, repetitive behaviors	Hallucinations and delusions; thought disorder
Adaptive functioning	Impaired	Deterioration in functioning
Level of intelligence Disabled (30%)	Wide range, may be intellectually Usually within normal range, may be low average normal	
Pattern of IQ	Typical higher performance than verbal	More even
Grand mal seizures	4–32%	Low incidence

Reprinted from Sadock BJ, Sadock VA, Ruiz P, Sadock BJ. *Kaplan & Sadock's Concise Textbook of Clinical Psychiatry*. Philadelphia: Wolters Kluwer; 2017; and adapted from Magda Campbell, M.D. and Wayne Green, M.D.

Table 25-8
Autism Spectrum Disorder versus Language Disorder

Criteria	Autism Spectrum Disorder	Language Disorder
Incidence	1%	5 of 10,000
Sex ratio (M:F)	4:1	Equal or almost equal sex ratio
Family history of speech delay or language problems	<25% of cases	<25% of cases
Associated deafness	Very infrequent	Not infrequent
Nonverbal communication (e.g., gestures)	Impaired	Actively utilized
Language abnormalities (e.g., echolalia, stereotyped phrases out of context)	Present in a subset	Uncommon
Articulation problems	Infrequent	Frequent
Intellectual level	Impaired in a subset (about 30%)	Uncommon, less frequently severe
Patterns of intelligence quotient (IQ) tests	Typically lower on verbal scores than performance scores	Often verbal scores lower than performance scores
Impaired social communication, restricted and repetitive behaviors	Present	Absent or, if present, mild
Imaginative play	Often impaired	Usually in tact

Reprinted from Sadock BJ, Sadock VA, Ruiz P, Sadock BJ. *Kaplan & Sadock's Concise Textbook of Clinical Psychiatry*. Philadelphia: Wolters Kluwer; 2017; and adapted from Magda Campbell, M.D. and Wayne Green, M.D.

9 hr/day. Second-line agents include antidepressants such as bupropion (Wellbutrin, Wellbutrin SR), venlafaxine (Effexor, Effexor XR), and α-adrenergic receptor agonists clonidine (Catapres) and guanfacine (Tenex). Atomoxetine (Strattera), a norepinephrine reuptake inhibitor, is also used.

F. Disruptive behavior disorders. Includes two persistent constellations of disruptive symptoms categorized as oppositional defiant disorder and conduct disorder, which result in impaired social or academic function in a child.

1. Oppositional defiant disorder. Enduring pattern of negative, hostile behavior in absence of serious violation of societal norms or rules.

a. Diagnosis. A pattern of defiant, angry, and negative behavior enduring for at least 6 months. The child frequently loses his or her temper, is resentful and easily annoyed, and actively defies requests and rules in the presence of familiar adults and peers.

b. Epidemiology

Ranges from 2% to 16% in children.

Can begin as early as 3 years of age and typically noted by 8 years of age and usually not later than adolescence.

More common in males prior to puberty; sex ratio equal after puberty.

c. Etiology

Possible result of unresolved conflicts.

May be a reinforced, learned behavior.

d. Differential diagnosis

Developmentally appropriate oppositional behavior: Duration is shorter and is not as frequent or intense.

Adjustment disorder: Oppositional defiant behavior occurs temporarily in reaction to stress.

Conduct disorder: The basic rights of others are violated.

e. Course and prognosis. Course depends on severity of symptoms in the child and the ability of the child to develop more adaptive responses to authority. The stability over time is variable. Persistence of symptoms poses an increased risk of additional disorders such as conduct disorder and substance use disorders. Prognosis depends on the degree of functioning in the family and the development of comorbid psychopathology.

f. Treatment

Psychotherapy: Primary treatment is family intervention utilizing both direct training of parents in child management skills and careful assessment of family interactions. Behavior therapy focuses on selectively reinforcing and praising appropriate behavior and ignoring or not reinforcing undesired behavior. Individual psychotherapy is focused on adaptive responses.

Pharmacotherapy: Comorbid disorders (i.e., anxiety or depression) treated with appropriate anti-anxiety or antidepressant pharmacologic agents.

2. **Conduct disorder.** Characterized by aggression and violations of the rights of others. Three specific behaviors include bullying and threatening or intimidating others, beginning before age 13 years.

   a. **Diagnosis.** Patients show a repetitive pattern in which the basic rights of others or major societal norms or rules are violated. Antisocial behavior includes bullying, physical aggression, and cruel behavior toward peers. Children may be hostile, verbally abusive, and defiant. Persistent lying, truancy, and vandalism are also common. Severe cases demonstrate stealing and physical violence. Promiscuity and use of tobacco and illegal drugs begin unusually early. Suicidal thoughts, gestures, and acts are frequent.

   b. **Epidemiology**

   Prevalence ranges from 1% to 10% in studies.

   Male-to-female ratio ranges from 4:1 to 12:1.

   c. **Etiology**

   Multifactorial.

   Maladaptive aggressive behaviors are associated with family instability, physical and sexual victimization, socioeconomic factors, and negligent conditions.

   Often coexists with ADHD, learning disorders, or communication disorders.

   A subset may have low plasma levels of dopamine and B-hydroxylase. Abnormal serotonin levels have been implicated.

   d. **Differential diagnosis**

   Oppositional defiant disorder: Hostility and negativism fall short of seriously violating the rights of others.

   Mood disorders: Often present in those children who exhibit irritability and aggressive behavior.

   Major depressive disorder and bipolar I disorder must be ruled out.

   Attention-deficit/hyperactivity disorder: Impulsive and aggressive behavior is not as severe.

   e. **Course and prognosis.** Prognosis is guarded in younger age groups, those who exhibit a greater number of symptoms, and those who express symptoms more frequently. Severe cases are most vulnerable to comorbid disorders later in life, such as substance use disorders and mood disorders. Good prognosis is predicted in mild cases in the absence of coexisting psychopathology and normal intellectual functioning.

   f. **Treatment**

   Psychotherapy: Includes individual or family therapy, parenting classes, tutoring, and emphasis of special interests. Placement away from home may be necessary in some circumstances.

   Pharmacotherapy: Antipsychotics such as haloperidol (Haldol), risperidone, and olanzapine help control severe aggressive and assaultive behavior. Lithium (Eskalith) is helpful for some aggressive children with or without comorbid bipolar disorders. Stimulants may be used in comorbid ADHD.

G. **Feeding and eating disorders of infancy or early childhood.** Persistent symptoms of inadequate food intake, recurrent regurgitating and rechewing of food, or repeated ingestion of nonnutritive substances. Includes pica, rumination disorder, and feeding disorder of infancy or early childhood.

1. **Pica.** Repeated ingestion of a nonnutritive substance for at least 1 month. The behavior must be developmentally inappropriate, not culturally sanctioned, and sufficiently severe to merit clinical attention.

   a. **Diagnosis.** Ingestion of nonedible substances after 18 months of age. Nonedible substances include paint, plaster, string, hair, cloth, dirt, feces, stones, and paper. Onset is usually between the ages of 12 and 24 months, and incidences decline with age. The clinical implication can be benign or life threatening depending on the objects ingested.

   b. **Epidemiology**
   More common in preadolescents.
   Occurs in up to 15% of those with severe intellectual disability.
   Affects both sexes equally.

   c. **Etiology**
   Associated with intellectual disability, neglect, and nutritional deficiencies (e.g., iron or zinc).
   Onset usually between 1 and 2 years of age.
   Higher-than-expected incidences occur in relatives.

   d. **Differential diagnosis**
   Iron and zinc deficiencies.
   Can occur in conjunction with schizophrenia, autism spectrum disorder, Kleine–Levin syndrome, and anorexia nervosa.

   e. **Course and prognosis.** Prognosis is variable. In children, pica usually resolves with increasing age; in pregnant women, it is usually limited to the term of pregnancy. In some adults, especially those who are mentally intellectually disabled, pica may continue for years.

   f. **Treatment.** In cases of neglect or maltreatment, such circumstances should be altered. Exposure to toxic substances (i.e., lead) should be eliminated. Treatments emphasize psychosocial, environmental, behavioral, and family guidance approaches. Mild aversion therapy or negative reinforcement (i.e., a mild electric shock, an unpleasant noise, or an emetic drug) has been successful. Positive reinforcement, modeling, and behavioral shaping have also been used.

2. **Rumination disorder.** Repeated regurgitation and rechewing of food after a period of normal eating. Symptoms last at least 1 month, are not caused by a medical condition, and are severe enough for clinical attention.

   a. **Diagnosis.** Essential feature is the repeated regurgitation of food occurring at least 1 month following a period of normal eating. It is not due to a gastrointestinal condition or secondary to anorexia nervosa or bulimia nervosa. Swallowed food is forced back into the mouth without nausea, retching, or disgust. Subsequently it is ejected, or rechewed and swallowed.

   b. **Epidemiology**
   Rare. Occurs between 3 and 12 months.
   May be more common in males.

   c. **Etiology**
   Associated with immature, emotionally neglectful mothers.
   Implication of a dysfunctional autonomic nervous system.
   Possible link to gastroesophageal reflux or hiatal hernia.
   Overstimulation and tension have been suggested.

   d. **Differential diagnosis.** Pyloric stenosis is associated with projectile vomiting and typically manifests prior to 3 months.

   e. **Course and prognosis.** There are high rates of spontaneous remission. Course may also include malnutrition, failure to thrive, and even death.

   f. **Treatment.** Often involves parental guidance and behavioral techniques. Evaluation of the mother–child relationship may reveal deficits that can be influenced by offering guidance to the mother. Behavioral interventions, such as squirting lemon juice into the infant's mouth, can be effective in diminishing the behavior. Medications such as metoclopramide (Reglan), cimetidine (Tagamet), and antipsychotics (i.e., haloperidol) have seen success.

3. **Avoidant/restrictive food intake disorder.** Persistent failure to eat adequately for at least 1 month.

   a. **Diagnosis.** Failure to eat adequately for at least 1 month in the absence of a general medical or mental condition with a subsequent failure to gain weight or subsequent loss of weight.

   b. **Epidemiology**
   Occurs in 1.5% of infants, 3% of infants with failure to thrive syndromes, and 50% of infants with feeding disorders.
   Onset is before 6 years of age.

   c. **Etiology.** Genetic studies indicate a high concordance among monozygotic twins.

   d. **Differential diagnosis.** Must be differentiated from gastrointestinal structural abnormalities contributing to discomfort during feeding.

   e. **Course and prognosis.** With intervention, failure to thrive may not develop. Children with later onset may develop deficits in growth and development when the disorder lasts for several months. Seventy percent persistent with the disorder in their first year will continue to have some feeding problems during childhood.

   f. **Treatment.** Counseling of the caregiver is crucial if there are comorbid developmental delays or difficult temperament. Cognitive behavioral intervention can be useful.

H. **Elimination disorders.** These disorders are considered when a child is chronologically and developmentally beyond the point at which it is expected that elimination functions can be mastered. These include encopresis and enuresis.

1. **Encopresis.** An involuntary or intentional pattern of passing feces into inappropriate places.
   a. **Diagnosis.** Repeated passage of feces into inappropriate places whether involuntary or intentional, occurring at at least 4 years of age on a regular basis (at least once a month) for 3 months. There are two types: with constipation and overflow incontinence and without constipation and overflow incontinence.
   b. **Epidemiology**
   Prevalence is about 1% of 5-year-old children.
   It is three to four times more common in males in all age groups.
   c. **Etiology**
   Constipation with overflow incontinence can be caused by faulty nutrition; structural disease of the anus, rectum, or colon; medical side effects; or endocrine disorders.
   Children without constipation and overflow incontinence (with control) often have oppositional defiant or conduct disorder.
   Inadequate training or emotional reasons may contribute to inefficient sphincter control. This can be precipitated by birth of a sibling or parental separation.
   d. **Differential diagnosis**
   Hirschsprung's disease: Patient may have an empty rectum and have no desire to defecate, but still have an overflow of feces; shows symptoms shortly after birth.
   Physiologic effects of a substance such as a laxative.
   e. **Course and prognosis.** Outcome depends on the cause, the chronicity of the symptoms, and coexisting behavioral problems. Many cases are self-limiting, rarely continuing beyond mid-adolescence.
   f. **Treatment.** Individual psychotherapy and relaxation techniques are used to address the cause and embarrassment. Behavioral techniques may be useful. Parental guidance and family therapy often are needed. Conditions such as impaction and anal fissures require a consultation with a pediatrician.
2. **Enuresis.** Repeated voiding of urine into bed or clothing.
   a. **Diagnosis.** Repeated voiding of urine into bed or clothes whether involuntary or intentional, occurring at at least 5 years of age. Behavior must occur twice weekly for a period of at least 3 months. Is broken down into three types: nocturnal only, diurnal only, and nocturnal and diurnal.
   b. **Epidemiology**
   By age 5, 7%; age 10, 3%; age 18, 1%.
   Much more common in males.
   The diurnal subtype is least prevalent and more common in females.
   Mental disorders are present in 20% of patients.
   c. **Etiology**
   Strong genetic component; concordance is greater in monozygotic than dizygotic twins.

Toilet training may be inadequate and some may have small bladders requiring frequent voiding.

Psychosocial stressors such as birth of a sibling or parental separation may precipitate cases.

d. Differential diagnosis

Genitourinary pathology such as obstructive uropathy, spina bifida occulta, and cystitis.

Diabetes insipidus and diabetes mellitus.

Seizures, sleepwalking disorder, and side effects of medication, such as antipsychotics or diuretics.

e. Course and prognosis. Usually self-limited; remissions are frequent between 6 and 8 years and puberty.

f. Treatment

Behavioral therapy: Classic conditioning with a bell or pad apparatus is the most effective treatment. Other approaches include rewards for delaying micturition and restricting fluids before bed.

Psychotherapy: Not an effective treatment alone, but can be useful in dealing with coexisting psychiatric problems and emotional and family difficulties.

Pharmacotherapy: Medications are not first line considering the high rate of spontaneous remissions and success of behavioral approaches. Imipramine (Tofranil) and desmopressin (DDAVP) have shown success in reducing or eliminating bed-wetting.

I. Childhood anxiety disorders

1. Separation anxiety disorder

a. Diagnosis. Must be characterized by three of the following symptoms for at least 4 weeks: (1) persistent and excessive worry about losing or possible harm befalling major attachment figures, (2) persistent and excessive worry that an untoward event can lead to separation from a major attachment figure, (3) persistent reluctance to be without attachment figures (i.e., refusal to go to school), (4) persistent and excessive fear or reluctance to be alone or without major attachment figures, (5) repeated nightmares involving the theme of separation, (6) repeated complaints of physical symptoms (i.e., headaches, stomachaches) in anticipation of separation, and (7) recurrent excessive distress when separation is anticipated or involved. Anticipation of separation can manifest as nausea, vomiting, stomachaches, dizziness, faintness, or flulike symptoms.

b. Epidemiology

Estimated prevalence is 4% of school-aged children.

More common in 7- and 8-year olds than adolescents or preschoolers.

It found in equal rates among females and males.

c. Etiology

Clusters in families but genetic transmission is unclear.

Biologic offspring of adults with anxiety disorders and panic disorder with agoraphobia are prone to separation anxiety disorder.

There is a neurophysiologic correlation of behavioral inhibition (extreme shyness).

Increased autonomic nervous system activity has been demonstrated.

d. Differential diagnosis

Generalized anxiety disorder (GAD): Anxiety is not focused on separation.

Panic disorder with agoraphobia: Typically does not manifest until 18 years of age.

e. Course and prognosis. Course and prognosis are variable and are related to age of onset, the duration of the symptoms, and the development of comorbid anxiety and depressive disorders. Slower recovery found in those with earlier onset and later age at diagnosis. Prognosis is guarded when there is coexistent depression.

f. Treatment

Psychotherapy: Cognitive–behavioral therapy is widely recommended as a first-line treatment. Attitudes and feelings about exaggerated environmental dangers are focused on. Family intervention is crucial, especially in children who refuse to attend school. Behavioral modification includes gradual adjustment strategies to achieve a return to school and separation from parents.

Pharmacotherapy: SSRIs are currently recommended as first-line medications in the treatment of childhood anxiety disorders. Diphenhydramine (Benadryl) may be used in the short-term to control sleep disturbances but with caution because some children show a paradoxical reaction of excitement. The benzodiazepine alprazolam (Xanax) may be helpful in controlling anxiety symptoms. Clonazepam (Klonopin) may be used in controlling symptoms of panic.

2. **Selective mutism.** A childhood condition in which a child who can speak and understand refuses to talk in social situations for at least 1 month.

   a. Diagnosis. Failure to speak in social situations for a duration of at least 1 month when it is clear that the child has adequate language skills in other environments. Mutism may develop gradually or suddenly after a disturbing experience. It is most commonly manifested in school and rarely at home. Child will commonly demonstrate social anxiety, separation anxiety disorder, and delayed language acquisition. See Table 25-9 for characteristics of anxiety disorder.

   b. Epidemiology

   Prevalence estimated to range between three and eight per 10,000 children but may be as high as 0.5%.

   More common in females and young children.

   Begins between ages 4 and 8.

   c. Etiology

   Many children have histories of delayed onset of speech or speech abnormalities.

Table 25-9
Common Characteristics in Childhood Anxiety Disorders

Criteria	Separation Anxiety Disorder	Social Anxiety Disorder	Generalized Anxiety Disorder
Minimum duration to establish diagnosis	At least 4 wks	Persistent, typically at least 6 mos	At least 6 mos
Age of onset Precipitating stressors	Not specified Separation from home or attachment figures	Not specified Social situations with peers or specific	Not specified Pressure for any type of performance, activities which are scored, school performance
Peer relationships	Good when no separation is involved	Tentative, overly inhibited	May appear overly eager to please, peers sought out for reassurance
Sleep	Reluctance or refusal to sleep away from home or not near attachment figure	May experience insomnia	Often difficulty falling asleep
Psychophysiologic symptoms	Stomachaches, headaches nausea, vomiting, palpitations, dizziness when anticipating separation	May exhibit blushing, inadequate eye contact, soft voice, or rigid posture	Stomachaches, nausea, lump in the throat, shortness of breath, dizziness, palpitations when anticipating performing an activity
Differential diagnosis	GAD, Soc AD, major depressive disorder, panic disorder with agoraphobia, PTSD, oppositional defiant disorder	GAD, Soc AD, major depressive disorder, dysthymic disorder, selective mutism, agoraphobia	SAD, Soc AD, attention-deficit/hyperactivity disorder, obsessive-compulsive disorder, major depressive disorder, PTSD

GAD, generalized anxiety disorder; Soc AD, social anxiety disorder; PTSD, posttraumatic stress disorder.
Reprinted from: Sadock BJ, Sadock VA, Ruiz P, Sadock BJ. *Kaplan & Sadock's Concise Textbook of Clinical Psychiatry.* Philadelphia: Wolters Kluwer; 2017; and adapted from Sidney Werkman, M.D.

Ninety percent met the criteria of social phobia, making it a possible subtype of social phobia.

d. Differential diagnosis

Shyness: Child exhibits a transient muteness in new, anxiety-provoking situations and has a history of not speaking in the presence of strangers and clinging to his or her mother.

Mutism: Child improves spontaneously upon entering school.

Intellectual disability, autism, and expressive language disorder: Symptoms are widespread and the child is unable to communicate normally.

Mutism Secondary to conversion disorder: The mutism is pervasive.

e. Course and prognosis. The disorder usually remits with or without treatment. Most cases last for only a few weeks or months. Children who do not improve by age 10 have a long-term course and a worse prognosis. One-third of children with the disorder, with or without treatment, may develop other psychiatric disorders, particularly other anxiety disorders and depression.

f. Treatment

Psychotherapy: A multimodal approach using individual, cognitive–behavioral, and family interventions is recommended. A therapeutic nursery is beneficial for preschool children. Individual cognitive–behavioral therapy is a first-line treatment for school-aged children. Family education and cooperation are beneficial.

Pharmacotherapy: SSRIs were an accepted component of treatment; however, their use in children is no longer warranted.

3. **Reactive attachment disorder and disinhibited social engagement disorder.** An inappropriate social relatedness that occurs in most contexts. Includes two subtypes: the inhibited type, in which the disturbance takes the form of constantly failing to initiate and respond to most social interactions, and the disinhibited type, in which the disturbance takes the form of undifferentiated, unselective social readiness.

a. **Diagnosis.** Markedly disturbed social relatedness in a child younger than 5 years old in the context of persistent disregard of physical or emotional needs or repeated change of caretaker. Expected social interaction and liveliness are not present. Infants demonstrate nonorganic failure to thrive. Physically, head circumference is normal, weight very low, and height somewhat short. Associated with low socioeconomic status and mothers who are depressed or isolated or have experienced abuse.

b. **Epidemiology.** There is no specific data on prevalence, sex ratio, or familial pattern. Often diagnosed and treated by pediatricians.

c. **Etiology.** Linked to maltreatment, including neglect and physical abuse.

d. **Differential diagnosis**

Autism spectrum disorder: The child is typically well nourished, of age-appropriate size and weight, alert and active, and does not improve rapidly if removed from home.

Intellectual disability: Children show appropriate social readiness for their mental age and a sequence of development similar to that of normal children.

e. **Course and prognosis.** Course and prognosis depend on the duration and severity of the neglectful and pathogenic parenting and on associated complications such as failure to thrive. Outcomes range from the extremes of death to the developmentally healthy child. Generally, the earlier the intervention the more reversible is the disorder.

f. **Treatment.** Removal of the child is necessary in most cases. Malnourishment and other medical problems may require hospitalization. Parent education and provision of a homemaker or financial aid may improve conditions so child can return.

J. Mood disorders in children and adolescents. Core features are similar to those in adults with expression of features modified to match the age and maturity of the individual.

1. **Diagnosis**
    a. **Major depressive disorder.** It is most easily diagnosed in children when it is acute and occurs in a child without previous psychiatric symptoms. Onset is usually insidious, and the disorder occurs in a child who has had several years of difficulties with hyperactivity, separation anxiety disorder, or intermittent depressive symptoms. Symptoms include depressed or irritable mood, loss of interest or pleasure, failure to gain weight, daily insomnia or hypersomnia, psychomotor agitation or retardation, diminished ability to think or concentrate, and recurrent thoughts of death. Anhedonia, hopelessness, psychomotor retardation, and delusions are more common in adolescents and adults.

    b. **Dysthymic disorder (persistent depressive disorder).** Onset in children and adolescents consists of a depressed or irritable mood for most of the day, for more days than not, over a period of at least 1 year. Patients may have a previous major depressive episode. The average age of onset is several years earlier than that of major depressive disorder.

    c. **Early-onset bipolar disorder.** Diagnostic criteria in children and adolescents are the same as for adults. Features include extreme mood variability, intermittent aggressive behavior, high levels of distractibility, and poor attention span. Patients may function poorly, require hospitalization, exhibit symptoms of depression, and often have a history of ADHD. When mania appears in adolescents, there is a higher incidence than in adults of psychotic features.

2. **Epidemiology**
    Extremely rare in preschool children. Prevalence increases with increasing age.
    Mania typically appears for the first time in adolescence.

3. **Etiology**
    Increased incidence among children of parents with mood disorder and relatives of children with mood disorder.
    Increased secretion of growth hormones during sleep in children with depressive disorder.
    Possible link to a decrease in thyroid hormones and depression.
    A dysfunction in the hypothalamic pituitary axis may contribute to depression in adolescents.

4. **Differential diagnosis**
    Differentiate psychotic forms of mood disorders from schizophrenia.
    Distinguish between agitated depressive or manic episodes and ADHD, which demonstrates persistent and excessive activity.

5. **Course and prognosis.** A young age of onset and multiple disorders predict a poorer prognosis. The mean length of an episode of major

depression in children and adolescents is about 9 months. Recurrence of a major depressive episode is 40% by 2 years and 70% by 5 years. Dysthymic episodes last on average 4 years and are associated with major depression (70%), bipolar disorder (13%), substance abuse (15%), and suicide (12%).

6. **Treatment.** Delusions, hallucinations, and thought disorders are difficult to diagnose in children. Onset is insidious, and all symptoms included in adult-onset schizophrenia may be found. The child may experience deterioration in function along with emergence of psychotic symptoms and might not reach developmental milestones. Auditory hallucinations, visual hallucinations, and delusions are frequent. The child may hear several voices making ongoing critical commentary, or command hallucinations may tell children to kill themselves. Visual hallucinations are often frightening.

Hospitalization: Hospitalization is indicated when a patient is suicidal or has a coexisting substance abuse or dependence.

Psychotherapy: Cognitive–behavioral therapy for moderately severe depression aims to challenge maladaptive beliefs and enhance problem-solving abilities and social competence. "Active" treatments such as relaxation techniques are helpful for mild or moderate depression. Family education and participation are necessary for depression. Modeling and role-playing techniques can be useful in fostering good problem-solving skills.

Pharmacotherapy: The SSRIs currently are the drugs of choice in the pharmacologic treatment of depressive disorders in children and adolescents. Given the FDA placement of the "black-box" warning in 2004 on all antidepressants used in children and adolescents because of the slightly increased risk of suicidal behaviors, it is imperative that close monitoring of suicidal ideation and behavior is achieved by all clinicians who prescribe these medications. Bupropion (Wellbutrin) is useful for depression as well as ADHD. Venlafaxine (Effexor) is used in treating adolescent depression. Lithium (Eskalith) has been used in the treatment of bipolar I and bipolar II disorder in childhood and adolescents. Divalproex (Depakote) is currently used frequently to treat bipolar disorder in children and adolescents. Few case reports and open label studies of atypical antipsychotics support the effectiveness of these medications in pediatric bipolar disorder. Many double and open label studies of olanzapine, risperidone, and quetiapine have demonstrated efficacy of these medications.

K. **Disruptive mood dysregulation disorder.** A new diagnosis classified as a mood disorder in DSM-5 characterized by recurrent temper tantrums with a persistent angry mood. The diagnosis was conceptualized because too many children were being misdiagnosed with early-onset bipolar disorder based upon volatile episodes of mood dysregulation.

1. **Diagnosis.** The child shows easily provoked temper tantrums accompanied by verbal or physical aggression. Symptoms occur both at home and

in school. The child's mood is irritable and persistently angry. Temper outburst occur at least three times per week to make the diagnosis.

2. Epidemiology. A lifetime prevalence of 2% to 5%. Mean age of onset is 5 to 11 years of age. More common in males.

3. Etiology. Genetic and neurobiologic factors play a role although no specific data has accumulated because this is a new diagnosis. There may be some overlap with the neurobiologic abnormalities found in bipolar disorder.

4. Differential diagnosis

Bipolar disorder: A more longitudinal course is present, manic phases are more discrete with elevated or expansive mood, episodes occur without precipitating events and persistent irritability is not common.

Oppositional defiant disorder: recurrent outburst of temper not present to the same extent and persistent irritability not as common.

Attention-deficit/hyperactivity disorder (ADHD): Generalized hyperactivity and inattentiveness more common. May be comorbid with disruptive mood dysregulation disorder.

Anxiety disorder: Symptoms generally occur only in anxiety provoking situations

5. Course and prognosis. Symptoms become less common as child approaches adolescence but in 50% of cases, symptoms persist for about one year after diagnosis is made. Some cases transition into bipolar disorder later in life.

6. Treatment

Pharmacotherapy: Mood stabilizers, such as divalproex, have been used with some success. Antipsychotic medication is severe cases; but should be used cautiously in children.

Psychosocial treatment: Sessions involving whole family with focus on current stresses and mood management. Individual therapy of use in socializing child so that they communicate with words instead of action.

L. Early-onset schizophrenia. Characterized by onset of psychotic symptoms before the age of 13 years. Has a chronic course with negative symptoms predominating.

1. Diagnosis. Essential features of schizophrenia same as in adulthood with delusions and hallucinations less well formed. Disorganized speech and behavior are common. Negative symptoms are pervasive.

2. Epidemiology

Less frequent than autism spectrum disorder (0.05%).

More common in males.

3. Etiology

Prevalence is greater in first-degree relatives, and monozygotic twins demonstrate higher concordance rates than dizygotic twins.

Psychosocial stressors may also interact with mechanisms of biologic vulnerability to produce symptoms.

4. Differential diagnosis

Schizotypal personality disorder: Overt psychotic symptoms are not present.

Major depressive disorder: Delusions and hallucinations are not as bizarre.

Autism spectrum disorders: Hallucinations, delusions, and formal thought disorder are not present.

5. **Course and prognosis.** Children with developmental delays, learning disorders, and premorbid behavioral disorders such as ADHD and conduct disorder are poor responders to medication treatment of schizophrenia and are more likely to have guarded prognoses. Some children given a diagnosis of schizophrenia will later be diagnosed with mood disorder when followed to adolescence.

6. **Treatment**

Psychotherapy: Family education and ongoing family interventions are critical. Proper educational setting is also important. Long-term intensive and supportive psychotherapy combined with pharmacotherapy is the most effective form of treatment. Psychotherapists must take into account a child's developmental level. They must continually support the child's good reality testing and have sensitivity to the child's sense of self.

Pharmacotherapy: Serotonin–dopamine agonists, including risperidone, olanzapine, and clozapine (Clozaril), have replaced dopamine receptor antagonists in the treatment of early-onset schizophrenia.

M. **Adolescent substance abuse (see Chapter 8 for further discussion)**

1. **Diagnosis.** Includes substance dependence, substance abuse, substance intoxication, and substance withdrawal diagnosed in adulthood. Diagnosis is made through careful interview, laboratory findings, and history provided by a reliable source.

2. **Epidemiology**

a. **Alcohol**

A significant problem in 10% to 20% of adolescents.

By 12th grade, 88% of high school students reported drinking, with the gap between male and female consumers decreasing.

b. **Marijuana**

The strongest predictor of cocaine use.

Ten percent, 23%, and 36% reported use in 8th, 10th, and 12th grade, respectively.

Prevalence rates are highest among Native American and white males and females. The lowest rates are seen in Latin American females, African American females, and Asian American males and females.

c. **Cocaine**

Annual cocaine use for high school seniors decreased more than 30% between 1990 and 2000.

Daily use of 0.1% and 0.05% was reported for cocaine and crack, respectively.

d. **Lysergic acid diethylamide (LSD)**

Current LSD rates are the lowest in two decades.

Among 8th-, 10th-, and 12th-grade students, 2.7%, 5.6%, and 8.8%, respectively, reported use at some time.

e. Inhalants

More common in younger than older adolescents.

Among 8th-, 10th-, and 12th-grade students, 17.6%, 15.7% and 17.6%, respectively, reported use.

3. Etiology

Concordance for alcoholism is higher in monozygotic than dizygotic twins.

Low parental supervision has also been associated with earlier drug use.

4. Treatment

Psychotherapy: Treatment setting and strategy should be decided after a screening process determines type and severity of substance(s) abused. Treatment settings include inpatient units, residential treatment facilities, halfway houses, group homes, partial hospital programs, and outpatient settings. Basic components include individual psychotherapy, drug-specific counseling, self-help groups (e.g., Alcoholics Anonymous [AA], Narcotics Anonymous [NA]), substance abuse education and relapse prevention programs, and random urine drug testing. Cognitive–behavioral therapy generally requires that adolescents be motivated to participate in treatment and refrain from further substance use. Family therapy may be added.

Pharmacotherapy: When mood disorders are present, antidepressants can be used. In some cases, medication can be administrated to block the reinforcing effect of the illicit drug (i.e., naltrexone [ReVia] for opioid abuse). Clonidine (Catapres) has been used in heroin withdrawal. Efficacious treatments for cigarette smoking cessation include nicotine-containing gum, patches, or nasal spray or inhaler. Bupropion (Zyban) is beneficial for smoking cessation.

N. Other childhood issues

1. Child abuse and neglect. An estimated one million children are abused or neglected annually in the United States, a problem that results in 2,000 to 4,000 deaths per year. The abused are apt to be of low birth weight or born prematurely (50% of all abused children), handicapped (e.g., mental retardation, cerebral palsy), or troubled (e.g., defiant, hyperactive). The abusing parent is usually the mother, who likely was abused herself. Abusing parents often are impulsive, substance abusers, depressed, antisocial, or narcissistic.

Each year, 150,000 to 200,000 new cases of sexual abuse are reported. Of these allegations, 2% to 8% appear to be false, and many other allegations cannot be substantiated. In 8 of 10 sexually abused children, the perpetrator, usually male, is known to the child. In 50%, the offender is a parent, parent surrogate, or relative.

2. Borderline intellectual functioning. A child has an IQ in the range of 71 to 84 and presents impaired adaptive functioning.

3. Academic problem. A child or adolescent has significant academic difficulties that are not deemed to be due to a specific learning or communication disorder or directly related to a mental or psychiatric disorder.

4. **Childhood or adolescent antisocial behavior.** A child or adolescent presents behavior that is not caused by a mental disorder and includes isolated antisocial acts, not a pattern of behavior. The acts violate the rights of others, such as overt acts of aggression and violence and covert acts of lying, stealing, truancy, and running away from home.

5. **Identity problem.** DSM-5 does not recognize this as a mental disorder, but it can manifest in mental disorders such as mood disorders, psychotic disorders, and borderline personality disorders. It refers to uncertainty about issues relating to identity, such as goals, career choice, friendships, sexual behavior, moral values, and group loyalties.

6. **Obesity.** Present in 5% to 20% of children and adolescents. A small percentage present with an obesity–hypoventilation syndrome that is similar to adult Pickwickian syndrome. These children can have dyspnea, and their sleep is characterized by snoring, stridor, perhaps apnea, and hypoxia with oxygen desaturation. Death can result. Other conditions, such as hypothyroidism or Prader–Willi syndrome, should be ruled out.

7. **AIDS.** AIDS has presented child and adolescent psychiatrists with a multitude of difficult problems. For example, the care of young patients from lower socioeconomic groups, already grossly inadequate because of insufficient resources, is further burdened by HIV-related illness or the death of parents and relatives. Young psychiatric patients who have concomitant nonsymptomatic positive serology and require residential treatment are rejected for fear of transmission of the disease. In adolescence, AIDS has further complicated sexuality and the problem of substance abuse.

For more detailed discussion of this topic, see Child Psychiatry, Ch 36, p. 3375; Psychiatric Examination of the Infant, Child, and Adolescent, Ch 36.1, p. 3375; Intellectual Disability, Ch 40, p. 3491; Learning Disorders, Ch 41, p. 3520; Motor Skills Disorder: Developmental Coordination Disorder, Ch 42, p. 3537; Communication Disorders, Ch 43, p. 3545; Autism Spectrum Disorder and Social Communication Disorder, Ch 44, p. 3571; Attention-Deficit Disorders, Ch 45, p. 3587; Disruptive Behavior Disorders, Ch 46, p. 3605; Feeding and Eating Disorders of Infancy and Early Childhood, Ch 47, p. 3622; Tic Disorders, Ch 48, p. 3635; Elimination Disorders, Ch 49, p. 3650; Other Disorders of Infancy, Childhood, and Adolescence, Ch 50, p. 3662; Mood Disorders in Children and Adolescents, Ch 51, p. 3674; Anxiety Disorders in Children, Ch 52, p. 3695; Early-Onset Psychotic Disorders, Ch 53, p. 3725; Child Psychiatry: Psychiatric Treatment, Ch 54, p. 3734; and Child Psychiatry: Special Areas of Interest, Ch 55, p. 3817, in CTP/X.

26

Geriatric Psychiatry

I. Introduction

Old age, or late adulthood, is not a disease and usually refers to the stage of the life cycle that begins at age 65. It is mirrored by a shift from the pursuit of wealth to the maintenance of health, loss of physical agility and mental acuity, friends and loved ones, and status and power. However, there are elderly persons with mental or physical disorders, or both, that impair their ability to function or even survive, known as the sick-old. Despite these occurrences, the body in late adulthood can still be a source of considerable pleasure and can convey a sense of competence, particularly if attention is paid to regular exercise, healthy diet, adequate rest, and preventive maintenance medical care. Geriatric psychiatry is concerned with preventing, diagnosing, and treating psychological disorders in older adults and promoting longevity. Persons with a healthy mental adaptation to life have been found to live longer than those stressed with emotional problems.

II. Demographics

A. Late adulthood or old age considered to begin at age 65. Divided into young-old, ages 65 to 74; old-old, ages 75 to 84; and oldest-old, age 85 and beyond. Also, divided into well-old (those who are healthy) and sick-old (persons with an infirmity that interferes with daily functioning and that requires medical or psychiatric care).

B. The life expectancy in the United States is approaching 80 years, with an average of 74 for men and 81 for women. Women outlive men by about 7 years. People at least 85 years old now constitute 10% of those 65 and older and is the most rapidly growing segment of the older population. The developmental tasks of late adulthood that lead to mental health are listed in Table 26-1.

III. Biology of Aging

A. The aging process (senescence) is characterized by a gradual decline in the functioning of all the body's systems—cardiovascular, respiratory, endocrine, and immune, among others. An overview of all the biologic changes is given in Table 26-2.

B. Cognition

1. Mild memory loss common—called benign senescent forgetfulness. New material can be learned; however, it requires more repetition and practice than in younger persons. IQ does not decrease.

2. Persons of low socioeconomic status are at a higher risk for cognitive decline than persons in higher groups. Cognitive decline slowed in persons who are involved in continual learning and stimulation.

Table 26-1
Developmental Tasks of Late Adulthood

To maintain the body image and physical integrity
To conduct the life review
To maintain sexual interests and activities
To deal with the death of significant loved ones
To accept the implications of retirement
To accept the genetically programmed failure of organ systems
To divest oneself of the attachment to possessions
To accept changes in the relationship with grandchildren

Table 26-2
Biologic Changes Associated with Aging

Cellular level
  Change in cellular DNA and RNA structures: intracellular organelle degeneration
  Neuronal degeneration in central nervous system, primarily in superior temporal precentral and
    inferior temporal gyri; no loss in brainstem nuclei
  Receptor sites and sensitivity altered
  Decreased anabolism and catabolism of cellular transmitter substances
  Intercellular collagen and elastin increase
Immune system
  Impaired T-cell response to antigen
  Increase in function of autoimmune bodies
  Increased susceptibility to infection and neoplasia
  Leukocytes unchanged, T lymphocytes reduced
  Increased erythrocyte sedimentation (nonspecific)
Musculoskeletal
  Decrease in height because of shortening of spinal column (2-in loss in both men and women from
    the second to the seventh decade)
  Reduction in lean muscle mass and muscle strength; deepening of thoracic cage
  Increase in body fat
  Elongation of nose and ears
  Loss of bone matrix, leading to osteoporosis
  Degeneration of joint surfaces may produce osteoarthritis
  Risk of hip fracture is 10–25% by age 90
  Continual closing of cranial sutures (parietomastoid suture does not attain complete closure until
    age 80)
  Men gain weight until about age 60, then lose; women gain weight until age 70, then lose
Integument
  Graying of hair results from decreased melanin production in hair follicles (by age 50, 50% of all
    persons male and female are at least 50% gray; pubic hair is last to turn gray)
  General wrinkling of skin
  Less active sweat glands
  Decrease in melanin
  Loss of subcutaneous fat
  Nail growth slowed
Genitourinary and reproductive
  Decreased glomerular filtration rate and renal blood flow
  Decreased hardness of erection, diminished ejaculatory spurt
  Decreased vaginal lubrication
  Enlargement of prostate
  Incontinence
Special senses
  Thickening of optic lens, reduced peripheral vision
  Inability to accommodate (presbyopia)
  High-frequency sound hearing loss (presbycusis)—25% show loss by age 60, 65% by age 80
  Yellowing of optic lens
  Reduced acuity of taste, smell, and touch
  Decreased light–dark adaption

(continued)

Table 26-2
Biologic Changes Associated with Aging *(Continued)*

Neuropsychiatric
Takes longer to learn new material, but complete learning still occurs
IQ remains stable until age 80
Verbal ability maintained with age
Psychomotor speed declines

Memory
Tasks requiring shifting attentions performed with difficulty
Encoding ability diminishes (transfer of short-term to long-term memory and vice versa)
Recognition of right answer on multiple-choice tests remains intact
Simple recall declines

Neurotransmitters
Norepinephrine decreases in central nervous system
Increased monoamine oxidase and serotonin in brain

Brain
Decrease in gross brain weight, about 17% by age 80 in both sexes
Widened sulci, smaller convolutions, gyral atrophy
Ventricles enlarge
Increased transport across blood-brain barrier
Decreased cerebral blood flow and oxygenation

Cardiovascular
Increase in size and weight of heart (contains lipofuscin pigment derived from lipids)
Decreased elasticity of heart valves
Increased collagen in blood vessels
Increased susceptibility to arrhythmias
Altered homeostasis of blood pressure
Cardiac output maintained in absence of coronary heart disease

Gastrointestinal (GI) system
At risk for atrophic gastritis, hiatal hernia, diverticulosis
Decreased blood flow to gut, liver
Diminished saliva flow
Altered absorption from GI tract (at risk for malabsorption syndrome and avitaminosis)
Constipation

Endocrine
Estrogen levels decrease in women
Adrenal androgen decreases
Testosterone production declines in men
Increase in follicle-stimulating hormone (FSH) and luteinizing hormone (LH) in postmenopausal women
Serum thyroxine (T_4) and thyroid-stimulating hormone (TSH) normal, triiodothyronine (T_3) reduced
Glucose tolerance test result decreases

Respiratory
Decreased vital capacity
Diminished cough reflex
Decreased bronchial epithelium ciliary action

IV. Medical Illness

The leading five causes of death in the elderly are heart disease, cancer, stroke, Alzheimer's disease, and pneumonia. Central nervous system (CNS) changes and psychopathology are frequent causes of morbidity, as are arthritis and related symptoms. Benign prostatic hyperplasia affects three-fourths of men over age 75. Urinary incontinence is believed to occur in as many as one-fifth of the elderly, sometimes in association with dementia. These common disorders result in behavior modification. Arthritis, for example, may restrict activity and alter lifestyle. The elderly, like other adults, are profoundly embarrassed by urinary difficulties and will restrict activities and hide or deny their disability to maintain self-esteem. Cardiovascular disease is a prominent cause of morbidity and mortality in the elderly. Hypertension may be present in 40% of the elderly, many of whom are receiving diuretics or antihypertensive medications. Hypertension itself can result in CNS effects ranging from headaches to stroke, and pharmacotherapy for this condition can result in mood and cognitive disorders (e.g., electrolyte disturbances due to diuretic treatment). Atherosclerosis, associated with both cardiovascular disease and hypertension, has been related to the occurrence of the major forms of dementia—not only vascular dementia but also Alzheimer's disease. Sensory changes also accompany the aging process. One-third of the aged have some degree of auditory disability. In one study, nearly one-half of persons 75 to 85 years of age had lens cataracts, and more than 70% had glaucoma. Difficulties with convergence, accommodation, and macular degeneration also are sources of visual disability in the aged. These sensory changes frequently interact with psychopathologic disabilities, serving to magnify psychopathologic deficit and color symptoms.

V. **Psychiatric Illness**

Prevalence data for mental disorders in elderly persons vary widely, but a conservatively estimated 25% have significant psychiatric symptoms. The most common disorders of old age are depressive disorder, cognitive disorders (dementia), phobic disorders, and alcohol use disorders. Older adults (over age 75) also have one of the highest risks for suicide. Many mental disorders of old age can be prevented, ameliorated, or even reversed. Of special importance are the reversible causes of delirium and dementia; if not diagnosed accurately and treated in a timely fashion, these conditions can progress to an irreversible state requiring a patient's institutionalization.

A. **Dementing disorders.** About 5% of persons in the United States older than age 65 have severe dementia, and 15% have mild dementia. Of persons older than age 80, about 20% have severe dementia. Known risk factors for dementia are age, family history, and female sex. Characteristic changes of dementia involve cognition, memory, language, and visuospatial functions, but behavioral disturbances are common as well and include agitation, restlessness, wandering, rage, violence, shouting, social and sexual disinhibition, impulsiveness, sleep disturbances, and delusions. Delusions and hallucinations occur during the course of the dementias in nearly 75% of patients. About 10% to 15% of all patients who exhibit symptoms of dementia have potentially treatable conditions. See Table 26-3.

1. **Dementia of the Alzheimer's type**

a. **Diagnosis, signs, and symptoms.** Most common type of dementia. It is higher in women than in men. Characterized by the gradual onset and progressive decline of cognitive functions. Memory is impaired, and at least one of the following is seen: aphasia, apraxia, agnosia, and disturbances in executive functioning. Neurologic defects (e.g., gait disturbances, aphasia, apraxia, and agnosia) eventually

Table 26-3
Some Potentially Reversible Conditions That May Resemble Dementia

Substances
  Anticholinergic agents
  Antihypertensives
  Antipsychotics
  Corticosteroids
  Digitalis
  Narcotics
  Nonsteroidal anti-inflammatory agents
  Phenytoin
  Polypharmacotherapy
  Sedative hypnotics

Psychiatric disorders
  Anxiety
  Depression
  Mania
  Delusional (paranoid) disorders

Metabolic and endocrine disorders
  Addison's disease
  Cushing's syndrome
  Hepatic failure
  Hypercarbia (chronic obstructive pulmonary disease)
  Hypernatremia
  Hyperparathyroidism
  Hyperthyroidism
  Hypoglycemia
  Hyponatremia
  Hypothyroidism
  Renal failure
  Volume depletion

Miscellaneous conditions
  Fecal impaction
  Hospitalization
  Impaired hearing or vision

Courtesy of Gary W. Small, M.D.

appear. About 50% of patients with Alzheimer's disease experience psychotic symptoms. See Table 26-4 to differentiate the two.

  b. **Etiology.** Selective loss of cholinergic neurons. Reduced gyral volume in the frontal and temporal lobes. Microscopic alterations include senile plaques and neurofibrillary tangles.

  c. **Treatment.** There is no known prevention or cure. Treatment is palliative. Some patients with dementia of the Alzheimer's type show improvement in cognitive and functional measures when treated with donepezil (Aricept). Drugs such as memantine (Namenda) that project neurons from excessive glutamate stimulation are also of use. Psychosis of Alzheimer's type is treated pharmacologically. See Table 26-5.

2. **Vascular dementia**. The second most common type of dementia is vascular dementia. It has focal neurologic signs and symptoms. It also has an abrupt onset and a stepwise, deteriorating course.

Table 26-4
Psychosis of AD Versus Schizophrenia in the Elderly: Clinical Characteristics

Characteristic	Schizophrenia	Psychosis of AD
Prevalence	1% of general population	50% of AD patients
Bizarre or complex delusions	Frequent	Rare
Common hallucinations	Auditory	Visual
First-rank symptoms	Frequent	Rare
Active suicidal ideation	Frequent	Rare
Past history of psychosis	Very common	Rare
Family history of psychosis	Sometimes	Uncommon
Eventual remission of psychosis	Uncommon	Frequent
Need for years of antipsychotic use	Very common	Uncommon
Optimal antipsychotic dose (% of dose for young adult with schizophrenia)	50%	20%

AD, Alzheimer's disease.
From Forester BP, Dukoff R. *Primary Psychiatry*. 2004, 11(1):48, 51–55.

3. **Other dementias.** Dementias due to Huntington's disease, dementia due to normal pressure hydrocephalus, Parkinson's disease, and other causes are covered in Chapter 5.

B. **Depressive disorders.** Present in about 15% of all older adult community residents and nursing home patients. Common signs and symptoms of depressive disorders include reduced energy and concentration, sleep problems (especially early morning awakening and multiple awakenings), decreased appetite, weight loss, and somatic complaints. Cognitive impairment in depressed geriatric patients is referred to as the *dementia syndrome of depression* (*pseudodementia*), which can be confused easily with true dementia. Pseudodementia occurs in about 15% of depressed older patients, and 25% to 50% of patients with dementia are depressed.

C. **Bipolar I disorder**

1. **Diagnosis, signs, and symptoms.** Usually begins in middle adulthood. A vulnerability to recurrence remains, so patients with a history of bipolar I disorder may display a manic episode late in life. Signs and symptoms in older persons are similar to those in younger adults and include an elevated, expansive, or irritable mood; a decreased need to sleep; distractibility; impulsivity; and often, excessive alcohol intake. Hostile or paranoid behavior is usually present.

Table 26-5
Second Generation Antipsychotic Used in Treatment of Psychosis of Alzheimer's Disease

Drug	Initial Dose (mg/day)	Maintenance Dose
Clozapine (Clozaril)	6.25–12.5	25–75
Risperidone (Risperdal)	0.025–0.5	0.5–1.5
Olanzapine (Zyprexa)	2.5–5	5–10
Paliperidone (Invega)	3–12	3–6
Quetiapine (Seroquel)	12.5–5	50–150
Ziprasidone (Geodon)	40	60–180
Aripiprazole (Abilify)	10	10–15

Table 26-6
Geriatric Dosages of Drugs Commonly Used to Treat Bipolar Disorder

Generic Name	Trade Name	Geriatric Dosage Range (mg/day)
Lithium carbonate	Eskalith, Lithotabs, Lithonate, Lithobid	75–900
Carbamazepine	Tegretol	200–1,200
Valproate (valproic acid, divalproex)	Depakene, Depakote	250–1,000

    2. Treatment. Lithium (Eskalith) remains the treatment choice for mania, but its use by older patients must be monitored carefully, because their reduced renal clearance makes lithium toxicity a significant risk. Neurotoxic effects are also more common in older persons than in younger adults. Other drugs used to treat elderly patients with bipolar disorder are listed in Table 26-6.

D. Schizophrenia

    1. Diagnosis, signs, and symptoms. Psychopathology becomes less marked as the patient ages. Signs and symptoms include emotional blunting, social withdrawal, eccentric behavior, and illogical thinking. Delusions and hallucinations are uncommon.

    2. Epidemiology. Usually begins in late adolescence or young adulthood and persists throughout life. Women are more likely to have a late onset of schizophrenia than men. About 20% of persons with schizophrenia show no active symptoms by age 65; 80% show varying degrees of impairments.

    3. Treatment. Older persons with schizophrenic symptoms respond well to antipsychotic drugs. Medication must be administered judiciously, and lower-than-usual dosages are often effective for older adults. See Table 26-7.

E. Delusional disorder

    1. Diagnosis, signs, and symptoms. Can occur under physical or psychological stress and may be precipitated by the death of a spouse, loss of a job, retirement, social isolation, adverse financial circumstances, debilitating medical illness or surgery, visual impairment, and deafness.

    2. Epidemiology. Usually occurs between ages 40 and 55. Delusions take many forms; the most common is persecutory—patients believe that they are being spied on, followed, poisoned, or harassed in some way.

    3. Etiology. May result from prescribed medications or be early signs of a brain tumor.

Table 26-7
Second-Generation Antipsychotics: Schizophrenia in the Elderly

Drug	Initial Dose (mg/day)	Maintenance Dose (mg/day)
Clozapine (Clozaril)	12.5–25	50–150
Risperidone (Risperdal)	0.5–1	1–3
Olanzapine (Zyprexa)	5–7.5	10–15
Paliperidone (Invega)	3–12	3–6
Quetiapine (Seroquel)	25–50	100–250
Ziprasidone (Geodon)	40	60–180
Aripiprazole (Abilify)	10	10–15

F. **Anxiety disorder.** Includes panic disorder, phobias, obsessive–compulsive disorder, generalized anxiety disorder, acute stress disorder, and posttraumatic stress disorder.

1. **Diagnosis, signs, and symptoms.** Signs and symptoms of phobia in older adults are less severe than in those that occur in younger persons, but the effects are equally, if not more, debilitating for older patients. Obsessions and compulsions may appear for the first time in older adults, although older adults with obsessive-compulsive disorder usually had demonstrated evidence of the disorder (e.g., being orderly, perfectionistic, punctual, and parsimonious) when they were younger. When symptomatic, patients become excessive in their desire for orderliness, rituals, and sameness.

2. **Epidemiology.** Anxiety disorders begin in early or middle adulthood, but some appear for the first time after age 60. The most common disorders are phobias (4% to 8%). The rate for panic disorder is 1%.

3. **Treatment.** Treatment must be tailored to individual patients and must take into account the biopsychosocial interplay producing the disorder. Both pharmacotherapy and psychotherapy are required.

G. **Somatoform disorders**

1. **Diagnosis, signs, and symptoms.** Characterized by physical symptoms resembling medical diseases, and are relevant to geriatric psychiatry because somatic complaints are common among older adults.

2. **Epidemiology.** More than 80% of persons over 65 years of age have at least one chronic disease—usually arthritis or cardiovascular problems. After age 75, 20% have diabetes and an average of four diagnosable chronic illnesses that require medical attention. Hypochondriasis is common in persons over 60 years of age, although the peak incidence is in the 40- to 50-year-old age group.

3. **Treatment.** The disorder is usually chronic, and the prognosis guarded. Repeated physical examinations help reassure patients that they do not have a fatal illness, but invasive and high-risk diagnostic procedures should be avoided unless medically indicated. Clinicians should acknowledge that the complaint is real, the pain is really there and perceived as such by the patients, and a psychological or pharmacologic approach to the problem is indicated.

H. **Alcohol and other substance use disorders**

1. **Diagnosis, signs, and symptoms.** Older adults with alcohol dependence usually give a history of excessive drinking that began in young or middle adulthood. They usually are medically ill, primarily with liver disease, and are either divorced, widowers, or men who never married. The clinical presentation of older patients with alcohol and other substance use disorders varies and includes confusion, poor personal hygiene, depression, malnutrition, and the effects of exposure and falls. Unexplained gastrointestinal, psychological, and metabolic problems should alert clinicians to over-the-counter substance abuse.

2. **Epidemiology.** Twenty percent of nursing home patients have alcohol dependence. Alcohol and other substance use disorders account for

10% of all emotional problems in older persons, and dependence on such substances such as hypnotics, anxiolytics, and narcotics is more common in old age than is generally recognized. Thirty-five percent use over-the-counter analgesics, and 30% use laxatives.

I. Sleep disorders

1. **Diagnosis, signs, and symptoms.** As a result of the decreased length of their daily sleep–wake cycle, older persons without daily routines, especially patients in nursing homes, may experience an advanced sleep phase, in which they go to sleep early and awaken during the night. Changes in sleep structure among persons over 65 years of age involve both rapid eye movement (REM) sleep and nonrapid eye movement (NREM) sleep. The REM changes include the redistribution of REM sleep throughout the night, more REM episodes, shorter REM episodes, and less total REM sleep. The NREM changes include the decreased amplitude of delta waves, a lower percentage of stages III and IV sleep, and a higher percentage of stages I and II sleep.

2. **Epidemiology.** Reported more frequently by older than by younger adults are sleeping problems, daytime sleepiness, daytime napping, and the use of hypnotic drugs. Among the primary sleep disorders, dyssomnias are the most frequent, especially primary insomnia, nocturnal myoclonus, restless legs syndrome, and sleep apnea.

3. **Etiology.** Deterioration in the quality of sleep in older persons is due to the altered timing and consolidation of sleep. Causes of sleep disturbances in older persons include primary sleep disorders, other mental disorders, general medical disorders, and social and environmental factors. Alcohol usage can also interfere with the quality of sleep and can cause sleep fragmentation and early morning awakening.

J. Suicide risk

1. **Diagnosis, signs, and symptoms.** Older patients with major medical illnesses or a recent loss should be evaluated for depressive symptomatology and suicidal ideation or plans. There should be no reluctance to question patients about suicide, because there is no evidence that such questions increase the likelihood of suicidal behavior.

2. **Epidemiology.** Elderly persons have a higher risk for suicide than any other population. The suicide rate for white men over the age of 65 is five times higher than that of the general population. One-third of elderly persons report loneliness as the principal reason for considering suicide. Approximately 10% of elderly individuals with suicide ideation report financial problems, poor medical health, or depression as reasons for suicidal thoughts. Seventy percent of suicide attempters take a drug overdose, and 20% cut or slash themselves. More elderly suicide victims are widowed and fewer are single, separated, or divorced than is true of younger adults.

K. Other conditions of old age

1. **Vertigo.** Feelings of vertigo or dizziness, a common complaint of older adults, cause many older adults to become inactive because they fear falling. The causes of vertigo vary and include anemia, hypotension,

cardiac arrhythmia, cerebrovascular disease, basilar artery insufficiency, middle ear disease, acoustic neuroma, and Ménière's disease. The overuse of anxiolytics can cause dizziness and daytime somnolence. Treatment with meclizine (Antivert), 25 to 100 mg daily, has been successful in many patients with vertigo.

2. **Syncope.** The sudden loss of consciousness associated with syncope results from a reduction of cerebral blood flow and brain hypoxia. A thorough medical workup is required to rule out the various causes listed in Table 26-8.

3. **Hearing loss.** About 30% of persons over age 65 have significant hearing loss (presbycusis). After age 65, that figure rises to 50%. Causes vary. Clinicians should be sensitive to hearing loss in patients who complain they can hear but cannot understand what is being said or

Table 26-8
Causes of Syncope

Cardiac disorders
  Anatomic/valvular
    Aortic stenosis
    Mitral prolapse and regurgitation
    Hypertrophic cardiomyopathy
    Myxoma
  Electrical
    Tachyarrhythmia
    Bradyarrhythmia
    Heart block
    Sick sinus syndrome
  Functional
    Ischemia and infarct

Situational hypotension
  Dehydration (diarrhea, fasting)
  Orthostatic hypotension
  Postprandial hypotension
  Micturition, defecation, coughing, swallowing

Abnormal cardiovascular reflexes
  Carotid sinus syndrome
  Vasovagal syncope

Drugs
  Vasodilators
  Calcium channel blockers
  Diuretics
  Beta blockers

Central nervous system abnormalities
  Cerebrovascular insufficiency
  Seizures

Metabolic abnormalities
  Hypoxemia
  Hypoglycemia or hyperglycemia
  Anemia

Pulmonary disorders
  Chronic obstructive pulmonary disease
  Pneumonia
  Pulmonary embolus

who ask that questions be repeated. Most elderly patients with hearing loss can be treated with hearing aids.

4. **Elder abuse.** An estimated 10% of persons above 65 years of age are abused. *Elder abuse* is defined by the American Medical Association as "an act or omission which results in harm or threatened harm to the health or welfare of an elderly person." Mistreatment includes abuse and neglect—physically, psychologically, financially, and materially. Sexual abuse does occur. The types of elder abuse are listed in Table 26-9.

5. **Spousal bereavement.** Demographic data suggest that 51% of women and 14% of men over the age of 65 will be widowed at least once. Spousal loss is among the most stressful of all life experiences. Elderly survivors of spouses who committed suicide are especially vulnerable, as are those with psychiatric illness.

VI. Psychotherapy in the Elderly

Fundamental psychological processes in the elderly do not differ from those of younger adults. However, the aging process and associated pathologic changes do result in psychological issues that are relatively particular to this age group. Common issues in therapy include evolving and changing relationships of the elderly with their adult children. For example, in the presence of disease, the elderly may have both a desire for independence and, in the present social context, unrealistic expectations with regard to their adult children. Adult children, in turn, may harbor resentments toward their parents continued from childhood, or, conversely, they may experience unrealistic feelings of guilt in regard to what they should be doing for their parents in the event of illness or other traumatic events.

Family therapy, consequently, can be of particular value in the elderly, sometimes in conjunction with group or individual psychotherapy. Other goals of individual therapy particular to the elderly include the maintenance of self-esteem despite physical, marital, and social change; the meaningful use of unaccustomed leisure time; and clarification of options in the context of more or less overwhelming physical and social change. In general, psychotherapy in the elderly is relatively situation- and problem-oriented, and seeks solutions within the established personality framework rather than overwhelming personality change. Many elderly persons, however, respond remarkably well to seemingly overwhelming changes and personal tragedies (e.g., loss of health, loss of a spouse) and display hitherto unseen social strengths and adaptive capacities.

Dementia poses special psychotherapeutic challenges. In a phenomenon termed *retrogenesis,* which occurs in Alzheimer's dementia and to a variable extent in other dementing conditions, the patient's cognitive, functional, and physiologic changes reverse the patterns of normal human development. This is illustrated for the functional changes in Alzheimer's disease in Table 26-10. Consequently, each functional stage of Alzheimer's disease can be formulated as a corresponding developmental age of childhood. The developmental age of the Alzheimer's patient provides a rapid appreciation of his or her overall management and care needs (Table 26-11). Thus, a stage 7 patient with severe Alzheimer's disease requires approximately the same amount of care

Table 26-9
Types of Elder Abuse

Physical or sexual abuse
Bruises (bilateral and at various stages of healing)
Welts
Lacerations
Punctures
Fractures
Evidence of excessive drugging
Burns
Physical restraints (tying to beds, etc.)
Malnutrition and dehydration
Lack of personal care
Inadequate heating
Lack of food and water
Unclean clothes or bedding
Lack of needed medication
Lack of eyeglasses, hearing aids, false teeth
Difficulty walking or sitting
Venereal disease
Pain or itching, bruises, or bleeding of external genitalia, vaginal area, or anal area

Psychological abuse (vulnerable adults react by exhibiting resignation, fear, depression, mental
confusion, anger, ambivalence, insomnia)
Threats
Insults
Harassment
Withholding of security and affection
Harsh orders
Refusal on the part of the family or those caring for the adult to allow travel, visits by friends or
other family members, attendance at church

Exploitation
Misuse of vulnerable adult's income or other financial resources (victim is best source of
information but in most cases has turned management of financial affairs over to another
person; as a result, there may be some confusion about finances)

Medical abuse
Withholding or improper administration of medications or necessary medical treatments for a
condition or the withholding of aids the person would medically require, such as false teeth, glasses,
hearing aids
May be a cause of:
Confusion
Disorientation
Memory impairment
Agitation
Lethargy
Self-neglect

Neglect
Conduct of vulnerable adult or others that results in deprivation of care necessary to maintain
physical and mental health
May be manifest by:
Malnutrition
Poor personal hygiene
Any of the indicators for medical abuse

Reprinted with permission from Washington State Medical Association. *Elder Abuse: Guidelines
for Intervention by Physicians and Other Service Providers.* Seattle, WA: Washington State Medical
Association; 1985.

Table 26-10
Functional Stages in Normal Human Development and Alzheimer's Disease

Approximate Age	Acquired Abilities	Lost Abilities	Alzheimer's Stage
12+ yrs	Hold a job	Hold a job	3 INCIPIENT
8–12 yrs	Handle simple finances	Handle simple finances	4 MILD
5–7 yrs	Select proper clothing	Select proper clothing	5 MODERATE
5 yrs	Put on clothes unaided	Put on clothes unaided	6a MODERATELY SEVERE
4 yrs	Shower unaided	Shower unaided	b
4 yrs	Toilet unaided	Toilet unaided	c
3–4½ yrs	Control urine	Control urine	d
2–3 yrs	Control bowels	Control bowels	e
15 mos	Speak five or six words	Speak five or six words	7a SEVERE
1 yr	Speak one word	Speak one word	b
1 yr	Walk	Walk	c
6–10 mos	Sit up	Sit up	d
2–4 mos	Smile	Smile	e
1–3 mos	Hold up head	Hold up head	f

From Reisberg B. Dementia: a systematic approach to identifying reversible causes. *Geriatrics*. 1986; 41(4):30–46; Reisberg B. Functional assessment staging (FAST). *Psychopharmacol Bull*. 1988;24:653–659; and Reisberg B, Franssen EH, Souren LEM, Auer S, Kenowsky S. Progression of Alzheimer's disease: variability and consistency; ontogenic models, their applicability and relevance. *J Neural Transm Suppl*. 1998;54:9–20, with permission.

as an infant. Similarly, one can leave a stage 4 patient with mild Alzheimer's disease alone to a large extent, just as an 8- to 12-year-old child may require only limited supervision. The developmental age of the Alzheimer's patient is also useful in understanding his or her emotional needs, behavioral disturbances, and physical needs. As noted, these principles are also to some extent applicable to dementing disorders other than Alzheimer's disease.

VII. Psychopharmacologic Treatment in the Elderly

The major goals of the pharmacologic treatment of older persons are to improve the quality of life, maintain persons in the community, and delay or avoid their placement in nursing homes. Individualization of dosing is the basic tenet of geriatric psychopharmacology. Alterations in drug doses

Table 26-11
Management Needs in Normal Development and of the Alzheimer's Patient at the Corresponding Developmental Age

Global Deterioration and Functional Stage of Aging and Alzheimer's Disease	Development Age	Management Needs of Aged and Alzheimer's Patient
1	Adult	None
2	Adult	None
3	12+ yrs	None
4	8–12 yrs	Independent survival still attainable
5	5–7 yrs	Patient can no longer survive in the community without part-time assistance
6	2–5 yrs	Patient requires full-time supervision
7	0–2 yrs	Patient requires continuous care

Adapted from Reisberg B, Franssen EH, Souren LEM, Auer S, Kenowsky S. Progression of Alzheimer's disease: variability and consistency; ontogenic models, their applicability and relevance. *J Neural Transm Suppl*. 1998;54:9–20, with permission.

are required because of the physiologic changes that occur as persons age. Renal disease is associated with decreased renal clearance of drugs; liver disease results in a decreased ability to metabolize drugs; cardiovascular disease and reduced cardiac output can affect both renal and hepatic drug clearance; and gastrointestinal disease and decreased gastric acid secretion influence drug absorption. As a general rule, the lowest possible dose should be used to achieve the desired therapeutic response. Clinicians must know the pharmacodynamics, pharmacokinetics, and biotransformation of each drug prescribed and the effects of the interaction of the drug with other drugs that a patient is taking.

For more detailed discussion of this topic, see Geriatric Psychiatry, Chapter 57, p. 3947, in CTP/X.

27

End-of-Life Care Issues

I. End-of-Life Care

End-of-life refers to death and dying. Whereas *death* may be considered the absolute cessation of vital functions, *dying* is the process of losing these functions. This phase involves all who care for the terminally ill, and it begins when curative therapy ceases. Palliative care is the most important part of end-of-life care. Also included are other complex issues such as euthanasia, physician-assisted suicide, and ethical issues.

    A. Palliative care. Palliative care (from Latin *palliere*, "to cloak") is concerned with treating the dying patient. It is geared to the relief of pain and suffering; it is not designed to cure. While this is most commonly associated with analgesic drug administration, many other medical interventions and surgical procedures fall under the umbrella of palliative care because they can make the patient more comfortable. Such care provides pain relief and emotional, social, and spiritual support, including psychiatric treatment if indicated. Psychiatric consultation is indicated for patients who become severely anxious, suicidal, depressed, or overtly psychotic. In each instance, appropriate psychiatric medication can be prescribed to provide relief. Palliative care physicians must also be skilled in pain management, especially in the use of powerful opioids—the gold standard of drugs used for pain relief. Pain management is discussed in further detail at the end of this chapter.

    B. Euthanasia and physician-assisted suicide. Euthanasia is defined as a physician's deliberate act to cause a patient's death by directly administering a lethal dose of medication or other agent (sometimes called *mercy killing*). It is illegal and unethical. Physician-assisted suicide is defined as a physician's imparting information or providing means that enable a person to take his or her own life deliberately. Physician-assisted suicide and euthanasia should not be confused with palliative care designed to alleviate the suffering of dying patients.

    C. Ethical issues. Euthanasia and physician-assisted suicide are opposed by the American Medical Association and the American Psychiatric Association. In Oregon, physicians are legally permitted to prescribe lethal medication for patients who are terminally ill (1994 Oregon Death with Dignity Law [Table 27-1]).

    D. End-of-life decisions. The principle of patient autonomy requires that physicians respect the decision of a patient to forego life-sustaining treatment. Life-sustaining treatment is defined as any medical treatment that serves to prolong life without reversing the underlying medical condition. It includes, but is not limited to, mechanical ventilation, renal dialysis, blood

Table 27-1
Oregon's Assisted Suicide Law

- Oregon residents whose physicians determine they have less than 6 months to live are eligible to ask for suicide medication.
- A second doctor must determine if the patient is mentally competent to make the decision and is not suffering from mental illness such as depression.
- The law does not compel doctors to comply with patients' requests for suicide medication.
- Doctors who agree to provide medication must receive a request in writing from the patient, signed by two witnesses. The written request must be made 48 hours before the doctor delivers the prescription. A second oral request is made just before the doctor writes the prescription.
- Pharmacists who are opposed to suicide may refuse to fill the prescriptions.
- The law does not specify which medication may be used. Supporters of the law say an overdose of barbiturates combined with antinausea medication would probably be used.

transfusions, chemotherapy, antibiotics, and artificial nutrition and hydration. Patients *in extremis* should never be forced to endure intolerable, prolonged suffering in an effort to prolong life.

II. Grief, Mourning, and Bereavement

Generally synonymous terms that describe a syndrome precipitated by the loss of a loved one. Attempts have been made to characterize the stages of grief, which are listed in Table 27-2. Characteristics of bereavement in parents and children are listed in Table 27-3.

Table 27-2
Grief and Bereavement

Stage	John Bowlby	Stage	CM Parkes
1	**Numbness or protest.** Characterized by distress, fear, and anger. Shock may last moments, days, or months.	1	**Alarm.** A stressful state characterized by physiologic changes (e.g., rise in blood pressure and heart rate); similar to Bowlby's first stage.
2	**Yearning and searching for the lost figure.** World seems empty and meaningless, but self-esteem remains intact. Characterized by preoccupation with lost person, physical restlessness, weeping, and anger. May last several months or even years.	2	**Numbness.** Person appears superficially affected by loss but is actually protecting himself or herself from acute distress.
3	**Disorganization and despair.** Restlessness and aimlessness. Increase in somatic preoccupation, withdrawal, introversion, and irritability. Repeated reliving of memories.	3	**Pining (searching).** Person looks for or is reminded of the lost person. Similar to Bowlby's second stage.
		4	**Depression.** Person feels hopeless about future, cannot go on living, and withdraws from family and friends
4	**Reorganization.** With establishment of new patterns, objects, and goods, grief recedes and is replaced by cherished memories. Healthy identification with deceased occurs.	5	**Recovery and reorganization.** Person realizes that his or her life will continue with new adjustments and different goods.

Table 27-3
Bereavement in Patients and Children

Loss of a Parent	Loss of a Child
Protest phase. Child has strong desire for the deceased parent.	May be a more intense experience than the death of an adult.
Despair phase. Child experiences hopelessness, withdrawal, and apathy.	Feelings of guilt and helplessness may be overwhelming.
Detachment phase. Child relinquishes emotional attachment to dead parent.	Stages of shock, denial, anger, bargaining, and acceptance occur.
Child may transfer need for a parent to one or more adults.	Manifestations of grief may last a lifetime.
	Up to 50% of marriages in which a child dies end in divorce.

Grief can occur for reasons other than the actual death of a loved one. These reasons include (1) loss of a loved one through separation, divorce, or incarceration; (2) loss of an emotionally charged object or circumstance (e.g., a prized possession or valued job or position); (3) loss of a fantasized love object (e.g., therapeutic abortion or death of an intrauterine fetus); and (4) loss resulting from narcissistic injury (e.g., amputation, mastectomy).

Grief is normal and differs from depression in a number of ways, described in Table 27-4. Risk factors for a major depressive episode after the death of a spouse are listed in Table 27-5. Complications of bereavement are listed in Table 27-6.

CLINICAL HINTS: GRIEF MANAGEMENT AND THERAPY

- *Encourage the ventilation of feelings. Allow the patient to talk about loved ones. Reminiscing about positive experiences can be helpful.*
- *Do not tell a bereaved person not to cry or get angry.*
- *Try to have a small group of people who knew the deceased talk about him or her in the presence of the grieving person.*
- *Do not prescribe antianxiety or antidepressant medication on a regular basis. If the person becomes acutely agitated, it is better to offer verbal comfort than a pill. However, small doses of medications (5 mg of diazepam [Valium]) may help in the short term.*
- *Frequent short visits are better than a few long visits.*
- *Be aware of delayed grief reaction, which occurs some time after a death and may be marked by behavioral changes, agitation, lability of mood, and substance abuse. Such reactions may occur close to the anniversary of a death (anniversary reaction).*
- *An anticipatory grief reaction occurs in advance of loss and can mitigate acute grief reaction at the actual time of loss. This can be a useful process if it is recognized when occurring.*
- *Be aware that the person grieving for a family member who died by suicide may not want to talk about his or her feelings of being stigmatized.*

Table 27-4
Grief Versus Depression

Grief	Depression
Normal identification with deceased. Little ambivalence toward deceased.	Abnormal overidentification with deceased. Increased ambivalence and unconscious anger toward deceased.
Crying, weight loss, decreased libido, withdrawal, insomnia, irritability, decreased concentration, and attention.	Similar.
Suicidal ideas rare.	Suicidal ideas common.
Self-blame relates to how deceased was treated.	Self-blame is global. Person thinks he or she is generally bad or worthless.
No global feelings of worthlessness.	Usually evokes interpersonal annoyance or irritation.
Evokes empathy and sympathy.	
Symptoms abate with time. Self-limited. Usually clears within 6 months to 1 year.	Symptoms do not abate and may worsen. May still be present after years.
Vulnerable to physical illness.	Vulnerable to physical illness.
Responds to reassurance and social contacts.	Does not respond to reassurance and pushes away social contacts.
Not helped by antidepressant medication.	Helped by antidepressant medication.

Table 27-5
Risk Factors for Major Depressive Episode After Death of a Spouse

History of depression, major depressive disorder, dysthymic disorder, depressive personality disorder, bipolar disorder
Under 30 years of age
Poor general health
Limited social support system
Unemployment
Poor adaptation to the loss

Table 27-6
Complications of Bereavement

Disturbance in the process of grief
   Absent or delayed grief
   Exaggerated grief
   Prolonged grief
Increased vulnerability to adverse effects
   General medical morbidity
   Mortality
   Psychiatric disorders
     Anxiety disorders
     Substance use disorders
     Depressive disorders

Adapted from and courtesy of Sidney Zisook, M.D.

Table 27-7
Death and Dying (Reactions of Dying Patients): Elisabeth Kübler-Ross

Stage 1	**Shock and denial.** Patient's initial reaction is shock, followed by denial that anything is wrong. Some patients never pass beyond this state and may go doctor shopping until they find one who supports their position.
Stage 2	**Anger.** Patients become frustrated, irritable, and angry that they are ill; they ask. "Why me?" Patients in this stage are difficult to manage because their anger is displaced onto doctors, hospital staff, and family. Sometimes anger is directed at themselves in the belief that illness has occurred as punishment for wrongdoing.
Stage 3	**Bargaining.** Patient may attempt to negotiate with physicians, friends, or even God, that in return for a cure, he or she will fulfill one or many promises (e.g., give to charity, attend church regularly).
Stage 4	**Depression.** Patient shows clinical signs of depression, withdrawal, psychomotor retardation, sleep disturbances, hopelessness, and possibly suicidal ideation. The depression may be a reaction to the effects of illness on his or her life (e.g., loss of job, economic hardship, isolation from friends and family), or it may be in anticipation of the actual loss of life that will occur shortly.
Stage 5	**Acceptance.** Person realizes that death is inevitable and accepts its universality.

III. Death and Dying

The reactions of patients to being told by a physician that they have a terminal illness vary. The reactions are described as a series of stages by thanatologist Elisabeth Kübler-Ross (Table 27-7).

Be aware that stages do not always occur in sequence. Shifts from one stage to another may occur. Moreover, children under 5 years of age do not appreciate death; they see it as a separation, similar to sleep. Between 5 and 10 years of age, they become increasingly aware of death as something that happens to others, particularly parents. After 10 years of age, children conceptualize death as something that can happen to them. Table 27-8 summarizes some essential features in the management of the dying patient.

Table 27-8
Essential Features in the Management of the Dying Patient

- **Concern:** Empathy, compassion, and involvement are essential; concern is ranked as the quality most appreciated by patients.
- **Competence:** Skills and knowledge can be as reassuring as warmth and concern. In particular, health care providers must adeptly manage the main medical and psychiatric complications of terminal illness: pain, nausea, shortness of breath, and hopelessness. Patients benefit immeasurably from the reassurance that their providers will not allow them to live or die in pain.
- **Communication:** Open lines of communication are essential in every stage of illness and dying, without exception.
- **Children:** Allowing children or family members who want to visit the dying patient to do so is generally advisable; family provides consolation to dying patients.
- **Cohesion:** Cohesion between the patient, family members, and caretakers maximizes patient support and helps the family through bereavement.
- **Cheerfulness:** A gentle, appropriate sense of humor can be palliative; a somber or anxious demeanor should be avoided.
- **Consistency:** Continuing, persistent attention is highly valued by patients, who often fear that they are a burden and will be abandoned; consistent physician involvement mitigates these fears.

CLINICAL HINTS: BREAKING BAD NEWS

- *Do not have a rigid attitude (e.g., "I always tell the patient"); let the patient be your guide. Many patients will want to know the diagnosis, whereas others will not. Determine what the patient already knows and understands about the prognosis.*
- *Do not stifle hope or break through a patient's denial if that is the major defense. If the patient refuses to obtain help as a result of denial, gently and gradually help the patient to understand that help is necessary and available.*
- *Reassure the patient that he or she will be taken care of regardless of behavior.*
- *Stay with the patient for a period of time after informing him or her of the condition or diagnosis. Encourage the patient to ask questions and provide truthful answers. Indicate that you will return to answer any questions that the patient or family may have.*
- *Make a return visit after a few hours, if possible, to check on the patient's reaction. If the patient exhibits anxiety that cannot be coped with, 5 mg of diazepam can be prescribed as needed for 24 to 48 hours.*
- *Advise family members of the medical facts. Encourage them to visit and allow the patient to talk of his or her fears.*
- *Always check for the presence of living will or do not resuscitate (DNR) wishes of the patient or family. Try to anticipate their wishes regarding life-sustaining procedures.*
- *Alleviate pain and suffering. There is no reason for withholding narcotics for fear of dependence in a dying patient. Pain management should be vigorous.*

IV. Pain

Pain is a complex symptom consisting of a sensation underlying potential disease and an associated emotional state. Acute pain is a reflex biologic response to injury. By definition, chronic pain is pain that lasts at least 6 months. A physiologic classification of pain is listed in Table 27-9, and characteristics of pain are listed in Table 27-10.

V. Pain Management

Patients who fear death fear pain most of all. Those who fear death less also wish for a painless (i.e., peaceful death). Thus, it cannot be overemphasized that pain management is essential. A good pain regimen may require several drugs or the same drug used in different ways and administered via different routes. For example, intravenous morphine may be supplemented by self-administered oral "rescue" doses, or a continuous epidural drip may be supplemented by bolus intravenous doses. Transdermal patches may provide baseline concentrations in patients for whom intravenous or oral intake is difficult.

VI. Analgesia

Analgesia is the loss or absence of pain. The most effective analgesics are the narcotics (drugs derived from opium or an opiumlike substance), which relieve pain, alter mood and behavior, and have the potential to cause dependence and

Table 27-9
Physiologic Classification of Pain

Type	Subtypes	Example	Comment
Nociceptive	Somatic Visceral	Bone metastasis Intestinal obstruction	Caused by activation of pain- sensitive fibers; usually aching or pressure.
Neuropathic	Peripheral Central Somatic Visceral Sympathetic-dependent Non-sympathetic- dependent	Causalgia Thalamic pain Causalgia Visceral pain in paraplegics Postherpetic pain Phantom pain	Caused by interruption of afferent pathways. Pathophysiology poorly understood, with most syndromes probably involving both peripheral and central nervous system changes. Usually dysesthetic, often burning and lancinating.
Psychogenic	Somatization disorder Psychogenic pain Hypochondriasis Specific pain diagnoses with organic contribution	Failed low back Atypical facial pain Chronic headache	Does not include factitious disorders (i.e., malingering, Munchausen's syndrome).

Adapted from Berkow R, ed. *Merck Manual.* 15th ed. Rahway, NJ: Merck, Sharp & Dohme Research
Laboratories, 1987:1341, with permission.

tolerance. *Opioids* is a generic term that includes drugs that bind to opioid receptors and produce a narcotic effect. They are most useful in the short-term management of severe, acute, serious pain. A goal should be to lower the pain level so that the patient can eat and sleep with minimal upset. A guideline should be to give the drug at the request of the patient. The self-administration by patients with pain of measured amounts of narcotics through an intravenous pump, when carried out in a hospital, is a new approach to pain control that is proving effective. The major opioid analgesics are listed in Table 27-11.

A. Nonnarcotic analgesics. Typical of this group is aspirin. Unlike narcotic analgesics, which act on the central nervous system (CNS), salicylates act at the peripheral or local level—the site of origin of the pain. Usually taken every 3 hours.

With most analgesics, peak plasma concentrations occur in 45 minutes, and analgesic effects last 3 to 4 hours. Other nonsteroidal anti-inflammatory drugs (NSAIDs) can also be used for analgesia (200 to 400 mg of ibuprofen every 4 hours). Drug equivalents: 650 mg of aspirin = 32 mg of codeine = 65 mg of propoxyphene (Darvon) = 50 mg of oral pentazocine (Talwin).

Table 27-10
Characteristics of Somatic and Neuropathic Pain

Somatic Pain	Neuropathic Pain
Nociceptive stimulus usually evident	No obvious nociceptive stimulus
Usually well localized; visceral pain may be referred	Often poorly localized
Similar to other somatic pains in patient's experience	Unusual, dissimilar from somatic pain
Relieved by anti-inflammatory or narcotic analgesics	Only partially relieved by narcotic analgesics

Adapted from Braunwald E, Isselbacher K, Petersdorf RG, et al. *Harrison's Principles of Internal
Medicine,* 11th ed. *Companion Handbook.* New York, McGraw-Hill, 1988:1.

Table 27-11
Opioid Analgesics for Management of Pain

Drug and Equianalgesic Dose Relative Potency	Dose (mg IM or oral)	Plasma Half-Life (hours)	Starting Oral Dose[a] (mg)	Commercial Available Preparations
Opioid agonists				
Morphine	10 IM 60 oral	3–4	30–60	Oral: tablet, liquid, slow-release tablet Rectal: 5–30 mg Injectable: SC, IM, IV, epidural, intrathecal
Hydromorphone	1.5 IM 7.5 oral	2–3	2–48	Oral: tablets—1, 2, 4 mg Injectable: SC, IM, IV 2, 3, and 10 mg/mL
Methadone	10 IM 20 oral	12–24	5–10	Oral: tablets, liquid Injectable: SC, IM, IV
Levorphanol	2 IM 4 oral	12–16	2–4	Oral: tablets Injectable: SC, IM, IV
Oxymorphone	1 IM	2–3	NA	Rectal: 10 mg Injectable: SC, IM, IV
Heroin	5 IM 60 oral	3–4	NA	NA
Meperidine	75 IM 300 oral	3–4 (normeperidine 12–16)	75	Oral: tablets Injectable: SC, IM, IV
Codeine	30 IM 200 oral	3–4	60	Oral; tablets and combination with acetylsalicylic acid, acetaminophen, liquid
Oxycodone	15 oral 30 oral 80 oral	— Long-acting (12-hour OxyContin)	5	Oral: tablets, liquid, oral formulation in combination with acetaminophen (tablet and liquid) and aspirin (tablet)

The time of peak analgesia in nontolerant patients ranges from ½ to 1 hour, and the duration from 4 to 6 hours. The peak analgesic effect is delayed, and the duration is prolonged after oral administrations.
[a]Recommended starting IM doses; the optimal dose for each patient is determined by titration, and the maximal dose is limited by adverse effects.

B. Placebos. Substances with no known pharmacologic activity that act through suggestion rather than biologic action. It has recently been demonstrated, however, that naloxone (Narcan), an opioid antagonist, can block the analgesic effects of a placebo, which suggests that a release of endogenous opioids may explain some placebo effects.

Long-term treatment with placebos should never be undertaken when patients have clearly stated an objection to such treatment. Furthermore, deceptive treatment with placebos seriously undermines patients' confidence in their physicians. Finally, placebos should not be used when an effective therapy is available.

For more detailed discussion of this topic, see Chapter 27, Section 27.9, End-of-Life and Palliative Care, p. 2288 and Section 27.15, Management of Chronic Pain, p. 2387, in CTP/X.

28

Psychotherapies

I. Definition

Psychotherapy is a therapeutic process to treat psychological problems by way of establishing a relationship between a trained professional and an individual. This treatment modality is established through therapeutic communication, both verbal and nonverbal, attempts to alleviate the emotional disturbance, reverse or change maladaptive patterns of behavior, and encourage personality growth and development. It is distinguished from other forms of psychiatric treatment such as somatic therapies (e.g., psychopharmacology and convulsive therapies).

II. Psychoanalysis and Psychoanalytic Psychotherapy

These two forms of treatment are based on Sigmund Freud's theories of a dynamic unconscious and psychological conflict. The major goal of these forms of therapy is to help the patient develop insight into unconscious conflicts, based on unresolved childhood wishes and manifested as symptoms, and to develop more adult patterns of interacting and behaving.

A. Psychoanalysis. Psychoanalysis is a theory of human mental phenomena and behavior, a method of psychic investigation and research, and a form of psychotherapy originally formulated by Freud. As a method of treatment, it is the most intensive and rigorous of this type of psychotherapy. The patient is seen three to five times a week, generally for a minimum of several hundred hours over a number of years. The patient lies on a couch with the analyst seated behind, out of the patient's visual range. The patient attempts to say freely and without censure whatever comes to mind, to associate freely, so as to follow as deeply as possible the train of thoughts to their earliest roots. As a technique for exploring the mental processes, psychoanalysis includes the use of free association and the analysis and interpretation of dreams, resistances, and transferences. The analyst uses interpretation and clarification to help the patient work through and resolve conflicts that have been affecting the patient's life, often unconsciously. Psychoanalysis requires that the patient be stable, highly motivated, verbal, and psychologically minded. The patient also must be able to tolerate the stress generated by analysis without becoming overly regressed, distraught, or impulsive. As a form of psychotherapy, it uses the investigative technique, guided by Freud's libido and instinct theories and by ego psychology, to gain insight into a person's unconscious motivations, conflicts, and symbols and thus to effect a change in maladaptive behavior.

B. Psychoanalytically psychotherapy. Based on the same principles and techniques as classic psychoanalysis, but less intense. There are two types: (1) insight-oriented or expressive psychotherapy and (2) supportive or relationship psychotherapy.

1. **Expressive psychotherapy.** Patients are seen one to two times a week and sit up facing the psychiatrist. The goal of resolution of unconscious psychological conflict is similar to that of psychoanalysis, but a greater emphasis is placed on day-to-day reality issues and a lesser emphasis on the development of transference issues. Patients suitable for psychoanalysis are suitable for this therapy, as are patients with a wider range of symptomatic and characterologic problems. Patients with personality disorders are also suitable for this therapy. A comparison of psychoanalysis and psychoanalytically oriented psychotherapy is presented in Table 28-1.

2. **Supportive psychotherapy.** In supportive psychotherapy, the essential element is support rather than the development of insight. This type of therapy often is the treatment of choice for patients with serious ego vulnerabilities, particularly psychotic patients. Patients in a crisis situation, such as acute grief, also are suitable. This therapy can be continued on a long-term basis and last many years, especially in the case of patients with chronic problems. Support can take the form of limit setting, increasing reality testing, reassurance, advice, and help with developing social skills.

C. **Brief psychodynamic psychotherapy.** A short-term treatment, generally consisting of 10 to 40 sessions during a period of less than 1 year. The goal, based on psychodynamic theory, is to develop insight into underlying conflicts; such insight leads to psychological and behavioral changes.

   This therapy is more confrontational than the other insight-oriented therapies in that the therapist is very active in repeatedly directing the patient's associations and thoughts to conflictual areas. The number of hours is explicitly agreed on by the therapist and patient before the beginning of therapy, and a specific, circumscribed area of conflict is chosen to be the focus of treatment. More extensive change is not attempted. Patients suitable for this therapy must be able to define a specific central problem to be addressed and must be highly motivated, psychologically minded, and able to tolerate the temporary increase in anxiety or sadness that this type of therapy can evoke. Patients who are not suitable include those with fragile ego structures (e.g., suicidal or psychotic patients) and those with poor impulse control (e.g., borderline patients, substance abusers, and antisocial personalities).

   There are several methods, each having its own treatment technique and specific criteria for selecting patients; however, they are more similar than different. Some of the types of brief psychodynamic therapy are:

1. **Brief focal psychotherapy (Tavistock—Malan)**
   Therapists should formulate a circumscribed focus and set a termination date in advance, and patients should work through grief and anger about termination.

Table 28-1
Scope of Psychoanalytic Practice: A Clinical Continuum[a]

Feature	Psychoanalysis	Psychoanalytic Psychotherapy	
		Expressive Mode	**Supportive Mode**
Frequency	Regular, 4–5 times a week, 30- to 50-min session.	Regular, 1–3 times a week, half to full hour.	Flexible, once a week or less or as needed, half to full hour.
Duration	Long term, usually 3–5+ yrs.	Short term or long term, several sessions to months of years.	Short term or intermittent long term; single session to lifetime.
Setting	Patient primarily on couch with analyst out of view.	Patient and therapist face to face; occasional use of couch.	Patient and therapist face to face; couch contraindicated.
Modus operandi	Systematic analysis of all (positive and negative) transference and resistance; primary focus on analyst and intrasession events; transference neurosis facilitated; regression encouraged.	Partial analysis of dynamics and defenses; focus on current interpersonal events and transference to others outside sessions; analysis of negative transference; positive transference left unexplored unless it impedes progress; limited regression encouraged.	Formation of therapeutic alliance and real object relationship; analysis of transference contraindicated with rare exceptions; focus on conscious external events; regression discouraged.
Analyst– therapist role	Absolute neutrality; frustration of patient; reflector–minor role.	Modified neutrality; implicit gratification of patient and great activity.	Neutrality suspended; limited explicit gratification, direction, and disclosure.
Putative change agents	Insight predominates within relatively deprived environment.	Insight within empathic environment; identification with benevolent object.	Auxiliary or surrogate ego as temporary substitute; holding environment; insight to degree possible.
Patient population	Neuroses; mild character psychopathology.	Neuroses; mild to moderate character psychopathology, especially narcissistic and borderline personality disorders.	Severe character disorders; latent or manifest psychoses; acute crises; physical illness.
Patient requisites	High motivation; psychological- mindedness; good previous object relationships; ability to maintain transference neurosis; good frustration tolerance.	High to moderate motivation and psychological- mindedness; ability to form therapeutic alliance; some frustration tolerance.	Some degree of motivation and ability to form therapeutic alliance.
Basic goals	Structural reorganization of personality; resolution of unconscious conflicts; insight into intrapsychic events; symptom relief an indirect result.	Partial reorganization of personality and defenses; resolution of preconscious and conscious derivatives of conflicts; insight into current interpersonal events; improved object relations; symptom relief a goal or prelude to further exploration.	Reintegration of self and ability to cope; stabilization or restoration of preexisting equilibrium; strengthening of defenses; better adjustment or acceptance of pathology; symptom relief and environmental restructuring as primary goals.

(continued)

Table 28-1
Scope of Psychoanalytic Practice: A Clinical Continuum [a] *(Continued)*

		Psychoanalytic Psychotherapy	
Feature	**Psychoanalysis**	**Expressive Mode**	**Supportive Mode**
Major techniques	Free association method predominates; fully dynamic interpretation (including confrontation, clarification, and working through), with emphasis on genetic reconstruction.	Limited free association; confrontation, clarification, and partial interpretation predominate, with emphasis on here-and-now interpretation and limited genetic interpretation.	Free association method contraindicated; suggestion (advice) predominates; abreaction useful; confrontation, clarification, and interpretation in the here and now secondary; genetic interpretation contraindicated.
Adjunct treatment	Primarily avoided; if applied, all negative and positive meanings and implications thoroughly analyzed.	May be necessary (e.g., psychotropic drugs as temporary measure); if applied, negative implications explored and diffused.	Often necessary (e.g., psychotrophic drugs, family therapy, rehabilitative therapy, or hospitalization); If applied, positive implications are emphasized.

[a]This division is not categoric; all practices reside on a clinical continuum.
From Toksoz Byram Karasu, M.D.

2. **Time-limited psychotherapy (Boston University—Mann)**

A psychotherapeutic model of exactly 12 interviews focusing on a specified central issue and determining a patient's central conflict reasonably correctly and exploring young persons' maturational crises with many psychological and somatic complaints.

3. **Short-term dynamic psychotherapy (McGill University—Davanloo)**

This encompasses nearly all varieties of brief psychotherapy and crisis intervention. This includes flexibility (therapists should adapt the technique to the patient's needs), control, the patient's regressive tendencies, active intervention to avoid having the patient develop overdependence on a therapist, and the patient's intellectual insight and emotional experiences in the transference. These emotional experiences become corrective as a result of the interpretation.

4. **Short-term anxiety-provoking psychotherapy (Harvard University—Sifneos)**

Treatment can be divided into four major phases: patient–therapist encounter, early therapy, height of treatment, and evidence of change and termination.

The final phase of the therapy emphasizes the tangible demonstration of change in the patient's behavior outside therapy, evidence that adaptive patterns of behavior are being used, and initiation of talk about terminating the treatment.

III. Behavior Therapy

Behavior therapy focuses on overt and observable behavior and uses various conditioning techniques derived from learning theory to directly modify the patient's behavior. This therapy is directed exclusively toward symptomatic improvement, without addressing psychodynamic causation. Behavior therapy is based on the principles of learning theory, including operant and classical conditioning. Operant conditioning is based on the premise that behavior is shaped by its consequences; if behavior is positively reinforced, it will increase; if it is punished, it will decrease; and if it elicits no response, it will be extinguished. Classical conditioning is based on the premise that behavior is shaped by being coupled with or uncoupled from anxiety-provoking stimuli. Just as Ivan Pavlov's dogs were conditioned to salivate at the sound of a bell once the bell had become associated with meat, a person can be conditioned to feel fear in neutral situations that have come to be associated with anxiety. Uncouple the anxiety from the situation, and the avoidant and anxious behavior will decrease.

Behavior therapy is believed to be most effective for clearly delineated, circumscribed maladaptive behaviors (e.g., phobias, compulsions, overeating, cigarette smoking, stuttering, and sexual dysfunctions). In the treatment of conditions that can be strongly affected by psychological factors (e.g., hypertension, asthma, pain, and insomnia), behavioral techniques can be used to induce relaxation and decrease aggravating stresses (Table 28-2). There are several behavior therapy techniques.

A. **Token economy.** A form of *positive reinforcement* used with inpatients who are rewarded with various tokens for performing desired behaviors (e.g., dressing in street clothes, attending group therapy). Has been used to treat schizophrenia, especially in hospital settings. The tokens can be exchanged for a variety of positive reinforcers, such as food, television time, or a weekend pass.

B. **Aversion therapy.** A form of conditioning that involves the repeated coupling of an unpleasant or painful stimulus, such as an electric shock, with an undesirable behavior. In a less controversial form of aversion therapy, the patient couples imagining something unpleasant with the undesired behavior. Has been used to treat substance abuse.

C. **Systematic desensitization.** This technique is based on the behavioral principle of counterconditioning, whereby a person overcomes maladaptive anxiety elicited by a situation or object by approaching the feared situation gradually and in a psychophysiologic state that inhibits anxiety. Rather than use actual situations or objects that elicit fear, patients and therapists prepare a graded list or hierarchy of anxiety-provoking scenes associated with a patient's fears. The learned relaxation state and the anxiety-provoking scenes are systematically paired in treatment. Thus, the three steps are relaxation training, hierarchy construction, and desensitization of the stimulus. When this procedure is performed in real life rather in the imagination, it is called *graded exposure.*

D. **Therapeutic-graded exposure.** Similar to systematic desensitization, except that relaxation training is not involved and treatment is usually carried out in a real-life context. Exposure is graded according to a hierarchy. Patients afraid of cats, for example, might progress from looking at a picture of a cat to holding one.

Table 28-2
Some Common Clinical Applications of Behavior Therapy

Disorder	Comments
Agoraphobia	Graded exposure and flooding can reduce the fear of being in crowded places. About 60% of patients so treated are improved. In some cases, the spouse can serve as the model while accompanying the patient into the fear situation; however, the patient cannot get a secondary gain by keeping the spouse nearby and displaying symptoms.
Alcohol dependence	Aversion therapy, in which the alcohol-dependent patient is made to vomit (by adding an emetic to the alcohol) every time a drink is ingested, is effective in treating alcohol dependence. Disulfiram (Antabuse) can be given to alcohol-dependent patients when they are alcohol-free. Such patients are warned of the severe physiologic consequences of drinking (e.g., nausea, vomiting, hypotension, collapse) with disulfiram in the system.
Anorexia nervosa	Observe eating behavior; contingency management; record weight.
Bulimia nervosa	Record bulimic episodes; log moods.
Hyperventilation	Hyperventilation test; controlled breathing; direct observation.
Other phobias	Systematic desensitization has been effective in treating phobias, such as fears of heights, animals, and flying. Social skills training has also been used for shyness and fear of other people.
Paraphilias	Electric shocks or other noxious stimuli can be applied at the time of a paraphilic impulse, and eventually the impulse subsides. Shocks can be administered by either the therapist or the patient. The results are satisfactory but must be reinforced at regular intervals.
Schizophrenia	The token economy procedure, in which tokens are awarded for desirable behavior and can be used to buy ward privileges, has been useful in treating schizophrenic inpatients. Social skills training teaches schizophrenic patients how to interact with others in a socially acceptable way so that negative feedback is eliminated. In addition, the aggressive behavior of some schizophrenic patients can be diminished through those methods.
Sexual dysfunctions	Sex therapy, developed by William Masters and Virginia Johnson, is a behavior therapy technique used for various sexual dysfunctions, especially male erectile disorder, orgasm disorders, and premature ejaculation. It uses relaxation desensitization, and graded exposure as the primary techniques.
Shy bladder	Inability to void in a public bathroom; relaxation exercises.
Type A behavior	Physiologic assessment muscle relaxation, biofeedback (on electromyogram).

E. Flooding. A technique in which the patient is exposed immediately to the most anxiety-provoking stimulus (e.g., the top of a tall building if he or she is afraid of heights) instead of being exposed gradually or systematically to a hierarchy of feared situations. If this technique is carried out in the imagination rather than in real life, it is called *implosion*. Flooding is thought to be an effective behavioral treatment of such disorders as phobias, provided the patient can tolerate the associated anxiety. A great deal of experimental work is being done with exposure to the feared situations using virtual reality. Beneficial effects have been reported with computer-generated virtual reality exposure of patients with height phobia, fear of flying, arachnophobia, and claustrophobia.

F. Assertiveness training. A variety of techniques, including role modeling, desensitization, and positive reinforcement, are used to increase assertiveness. To be assertive requires that people have confidence in their judgment and sufficient self-esteem to express their opinions. Social skills training deals with assertiveness but also attends to a variety of real-life tasks, such as food shopping, looking for work, interacting with other people, and overcoming shyness.

G. **Eye movement desensitization and reprocessing (EMDR).** Saccadic eye movements are rapid oscillations of the eyes that occur when a person tracks an object that is moved back and forth across a line of vision. If the saccades are induced while the person is imagining or thinking about an anxiety-producing event, a few studies have demonstrated that a positive thought or image can be induced that results in decreased anxiety.

H. **Participant modeling.** Patients learn a new behavior by imitation, primarily by observation, without having to perform the behavior until they feel ready. It is useful with phobic children and used successfully with agoraphobia by having a therapist accompany a patient into the feared situation.

I. **Exposure to stimuli presented in virtual reality.** Beneficial effects have been reported with virtual reality exposure of patients with height phobia, fear of flying, spider phobia, and claustrophobia.

J. **Social skills training.** Most used in patients with Schizophrenia or schizophrenic like disorders, this type of therapy improves social skills. Social dysfunction is normalized by teaching the patient how to accurately read or decode social inputs. Role-playing is used to decrease social anxiety and improve social and conversational skills. It is usually done in groups.

IV. Cognitive–Behavioral Therapy

This therapy is based on the theory that behavior is determined by the way in which persons think about themselves and their roles in the world. Maladaptive behavior is secondary to ingrained, stereotyped thoughts, which can lead to cognitive distortions or errors in thinking. The theory is aimed at correcting cognitive distortions and the self-defeating behaviors that result from them. Therapy is on a short-term basis, generally lasting for 15 to 20 sessions during a period of 12 weeks. Patients are made aware of their own distorted cognitions and the assumptions on which they are based. Homework is assigned; patients are asked to record what they are thinking in certain stressful situations (e.g., "I'm no good" or "No one cares about me") and to ascertain the underlying, often relatively unconscious, assumptions that fuel the negative cognitions. This process has been referred to as "recognizing and correcting automatic thoughts." The cognitive model of depression includes the cognitive triad, which is a description of the thought distortions that occur when a person is depressed. The triad includes (1) a negative view of the self, (2) a negative interpretation of present and past experience, and (3) a negative expectation of the future (Table 28-3).

Cognitive therapy has been most successfully applied to the treatment of mild to moderate nonpsychotic depressions. It also has been effective as an adjunctive treatment in substance abuse and in increasing compliance with medication. It has been used recently to treat schizophrenia.

Table 28-3
General Assumptions of Cognitive Therapy

Perception and experiencing in general are active processes that involve both inspective and introspective data.
The patient's cognitions represent a synthesis of internal and external stimuli.
How persons appraise a situation is generally evident in their cognitions (thoughts and visual images).
Those cognitions constitute their stream of consciousness or phenomenal field, which reflects their configuration of themselves, their world, their past and future.
Alterations in the content of their underlying cognitive structures affect their affective state and behavioral pattern.
Through psychological therapy, patients can become aware of their cognitive distortions.
Correction of those faulty dysfunctional constructs can lead to clinical improvement.

Adapted from Beck AT, Rush AJ, Shaw BF, Emery G. *Cognitive Therapy of Depression.* New York: Guilford, 1979:47, with permission.

V. Family Therapy

Family therapy is based on the theory that a family is a system that attempts to maintain homeostasis, regardless of how maladaptive the system may be. This theory has been referred to as a "family systems orientation," and the techniques include focusing on the family rather than on the identified patient. The family therefore becomes the patient, rather than the individual family member who has been identified as sick. One of the major goals of a family therapist is to determine what homeostatic role, however pathologic, the identified patient is serving in the particular family system. A family therapist's goal is to help a family understand that the identified patient's symptoms in fact serve the crucial function of maintaining the family's homeostasis. One example is the triangulated child—the child who is identified by the family as the patient is actually serving to maintain the family system by becoming involved in a marital conflict as a scapegoat, referee, or even surrogate spouse. The therapist's job is to help the family understand the triangulation process and address the deeper conflict that underlies the child's apparent disruptive behavior. Techniques include reframing and positive connotation (a relabeling of all negatively expressed feelings or behaviors as positive); for example, "This child is impossible" becomes "This child is desperately trying to distract and protect you from what he or she perceives is an unhappy marriage."

Other goals of family therapy include changing maladaptive rules that govern a family, increasing awareness of cross-generational dynamics, balancing individuation and cohesiveness, increasing one-on-one direct communication, and decreasing blaming and scapegoating. Table 28-4 summarizes the principles in which the history of the family is examined in an effort to understand how that history informs the current familial interactions.

VI. Interpersonal Therapy

This is a short-term psychotherapy, lasting 12 to 16 weeks, developed specifically for the treatment of nonbipolar, nonpsychotic depression. Sessions 1 to

Table 28-4
Rationale for Family-Life Chronology

The family therapist enters a session knowing little or nothing about the family.
The therapist may know who the identified patient is and what symptoms the patient manifests, but that is usually all. So the therapist must get clues about the meaning of the symptom.
The therapist may know that pain exists in the marital relationship, but needs to get clues about how the pain shows itself.
The therapist needs to know how the mates have tried to cope with their problems.
The therapist may know that the mates both operate from models (from what they saw going on between their own parents), but needs to find out how those models have influenced each mate's expectations about how to be a mate and how to be a parent.
The family therapist enters a session knowing that the family, in fact, has had a history, but that is usually all.
Every family, as a group, has gone through or jointly experienced many events. Certain events (e.g., deaths, childbirth, sickness, geographical moves, and job changes) occur in almost all families.
Certain events primarily affect the mates and only indirectly the children. (Maybe the children were not born yet or were too young to fully comprehend the nature of an event as it affected their parents. They may have only sensed periods of parental remoteness, distraction, anxiety, or annoyance.)
The therapist can profit from answers to just about every question asked.
Family members enter therapy with a great deal of fear.
Therapist structuring helps decrease the threats. It says, "I am in charge of what will happen here. I will see to it that nothing catastrophic happens here."
All members are covertly feeling to blame that nothing seems to have turned out right (even though they may overtly blame the identified patient or the other mate).
Parents, especially, need to feel that they did the best they could as parents. They need to tell the therapist, "This is why I did what I did. This is what happened to me."
A family-life chronology that deals with such facts as names, dates, labeled relationships, and moves, seems to appeal to the family. It asks questions that members can answer, questions that are relatively nonthreatening. It deals with life as the family understands it.
Family members enter therapy with a great deal of despair.
Therapist structuring helps stimulate hope.
As far as family members are concerned, past events are part of them. They now can tell the therapist, "I existed." And they can also say, "I am not just a big blob of pathology. I succeeded in overcoming many handicaps."
If the family knew what questions needed asking, they would not need to be in therapy. So the therapist does not say, "Tell me what you want to tell me." Family members will simply tell the therapist what they have been telling themselves for years. The therapist's questions say, "I know what to ask. I take responsibility for understanding you. We are going to go somewhere."
The family therapist also knows that, to some degree, the family has focused on the identified patient to relieve marital pain. The therapist also knows that, to some degree, the family will resist any effort to change that focus. A family-life chronology is an effective, nonthreatening way to change from an emphasis on the "sick" or "bad" family member to an emphasis on the marital relationship.
The family-life chronology serves other useful therapy purposes, such as providing the framework within which a reeducation process can take place. The therapist serves as a model in checking out information or correcting communication techniques and placing questions and eliciting answers to begin the process. In addition, when taking the chronology, the therapist can introduce in a relatively nonfrightening way some of the crucial concepts to induce change.

Adapted from Satir V. *Conjoint Family Therapy*. Palo Alto, CA: Science and Behavior; 1967:57, with permission.

5 are initial phase, sessions 6 to 15 intermediate, and sessions 16 to 20 are the termination phase. Intrapsychic conflicts are not addressed. Emphasis is on current interpersonal relationships and on strategies to improve the patient's interpersonal life. Antidepressant medication is often used as an adjunct to interpersonal therapy. The therapist is very active in helping to formulate the patient's predominant interpersonal problem areas, which define the treatment focus (Table 28-5).

Table 28-5
Interpersonal Psychotherapy

Goal	Improvement in current interpersonal skills
Selection criteria	Outpatient, nonbipolar disorder, nonpsychotic depressive disorder
Duration	12–16 wks, usually once-weekly meetings
Technique	Reassurance
	Clarification of feeling states
	Improvement of interpersonal communication
	Testing perceptions
	Development of interpersonal skills
	Medication

From Ursano RJ, Silberman EK. Individual psychotherapies. In: Talbott JA, Hales RE, Yudofsky SC, eds. *The American Psychiatric Press Textbook of Psychiatry.* Washington, DC: American Psychiatric Press, 1988:868, with permission.

VII. Group Therapy

Group therapies are based on as many theories as are individual therapies. Groups range from those that emphasize support and an increase in social skills, to those that emphasize specific symptomatic relief, to those that work through unresolved intrapsychic conflicts. Compared with individual therapies, two of the main strengths of group therapy are the opportunity for immediate feedback from a patient's peers and the chance for both patient and therapist to observe a patient's psychological, emotional, and behavioral responses to a variety of people, who elicit a variety of transferences. Both individual and interpersonal issues can be resolved. Therapeutic factors in group therapy are listed in Table 28-6.

Groups tend to meet one to two times a week, usually for 1½ hours. They may be homogeneous or heterogeneous, depending on the diagnosis. Examples of homogeneous groups include those for patients attempting to lose weight or stop smoking, and groups whose members share the same medical or psychiatric problem (e.g., AIDS, posttraumatic stress disorder, substance use disorders). Certain types of patients do not do well in certain types of groups. Psychotic patients, who require structure and clear direction, do not do well in insight-oriented groups. Paranoid patients, antisocial personalities, and substance abusers can benefit from group therapy but do not do well in heterogeneous, insight-oriented groups. In general, acutely psychotic or suicidal patients do not do well in groups.

Table 28-6
Twenty Therapeutic Factors in Group Psychotherapy

Factor	Definition
Abreaction	A process by which repressed material, particularly a painful experience or conflict, is brought back to consciousness. In the process, the person not only recalls but relives the material, which is accompanied by the appropriate emotional response; insight usually results from the experience.
Acceptance	The feeling of being accepted by other members of the group; differences of opinion are tolerated; there is an absence of censure.

(continued)

Table 28-6
Twenty Therapeutic Factors in Group Psychotherapy *(Continued)*

Factor	Definition
Altruism	The act of one member's being of help to another; putting another person's need before one's own and learning that there is value in giving to others. The term was originated by Auguste Comte (1738–1857), and Sigmund Freud believed it was a major factor in establishing group cohesion and community feeling.
Catharsis	The expression of ideas, thoughts, and suppressed material that is accompanied by an emotional response that produces a state of relief in the patient.
Cohesion	The sense that the group is working together toward a common goal; also referred to as a sense of "we-ness"; believed to be the most important factor related to positive therapeutic effects.
Consensual validation	Confirmation of reality by comparing one's own conceptualizations with those of other group members; interpersonal distortions are thereby corrected. The term was introduced by Harry Stack Sullivan. Trigant Burrow had used the phrase *consensual observation* to refer to the same phenomenon.
Contagion	The process in which the expression of emotion by one member stimulates the awareness of a similar emotion in another member.
Corrective familial experience	The group recreates the family of origin for some members who can work through original conflicts psychologically through group interaction (e.g., sibling rivalry, anger toward parents).
Empathy	The capacity of a group member to put himself or herself into the psychological frame of reference of another group member and thereby understand his or her thinking, feeling, or behavior.
Identification	An unconscious defense mechanism in which the person incorporates the characteristics and the qualities of another person or object into his or her ego system.
Imitation	The conscious emulation or modeling of one's behavior after that of another (also called *role modeling*); also known *as spectator therapy,* as one patient learns from another.
Insight	Conscious awareness and understanding of one's own psychodynamics and symptoms of maladapting behavior. Most therapists distinguish two types: (1) intellectual insight—knowledge and awareness without any changes in maladaptive behavior; (2) emotional insight—awareness and understanding leading to positive changes in personality and behavior.
Inspiration	The process of imparting a sense of optimism to group members; the ability to recognize that one has the capacity to overcome problems; also known as *instillation of hope.*
Interaction	The free and open exchange of ideas and feelings among group members; effective interaction is emotionally charged.
Interpretation	The process during which the group leader formulates the meaning or significance of a patient's resistance, defenses, and symbols; the result is that the patient has a cognitive framework within which to understand his or her behavior.
Learning	Patients acquire knowledge about new areas, such as social skills and sexual behavior; they receive advice, obtain guidance, and attempt to influence and are influenced by other group members.
Reality testing	Ability of the person to evaluate objectively the world outside the self; includes the capacity to perceive oneself and other group members accurately. *See also consensual validation.*
Transference	Projection of feelings, thoughts, and wishes onto the therapist, who has come to represent an object from the patient's past. Such reactions, while perhaps appropriate for the condition prevailing in the patient's earlier life, are inappropriate and anachronistic when applied to the therapist in the present. Patients in the group may also direct such feelings toward one another, a process called *multiple transferences.*
Universalization	The awareness of the patient that he or she is not alone in having problems; others share similar complaints or difficulties in learning; the patient is not unique.
Ventilation	The expression of suppressed feelings, ideas, or events to other group members; the sharing of personal secrets that ameliorate a sense of sin or guilt (also referred to as *self-disclosure*).

A. **Alcoholics Anonymous (AA).** An example of a large, highly structured, peer-run group that is organized around persons with a similar central problem. AA emphasizes sharing experiences, role models, ventilation of feelings, and a strong sense of community and mutual support. Similar groups include Narcotics Anonymous (NA) and Sex Addicts Anonymous (SAA).

B. **Milieu therapy.** The multidisciplinary therapeutic approach used on inpatient psychiatric wards. The term *milieu therapy* reflects the idea that all activities on a ward are oriented toward increasing a patient's ability to cope in the world and relate appropriately to others. The treatment emphasizes appropriate socio-environmental manipulation for the benefit of the patient.

C. **Multiple family groups.** Composed of families of schizophrenic patients. The groups discuss issues and problems related to having a schizophrenic person in the family and share suggestions and means of coping. Multiple family groups are an important factor in decreasing relapse rates among the schizophrenic patients whose families participate in the groups.

VIII. Couple and Marital Therapy

As many as 50% of patients are estimated to enter psychotherapy primarily because of marital problems; another 25% experience marital problems along with their other presenting problems. Couple or marital therapy is designed to psychologically modify the interaction of two people who are in conflict with each other over one parameter or a variety of parameters—social, emotional, sexual, or economic. As in family therapy, the relationship rather than either of the individuals is viewed as the patient.

A. **Types of therapies**

1. **Individual therapy.** Partners may consult different therapists, who do not necessarily communicate with each other and the goal of treatment is to strengthen each partner's adaptive capacities.

2. **Individual couples therapy.** Each partner is in therapy, which is either concurrent, with the same therapist, or collaborative, with each partner seeing a different therapist.

3. **Conjoint therapy.** It is the most common treatment method in couples therapy and either one or two therapists treat the partners in joint sessions.

4. **Four-way session.** Each partner is seen by a different therapist in regular joint sessions and all four persons participate. A variation developed by William Masters and Virginia Johnson is used for the rapid treatment of sexually dysfunctional couples.

5. **Group psychotherapy.** Consists of three to four couples and two therapists. They explore sexual attitudes and have an opportunity to gain new information from their peer groups, and each receives specific feedback about his or her behavior, either negative or positive.

6. **Combined therapy.** Refers to all or any of the preceding techniques used concurrently or in combination.

IX. Dialectical Behavior Therapy

This form of therapy has been used successfully in patients with border-line personality disorder and parasuicidal behavior. It is eclectic, drawing on methods from supportive, cognitive, and behavioral therapies. Some elements are derived from Franz Alexander's view of therapy as a corrective emotional experience, and also from certain Eastern philosophical schools (e.g., Zen). Patients are seen weekly, with the goal of improving interpersonal skills and decreasing self-destructive behavior by means of techniques involving advice, use of metaphor, storytelling, and confrontation, among many others. Borderline patients especially are helped to deal with the ambivalent feelings that are characteristic of the disorder.

X. Hypnosis

Hypnosis is a complex mental state in which consciousness is altered in such a way that the subject is amenable to suggestion and receptive to direction by the therapist. When hypnotized, the patient is in a trance state, during which memories can be recalled and events experienced. The material can be used to gain insight into the makeup of a personality. Hypnosis is used to treat many disorders, including obesity, substance-related disorders (especially nicotine dependence), sexual disorders, and dissociative states.

XI. Guided Imagery

Used alone or with hypnosis. The patient is instructed to imagine scenes with associated colors, sounds, smells, and feelings. The scene may be pleasant (used to decrease anxiety) or unpleasant (used to master anxiety). Imagery has been used to treat patients with generalized anxiety disorders, posttraumatic stress disorder, and phobias, and as an adjunct therapy for medical or surgical disease.

XII. Biofeedback

Biofeedback provides information to a person about his or her physiologic functions, usually related to the autonomic nervous system (e.g., blood pressure), with the goal of producing a relaxed, euthymic mental state. It is based on the idea that the autonomic nervous system can be brought under voluntary control through operant conditioning. It is used in the management of tension states associated with medical illness (e.g., to increase hand temperature in patients with Raynaud's syndrome and to treat headaches and hypertension) (Table 28-7).

XIII. Paradoxical Therapy

In this approach, the therapist suggests that the patient intentionally engages in an unwanted or undesirable behavior (called *paradoxical injunction*)—for example, avoiding a phobic object or performing a compulsive ritual. This approach can create new insights for some patients.

Table 28-7
Biofeedback Applications

Condition	Effects
Asthma	Both frontal EMG and airway resistance biofeedback have been reported as producing relaxation from the panic associated with asthma, as well as improving air flow rate.
Cardiac arrhythmias	Specific biofeedback of the ECG has permitted patients to lower the frequency of premature ventricular contractions.
Fecal incontinence and enuresis	The timing sequence of internal and external anal sphincters has been measured with triple–lumen rectal catheters providing feedback to incontinent patients for them to reestablish normal bowel habits in a relatively small number of biofeedback sessions. An actual precursor of biofeedback dating to 1938 was the sounding of a buzzer for sleeping enuretic children at the first sign of moisture (the pad and bell).
Grand mal epilepsy	A number of EEG biofeedback procedures have been used experimentally to suppress seizure activity prophylactically in patients not responsive to anticonvulsant medication. The procedures permit patient to enhance the sensorimotor brain wave rhythm or to normalize brain activity as computed in real-time power spectrum displays.
Hyperactivity	EEG biofeedback procedures have been used on children with attention-deficit/hyperactivity disorder to train them to reduce their motor restlessness.
Idiopathic hypertension and orthostatic hypotension	A variety of specific (direct) and nonspecific biofeedback procedures—including blood pressure feedback, galvanic skin response, and foot-hand thermal feedback combined with relaxation procedures—have been used to teach patients to increase or decrease their blood pressure. Some follow-up data indicate that the changes may persist for years and often permit the reduction or elimination of antihypertensive medications.
Migraine	The most common biofeedback strategy with classic or common vascular headaches has been thermal biofeedback from a digit accompanied by autogenic self-suggestive phrases encouraging hand warming and head cooling. The mechanism is thought to help prevent excessive cerebral artery vasoconstriction, often accompanied by an ischemic prodromal symptom, such as scintillating scotomata, followed by rebound engorgement of arteries and stretching of vessel wall pain receptors.
Myofacial and temporomandibular joint pain	High levels of EMG activity over the powerful muscles associated with bilateral temporomandibular joints have been decreased by means of biofeedback in patients who are jaw clenchers or have bruxism.
Neuromuscular rehabilitation	Mechanical devices or an EMG measurement of muscle activity displayed to a patient increases the effectiveness of traditional therapies, as documented by relatively long clinical histories in peripheral nerve–muscle damage, spasmodic torticollis, selected cases of tardive dyskinesia, cerebral palsy, and upper motor neuron hemiplegias.
Raynaud's syndrome	Cold hands and cold feet are frequent concomitants of anxiety and also occur in Raynaud's syndrome, caused by vasospasm of arterial smooth muscle. A number of studies report that thermal feedback from the hand, an inexpensive and benign procedure compared with surgical sympathectomy, is effective in about 70% of cases of Raynaud's syndrome.
Tension headaches	Muscle contraction headaches are most frequently treated with two large active electrodes spaced on the forehead to provide visual or auditory information about the levels of muscle tension. The frontal electrode placement is sensitive to EMG activity in the frontalis and occipital muscles, which the patient learns to relax.

ECG, electrocardiogram; EMG, electromyogram.

XIV. Sex Therapy

In sex therapy, the therapist discusses the psychological and physiologic aspects of sexual functioning in great detail. Therapists adopt an educative attitude, and aids such as models of the genitalia and videotapes may be used. Treatment is on a short-term basis and behaviorally oriented. Specific exercises are prescribed, depending on the disorder being treated (e.g., graduated dilators for vaginismus). Usually, the couple is treated, but individual sex therapy is also effective.

XV. Narrative Psychotherapy

Narrative psychotherapy emerges out of increased interest in clinical stories. This therapy emerges from two different sides of psychiatry: narrative medicine and narrative psychotherapy. Narrative medicine uses narrative approaches to augment scientific understandings of illness. A major task of narrative psychotherapy is to be a good listener and to connect empathically with the patient's story. Narrative approaches are invaluable for psychotherapy integration because they provide a metatheoretical orientation from which to understand and practice psychotherapy.

XVI. Vocational Rehabilitation

Vocational rehabilitation is a centerpiece of psychiatric rehabilitation. It emphasizes independence rather than reliance on professionals, community integration rather than isolation in segregated settings for persons with disabilities, and patient preferences rather than professional goals. It includes a wide range of interventions designed to help people with disabilities caused by mental illness improve their functioning and quality of life by enabling them to acquire the skills and supports needed to be successful in usual adult roles and in the environments of their choice. Normative adult roles include living independently, attending school, working in competitive jobs, relating to family, having friends, and having intimate relationships.

XVII. Combined Therapy

Concurrent use of psychotropic drugs and psychotherapy is widespread and become the standard of care. In this therapeutic approach, psychotherapy is augmented by the use of pharmacologic agents. The term *pharmacotherapy-oriented psychotherapy* is used by some practitioners to refer to the combined approach. Whenever more than one clinician is involved in treatment, there should be regular exchanges of information. When a patient is in psychotherapy with someone other than the clinician prescribing medication, it is important to recognize treatment bias and to avoid contentious turf battles that put the patient in the middle of such conflict.

For more detailed discussion of this topic, see Chapter 33, Psychotherapies, p. 2638, in CTP/X.

29

Psychopharmacological Treatment and Nutritional Supplements

I. Introduction

 CLINICAL HINT:
Do not be the first doctor to prescribe a new drug or the last doctor to prescribe an old drug.

In recent years, psychiatric disorders and their impact on cognition has been a focus of interest. The discovery of new receptor subtypes, brain imaging and modulation of gene expression have led to greater understanding of the role that neurotransmitters and neural pathway play in the brain and consequently the development of receptor-specific targeted psychotropic drugs that are more efficacious, less toxic, and better tolerated. The term neuropsychopharmacology may be a more accurate and appropriate term to use considering the role of neurotransmitters, ligands, neuropeptides, and specific drugs being developed to target and manipulate these systems.

Medications for psychiatric disorders are called *psychotropic drugs* and are described by their major clinical application: *antidepressants, antipsychotics, mood stabilizers,* and *anxiolytics.* During the last decade, the definition of psychotropic drugs has evolved and instead of describing them by their clinical indication, the better approach has been to classify them based on mechanism of action. This is a fundamental shift in psychiatric thinking and conceptualization, and hence, it is preferable to think of drugs in terms of their pharmacologic actions rather than their therapeutic indications, which often change and overlap.

II. Basic Principles of Psychopharmacology

A. **Pharmacologic actions.** Pharmacologic actions are divided into two categories: pharmacokinetic and pharmacodynamic. In simple terms, *pharmacokinetics* describes *what the body does to the drug* and *pharmacodynamics* describes *what the drug does to the body*. Pharmacokinetic data trace the absorption, distribution, metabolism, and excretion of a drug in the body. Pharmacodynamic data measure the effects of a drug on cells in the brain and other tissues of the body.

1. **Pharmacokinetics**

a. **Absorption.** Orally administered drugs dissolve in the fluid of the gastrointestinal (GI) tract and then reach the brain through the bloodstream. Some drugs are available in *depot* preparations, which are injected intramuscularly (IM) once every 1 to 4 weeks. Intravenous (IV) administration is the quickest route for achieving therapeutic blood concentrations, but it also carries the highest risk for sudden and life-threatening adverse effects. Few drugs, however, are given in IV form.

b. **Distribution and bioavailability.** Drugs that circulate bound to plasma proteins are *protein-bound,* and those that circulate unbound are said to be *free*. Only the free fraction can pass through the blood–brain barrier. The *distribution* of a drug to the brain is promoted by high rates of cerebral blood flow, lipid solubility, and receptor affinity.

Bioavailability refers to the fraction of administered drug that can eventually be recovered from the bloodstream.

c. **Metabolism and excretion.** The four metabolic routes—*oxidation, reduction, hydrolysis,* and *conjugation*—usually produce metabolites that are readily excreted. Metabolism usually yields inactive metabolites that are more polar and therefore more readily excreted. However, metabolism also transforms many inactive prodrugs into therapeutically active metabolites. The liver is the principal site of *metabolism* (Table 29-1), and bile, feces, and urine are the major routes of *excretion*. Psychotherapeutic drugs are also excreted in body fluids such as sweat and saliva.

 CLINICAL HINT:
Drugs are excreted in breast milk, an important fact to be considered for mothers who want to nurse their children.

The *half-life* of a drug is the amount of time it takes for its plasma concentration to be reduced by half during metabolism and excretion. A greater number of daily doses are required for drugs with shorter half-lives than for drugs with longer half-lives. Drug interactions or disease states that inhibit the metabolism of psychoactive drugs can produce toxicity.

d. **Cytochrome P450 enzymes.** Most psychotherapeutic drugs are oxidized by the hepatic cytochrome P450 (CYP) enzyme system, which is so named because it absorbs light strongly at a wavelength of 450 nm.

The CYP enzymes are responsible for the inactivation of most psychotherapeutic drugs (see Table 29-1). Expression of the CYP genes may be induced by alcohol, by certain drugs (barbiturates, anticonvulsants), or by smoking. For example, an inducer of CYP 3A4, such as cimetidine, may increase the metabolism and decrease the plasma concentrations of a substrate of 3A4, such as alprazolam (Xanax). Administration of a CYP 2D6 inhibitor, such as fluoxetine (Prozac),

Table 29-1
Representative Psychotropic Drug Substrates of Human Cytochromes P450, Along With Representative Inhibitors

CYP 3A	CYP 2D6	CYP 2C19
Substrates	**Substrates**	**Substrates**
Triazolam (Halcion)	Desipramine (Norpramin)	Diazepam^a
Alprazolam (Xanax)	Nortriptyline (Aventyl)	Amitriptyline^a
Midazolam (Versed)	Paroxetine (Paxil)	Citalopram^a
Quetiapine (Seroquel)	Venlafaxine (Effexor)	
Nefazodone (Serzone)	Tramadol (Ultram)	**Inhibitors**
Buspirone (BuSpar)	Fluoxetine^a (Prozac)	Fluvoxamine
Trazodone (Desyrel)	Citalopram^a	Omeprazole (Prilosec)
Zolpidem^a (Ambien)		
Amitriptyline^a (Endep)	**Inhibitors**	
Imipramine^a (Tofranil)	Quinidine (Cardioquin)	
Haloperidol^a (Haldol)	Fluoxetine	
Citalopram^a (Celexa)	Paroxetine (Paxil)	
Clozapine^a (Clozaril)	Bupropion (Wellbutrin)	
Diazepam^a (Valium)	Terbinafine (Lamisil)	
	Diphenhydramine (Benadryl)	
Inhibitors		
Ritonavir (Norvir)		
Ketoconazole (Nizoral)		
Itraconazole (Sporanox)		
Nefazodone		
Fluvoxamine (Luvox)		
Erythromycin (E-Mycin)		
Clarithromycin (Biaxin)		

^{a}Indicates partial substrate.

may inhibit the metabolism and thus raise the plasma concentrations of CYP 2D6 substrates, including amitriptyline (Elavil).

e. Pharmacogenetics and pharmacogenomic testing. Genetics play a pivotal role in understanding illnesses and response to medications. Pharmacogenomics is defined as an individual's genetic variability to drug response and is an emerging and evolving field in psychiatry. The field of genetics in behavioral health so far has mostly been limited to epidemiology. Its utility in clinical practice is limited though it has some utility for psychotropic drugs. The principles of pharmacogenomic testing are categorized into pharmacodynamic and pharmacokinetic genes. The former set of genes illustrate the effect of the drug on the body and help in identifying drug candidate selection while the latter indicates the effect of the body on the drug through metabolism and determines drug dosage.

2. Pharmacodynamics. The major pharmacodynamic considerations include the molecular site of action, dose–response curve, therapeutic index, and development of tolerance, dependence, and withdrawal symptoms.

a. Molecular site of action. The *molecular site of action* is determined in laboratory assays and may or may not correctly identify the drug–receptor interactions responsible for a drug's clinical effects, which are identified empirically in clinical trials.

b. **Dose–response curve.** The *dose–response curve* plots the effects of a drug against its plasma concentration. *Potency* refers to the ratio of drug dosage to clinical effect. For example, risperidone (Risperdal) is more potent than olanzapine (Zyprexa) because about 4 mg of risperidone is required to achieve the comparable therapeutic effect of 20 mg of olanzapine. However, because both are capable of eliciting a similar beneficial response at their respective optimal dosages, the *clinical efficacies* of risperidone and olanzapine are equivalent.

c. **Therapeutic index.** The *therapeutic index* is the ratio of a drug's toxic dosage to its maximally effective dosage. Pharmacogenetic studies are beginning to identify genetic polymorphisms linked to individual differences in treatment response and sensitivity to side effects.

 CLINICAL HINT:
Lithium has a low therapeutic index, so that close monitoring of plasma concentrations is required to avoid toxicity.

---

d. **Tolerance, dependence, and withdrawal symptoms.** When a person becomes less responsive to a particular drug with time, *tolerance* to the effects of the drug has developed. The development of tolerance can be associated with the appearance of physical *dependence,* which is the need to continue taking a drug to prevent the appearance of *withdrawal symptoms.*

III. Clinical Guidelines

Optimizing the results of psychotropic drug therapy involves consideration of the six *D*s: diagnosis, drug selection, dosage, duration, discontinuation, and dialogue.

A. **The six *D*s**

1. **Diagnosis.** A careful diagnostic investigation should identify specific target symptoms with which the drug response can be objectively assessed.

2. **Drug selection.** Factors that determine drug selection include diagnosis, past personal and family history of response to a particular agent, and the overall medical status of the patient. Certain drugs will be excluded because concurrent drug treatment of medical and other psychiatric disorders creates a risk for drug–drug interactions. Other drugs will be excluded because they have unfavorable adverse effect profiles. A choice of the ideal drug should emerge based on the clinician's experience and preferences.

The Drug Enforcement Administration (DEA) has classified drugs according to their potential for abuse (Table 29-2), and clinicians are advised to use caution when prescribing controlled substances.

Table 29-2
Characteristics of Drugs at Each Drug Enforcement Agency Level

DEA Control Level (Schedule)	Characteristics of Drug at Each Control Level	Examples of Drugs at Each Control Level
I	High abuse potential No accepted use in medical treatment in the United States at the present time and, therefore, not for prescription use Can be used for research	Lysergic acid diethylamide (LSD), heroin, marijuana, peyote, 3,4-methylenedioxymethamphetamine (MDMA), methcathinone, gamma hydroxybutyrate (GHB), phencyclidine (PCP), mescaline, psilocybin, nicocodeine, nicomorphine
II	High abuse potential Severe physical dependence liability Severe psychological dependence liability No refills; no telephone prescriptions	Amphetamine, opium, morphine, codeine, hydromorphone, phenmetrazine, amobarbital, secobarbital, pentobarbital, methylphenidate, ketamine
III	Abuse potential less than levels I and II Moderate or low physical dependence liability High psychological liability Prescriptions must be rewritten after 6 months or five refills	Glutethimide, methyprylon, nalorphine, sulfonmethane, benzphetamine, phendimetrazine, chlorphentermine; compounds containing codeine, morphine, opium, hydrocodone, dihydrocodeine, naltrexone, diethylpropion, dronabinol
IV	Low abuse potential Limited physical dependence liability Limited psychological dependence Prescriptions must be rewritten after 6 months or five refills	Phenobarbital, benzodiazepines,[a] chloral hydrate, ethchlorvynol, ethinamate, meprobamate, paraldehyde, phentermine
V	Lowest abuse potential of all controlled substances	Narcotic preparations containing limited amounts of nonnarcotic active medicinal ingredients

[a]In New York State benzodiazepines are treated as schedule II substances, which require a triplicate prescription for a maximum of 1 month's supply.

3. **Dosage.** The two most common causes of failure of psychotropic drug treatment are inadequate dosing and an incomplete therapeutic trial of a drug.

4. **Duration**. For antipsychotic, antidepressant, and mood-stabilizing drugs, a therapeutic trial should continue for 4 to 6 weeks. In the treatment of these conditions, drug efficacy tends to improve with time, whereas drug discontinuation is frequently associated with relapses. In contrast, for most anxiolytic and stimulant drugs, the maximum therapeutic benefit is usually evident within an hour of administration.

5. **Discontinuation.** Many psychotropic agents are associated with a discontinuation syndrome when they are stopped. Drugs with a short-half life are most prone to causing these withdrawal symptoms, especially if they are stopped abruptly after extended use. It is thus important to discontinue all drugs as slowly as possible, if clinical circumstances permit.

6. **Dialogue.** Informing patients about likely side effects at the outset of treatment, as well as the reasons they are taking a specific drug, serves to improve treatment compliance. Clinicians should distinguish between probable or expected adverse effects and rare or unexpected adverse effects.

B. Special considerations

1. Children. Begin with a small dosage and increase until clinical effects are observed. Do not hesitate to use adult dosages in children if the dosage is effective and no adverse effects develop. Some children need higher doses because their livers metabolize drugs more quickly than adults. Special caution should be used when prescribing selective serotonin reuptake inhibitors (SSRIs) in children because of the risk suicidality, which is discussed below.

2. The elderly. Begin treating elderly patients with a small dosage, usually approximately one-half the usual dosage. The dosage should be increased in small amounts, until either a clinical benefit is achieved or unacceptable adverse effects appear.

3. Pregnant and nursing women. Clinicians are best advised to avoid administering any drug to a woman who is pregnant (particularly during the first trimester) or nursing a child. This rule, however, occasionally needs to be broken when the mother's psychiatric disorder is severe. It has been suggested that withdrawing a drug during pregnancy could cause a discontinuation syndrome in both mother and fetus. Most psychotropic drugs have not been linked to an increased rate of specific birth defects.

4. Medically ill persons. Medically ill persons should be treated conservatively, which means beginning with a small dosage, increasing it slowly, and watching for both clinical and adverse effects. If applicable, plasma drug concentrations are helpful during the treatment of these persons.

IV. Anxiolytics and Hypnotics

A. Treatment recommendations

1. Treatment of acute anxiety. Acute anxiety responds best to either oral or parenteral administration of benzodiazepines. In the presence of mania or psychosis, a benzodiazepine in combination with antipsychotics is appropriate.

2. Treatment of chronic anxiety

a. Antidepressants. Selective serotonin reuptake inhibitors (SSRis) like (fluoxetine) and serotonin–norepinephrine reuptake inhibitors (SNRIs) such as venlafaxine (Effexor) and duloxetine (Cymbalta) are antidepressants that are used for the control of chronic anxiety disorders, including panic disorder and obsessive-compulsive disorder (OCD). All antidepressants may increase anxiety when they are started.

b. Benzodiazepines. Benzodiazepines may be used on a long-term basis for the treatment of generalized anxiety symptoms and panic disorder.

 CLINICAL HINT:
Careful monitoring of benzodiazepine use should be done with long-term use. If the patient starts to increase the dose, tolerance and dependence should be considered.

c. **Buspirone (BuSpar).** Buspirone is approved by the Food and Drug Administration (FDA) for the treatment of anxiety disorders, specifically generalized anxiety disorder.

d. **Mirtazapine (Remeron).** Mirtazapine is effective for the treatment of anxiety symptoms, but its utility is limited by its marked sedative qualities and the tendency for increased appetite and weight gain.

e. **Other treatments.** Monoamine oxidase inhibitors (MAOIs) and tricyclic and tetracyclic drugs are effective in treating anxiety, but are not used as first-line agents because of side effects and safety concerns.

3. **Treatment of insomnia**

a. **Nonbenzodiazepines.** The nonbenzodiazepine agents zolpidem (Ambien), eszopiclone (Lunesta), and zaleplon (Sonata) have a rapid onset of action, specifically target insomnia, lack muscle relaxant and anticonvulsant properties, are completely metabolized within 4 or 5 hours, and rarely cause withdrawal symptoms or rebound insomnia. The usual bedtime dose of each (zolpidem and eszopicline) is 10 mg. Zolpidem is said to be effective for 5 hours and zaleplon for 4 hours. The usual dose for eszopiclone is 2 mg that can be increased to 3 mg. Adverse events may include dizziness, nausea, and somnolence. Ramelteon (Rozerem) is another newly approved medication that acts at the melatonin receptor to help induce sleep. The usual starting and maintenance dose is 8 mg but some patients may need up to 16 mg. These medications are now considered "first-line" therapies for insomnia, and have advantages over benzodiazepines which cause tolerance and dependence.

b. **Benzodiazepines.** Benzodiazepines shorten sleep latency and increase sleep continuity, so that they are useful for the treatment of insomnia. The five benzodiazepines used primarily as hypnotics are flurazepam (Dalmane), temazepam (Restoril), quazepam (Doral), estazolam (ProSom), and triazolam (Halcion).

Benzodiazepines also curtail sleep stages III and IV (deep or slow-wave sleep) and are useful for sleepwalking and night terrors, which occur in those stages of sleep. Benzodiazepines suppress disorders related to rapid eye movement (REM) sleep, most notably violent behavior during REM sleep (REM behavior disorder).

c. **Trazodone (Desyrel).** Low-dose trazodone, 25 to 100 mg at bedtime, is widely used to treat insomnia. It has a favorable effect on sleep architecture.

d. **Quetiapine (Seroquel).** This serotonin dopamine antagonist is often used as an off-label medicine in a dosage of 25 to 100 mg for insomnia but may cause daytime somnolence and sedation.

e. **Ramelteon (Rozerem).** Ramelteon is an orally active hypnotic, and is indicated for the treatment of insomnia characterized by difficulty with sleep onset. It is a melatonin receptor agonist, with high binding affinity at the melatonin MT1 and MT2 receptors, and mimics and enhances the action of endogenous melatonin, which has been associated with maintenance of circadian sleep rhythm. It should be used with caution in patients taking other medicines that inhibit CYP 1A2, 2C9 and 3A4 activity, as this may increase the AUC of Ramelteon many 50- to 200-fold. The most commonly observed adverse effects are somnolence, dizziness, nausea, fatigue, headache, and insomnia. It is recommended that it should not be taken with or immediately after a high-fat meal.

A number of clinical and animal trials of Ramelteon did not yield evidence of formation of physical dependence or abuse potential, and it is not a controlled substance. Recently the FDA issued a warning for patients taking Ramelteon. Severe anaphylactic and anaphylactoid reactions with angioedema involving the tongue, glottis or larynx have been reported leading to airway obstruction and could be fatal. Patients who develop angioedema after treatment with Ramelteon should not be rechallenged with the drug. As with other hypnotics, patients are advised to avoid hazardous activities (including the operation of heavy machinery or vehicles) and tasks requiring concentration following dosing. Complex behaviors such as "sleep-driving" (i.e., driving while not fully awake) and other complex behaviors (e.g., preparing and eating food, making phone calls, or having sex), with amnesia for the event, have been reported in association with hypnotic use. It is available in an 8-mg strength tablet, and the usual dose is 8 mg taken within 30 minutes of going to bed.

f. **Suvorexant (Belsomra).** It is indicated for the treatment of insomnia characterized by difficulties with sleep onset and/or sleep maintenance. Its therapeutic effect is through highly selective antagonism of orexin receptors OX1R and OX2R. It can be taken with or without food but for faster sleep onset should not be taken with or soon after a meal. It is metabolized through CYP 3A4 with steady-state achieved in 3 days. The recommended dose is 10 mg, taken no more than once per night and within 30 minutes of going to bed, with at least 7 hours remaining before the planned time of awakening. Exposure is increased in obese patients and dose should be halved when used with CYP 3A4 inhibitors. The most common side effects are somnolence, amnesia, anxiety, hallucinations, as well as worsening of depression and suicidal ideation. It is contraindicated in narcolepsy. Coadministration with central nervous system (CNS) depressants may increase risk for CNS depression.

g. **Gabapentin (Neurontin).** Gabapentin was first introduced as an antiepileptic drug and was found to have sedative effects that were useful in some psychiatric disorders, especially insomnia. It is used as an off-label drug for anxiety conditions and insomnia. Gabapentin circulates in the blood largely unbound and is not appreciably metabolized in humans. It is eliminated unchanged by renal excretion and can be removed by hemodialysis. Food only moderately affects the rate and extent of absorption. Clearance is decreased in elderly persons, requiring dosage adjustments. Most common side effects are daytime somnolence, ataxia, and fatigue. The usual hypnotic dose range is between 600 and 900 mg.

B. Benzodiazepine agonists and antagonists. Fifteen benzodiazepines are available for clinical use in the United States (Table 29-3). They are widely prescribed, with at least 10% of the population using one of these drugs each year. They are safe, effective, and well tolerated in both short- and long-term use. The pharmacologic effects of the benzodiazepines are listed in Table 29-4.

1. Indications. Benzodiazepines are often used to augment the effects of antidepressant drugs during the first month of use, before the antidepressant drug has begun to exert its anxiolytic effects; they are then tapered once the antidepressant becomes effective.

2. Choice of drug. The most important differences among the benzodiazepines relate to potency and elimination half-life.

a. Potency. High-potency benzodiazepines, such as alprazolam (Xanax), alprazolam XR, and clonazepam (Klonopin), are effective in suppressing panic attacks. In general, at doses needed to control panic attacks, low-potency benzodiazepines, such as diazepam, may produce unwanted sedation.

b. Duration of action. Diazepam (Valium) and triazolam (Halcion) are readily absorbed and have a rapid onset; chlordiazepoxide (Librium) and oxazepam (Serax) work more slowly.

Compounds with a long half-life tend to accumulate with repeated dosing, so that the risk for excessive daytime sedation, difficulties with concentration and memory, and falls is increased. Rates of hip fractures resulting from falls are higher in elderly persons taking long-acting drugs than in those taking more rapidly eliminated compounds. Benzodiazepines with short half-lives also have the advantage of causing less impairment with regular use. However, they appear to produce a more severe withdrawal syndrome. Drugs affecting the rate of elimination of benzodiazepines are listed in Table 29-5.

c. Dependence and withdrawal symptoms. A major concern with long-term benzodiazepine use is the development of dependence, particularly with high-potency agents. Not only can discontinuation of benzodiazepines result in symptom recurrence and rebound, but it can also precipitate withdrawal symptoms. Several factors contribute to the development of benzodiazepine withdrawal symptoms (Table 29-6). Drug type and duration of use are the most significant factors, but other considerations such as personality makeup are also important. Despite these concerns benzodiazepines can be used long-term in select groups of patients with close and careful monitoring.

Table 29-3
Half-Lives, Doses, and Preparations of Benzodiazepine Receptor Agonists and Antagonists

Drug	Dose Equivalents	Half-Life (hours)	Rate of Absorption	Usual Adult Dosage	Dose Preparations
Agonists					
Clonazepam	0.5	Long (metabolite, >20)	Rapid	1–6 mg b.i.d.	0.5-, 1.0-, and 2.0-mg tablets
Diazepam	5	Long (>20) (nordiazepam—long, >20)	Rapid	4–40 mg b.i.d. to q.i.d.	2-, 5-, and 10-mg tablets (slow-release 15-mg capsules)
Alprazolam	0.25	Intermediate (6–20)	Medium	0.5–10 mg b.i.d. to q.i.d.	0.25-, 0.5-, 1.0-, and 2.0-mg tablets
Lorazepam	1	Intermediate (6–20)	Medium	1–6 mg t.i.d.	0.5-, 1.0-, and 2.0-mg tablets, 2 mg/mL, 4 mg/mL parenteral
Oxazepam	15	Intermediate (6–20)	Slow	30–120 mg t.i.d. or q.i.d.	10-, 15-, and 30-mg capsules (15-mg)
Temazepam	5	Intermediate (6–20)	Medium	7.5–30 mg hs	7.5-, 15-, and 30-mg capsules
Chlordiazepoxide	10	Intermediate (6–20) (demethyl-chlordiazepoxide–intermediate, 6–20) (demoxapam—long, >20) (nordiazepam—long, >20)	Medium	10–150 mg t.i.d. or q.i.d.	5-, 10-, and 25-mg tablets and capsules
Flurazepam	5	Short (<6) (N-hydroxyethyl-flurazepam—short, <6) (N-desalkylflurazepam—long, >20)	Rapid	15–30 mg hs	15- and 30-mg capsules
Triazolam	0.1–0.03	Short (<6)	Rapid	0.125 mg or 0.250 mg hs	0.125- or 0.250-mg tablets
Clorazepate	7.5	Short (<6) (nordiazepam—long, >20)	Rapid	15–60 mg b.i.d. or q.i.d.	3.75-, 7.5-, and 15-mg tablets (slow-release 11.25- and 22.5-mg tablets)
Halazepam	20	Short (<6) (nordiazepam—long, >20)	Medium	60–160 mg t.i.d. or q.i.d.	20- and 40-mg tablets
Prazepam	10	Short (<6) (nordiazepam—long, >20)	Slow	30 mg (20–60 mg) q.i.d. or t.i.d.	5-, 10-, or 20-mg capsules
Estazolam	0.33	Intermediate (6–20) (4-hydroxye-stazolam— intermediate, 6–20)	Rapid	1.0 or 2.0 hs	1- and 2-mg tablets
Quazepam	5	Long (>20) (2-oxoquazepam-N-desalkylflurazepam—long, >20)	Rapid	7.5 or 15 mg hs	7.5- and 15-mg tablets
Midazolam	1.25–1.3	Short (<6)	Rapid	5–50 mg parenteral	5 mg/mL parenteral, 1-, 2-, 5-, and 10-mL vials
Zolpidem	2.5	Short (<6)	Rapid	5 mg or 10 mg hs	5- and 10-mg tablets
Zaleplon	2	Short (1)	Rapid	10 mg hs	5- and 10-mg capsules
Antagonist					
Flumazenil	0.06	Short (<6)	Rapid	0.2–0.5 mg/min injection over 3–10 min (total, 1–5 mg)	0.1 mg/mL (5- and 10-mL vials)

Table 29-4
Pharmacologic Effects of Benzodiazepines

Effects	Clinical Application/Consequences
Therapeutic effects	
Sedative	Insomnia, conscious sedation, alcohol withdrawal
Anxiolytic	Panic attacks, generalized anxiety
Anticonvulsant	Seizures
Muscle relaxant	Muscle tension, muscle spasm
Amnestic	Adjunct to chemotherapy or anesthesia
Antistress	Mild hypertension, irritable bowel syndrome, angina
Adverse effects	
Sedative	Daytime sleepiness, impaired concentration
Amnestic	Mild forgetfulness, anterograde memory impairment
Psychomotor	Accidents, falls
Behavioral	Depression, agitation
Decreased CO_2 response	Worsening of sleep apnea and other obstructive pulmonary disorders
Withdrawal syndrome	Dependence—anxiety, insomnia, excess sensitivity to light, excess sensitivity to sound, tachycardia, mild systolic hypertension, tremor, headache, sweating, abdominal distress, craving, seizures

d. Use during pregnancy. Benzodiazepine use in pregnancy has been a controversial issue and older studies and clinical data suggest increased risk of oral cleft. Recent data of pooled analyses show no association between fetal benzodiazepine exposure and oral cleft or other major congenital malformations. No long-term effects on IQ or neurodevelopment have been reported. At this time the risk of teratogenicity is insufficient but mothers should weigh risk benefits and provided with available conflicting information to make an informed decision.

CLINICAL HINT:
Withdrawal symptoms can mimic signs and symptoms of the underlying disorder. Do not unnecessarily continue the drug when this occurs.

Table 29-5
Drugs Affecting the Rate of Elimination of Oxidized Benzodiazepines

Increase Elimination Half-Life	Decrease Elimination Half-Life
Cimetidine	Chronic ethyl alcohol use
Propranolol	Rifampin
Oral contraceptives (estrogens)	
Chloramphenicol	
Propoxyphene	
Isoniazid	
Disulfiram	
Allopurinol	
Tricyclic antidepressants	
Acute ethyl alcohol use	

Table 29-6
Key Factors in the Development of Benzodiazepine Withdrawal Symptoms

Factor	Explanation
Drug type	High-potency, short half-life compounds (e.g., alprazolam, triazolam, lorazepam)
Duration of use	Risk increases with time
Dose level	Higher doses increase risk
Rate of discontinuation	Abrupt withdrawal instead of taper increases risk for severe symptoms, including seizures
Diagnosis	Panic disorder patients more prone to withdrawal symptoms
Personality	Patients with passive-dependent, histrionic, somatizing, or asthenic traits more likely to experience withdrawal.

3. **Benzodiazepine antagonist.** Flumazenil (Romazicon) is a benzodiazepine antagonist used to reverse the effects of benzodiazepine receptor agonists in overdose and in clinical situations such as sedation or anesthesia. It has also been used to reverse benzodiazepine effects immediately before the administration of ECT. Adverse effects include nausea, vomiting, and agitation. Flumazenil can precipitate seizures, particularly in persons who have seizure disorders, who are dependent on benzodiazepines, or who have taken large overdoses. The usual regimen is to give 0.2 mg intravenously over 30 seconds. If consciousness is not regained, an additional 0.3 mg can be given intravenously over 30 seconds. Most persons respond to a total of 1 to 3 mg. Doses larger than 3 mg are unlikely to add benefit.

V. Antipsychotic Drugs

These are classified into first-generation (conventional) antipsychotics or second-generation antipsychotics (SDAs, novel or atypical) antipsychotics. Historically, conventional antipsychotics were efficacious for treating the positive symptoms of schizophrenia with worsening of negative, cognitive, and mood symptoms. Atypical antipsychotics have been suggested to show improvement in (1) positive symptoms such as hallucinations, delusions, disordered thoughts, and agitation and (2) negative symptoms such as withdrawal, flat affect, anhedonia, poverty of speech, catatonia, and cognitive impairment. There has been controversy regarding the benefits of atypical antipsychotics compared to conventional antipsychotics. NIMH-funded research studies like the CATIE trial has brought attention to the long-term metabolic complications of atypical antipsychotics and showing no significant advantages over conventional antipsychotics. Overall atypical antipsychotic agents represent a major advance in the pharmacologic treatment for schizophrenia. The clinicians are advised to determine the best course of treatment based on individual patient taking into account risk–benefit analysis in the long-term.

A. **Second-generation antipsychotic drugs (SDAs, atypical antipsychotic drugs).** The original second-generation antipsychotic drugs include risperidone (Risperdal), risperidone consta (long acting), olanzapine, quetiapine (Seroquel), quetiapine XR (Seroquel XR), ziprasidone (Geodon), aripiprazole (Abilify), paliperidone (Invega), and clozapine (Clozaril). In recent times, newer agents have become available and are described in detail below. These drugs improve three classes of disability typical of schizophrenia: (1) positive symptoms (hallucinations, delusions, disordered thoughts, agitation); (2) negative symptoms (withdrawal, flat affect, anhedonia, catatonia); and (3) cognitive impairment (perceptual distortions, memory deficits, inattentiveness). Second-generation drugs have largely replaced the typical antipsychotics (dopamine receptor antagonists) because they are associated with a lower risk of extrapyramidal symptoms and eliminate the need for anticholinergic drugs. Second-generation drugs are also effective for the treatment of bipolar disorder and mood disorders with psychotic or manic features. A few are also approved for the treatment of bipolar depression, major depressive disorder (MDD), and will also have an indication in generalized anxiety disorder. All of these drugs except clozapine are FDA-approved for the treatment of bipolar I mania. Olanzapine is approved for bipolar I maintenance therapy.

1. **Pharmacologic actions**
   a. **Risperidone.** About 80% of risperidone is absorbed from the GI tract, and the combined half-life of risperidone averages 20 hours so that it is effective in once-daily dosing.
   b. **Olanzapine.** Approximately 85% of olanzapine is absorbed from the GI tract, and its half-life averages 30 hours. Therefore, it is also effective in once-daily dosing.
   c. **Quetiapine.** Quetiapine is rapidly absorbed from the GI tract. Its half-life is about 6 hours so that dosing two or three times per day is necessary. Quetiapine XR has a comparable bioavailability to equivalent dose of quetiapine administered two to three times daily. Quetiapine XR is given once daily preferable in the evening.
   d. **Ziprasidone.** Ziprasidone is well absorbed. Its half-life is 5 to 10 hours so that twice-daily dosing is optimal.
   e. **Clozapine.** Clozapine is absorbed from the GI tract. Its half-life is 10 to 16 hours and is taken twice daily.
   f. **Aripiprazole.** Aripiprazole is well absorbed from the GI tract. It has a long half-life of about 75 hours and can be given as a single daily dose. Aripiprazole extended-release injection reaches peak concentration in 5 to 7 days with a half-life of 30 days and given intradeltoid or intragluteal every 4 weeks.
   g. **Paliperidone.** Paliperidone has a peak plasma concentration of approximately 24 hours after dosing. It is available only in extended-release tablets, usually prescribed at 3 mg once daily. The paliperidone palmitate extended-release injection (Sustenna) reaches higher concentration in the deltoid muscle with a half-life of 25 to 49 days. It is given as an intramuscular injection on a monthly basis. Another injectable formulation (Trinza) has even longer duration of action and is given once every 3 months. Peak concentration

is reached in 30 days with elimination half-life of 84 to 140 days depending on site of injection.

h. Iloperidone. Iloperidone is well absorbed. Its elimination half-life varies based on CYP 2D6 metabolism. The dosing is twice daily, titrated slowly to prevent orthostatic hypotension and requires dose adjustment in CYP 2D6 poor metabolizers and with CYP 2D6 inhibitors.

i. Asenapine. Asenapine is rapidly absorbed with a half-life of 24 hours. Highly protein bound (95%), it is taken sublingually once daily.

j. Lurasidone. Lurasidone is rapidly absorbed with peak concentration in 1 to 3 and elimination half-life of 18 hours. It is given once daily with at least 350 calories of food for improved absorption. Dose adjustment is recommended in renal and hepatic impairment.

k. Brexpiprazole. Brexpiprazole is highly protein bound (99%), reaches peak concentration in 4 hours and has a half-life of 91 hours. It is taken once daily with titration over 8 days based on tolerability.

l. Cariprazine. Cariprazine reaches peak concentration in 3 to 6 hours and has a half-life of 2 to 4 days for cariprazine and 1 to 3 weeks for the metabolite. It is highly protein bound (97%), and is dosed once daily with titration over several days based on tolerability.

m. Pimavanserin. Pimavanserin has a half-life of 57 hours and reaches steady-state concentration in 12 days. It is taken once daily with no dose titration but dose adjustment is necessary with CYP 3A4 inhibitors or inducers.

2. Therapeutic indications. Second-generation drugs are effective for initial and maintenance treatment of psychosis in schizophrenia and schizoaffective disorders in both adults and adolescents. They are also effective in the acute treatment of manic or mixed episodes in bipolar disorder, bipolar depression, adjunctive therapy to antidepressants for MDD and for psychoses of all types—secondary to head trauma, dementia, and drug-induced psychosis. Aripiprazole (Abilify), quetiapine (Seroquel), and brexpiprazole (Rexulti) are the only medications approved by the FDA for add-on treatment to antidepressants for adults with MDD. Olanzapine and fluoxetine combination is indicated for use in treatment-resistant depression. Other SDAs are in the process of receiving this indication and extending it to GAD as well. Second-generation drugs are effective in acutely ill and treatment-refractory persons and prevent relapses. By comparison to persons treated with dopamine receptor antagonists, persons treated with second-generation drugs require less frequent hospitalization, fewer emergency room visits, less phone contact with mental health professionals, and less treatment in day programs.

The parenteral form of olanzapine is indicated for the treatment of acute agitation associated with schizophrenia and bipolar disorder, while ziprasidone is indicated for the treatment of agitation related to schizophrenia. Aripiprazole (Abilify) injection is indicated for the acute treatment of agitation associated with schizophrenia or bipolar disorder, manic or mixed in adults.

 CLINICAL HINT:
Because clozapine can cause severe agranulocytosis, it should be used only in refractory cases of schizophrenia. Clozapine provides a therapeutic niche for patients with severe tardive dyskinesias, unmanageable extrapyramidal symptoms, refractory bipolar disorder, and psychosis secondary to antiparkinsonian drugs.

---

3. **Clinical guidelines.** Dosing for the second-generation drugs vary considerably. Table 29-7 summarizes the usual dosing recommendations for these agents.

a. **Risperidone.** Risperidone is available in 0.25-, 0.5-, 1-, 2-, 3-, and 4-mg tablets, in M-tab form (rapidly dissolving), and as an oral solution with a concentration of 1 mg/mL. The initial dosage is usually 1 to 2 mg/day, taken at night. It can then be raised gradually (by 1 mg every 2 or 3 days) to 4 to 6 mg at night. Dosages higher than 6 mg/day are associated with increased adverse effects. Dosages below 6 mg/day have generally not been associated with extrapyramidal symptoms, but dystonic and dyskinetic reactions have been seen at dosages of 4 to 16 mg/day. The long-acting intramuscular form (Consta) should be initiated at 25 mg and the oral formulation should be continued for 2 weeks prior to discontinuation. The dosage may be increased to 37.5 mg depending on patient response and clinician discretion.

b. **Olanzapine.** Olanzapine is available in 2.5-, 5-, 7.5-, 10-, 15- and 20-mg oral and Zydis form (orally disintegrating) tablets. The initial dosage is usually 10 to 15 mg once daily. A starting dosage of 5 mg/day is recommended for elderly and medically ill persons and for persons with hepatic impairment or hypotension. The dosage can be raised to 20 mg/day after 5 to 7 days. Dosages in clinical use range from 5 to 20 mg/day, but benefit in both schizophrenia and bipolar mania is noted in most people at dosages of 10 to 15 mg/day. The intramuscular formulation for the treatment of agitation associated with schizophrenia and bipolar disorder is 10 mg. Coadministration with benzodiazepines is not approved. The higher dosages are occasionally associated with increased extrapyramidal and other adverse effects. Assessment of transaminases in patients with significant hepatic disease should be done periodically.

c. **Quetiapine.** Quetiapine is available in 25-, 100-, 200-, and 300-mg tablets. The dosage should begin at 25 mg twice daily and can be raised by 25 to 50 mg per dose every 2 to 3 days up to a target dosage of 400 to 500 mg/day, divided into two daily doses. Studies have shown efficacy in the range of 300 to 800 mg/day, with most people

Table 29-7
Comparison of Usual Dosing[a] for Some Available Second-Generation Antipsychotics in Schizophrenia

Antipsychotic	Typical Starting Dosage	Maintenance Therapy Dose Range	Titration	Maximum Recommended Dosage
Aripiprazole (Abilify)	10–15-mg tablets once a day	10–30 mg/day	Dosage increases should not be made before 2 weeks	30 mg/day
Asenapine (Saphris)	5 mg twice a day	0 mg twice a day	Titration not necessary	20 mg/day
Clozapine (Clozaril)	12.5-mg tablets once or twice a day	150–300 mg/day in divided doses or 200 mg as a single dose in the evening	The dosage should be increased to 25–50 mg on the second day. Further increases may be made in daily increments of 25–50 mg to a target dosage of 300–450 mg/day. Subsequent dosage increases should be made no more than once or twice weekly in increments of no more than 100 mg.	900 mg/day
Iloperidone (Fanapt)	1 mg twice a day	12–24 mg a day in divided dose	Start at 1 mg twice a day than move to 2, 4, 6, 8 and 12 mg twice a day. Do this over the course of 7 days	24 mg/day
Lurasidone (Latuda)	40 mg/day	40–80 mg/day	Titration not necessary	120 mg/day
Olanzapine (Zyprexa)	5–10-mg/day tablets or orally disintegrating tablets	10–20 mg/day	Dosage increments of 5 mg once a day are recommended when required at intervals of not less than 1 week.	20 mg/day
Paliperidone (Invega)	3–9-mg extended-release tablets once a day	3–6 mg/day	Plasma concentration rises to a peak approximately 24 hours after dosing	12 mg/day
Quetiapine (Seroquel)	25-mg tablets twice a day	Lowest dose needed to maintain remission	Increase in increments of 25–50 mg two or three times a day on the second and the third day, as tolerated, to a target dosage of 500 mg daily by the fourth day (given in two or three doses/day). Further dosage adjustments, if required, should be of 25–50 mg twice a day and occur at intervals of not fewer than 2 days.	800 mg/day

(continued)

Table 29-7

Comparison of Usual Dosing[a] for Some Available Second-Generation Antipsychotics in Schizophrenia *(Continued)*

Antipsychotic	Typical Starting Dosage	Maintenance Therapy Dose Range	Titration	Maximum Recommended Dosage
Risperidone (Risperdal)	1-mg tablet and oral solution once a day	2–6 mg once a day	Starting dose: 25 mg every 2 weeks	50 mg for 2 weeks
Risperidone IM long-acting (Consta)	25–50 mg IM injection every 2 weeks	Start with oral risperidone for 3 weeks	Increase to 2 mg once a day on the second day and 4 mg once a day on the third day. In some patients, a slower titration may be appropriate. When dosage adjustments are necessary, further dosage increments of 1–2 mg/day at intervals of not less than 1 week are recommended.	1–6 mg/day
Ziprasidone (Geodon)	20-mg capsules twice a day with food	20–80 mg twice a day	Dosage adjustments based on individual clinical status may be made at intervals of not fewer than 2 days.	80 mg twice a day
Ziprasidone (IM)	For acute agitation: 10–20 mg, as required, up to a maximum of 40 mg/day	Not applicable	For acute agitation: Doses of 10 mg may be administered every 2 hours, and doses of 20 mg may be administered every 4 hours up to a maximum of 40 mg/day.	For acute agitation: 40 mg/day, for not more than 3 consecutive days

[a]Dosage adjustments may be required in special populations.

Note: Information taken from U.S. Prescribing Information for individual agents.

IM, intramuscular.

receiving maximum benefit at 300 to 500 mg/day. Quetiapine XR is given once daily preferably in the evening without food or a light meal to prevent increase in Cmax. The usual starting dosage is 300 mg and may be increased to 400 to 800 mg.

d. Ziprasidone. Ziprasidone is available in 20-, 40-, 60-, and 80-mg capsules. Dosing should be initiated at 40 mg/day, divided into two daily doses. Studies have shown efficacy in the range of 40 to 200 mg, divided into two daily doses; taken with meals, the absorption is increased up to twofold.

e. Clozapine. Clozapine is available in 25- and 100-mg tablets. The initial dosage is usually 25 mg one or two times daily, although a conservative initial dosage is 12.5 mg twice daily. The dosage can then be raised gradually (by 25 mg every 2 or 3 days) to 300 mg/day, usually divided into two daily doses, with the higher dose in the evening. Dosages of up to 900 mg/day can be used, although most patients respond in the 600 mg/day range.

f. Aripiprazole. Aripiprazole is available in 2-, 5-, 10-, 15-, 20-, and 30-mg tablets. The recommended starting and target dose is 10 to 15 mg/day given once a day. Dosages higher than 10 to 15 mg/day have not shown increased efficacy in clinical trials. The recommended starting dose for aripiprazole as adjunctive treatment for patients already taking an antidepressant is 2 to 5 mg/day. The efficacy of aripiprazole as an adjunctive therapy for MDD was established within a dose range of 2 to 15 mg/day. Dose adjustments of up to 5 mg/day should occur gradually, at intervals of no less than 1 week. The most commonly reported dose-related adverse effect is somnolence.

Aripiprazole extended-release injectable (Maintena). It is available as 300 and 400 mg per vial. It is administered by intramuscular injection with starting and maintenance dose of 400 mg given every 4 weeks.

Aripiprazole Lauroxil extended-release injection (Aristada). It is available as 441, 662, and 882 mg per vial. It is administered either into deltoid muscle (441 mg only) or gluteal muscle (441, 662, or 882 mg). It is initiated at 441 or 662 mg and administered every 4 weeks or 882 mg every 6 weeks.

g. Paliperidone. Paliperidone is available in 3-, 6-, and 9-mg extended-release tablets. The usual dose is 3 to 6 mg/day. The maximum recommended dose is 12 mg/day.

Paliperidone Palmitate (Invega Sustenna). It is available as 39, 78, 117, 156, and 234 mg per vial. It is given IM and injection into a blood vessel should be avoided. It is administered slowly and deeply into the muscle. The starting dose is 234 mg followed by 156 mg given 1 week later. There after maintenance dose of 39 to 234 mg can be given every 4 weeks.

Paliperidone Palmitate (Trinza). It is available as 273, 410, and 546 mg per vial. It is given IM and injection into a blood vessel should be avoided. It is administered slowly and deeply into the deltoid or gluteal muscle every 3 months. Clinicians should be aware that 3-month injectable formulation (Trinza) could only be used once adequate treatment with Invega Sustenna (1-month Paliperidone Palmitate) has been established for at least 4 months.

h. Iloperidone (Fanapt). It is available in a titration pack, and the effective dose (12 mg) should be reached in approximately 4 days based on a twice-a-day dosing schedule. It is usually started on day 1 at 1 mg twice a day and increased daily on a twice-a-day schedule to reach 12 mg by day 4. The maximum recommended dose is 12 mg twice a day (24 mg a day), and it can be administered without regard to food.

i. Asenapine (Saphris). Asenapine is available as 5- and 10-mg sublingual tablets, and placed under the tongue. The bioavailability is less than 2% when swallowed, but 35% when absorbed sublingually. The recommended starting and target dose for schizophrenia is 5 mg twice a day. In bipolar disorder, it is 10 mg twice a day, and if necessary, the dosage may be lowered to 5 mg twice a day depending on the tolerability issues.

j. Lurasidone (Latuda). It is available as 20-, 40-, 80-, and 120-mg tablets. For the treatment of schizophrenia the initial dose titration is not required. The recommended starting dose is 40 mg once daily, and the medication should be taken with food (at least 350 calories). It has been shown to be effective in a dose range of 40 to 120 mg/day. Although there is no proven added benefit with the 120 mg per day dose, there may be a dose-related increase in adverse reactions. Still, some patients may benefit from the maximum recommended dose of 160 mg/day.

k. Brexpiprazole (Rexulti). It is available as 0.25-, 1-, 2-, 3-, and 4-mg tablets.

Dosing in schizophrenia;

Initial starting dose of 1 mg daily from day 1 to 4 and dose can be adjusted gradually based on response and tolerability to 2 mg daily for 3 days followed by 4 mg on day 8 with a maximum dose of 4 mg.

Dosing in major depressive disorder;

Initial starting dose is lower, 0.5 or 1 mg once daily and then adjust at weekly intervals based on response and tolerability to 1 mg once daily, followed by 2 mg once daily with a maximum daily dose of 3 mg.

l. Cariprazine (Vraylar). Cariprazine is available as a 1.5-, 3-, 4.5-, and 6-mg capsule and is given once daily orally with or without food. The usual starting dosage in schizophrenia and bipolar I disorder is 1.5 mg and can be increased to 3 mg on day 2. Further dose adjustments should be made based on response and tolerability in 1.5- or 3-mg increments up to a maximum dose of 6 mg. In patients with concomitant 3A4 inhibitors, dose should be reduced by half to one-third of the prescribed dosage.

m. **Pimavanserin (Nuplazid).** It is available as 17-mg tablet. The recommended dose is 34 mg taken as two 17-mg tablets together once daily. Dose adjustment is necessary with CYP 3A4 inhibitors or inducers.

4. **Pretreatment evaluation.** Before the initiation of treatment, an informed consent procedure should be documented. The patient's history should include information about blood disorders, epilepsy, cardiovascular disease, hepatic and renal diseases, and drug abuse. The presence of a hepatic or renal disease necessitates the use of low starting dosages. The physical examination should include supine and standing blood pressure measurements to screen for orthostatic hypotension. The laboratory examination should include an electrocardiogram (ECG); several complete blood cell counts including white blood cell counts, which can then be averaged; and tests of hepatic and renal function.

As second-generation drugs and SDAs have become the first-line treatment for various disorders, new controversies have arisen regarding their role in causing metabolic abnormalities (hyperglycemia, insulin resistance, and dyslipidemias). At this time, the American Psychiatric Association (APA) and American Diabetic Association (ADA) have developed a consensus guideline to help physicians monitor their patients. Olanzapine and clozapine have been the agents most often reported to be associated with treatment-emergent diabetes mellitus, a fact that may be linked to their propensity to cause marked weight gain.

The prevalence of diabetes in patients with schizophrenia and bipolar disorder is thought to be two to four times that of the general population. This is further complicated by the fact that obesity is on the rise and schizophrenics have an elevated risk of premature death from numerous medical problems. Obesity poses a serious health risk, contributing to such disorders as hypertension, dyslipidemia, cardiovascular disease, noninsulin-dependent diabetes, gallbladder disease, respiratory problems, gout, and osteoarthritis. Metabolic syndrome (disturbed glucose and insulin metabolism, obesity, dyslipidemia, and hypertension) is also more prevalent in patients with schizophrenia and numerous studies have suggested causal linkage to the use of antipsychotics particularly the second generations. There are differences among the antipsychotics in regards to the risk for weight gain, and diabetes but FDA has recommended the following guidelines for all second-generation antipsychotics.

a. **Baseline monitoring.**

(1) Personal and family history of obesity, diabetes, dyslipidemia, hypertension, and cardiovascular disease.

(2) Weight and height (so that body mass index [BMI] can be calculated).

(3) Waist circumference (at the level of the umbilicus).

(4) Blood pressure.

(5) Fasting plasma glucose.

(6) Fasting lipid profile.

Patients with pre-existing diabetes should have regular monitoring including, HgA1c and in some cases insulin levels. The oral glucose tolerance test (OGTT) is not recommended for routine clinical use, but may be required in the evaluation of patients with impaired fasting glucose or when diabetes is suspected despite normal fasting plasma glucose.

It is recommended that clinicians screen, evaluate, and monitor patients for metabolic changes irrespective of the antipsychotic class as these patients have an increased risk of metabolic syndrome and diabetes.

5. **Monitoring during treatment.** All patients on second-generation drugs should be routinely monitored for side effects. Although these drugs are presumed to have a lowered risk of tardive dyskinesia, some risk remains, so patients should be assessed for any movement abnormalities. According to FDA recommendations, all patients should have their blood glucose levels monitored, especially early in treatment or if weight gain occurs.

See Table 29-8 for guidelines of clinical management of clozapine-associated hematologic abnormalities.

a. **Clozapine risk evaluation and mitigation strategy (REMS)**

(1) Clozapine requires special monitoring. In 2015, FDA announced new requirements for prescribing and dispensing of clozapine. This led to the new clozapine REMS program and will replace the six existing clozapine registries. This will also centralize all the information and have patients, clinicians, and pharmacies enroll in one place.

(2) Patients will be monitored for neutropenia using the absolute neutrophil count (ANC) and WBC will no longer be acceptable. ANC threshold has also been lowered so more patients will be able to continue taking the drug.

(3) Treatment will be interrupted if the ANC drops below 1,000 cells/μL with special consideration to patients with African American origin who are more susceptible to develop benign ethnic neutropenia (BEN). These patients' treatment will be stopped if the ANC drops below 500 cells/μL. These changes allow clinicians to prescribe clozapine to patients who were previously ineligible to receive the medicine as well as continue treatment for a greater number of patients.

(4) During the first 6 months, weekly ANC counts are indicated to monitor for the development of agranulocytosis. If the ANC count remains normal, the frequency of testing can be decreased to every 2 weeks. Clozapine should be discontinued if the ANC count is below 1,000 cells per mm^3 or in case of BEN falls below 500 cells/μL. In addition, a hematologic consultation should be obtained, and obtaining bone marrow sample should be considered. FDA further stated, "Patients with agranulocytosis could

Clozapine Risk Evaluation and Mitigation Strategy (REMS)

Recommended Monitoring Frequency and Clinical Decisions by ANC Level

ANC Level	Treatment Recommendation	ANC Monitoring

Normal Range for a New Patient
• General Population (ANC ≥ 1500/μL)***
 	
BEN POPULATION
• BEN Population (ANC ≥ 1,000/μL)
• Obtain at least two baseline ANC* levels before initiating treatment
	• Initiate treatment
	• If treatment interrupted:
	  • < 30 days, continue monitoring as before
	  • ≥ 30 days, monitor as if new patient
	  • Discontinuation for reasons other than neutropenia
		• Weekly from initiation to 6 months
		• Every 2 weeks from 6 to 12 months
		• Monthly after 12 months

Mild Neutropenia (1000 to 1499/μL)***	**GENERAL POPULATION**
	• Continue treatment
	
	BEN POPULATION
	• Mild Neutropenia is normal range for BEN population, continue treatment
	• Obtain at least two baseline ANC levels before initiating treatment
	• If treatment interrupted
	  • < 30 days, continue monitoring as before
	  • ≥ 30 days, monitor as if new patient
	• Discontinuation for reasons other than neutropenia
		GENERAL POPULATION
		• Three times weekly until ANC* ≥ 1500/μL
		• Once ANC* ≥ 1500/μL return to patient's last "Normal Range" ANC* monitoring interval** (if clinically appropriate)
		
		BEN POPULATION
		• Weekly from initiation to 6 months
		• Every 2 weeks from 6 to 12 months
		• Monthly after 12 months

Moderate Neutropenia (500 to 999/μL)***	**GENERAL POPULATION** • Recommend hematology consultation • Interrupt treatment for suspected clozapine induced neutropenia • Resume treatment once ANC normalizes to ≥ 1000/μL **BEN** POPULATION • Recommend hematology consultation • Continue treatment	**GENERAL POPULATION** • Daily until ANC* ≥ 1000/μL then • Three times weekly until ANC* ≥ 1500/μL • Once ANC* ≥ 1500/μL, check ANC* weekly for 4 weeks, then return to patient's last "Normal Range" ANC* monitoring interval*** (if clinically appropriate) **BEN** POPULATION • Three times weekly until ANC* ≥ 1000/μL or ≥ patient's known baseline. • Once ANC* ≥ 1000/μL or patient's known baseline, then check ANC weekly for 4 weeks, then return to patient's last "Normal BEN** Range" ANC* monitoring interval** if clinically appropriate)
Severe Neutropenia (less than 500/μL)***	**GENERAL POPULATION** • Recommend hematology consultation • Interrupt treatment for suspected clozapine induced neutropenia • Do not rechallenge unless prescriber determines benefits outweigh risks **BEN** POPULATION • Recommend hematology consultation • Interrupt treatment for suspected clozapine induced neutropenia • Do not rechallenge unless prescriber determines benefits outweigh risks	**GENERAL POPULATION** • Daily until ANC* ≥ 1000/μL • Three times weekly until ANC* ≥ 1500/μL • If patient rechallenged, resume treatment as a new patient under "Normal Range" monitoring once ANC* ≥ 1500/μL **BEN** POPULATION • Daily until ANC* ≥ 500/μL • Three times weekly until ANC* ≥ patients established baseline • If patient rechallenged, resume treatment as a new patient under "Normal Range" monitoring once ANC ≥1000/μL or at patient's baseline

*ANC, Absolute Neutrophil Count; **BEN, Benign Ethnic Neutropenia; ***Confirm all initial reports of ANC less than 1500/μL (ANC < 1000/μL for BEN patients) with a repeat ANC measurement within 24 hours

Table 29-9
Maintenance Monitoring for SDAs

Parameters	Weeks
Weight	4, 8, 12, 16, 52
Waist circumference	52
Blood pressure	12, 52
Fasting glucose	12, 52
Fasting lipid	12; 5 years

be rechallenged if the prescriber determines the risk of psychiatric illness is greater than the risk of neutropenia." Patients exhibiting symptoms of chest pain, shortness of breath, fever, or tachypnea should be immediately evaluated for myocarditis or cardiomyopathy, an infrequent but serious adverse effect ending in death. Serial CPK-MB (creatine phosphokinase with myocardial band fractions), troponin levels, and EKG studies are recommended, with immediate discontinuation of clozapine.

   b. **Maintenance monitoring for SDAs.** Patients maintained on SDAs for prolonged periods should be monitored periodically as illustrated in Table 29-9.

6. **Switching from and to another antipsychotic drug.** The transition from a dopamine receptor antagonist to an SDA can be accomplished easily but should be done slowly. It is wise to overlap administration of the new drug with the old drug, lowering the dose of the former while raising the dose of the latter.

   Because the SDAs such as risperidone, quetiapine, and ziprasidone lack anticholinergic effects, the abrupt transition from a dopamine receptor antagonist to one of these agents may cause cholinergic rebound, which consists of excessive salivation, nausea, vomiting, and diarrhea. The risk for cholinergic rebound can be mitigated by initially augmenting the SDA with an anticholinergic drug, which is then tapered slowly.

   With depot formulations of a dopamine receptor antagonist, the first dose of the SDA is given on the day the next injection is due. At present, various SDAs are available in long-acting formulation.

7. **Adverse effects**
   a. **All second-generation drugs**
      (1) **Neuroleptic malignant syndrome.** The development of neuroleptic malignant syndrome is considerably rare with second-generation drugs than with dopamine receptor antagonists. This syndrome consists of muscular rigidity, fever, dystonia, akinesia, mutism, oscillation between obtundation and agitation, diaphoresis, dysphagia, tremor, incontinence, labile blood pressure, leukocytosis, and elevated creatine phosphokinase. Clozapine, especially if combined with lithium, and risperidone have been associated with neuroleptic malignant syndrome.

(2) **Tardive dyskinesias.** Second-generation drugs are significantly less likely than dopamine receptor antagonists to be associated with treatment-emergent tardive dyskinesias. Moreover, second-generation drugs, especially clozapine, relieve the symptoms of tardive dyskinesias and are especially indicated for psychotic persons with pre-existing tardive dyskinesias. For this reason, long-term maintenance treatment with dopamine receptor antagonists has become a questionable practice. A new drug valbenazine (Ingrezza) has been approved for the treatment of tardive dyskinesia and is discussed in more detail in Chapter 32.

b. **Risperidone.** Risperidone causes few adverse effects at the usual therapeutic dosages of 6 mg/day or less. The most common adverse effects include anxiety, insomnia, somnolence, dizziness, constipation, nausea, dyspepsia, rhinitis, rash, and tachycardia. At the rarely used higher dosages, it causes dosage-dependent extrapyramidal effects, hyperprolactinemia, sedation, orthostatic hypotension, palpitations, weight gain, decreased libido, and erectile dysfunction. Rare adverse effects associated with long-term use include neuroleptic malignant syndrome, priapism, thrombocytopenic purpura, and seizures in persons with hyponatremia.

c. **Olanzapine.** Olanzapine is generally well tolerated except for moderate somnolence and weight gain of 10 to 25 lb in up to 50% of persons on long-term therapy. Infrequent adverse effects include constipation, dizziness, hyperglycemia, orthostatic hypotension, transaminase elevations, and rarely extrapyramidal symptoms. More than other atypical antipsychotics, diabetes mellitus and acute-onset diabetic ketoacidosis have been reported in patients using olanzapine.

d. **Quetiapine.** The most common adverse effects of quetiapine are somnolence, dry mouth, asthenia, postural hypotension, and dizziness, which are usually transient and are best managed with initial gradual upward titration of the dose. Quetiapine appears no more likely than placebo to cause extrapyramidal symptoms. Quetiapine is associated with modest transient weight gain, transient rises in liver transaminases, small increases in heart rate, and constipation.

e. **Ziprasidone.** Adverse effects are unusual with ziprasidone. In particular, it is the only SDA not associated with weight gain. The most common adverse effects are somnolence, dizziness, nausea, and lightheadedness. Ziprasidone causes almost no significant effects outside the CNS, but it does have the capacity to prolong the QT/QTc interval and the associated risk of developing torsade de pointes.

f. **Clozapine.** Significant potential for the development of serious adverse effects is the reason that clozapine is reserved for use in only the most treatment-refractory persons. The most common adverse effects are sedation, seizures, dizziness, syncope, tachycardia, hypotension, ECG changes, nausea, vomiting, leukopenia, granulocytopenia, agranulocytosis, and fever. Weight gain can be marked. Diabetes mellitus has been linked to clozapine, regardless of any weight gain. Patients exhibiting symptoms of chest pain, shortness of breath, fever, or tachypnea should be immediately evaluated for myocarditis or cardiomyopathy, an infrequent but serious adverse effect ending in death. Serial CPK with MB fractions, troponin levels, and EKG are recommended with immediate discontinuation of clozapine. Other common adverse effects include fatigue, sialorrhea, various GI symptoms (most commonly constipation), anticholinergic effects, and subjective muscle weakness. Clozapine is best used in a structured setting.

Because of additive risks of agranulocytosis, clozapine should not be combined with carbamazepine (Tegretol) or other drugs known to cause bone marrow suppression.

g. Aripiprazole. Aripiprazole is well tolerated, and the discontinuation rate is similar to placebo. The most common treatment-emergent events are headache, nausea, vomiting, insomnia, lightheadedness, and somnolence. In short-term clinical trials, the incidence of extra pyramidal symptoms was similar to placebo. In clinical practice, some patients experience marked agitation and akathisia with aripiprazole.

h. Paliperidone and Paliperidone long-acting injectable. Paliperidone is well tolerated. Common side effects include dizziness, constipation, and lethargy. Akathisia may occur. The drug should be avoided in persons with a history of chronic arrhythmias.

i. Iloperidone. The most common adverse effects reported are dizziness, dry mouth, fatigue, sedation, tachycardia, and orthostatic hypotension (depending on dosing and titration). Iloperidone prolongs the QT interval by 9 milliseconds at dosages of 12 mg twice daily and may be associated with arrhythmia and sudden death.

j. Asenapine. The most common side effects observed are somnolence, dizziness, EPS other than akathisia, and increased weight, the mean weight gain after 52 weeks is 0.9 kg.

k. Lurasidone. The most common adverse effects are somnolence, akathisia, nausea, parkinsonism, and agitation.

l. Brexpiprazole. The most common side effects include akathisia (dose related), increased serum triglycerides, weight gain, headache, drowsiness, and EPS.

m. Cariprazine. The most common adverse reactions include extrapyramidal symptoms, akathisia, dyspepsia, vomiting, somnolence, insomnia, agitation, anxiety, and restlessness. Metabolic monitoring is required as 4% of patients with normal HgA1c developed elevated HgA1c above 6.5 and 8% of patients had a 7% weight increase or greater.

n. Pimavanserin. The most common adverse effects are peripheral edema, confusional state, nausea, and bloating.

8. Drug interactions. CNS depressants, alcohol, or tricyclic drugs coadministered with second-generation drugs may increase the risk for seizures, sedation, and cardiac effects. Antihypertensive medications may exacerbate the orthostatic hypotension caused by second-generation drugs. The coadministration of benzodiazepines and second-generation drugs may be associated with an increased incidence of orthostasis, syncope, and respiratory depression. Risperidone, olanzapine, quetiapine, and ziprasidone can antagonize the effects of levodopa and dopamine agonists. Long-term use of second-generation drugs together with drugs that induce hepatic cytochrome P450 (CYP) metabolic enzymes (e.g., carbamazepine, barbiturates, omeprazole [Prilosec], rifampin [Rifadin, Rifamate], glucocorticoids) may increase the clearance of second-generation drugs by 50% or more. Some significant drug–drug interactions are described below.

a. **Risperidone.** The concurrent use of risperidone and phenytoin or SSRIs may produce extrapyramidal symptoms. The use of risperidone by persons with opioid dependence may precipitate opioid withdrawal symptoms. The addition of risperidone to the regimen of a person taking clozapine can raise clozapine plasma concentrations by 75%.

b. **Olanzapine.** Fluvoxamine (Luvox) increases the serum concentrations of olanzapine.

c. **Quetiapine.** Phenytoin increases quetiapine clearance fivefold, and thioridazine (Mellaril) increases quetiapine clearance by 65%. Cimetidine reduces quetiapine clearance by 20%. Quetiapine reduces lorazepam (Ativan) clearance by 20%. A high-fat meal (800 to 1,000 calories) causes significantly increase in Cmax of quetiapine XR. It is suggested that quetiapine be taken without food or a light meal (300 calories).

d. **Ziprasidone.** Ziprasidone has a low potential for causing clinically significant drug interactions.

e. **Clozapine.** Clozapine should not be used with any other drug that can cause bone marrow suppression. Such drugs include carbamazepine, phenytoin, propylthiouracil, sulfonamides, and captopril (Capoten). The addition of paroxetine (Paxil) may precipitate clozapine-associated neutropenia. Lithium combined with clozapine may increase the risk for seizures, confusion, and movement disorders. Lithium should not be used in combination with clozapine by persons who have experienced an episode of neuroleptic malignant syndrome. Risperidone, fluoxetine, paroxetine, and fluvoxamine increase serum concentrations of clozapine.

f. **Aripiprazole.** Carbamazepine may lower the blood levels of aripiprazole. Fluoxetine and paroxetine can inhibit the metabolism and hence elimination of aripiprazole.

g. **Paliperidone.** Drugs such as paroxetine, fluoxetine, and other SSRIs can block the action of paliperidone. Combined use of SSRIs and paliperidone can result in significant elevation of prolactin in men and women. Paliperidone palmitate injectable may antagonize the effect of levodopa and dopamine agonists. When used with strong CYP 3A4 inducers the dose of paliperidone palmitate may need to be increased.

h. Iloperidone. Iloperidone is metabolized through CYP 2D6 and 3A4, so coadministration with drugs that inhibit 2D6 and 3A4 may increase its blood levels. It has a strong alpha-1 antagonism and may enhance effects of antihypertensive agents.

i. Asenapine. Asenapine is metabolized through glucuronidation and oxidative metabolism by CYP 1A2, so coadministration with fluvoxamine and other CYP 1A2 inhibitors should be done cautiously.

j. Lurasidone. When coadministration of lurasidone with a moderate CYP 3A4 inhibitor such as diltiazem is considered, the dose should not exceed 40 mg/day. Lurasidone should not be used in combination with a strong CYP 3A4 inhibitor (e.g., ketoconazole). Lurasidone also should not be used in combination with a strong CYP 3A4 inducer (e.g., rifampin), or grapefruit juice.

k. Brexpiprazole. Concomitant use of medications that are moderate to strong inhibitors of CYP 2D6 and CYP 3A4 require that dosage of brexpiprazole be reduced by 25% to 50%. Clinicians should consult drug interaction checker for an exhaustive list to prevent toxicity and adverse reactions.

l. Cariprazine. Clinicians should be aware of CYP 3A4 enzyme inhibition and make dosage adjustments especially when coadministered strong 3A4 inhibitor.

m. Pimavanserin. Dose should be reduced by one-half when used in combination with strong CYP 3A4 inhibitors and, increased in the presence of strong 3A4 inducers.

9. Use during pregnancy. Atypical antipsychotics are the mainstay of treatment in chronic psychotic conditions and the decision to continue during pregnancy should be discussed thoroughly as stopping these medicines may pose a high risk of relapse. Numerous studies suggest that medications including olanzapine, risperidone, and quetiapine pose no higher risk of complications like gestational diabetes, low birth weight, or preterm births. These medications have a higher risk for metabolic conditions but recent data showed no increase in pregnant mothers. In summary, atypical antipsychotics pose minimal risk to fetus and the pregnant mother. Clinicians should continue to weigh risk and benefits with close monitoring of pregnant mothers taking these drugs.

B. Dopamine receptor antagonists. The dopamine receptor antagonists are presently second-line agents for the treatment of schizophrenia and other psychotic disorders. Because of their immediate calming effects, however, dopamine receptor antagonists are often used for the management of acute psychotic episodes.

1. Choice of drug. Although dopamine receptor antagonist's potency varies widely (Table 29-10), all available typical dopamine receptor antagonists are equally efficacious in the treatment of schizophrenia. The dopamine receptor antagonists are available in a wide range of formulations and doses (Table 29-11).

Text continues on page 483.

Table 29-10
Dopamine Receptor Antagonists

Drug Name	Chemical Classification	Therapeutic Dose Equivalent Oral Dosage (mg)	Relative Potency	Therapeutically (mg/day)ᵃ	Sedation	Autonomicᵇ	Extrapyramidal Reactionsᶜ
						Side Effects	
Acetophenazine (Tindal)	Phenothiazine: piperazine compound	20	Med	20–100	++	+	++/+++
Chlorpromazine (Thorazine)	Phenothiazine: aliphatic compound	100	Low	150–2,000	+++	+++	++
Chlorprothixene (Taractan)	Thioxanthene	100	Low	100–600	+++	+++	+/++
Fluphenazine (Permitil) (Prolixin)	Phenothiazine: piperazine compound	2	High	5–60	+	+	+++
Haloperidol (Haldol)	Butyrophenone	2	High	2–100	+	+	+++
Loxapine (Loxitane)	Dibenzoxazepine	10	Med	30–250	++	+/++	++/+++
Mesoridazine (Serentil)	Phenothiazine: piperidine compound	50	—	—	+++	++	+
Molindone (Moban)	Dihydroindolone	10	—	—	+++	+	+
Perphenazine (Trilafon)	Phenothiazine: piperazine compound	8	Med	8–64	++	+	++/+++
Pimozide (Orap)ᵈ	Diphenylbutylpiperidine	1.5	High	2–20	+	+	+++
Prochlorperazine (Compazine)ᶜ	Phenothiazine: piperazine compound	15	—	—	++	+	+++
Thioridazine (Mellaril)	Phenothiazine: piperidine compound	100	Low	100–800	+++	+++	+
Thiothixene (Navane)	Thioxanthene	4	High	5–60	+	+	+++
Trifluoperazine (Stelazine)	Phenothiazine: piperazine compound	5	Med	5–60	++	+	++
Triflupromazine (Vesprin)	Phenothiazine: aliphatic compound	25	High	20–150	+++	++/+++	++

ᵃExtreme range.
ᵇAnti-α-adrenergic and anticholinergic effects.
ᶜExcluding tardive dyskinesia, which appears to be produced to the same degree and frequency by all agents with equieffective antipsychotic dosages.
ᵈPimozide is used principally in the treatment of Tourette's syndrome; prochlorperazine is used rarely, if ever, as an antipsychotic agent.
Adapted from American Medical Association. *AMA Drug Evaluations: Annual 1992.* Chicago: American Medical Association; 1992.

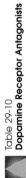

Table 29-11
Dopamine Receptor Antagonist Preparations

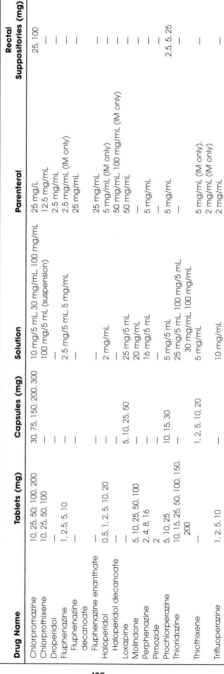

Drug Name	Tablets (mg)	Capsules (mg)	Solution	Parenteral	Rectal Suppositories (mg)
Chlorpromazine	10, 25, 50; 100, 200	30, 75, 150, 200, 300	10 mg/5 mL, 30 mg/mL, 100 mg/mL	25 mg/L	25, 100
Chlorprothixene	10, 25, 50, 100	—	100 mg/5 mL (suspension)	12.5 mg/mL	—
Droperidol	—	—	—	2.5 mg/mL	—
Fluphenazine	1, 2.5, 5, 10	—	2.5 mg/5 mL, 5 mg/mL	2.5 mg/mL (IM only)	—
Fluphenazine decanoate	—	—	—	25 mg/mL	—
Fluphenazine enanthate	—	—	—	—	—
Haloperidol	0.5, 1, 2, 5, 10, 20	—	2 mg/mL	5 mg/mL (IM only)	—
Haloperidol decanoate	—	—	—	50 mg/mL, 100 mg/mL (IM only)	—
Loxapine	—	5, 10, 25, 50	—	50 mg/mL	—
Molindone	5, 10, 25, 50, 100	—	25 mg/5 mL	—	—
Perphenazine	2, 4, 8, 16	—	20 mg/mL	5 mg/mL	—
Pimozide	2	—	16 mg/5 mL	—	—
Prochlorperazine	5, 10, 25	10, 15, 30	5 mg/5 mL	5 mg/mL	2.5, 5, 25
Thioridazine	10, 15, 25, 50, 100, 150, 200	—	25 mg/5 mL, 100 mg/5 mL, 30 mg/mL, 100 mg/mL	—	—
Thiothixene	—	1, 2, 5, 10, 20	5 mg/mL	5 mg/mL (IM only), 2 mg/mL (IM only)	—
Trifluoperazine	1, 2, 5, 10	—	10 mg/mL	2 mg/mL	—

a. **Short-term treatment.** The equivalent of 5 to 10 mg of haloperidol is a reasonable dose for an adult person in an acute psychotic state. An elderly person may benefit from as little as 1 mg of haloperidol.

Intramuscular administration of the dopamine receptor antagonists results in peak plasma concentrations in about 30 minutes versus 90 minutes with the oral route. Doses of dopamine receptor antagonists for intramuscular administration are about half the doses given by the oral route. The patient should be observed for 1 hour after the first dose. After that time, most clinicians administer a second dose or a sedative agent (e.g., a benzodiazepine) to achieve effective behavioral control. Possible sedatives include 2 mg of lorazepam IM and 50 to 250 mg of amobarbital (Amytal) intramuscularly. There have been reports of sudden death, QT prolongation, and torsades de pointes in patients receiving haldol. Higher and IV dosages appear to be associated with increased risk of QT prolongation and torsades de pointes.

CLINICAL HINT:
The administration of more than 50 mg of chlorpromazine in one injection may result in serious hypotension. It is safer to start with a dose of 25 mg.

There are two short-acting intramuscular formulations of atypical antipsychotics available that can be used in the treatment of acute agitation associated with schizophrenia or bipolar disorder (manic or mixed episode).

(1) **Olanzapine.** Available in 10-mg injection form and can be administered in a single dose to be repeated in 2 hours. A third dose can be given 4 hours after the second injection. It has a rapid onset of action occurring within 15 minutes in agitated schizophrenic patients and within 30 minutes in agitated bipolar patients. The most common observed side effect is somnolence.

CLINICAL HINT:
The coadministration of lorazepam and olanzapine should be avoided because fatalities have occurred.

(2) **Ziprasidone.** Indicated for the treatment of acute agitation associated with psychoses. It is available in 20-mg injection form and is administered in 10 to 20 mg as required to a maximum dose of 40 mg/day. Doses of 10 mg may be administered every 2 hours; doses of 20 mg may be given every 4 hours up to a maximum of 40 mg/day. The peak serum concentration typically occurs at approximately 60 minutes postdose, and the mean half-life ranges from 2 to 5 hours. The most common adverse effects are somnolence, nausea, and headache.

(3) **Aripiprazole.** The recommended dose in agitation associated with schizophrenia or bipolar mania (intramuscular injection) is 9.75 mg. The effectiveness of aripiprazole injection in controlling agitation in schizophrenia and bipolar mania was demonstrated over a dose range of 5.25 to 15 mg.

b. **Long-acting depot medications.** Because some persons with schizophrenia do not comply with oral dopamine receptor antagonist regimens, long-acting depot preparations may be needed. A clinician usually administers the intramuscular preparations once every 1 to 4 weeks. Depot dopamine receptor antagonists may be associated with an increase in adverse effects, including tardive dyskinesia.

(1) **Risperidone consta.** Risperidone consta was the first available long-acting formulation but is now joined by a host of other agents. It is administered every 2 weeks, and the recommended starting dose is 25 mg. To start the patient on consta, the patient needs to receive 3 weeks of oral antipsychotic supplementation. It is also available in doses of 37.5 and 50 mg. Dosing adjustment should not be made more frequently than once a month, and maximum dose should not exceed 50 mg over 2 weeks. Risperdal consta can now also be administered into deltoid muscle. This mode of administration is supposedly less painful than the gluteal administration as the needle is only 1 in long as compared to the 2-in needle. The most common adverse events reported are somnolence, akathisia, parkinsonism, dyspepsia, constipation, dry mouth, fatigue, and weight gain.

Paliperidone palmitate long-acting injectable is also available and approved for the treatment of schizophrenia. The two formulations include the monthly injection formulation (Sustenna) and (Trinza) injected every 3 months. The dosing details have been described above in the clinical guidelines section.

Aripiprazole long-acting formulation (Maintena) is an intramuscular injection given every 4 weeks while the second formulation Aripiprazole lauroxil (Aristada) can be given every 6 weeks. Details have been discussed in the clinical guidelines section.

(2) **Precautions and adverse reactions.** Low-potency dopamine receptor antagonists are most likely to cause nonneurologic adverse effects, and high-potency dopamine receptor antagonists are most likely to cause neurologic (i.e., extrapyramidal) adverse effects. Second-generation drugs are more likely to cause metabolic disturbances. Recent studies have suggested that atypical antipsychotic drugs had a similar, dose-related increased risk of sudden cardiac death as conventional antipsychotics. Clinicians should appropriately screen and monitor patients maintained on atypical antipsychotics for long periods of time.

Table 29-12
Antipsychotic Drug Interaction

Drug	Consequences
Tricyclic antidepressants	Increased concentration of both
Anticholinergics	Anticholinergic toxicity, decreased absorption of antipsychotics
Antacids	Decreased absorption of antipsychotics
Cimetidine	Decreased absorption of antipsychotics
Food	Decreased absorption of antipsychotics
Buspirone	Elevation of haloperidol levels
Barbiturates	Increased metabolism of antipsychotics, excessive sedation
Phenytoin	Decreased phenytoin metabolism
Guanethidine	Reduced hypotensive effect
Clonidine	Reduced hypotensive effect
α-Methyldopa	Reduced hypotensive effect
Levodopa	Decreased effects of both
Succinylcholine	Prolonged muscle paralysis
Monoamine oxidase inhibitors	Hypotension
Halothane	Hypotension
Alcohol	Potentiation of CNS depression
Cigarettes	Decreased plasma levels of antipsychotics
Epinephrine	Hypotension
Propranolol	Increased plasma concentration of both
Warfarin	Decreased plasma concentration of warfarin

2. **Drug interactions.** Because they produce numerous receptor effects and are for the most part metabolized in the liver, the dopamine receptor antagonists are associated with many pharmacokinetic and pharmacodynamic drug interactions (Table 29-12).

VI. Antidepressants

This section describes various antidepressants along with their indications, dosing guidelines, and adverse reactions.

A. **SSRIs.** Six SSRIs are now first-line agents for the treatment of depression. Fluoxetine (Prozac) was introduced in 1988, and it has since become the single most widely prescribed antidepressant in the world. During the subsequent decade, sertraline (Zoloft) and paroxetine (Paxil) became nearly as widely prescribed as fluoxetine. Citalopram (Celexa), paroxetine CR (Paxil CR), and escitalopram (Lexapro) are the other SSRIs approved for depression. A seventh SSRI, fluvoxamine (Luvox), while also effective as an antidepressant, is FDA approved only as a treatment for OCD. The SSRIs also are effective for a broad range of anxiety disorders.

1. **Pharmacologic actions**

   a. **Pharmacokinetics.** All SSRIs are well absorbed after oral administration and reach their peak concentrations in 4 to 8 hours. Fluoxetine has the longest half-life, 2 to 3 days; its active metabolite norfluoxetine has a half-life of 7 to 9 days. The half-life of sertraline is 26 hours, and its significantly less active metabolite has a half-life of 3 to 5 days. The half-lives of the other three SSRIs, which do not have metabolites with significant pharmacologic activity, are 35 hours for citalopram

Table 29-13
Pharmacokinetic Profiles of the Selective Serotonin Reuptake Inhibitors

Drug	Time to Peak Plasma Concentration (hours)	Half-Life	Half-Life Metabolite	Time to Steady State (days)	Plasma Protein Binding (%)
Citalopram (Celexa)	4	35 hours	3 hours	7	80
Escitalopram (Lexapro)	5	27–32 hours	—	7	56
Fluoxetine (Prozac)	6–8	4–6 days	4–16 days	28–35	95
Fluvoxamine (Luvox)	3–8	15 hours	—	5–7	80
Paroxetine (Paxil)	5–6	21 hours	—	5–10	95
Paroxetine CR (Paxil CR)	6–10	15–20 hours	—	<14	95
Sertraline (Zoloft)	4.5–8.5	26 hours	62–104 hours	7	95

and escitalopram, 21 hours for paroxetine and paroxetine CR, and 15 hours for fluvoxamine. (See Table 29-13.)

The administration of SSRIs with food has little effect on absorption and may reduce the incidence of nausea and diarrhea.

b. Pharmacodynamics. The clinical benefits of SSRIs are attributed to the relatively selective inhibition of serotonin reuptake, with little effect on the reuptake of norepinephrine and dopamine. The same degree of clinical benefit can usually be achieved through either steady use of a low dosage or more rapid escalation of the dosage. However, the clinical response varies considerably from person to person.

2. Therapeutic indications

a. Depression. Fluoxetine, sertraline, paroxetine, citalopram, paroxetine CR, and escitalopram are indicated for the treatment of depression in the general population, the elderly, the medically ill, and pregnant women. For severe depression and melancholia, several studies have found that the maximum efficacy of SNRIs, such as venlafaxine, duloxetine (Cymbalta), or tricyclic drugs, may exceed that of SSRIs.

(1) Choice of drug. Direct comparisons of the benefits of specific SSRIs have not shown any one to be generally superior to the others. However, responses to the various SSRIs can vary considerably within a given patient. A number of reports indicate that more than 50% of people who respond poorly to one SSRI will respond favorably to another. Thus, it is most reasonable to try other agents in the SSRI class for patients who do not respond to their first SSRI before shifting to non-SSRI antidepressants.

(2) Comparison with tricyclic antidepressants. The efficacy of the SSRIs is similar to that of the tricyclic antidepressants, but their adverse effect profile is markedly better. Some degree of nervousness or agitation, sleep disturbances, GI symptoms, and perhaps sexual adverse effects are more common in persons treated with SSRIs than in those treated with tricyclic drugs.

b. Suicide. In the overwhelming majority of people at risk for suicide, SSRIs reduce the risk. Some persons become especially anxious and agitated when given fluoxetine. The appearance of these symptoms in a suicidal person could conceivably aggravate the seriousness of their suicidal ideation.

 CLINICAL HINT:
Suicidal persons often act out their suicidal thoughts more effectively as they recover from their depression. Thus, potentially suicidal persons should be closely monitored during the first few weeks of SSRI therapy.

    c. Depression during and after pregnancy. The use of fluoxetine during pregnancy is not associated with increases in perinatal complications, congenital fetal anomalies, learning disabilities, language delays, or specific behavioral problems. Emerging data for sertraline, paroxetine, and fluvoxamine indicate that these agents are probably similarly safe when taken during pregnancy.

    d. Depression in the elderly and medically ill. All SSRIs are useful for elderly, medically frail persons.

    e. Chronic depression. Because discontinuation of SSRIs within 6 months after a depressive episode is associated with a high rate of relapse, a person with chronic depression should remain on SSRI therapy for several years. SSRIs are well tolerated in long-term use.

    f. Depression in children. SSRIs are increasingly prescribed to treat childhood depression and to forestall efforts by children and adolescents to self-medicate their depressed feelings with alcohol or illicit drugs. The adverse effect profile of SSRIs in children includes GI symptoms, insomnia, motor restlessness, social disinhibition, mania, hypomania, and psychosis. A recent FDA warning was issued to physicians regarding the potential risks of suicide in adolescents who are prescribed these antidepressants. Close monitoring of these medications by the physician is recommended.

    g. Premenstrual dysphoric disorder. SSRIs reduce the debilitating mood and behavioral changes that occur in the week preceding menstruation in women with premenstrual dysphoric disorder. Scheduled administration of SSRIs either throughout the cycle or only during the luteal phase (the 2-week period between ovulation and menstruation) is equally effective for this purpose.

3. Clinical guidelines
    a. Dosage and administration. See Table 29-14.
        (1) Fluoxetine. Fluoxetine is available in 10- and 20-mg capsules, in a scored 10-mg tablet, and as a liquid (20 mg/5 mL). For the treatment of depression, the initial dosage is usually 10 or 20 mg/day orally. The drug is generally taken in the morning because insomnia is a potential adverse effect. Fluoxetine may

Table 29-14
SSRI Dosage

	Starting (mg)	Maintenance (mg)	High Dosage (mg)
Paroxetine	5–10	20–60	>60
Paroxetine CR	25	25–62.5	>62.5
Fluoxetine	2–5	20–60	>80
Sertraline	12.5–25	50–200	>300
Citalopram	10	20–40	>60
Escitalopram	5	10–30	>30
Fluvoxamine	25	50–100	>300

be taken with food to minimize possible nausea. Because of the long half-lives of the drug and its metabolite, a 4-week period is required to reach steady-state concentrations. As with all available antidepressants, the antidepressant effects of fluoxetine may be seen in the first 1 to 3 weeks, but the clinician should wait until the patient has been taking the drug for 4 to 6 weeks before definitively evaluating its antidepressant activity.

Several studies indicate that 20 mg may be as effective as higher doses for the treatment of depression. The maximum daily dosage recommended by the manufacturer is 80 mg/day, and higher dosages may cause seizures. A reasonable strategy is to maintain a patient on 20 mg/day for 3 weeks. If the patient shows no signs of clinical improvement at that time, an increase to 40 mg/day may be warranted.

 CLINICAL HINT:
To minimize the early adverse effects of anxiety and restlessness, initiate fluoxetine at 5 to 10 mg/day, with use of the scored 10-mg tablets. Alternatively, because of the long half-life of fluoxetine, the drug can be initiated with an every-other-day administration schedule.

At least 2 weeks should elapse between the discontinuation of MAOIs and the initiation of fluoxetine. Fluoxetine must be discontinued for at least 5 weeks before the initiation of MAOI treatment.

(2) Sertraline. Sertraline is available in scored 25-, 50-, and 100-mg tablets. For the initial treatment of depression, sertraline should be initiated at a dosage of 50 mg taken once daily. To limit the GI effects, some clinicians begin at 25 mg/day and increase the dosage to 50 mg/day after 3 weeks. Persons who do not respond after 1 to 3 weeks may benefit from increases of 50 mg every week up to a maximum dosage of 200 mg taken once daily. Sertraline generally is given in the evening because it is somewhat more likely to cause sedation than insomnia. Persons who experience GI symptoms may benefit by taking the drug with food.

(3) Paroxetine. Paroxetine is available in scored 20-mg tablets, unscored 10-, 30-, and 40-mg tablets, and an orange-flavored oral suspension with a concentration of 10 mg/5 mL. Paroxetine is usually initiated for the treatment of depression at a dosage of 10 or 20 mg/day. An increase should be considered when an adequate response is not seen in 1 to 3 weeks. At that point, the clinician can initiate upward titration in 10-mg increments at weekly intervals to a maximum dosage of 50 mg/day. Dosages of up to 80 mg/day may be tolerated. Persons who experience GI symptoms may benefit by taking the drug with food.

Paroxetine should be taken initially as a single daily dose in the evening. Higher dosages may be divided into two doses per day. Persons with melancholic features may require dosages greater than 20 mg/day. The suggested therapeutic dosage range for elderly persons is 10 to 20 mg/day.

 CLINICAL HINT:
Paroxetine is the SSRI most likely to produce a discontinuation syndrome. To limit the development of symptoms of abrupt discontinuation, the dosage of paroxetine should be reduced by 10 mg each week until it is 10 mg/day, at which point it may be decreased to 5 mg/day and stopped after one more week.

(4) Paroxetine CR. Paroxetine CR (Paxil CR) is available as an enteric-coated tablet in 12.5-, 25-, and 37.5-mg doses. Paroxetine CR should be administered as a single daily dose, usually in the morning, with or without food. The recommended initial dose is 25 mg/day. Some patients not responding to a 25-mg dose may benefit from dose increases, in 12.5-mg/day increments, up to a maximum of 62.5 mg/day. Dose changes should occur at intervals of at least 1 week. Patients should be cautioned that paroxetine CR should not be chewed or crushed and should be swallowed whole.

(5) Citalopram. Citalopram is available in scored 20- and 40-mg tablets. The usual starting dosage is 20 mg/day for the first week, after which it is generally increased to 40 mg/day. Some persons may require 60 mg/day. For elderly persons or persons with hepatic impairment, a dosage of 20 mg/day is recommended, with an increase to 40 mg/day only if no response is noted at 20 mg/day. Tablets should be taken once daily, either in the morning or evening, with or without food.

(6) Escitalopram. Escitalopram (Lexapro) is available in 10- and 20-mg scored tablets. The medication should be initiated at 10 mg/day, taken in a single daily dose, with or without food. Patients not responding to this dosage may be increased to 20 mg/day after a minimum of 1 week.

b. Strategies for limiting adverse effects. Most adverse effects of SSRIs appear within the first 1 to 2 weeks and generally subside or resolve spontaneously if the drugs are continued at the same dosage. However, up to 15% of patients are not able to tolerate the lowest dosage. One approach for such persons is to fractionate the dose over a week, with one dose taken every 2, 3, or 4 days. Some people may tolerate a different SSRI or, if not, may have to take another class of antidepressant, such as a tricyclic drug.

c. **Augmentation strategies.** In depressed people with a partial response to SSRIs, augmentation strategies may be used. One such drug combination, SSRIs plus bupropion, has demonstrated marked added benefits. Some patients have also responded favorably to the addition of lithium, levothyroxine (Levoxine, Levothroid, Synthroid), or amphetamine (5 to 15 mg/day).

d. **Loss of efficacy.** Potential methods to manage attenuation of the response to an SSRI include increasing or decreasing the dosage; tapering the drug, then rechallenging with the same medication; switching to another SSRI or non-SSRI antidepressant; and augmenting with bupropion, thyroid hormone, lithium, sympathomimetics, buspirone, anticonvulsants, naltrexone (ReVia), or another non-SSRI antidepressant. A change in response to an SSRI should be explored in psychotherapy, which may reveal the underlying conflicts causing an increase in depressive symptoms.

4. **Precautions and adverse reactions**

a. **Sexual dysfunction.** Sexual inhibition is the most common adverse effect of SSRIs and may occur in up to 80% of patients. The most common complaints are inhibited orgasm and decreased libido, which are dosage-dependent. Unlike most of the other adverse effects of SSRIs, sexual inhibition does not resolve within the first few weeks of use but usually continues as long as the drug is taken.

Treatment for SSRI-induced sexual dysfunction includes decreasing the dosage or switching to bupropion, which does not cause sexual dysfunction. Other options include adding bupropion once or twice per day or adding sildenafil (Viagra). Small doses of amphetamines (2.5 mg) may also be of use.

b. **Gastrointestinal adverse effects.** The most common GI complaints are nausea, diarrhea, anorexia, vomiting, and dyspepsia. The nausea and loose stools are dosage-related and transient, usually resolving within a few weeks. Paroxetine CR is better tolerated due to its enteric coating, which delays dissolution until passing into the small intestine, and hence, potentially minimizes nausea. Anorexia is most common with fluoxetine, but some people gain weight while taking fluoxetine. Fluoxetine-induced loss of appetite and loss of weight begin as soon as the drug is taken and peak at 20 weeks, after which weight often returns to baseline.

c. **Weight gain.** Up to one-third of people taking SSRIs gain weight, sometimes more than 20 lb. Paroxetine is the SSRI most often associated with weight gain, but it can occur with any agent.

d. Headaches. The incidence of headache with SSRIs is about 18% to 20%. Fluoxetine is the most likely to cause headache. On the other hand, all SSRIs are effective prophylaxis against both migraine and tension-type headaches in many people.

 CLINICAL HINT:
Headaches usually occur in the morning and can be treated with aspirin or acetaminophen. They usually subside spontaneously after a few weeks.

e. CNS adverse effects
   (1) Anxiety. Fluoxetine is the most likely to cause anxiety, agitation, and restlessness, particularly in the first few weeks. These initial effects usually give way to an overall reduction in anxiety after the first month of use. Five percent of people discontinue taking fluoxetine because of increased nervousness. An increase in anxiety is caused considerably less frequently by the other SSRIs.

 CLINICAL HINT:
It may be useful to provide patients with a few 5-mg diazepam tablets that they can take if anxiety occurs when they first start the SSRI.

   (2) Insomnia and sedation. The major effect in this area attributable to SSRIs is improved sleep resulting from the treatment of depression and anxiety. However, as many as one-fourth of people taking SSRIs note either trouble sleeping or excessive somnolence. Fluoxetine is the most likely to cause insomnia, for which reason it is often taken in the morning. Sertraline is about equally likely to cause insomnia or somnolence; citalopram and especially paroxetine are more likely to cause somnolence than insomnia. With the latter agents, people usually report that taking the dose before retiring helps them sleep better and does not cause residual daytime somnolence.

     SSRI-induced insomnia can be treated with benzodiazepines, trazodone (clinicians must explain the risk for priapism), or other sedating medicines. The presence of significant SSRI-induced somnolence often requires switching to another SSRI or to bupropion.

   (3) Vivid dreams and nightmares. A minority of people taking SSRIs report recalling extremely vivid dreams or nightmares. A patient experiencing such dreams with one SSRI may derive the same therapeutic benefit without disturbing dream images by switching to another SSRI. This adverse effect often resolves spontaneously during several weeks.

   (4) Seizures. Seizures have been reported in 0.1% to 0.2% of all persons treated with SSRIs. This incidence is comparable with the incidence reported with other antidepressants and is not significantly different from that noted with placebo. Seizures are more frequent at the highest dosages of SSRIs (100 mg or more of fluoxetine per day).

(5) Extrapyramidal symptoms. Tremor is seen in 5% to 10% of people taking SSRIs. SSRIs may rarely cause akathisia, dystonia, tremor, cogwheel rigidity, torticollis, opisthotonos, gait disorders, and brady-kinesia. People with well-controlled Parkinson's disease may experience acute worsening of their motor symptoms when they take SSRIs. Extrapyramidal adverse effects are most closely associated with the use of fluoxetine; they are particularly noted at dosages in excess of 40 mg/day but may occur at any time during the course of therapy.

f. Anticholinergic effects. Paroxetine has mild anticholinergic activity that causes dry mouth, constipation, and sedation in a dosage-dependent fashion. However, the anticholinergic activity of paroxetine is perhaps only one-fifth that of nortriptyline, and most persons taking paroxetine do not experience cholinergic adverse effects. Although not considered to have anticholinergic activity, the other SSRIs are associated with dry mouth in about 20% of patients. This complaint may disappear with time.

g. Hematologic adverse effects. SSRIs affect platelet function but are rarely associated with increased bruisability. Paroxetine and fluoxetine are rarely associated with the development of reversible neutropenia, particularly if administered concurrently with clozapine.

h. Electrolyte and glucose disturbances. SSRIs are rarely associated with a decrease in glucose concentrations; therefore, persons with diabetes should be carefully monitored and the dosage of their hypoglycemic drug decreased as necessary. Rare cases of SSRI-associated hyponatremia and the secretion of inappropriate antidiuretic hormone (SIADH) have been seen in persons treated with diuretics who are also water-deprived.

i. Rash and allergic reactions. Various types of rashes may appear in about 4% of all persons; in a small subset, generalization of the allergic reaction and involvement of the pulmonary system result rarely in fibrotic damage and dyspnea. SSRI treatment may have to be discontinued in persons with drug-related rashes.

j. Galactorrhea. SSRIs may cause reversible galactorrhea, presumably a consequence of interference with dopaminergic regulation of prolactin secretion.

k. Serotonin syndrome. Serotonin syndrome is rare. Concurrent administration of an SSRI with an MAOI can raise plasma serotonin concentrations to toxic levels and produce a constellation of symptoms called *serotonin syndrome*. This serious and possibly fatal syndrome of serotonin overstimulation comprises, in order of appearance as the condition worsens, (1) diarrhea; (2) restlessness; (3) extreme agitation, hyperreflexia, and autonomic instability with possible rapid fluctuations of vital signs; (4) myoclonus, seizures, hyperthermia, uncontrollable shivering, and rigidity; and (5) delirium, coma, status epilepticus, cardiovascular collapse, and death.

Treatment of serotonin syndrome consists of removing the offending agents and promptly instituting comprehensive supportive care with nitroglycerine, cyproheptadine, methysergide (Sansert), cooling blankets, chlorpromazine (Thorazine), dantrolene (Dantrium), benzodiazepines, anticonvulsants, mechanical ventilation, and paralyzing agents.

l. SSRI discontinuation syndrome. The abrupt discontinuance of an SSRI, especially one with a relatively short half-life, such as paroxetine, has been associated with a syndrome that may include dizziness, weakness, nausea, headache, rebound depression, anxiety, insomnia, poor concentration, upper respiratory symptoms, paresthesias, and migrainelike symptoms. It usually does not appear until after at least 6 weeks of treatment and generally resolves spontaneously in 3 weeks. Persons who experience transient adverse effects in the first weeks of SSRI therapy are more likely to experience discontinuation symptoms. Fluoxetine is the least likely to be associated with this syndrome because the half-life of its metabolite is more than 1 week and it effectively tapers itself. Fluoxetine has therefore been used in some cases to treat the discontinuation syndrome associated with the termination of therapy with other SSRIs, although the syndrome itself is self-limited.

5. Drug interactions. See Table 29-15. SSRIs do not interfere with most other drugs. Serotonin syndrome can develop with concurrent administration of MAOIs, L-tryptophan, lithium, or other antidepressants that inhibit the reuptake of serotonin. Fluoxetine, sertraline, and paroxetine can raise the plasma concentrations of tricyclic antidepressants to levels that can cause clinical toxicity.

The combination of lithium and all serotonergic drugs should be used with caution because of the possibility of precipitating seizures. SSRIs may increase the duration and severity of zolpidem-induced hallucinations. Some significant interactions are discussed below.

a. Fluoxetine. Fluoxetine may slow the metabolism of carbamazepine, antineoplastic agents, diazepam, and phenytoin.

b. Sertraline. Sertraline may displace warfarin from plasma proteins and may increase the prothrombin time.

c. Paroxetine. Because of the potential for interference with the CYP 2D6 enzyme, the coadministration of paroxetine with other antidepressants, phenothiazine, and antiarrhythmic drugs should be undertaken with caution. Paroxetine may increase the anticoagulant effect of warfarin. Coadministration of paroxetine and tramadol (Ultram) may precipitate a serotonin syndrome in elderly persons.

d. Citalopram. Concurrent administration of cimetidine increases concentrations of citalopram by about 40%.

B. Venlafaxine (Effexor) and desvenlafaxine (Pristiq). Venlafaxine and desvenlafaxine are effective antidepressant drugs with a rapid onset of action. Venlafaxine is among the most efficacious drugs for the treatment of severe depression with melancholic features. For a list of non-SSRI antidepressants, see Table 29-16.

Table 29-15
Interactions of Drugs with the SSRIs

SSRI	Other Drugs	Effect	Clinical Importance
Fluoxetine	Desipramine	Inhibits metabolism	Possible
	Carbamazepine	Inhibits metabolism	Possible
	Diazepam	Inhibits metabolism	Not important
	Haloperidol	Inhibits metabolism	Possible
	Warfarin	No interaction	
	Tolbutamide	No interaction	
Fluvoxamine	Antipyrine	Inhibits metabolism	Not important
	Propranolol	Inhibits metabolism	Unlikely
	Tricyclics	Inhibits metabolism	Unlikely
	Warfarin	Inhibits metabolism	Possible
	Atenolol	No interaction	
	Digoxin	No interaction	
Paroxetine	Phenytoin	AUC increases by 12%	Possible
	Procyclidine	AUC increases by 39%	Possible
	Cimetidine	Paroxetine AUC increases by 50%	Possible
	Antipyrine	No interaction	
	Digoxin	No interaction	
	Propranolol	No interaction	
	Tranylcypromine	No interaction	Caution with combined treatment
Sertraline	Warfarin	No interaction	Not important
	Antipyrine	Increased clearance	
	Diazepam	Clearance decreased by 13%	Not important
	Tolbutamide	Clearance decreased by 16%	Not important
	Digoxin	No interaction	
	Lithium	No pharmacokinetic interaction	Caution with combined treatment
	Desipramine	No interaction	
	Atenolol	No pharmacokinetic interaction	
Citalopram	Cimetidine	Citalopram AUC increases	
	Metoprolol	May double blood concentration	

[a]Adapted from Warrington SJ. Clinical implications of the pharmacology of serotonin reuptake inhibitors. *Int Clin Psychopharmacol.* 1987;7(Suppl 2);13, with permission.
AUC, area under curve.

Table 29-16
Non-SSRI Antidepressants

Drugs	Time to Peak Plasma Concentration (hours)	Half-Life (hours)	Starting Dose (mg)	Maintenance Dose (mg)	High Dose (mg)
Venlafaxine	2.5	9	75	225	300–375
Venlafaxine XR	5	11	37.5–75	150	225
Bupropion	2	8	100	300	450
Bupropion SR	3	12	150	300	400
Bupropion XL	5	35	150	300	>300
Mirtazapine	2	20–40	15	45	60
Duloxetine	6	12	30–40	60	>60
Nefazodone	1	4–8	100–200	300–600	>600
Trazodone	1	10–12	150	400	600
Vilazodone	4–5	25	10	20	40
Levomilnacipran	6–8	12	20	40	80
Vortioxetine	7–11	66	10	20	-

1. **Pharmacologic actions.** Venlafaxine is well absorbed from the GI tract and reaches peak plasma concentrations within 2.5 hours. It has a half-life of about 3.5 hours, and its one active metabolite, *O*-desmethylvenlafaxine, has a half-life of 11 hours. Therefore, venlafaxine must be taken two to three times daily. Desvenlafaxine is an extended-release tablet and an active metabolite of venlafaxine. The peak plasma concentration is reached within 7.5 hours and has a half-life of 11 hours. It is formulated for once-a-day administration, and the usual dose is 50 mg with no further benefit seen at higher doses.

    Venlafaxine and desvenlafaxine are nonselective inhibitors of the reuptake of three biogenic amines—serotonin, norepinephrine, and, to a lesser extent, dopamine. They have no activity at muscarinic, nicotinic, histaminergic, opioid, or adrenergic receptors, and are not active as an MAOI.

2. **Therapeutic efficacy.** Venlafaxine is approved for the treatment of MDD and generalized anxiety disorder, while desvenlafaxine is indicated for the treatment of MDD. Many severely depressed persons respond to venlafaxine at a dosage of 200 mg/day and desvenlafaxine at a dosage of 50 mg/day within 2 weeks, a period of time somewhat shorter than 2 to 4 weeks usually required for SSRIs to take effect. Therefore, venlafaxine at high dosages may become a preferred drug for seriously ill persons in whom a rapid response is desired. However, sympathomimetics (e.g., amphetamines) and ECT appear to have the most rapid onset of antidepressant action, usually taking effect within 1 week. In direct comparison with fluoxetine for the treatment of seriously depressed persons with melancholic features, venlafaxine is considered superior.

3. **Clinical guidelines.** Venlafaxine is available in 25-, 37.5-, 50-, 75-, and 100-mg immediate-release tablets and in 37.5-, 75-, and 150-mg extended-release capsules (Effexor XR). The immediate-release tablets should be given in two or three daily doses, and the extended-release capsules are taken in a single dose before sleep up to a maximum dosage of 225 mg/day. The tablets and the extended-release capsules are equally potent, and persons stabilized with one can switch to an equivalent dosage of the other. Desvenlafaxine is available in 50- and 100-mg tablets. They are taken in a single dose of 50 mg with no further benefit observed at higher doses.

    The usual starting dosage for venlafaxine in depressed persons is 75 mg/day, given as tablets in two to three divided doses or as extended-release capsules in a single dose before sleep. Some persons require a starting dosage of 37.5 mg/day for 4 to 7 days to minimize adverse effects, particularly nausea, before titration up to 75 mg/day. In persons with depression, the dosage can be raised to 150 mg/day, given as tablets in two or three divided doses or as extended-release capsules once a day, after an appropriate period of clinical assessment at the lower dosage (usually 2 to 3 weeks). The dosage can be raised in increments of 75 mg/day every 4 days or more. Moderately depressed persons probably do not require dosages in excess of 225 mg/day, whereas severely depressed persons may require dosages of 300 to 375 mg/day for a satisfactory response.

A rapid antidepressant response—within 1 to 2 weeks—may result from the administration of a dosage of 200 mg/day from the beginning. The maximum dosage of venlafaxine is 375 mg/day. The dosage of venlafaxine should be halved in persons with significant diminished hepatic or renal function. If discontinued, venlafaxine should be gradually tapered during 2 to 4 weeks.

4. **Precautions and adverse reactions.** Venlafaxine and desvenlafaxine are generally well tolerated. The most common adverse reactions are nausea, somnolence, dry mouth, dizziness, and nervousness. The incidence of nausea is reduced somewhat with use of the extended-release capsules. The sexual adverse effects of these medicines can be treated like those of the SSRIs. Abrupt discontinuation may produce a discontinuation syndrome consisting of nausea, somnolence, and insomnia. Therefore, they should be tapered gradually during 2 to 4 weeks. The most potentially worrisome adverse effect associated with venlafaxine is an increase in blood pressure in some persons, particularly those treated with more than 300 mg/day. Thus, the drug should be used cautiously by persons with pre-existing hypertension, and then only at lower dosages.

Information about the use of venlafaxine by pregnant and nursing women is not available at this time. However, clinicians should avoid prescribing all newly introduced drugs to pregnant and nursing women until more clinical experience has been acquired.

5. **Drug interactions.** Venlafaxine may raise plasma concentrations of concurrently administered haloperidol. Like all antidepressant medications, venlafaxine and desvenlafaxine should not be used within 14 days of the use of MAOIs, and they may potentiate the sedative effects of other drugs that act on the CNS.

C. **Bupropion.** Bupropion is used for the treatment of depression and for smoking cessation. It generally is more effective against symptoms of depression than of anxiety, and it is quite effective in combination with SSRIs. Despite early warnings that it could cause seizures, clinical experience now shows that when used at recommended dosages, bupropion is no more likely to cause seizures than any other antidepressant drug. Smoking cessation is most successful when bupropion (called Zyban for this indication) is used in combination with behavioral modification techniques.

Bupropion is unique among antidepressants because of a highly favorable profile of adverse effects. Of particular note among antidepressants, the rates of sedation, sexual dysfunction, and weight gain are minor with this drug. Some patients, however, experience severe anxiety or agitation when starting bupropion.

1. **Pharmacologic actions.** Bupropion is well absorbed from the gastrointestinal tract. Peak plasma concentrations of the immediate-release formulation of bupropion are usually reached within 2 hours of oral administration,

and peak concentrations of the sustained-release formulation are seen after 3 hours. The half-life of the compound ranges from 8 to 40 hours (mean, 12 hours). The extended-release form reaches peak plasma concentration in about 5 hours and has a half-life of about 35 hours.

2. **Therapeutic efficacy.** The therapeutic efficacy of bupropion in depression is well established in both outpatient and inpatient settings.

3. **Dosage and administration.** There are three preparations of bupropion: (1) immediate-release bupropion is available in 75- and 100-mg tablets; (2) sustained-release bupropion (Wellbutrin SR) is available in 100-, 150-, and 200-mg tablets; and (3) extended-release bupropion is available in 150- and 300-mg tablets. Treatment in the average adult person should be initiated at 100 mg of the immediate-release version orally twice a day, or 150 mg of the sustained-release and extended-release version once a day. On the fourth day of treatment, the dosage can be raised to 100 mg of the immediate-release preparation orally three times a day, or 150 mg of the sustained-release preparation orally twice a day. The extended-release version can be raised to 300 mg once a day. Alternatively, 300 mg of the sustained-release version can be taken once each morning. The dosage of 300 mg/day should be maintained for several weeks before it is increased further. Because of the risk for seizures, increases in dosage should never exceed 100 mg in a 3-day period; a single dose of immediate-release bupropion should never exceed 150 mg, and a single dose of sustained-release bupropion should never exceed 300 mg; the total daily dose should not exceed 450 mg (immediate release or extended release) or 400 mg (sustained release).

4. **Precautions and adverse reactions.** The most common adverse effects associated with the use of bupropion are headache, insomnia, upper respiratory complaints, and nausea. Restlessness, agitation, and irritability may also occur. Most likely because of its potentiating effects on dopaminergic neurotransmission, bupropion has rarely been associated with psychotic symptoms (e.g., hallucinations, delusions, and catatonia) and delirium. Most notable about bupropion is the absence of significant drug-induced orthostatic hypotension, weight gain, daytime drowsiness, and anticholinergic effects. Some persons, however, may experience dry mouth or constipation, and weight loss may occur in about 25% of persons. Bupropion causes no significant cardiovascular or clinical laboratory changes.

A major advantage of bupropion over SSRIs is that bupropion is virtually devoid of any adverse effects on sexual functioning, whereas SSRIs are associated with such effects in up to 80% of all persons. Some people taking bupropion experience an increase in sexual responsiveness and even spontaneous orgasm.

At dosages of 300 mg/day or less, the incidence of seizures is about 0.1%, which is no worse, and in some cases superior, to the incidence of seizures with other antidepressants. The risk for seizures increases to about 5% in dosages between 450 and 600 mg/day. Risk factors for seizures, such as a past history of seizures, abuse of alcohol, recent benzodiazepine withdrawal, organic brain disease, head trauma, or epileptiform discharges on electroencephalogram (EEG), warrant critical examination of the decision to use bupropion.

Because high dosages (>450 mg/day) of bupropion may be associated with a euphoric feeling, bupropion may be relatively contraindicated in persons with a history of substance abuse. The use of bupropion by pregnant women has not been studied and is not recommended. Because bupropion is secreted in breast milk, its use in nursing women is not recommended.

Overdoses of bupropion are associated with a generally favorable outcome, except in cases of huge doses and overdoses of mixed drugs. Seizures occur in about one-third of all cases of overdose, and fatalities may result from uncontrollable seizures, bradycardia, and cardiac arrest. In general, however, overdoses of bupropion are less harmful than overdoses of other antidepressants, except perhaps SSRIs.

5. **Drug interactions.** Bupropion should not be used concurrently with MAOIs because of the possibility of inducing a hypertensive crisis, and at least 14 days should pass after an MAOI is discontinued before treatment with bupropion is initiated. Delirium, psychotic symptoms, and dyskinetic movements may be associated with the coadministration of bupropion and dopaminergic agents (e.g., levodopa [Laradopa], pergolide [Permax], ropinirole [Requip], pramipexole [Mirapex], amantadine [Symmetrel], and bromocriptine [Parlodel]).

D. **Duloxetine.** Duloxetine is a selective serotonin and norepinephrine reuptake inhibitor (SSNRI) effective in the treatment of MDD.

1. **Pharmacologic actions.** Duloxetine is well absorbed from the GI tract and reaches peak plasma concentration within 6 hours. Food delays the time to peak concentration from 6 to 10 hours and marginally decreases the extent of absorption by about 10%. It has a half-life of about 12 hours and steady-state plasma concentrations are achieved after 3 days. It is mainly metabolized through P450 isoenzymes, CYP 2D6, and CYP 1A2, and is highly protein-bound (>90%).

It is a potent inhibitor of neuronal serotonin and norepinephrine reuptake and a less potent inhibitor of dopamine reuptake.

2. **Therapeutic efficacy.** Duloxetine is approved for the treatment of MDD and diabetic peripheral neuropathic pain.

3. **Clinical guidelines.** Duloxetine is available in 20-, 30-, and 60-mg delayed-release capsules. The capsule should be administered preferably once a day without regard to meals, starting at a total dose of 40 mg/day (given as 20-mg b.i.d.) to 60 mg/day (given either once a day or as 30-mg b.i.d.). If starting at 30 to 40 mg/day, the dose should be titrated quickly to 60 mg/day. There is no evidence that doses greater than 60 mg/day are more beneficial. There is no need for dosage adjustment based on age or gender.

4. **Precautions and adverse reactions.** Duloxetine is usually well tolerated. The most common adverse events reported were nausea, dry

mouth, and insomnia. Of those reporting nausea, 60% had mild symptoms that lasted about 1 week.

Sexual dysfunction may occur, more frequently in males who have difficulty in attaining orgasm. Duloxetine can also affect urethral resistance, and this should be considered if symptoms develop. Discontinuation symptoms can develop, and gradual dose reduction is recommended.

There is a mean increase in blood pressure, averaging 2 mm Hg systolic and 0.5 mm Hg diastolic. Periodic measurements are recommended. It can cause mydriasis and should be used cautiously in patients with narrow-angle glaucoma.

There are no adequate studies in pregnant women and duloxetine should only be used if the benefit justifies the risk.

5. **Drug interactions.** Duloxetine is metabolized through both CYP 1A2 and CYP 2D6. When used concomitantly with fluvoxamine, a potent CYP 1A2 inhibitor, the dose of duloxetine should be decreased. Similarly, CYP 2D6 inhibitors can cause elevated duloxetine levels.

E. **Mirtazapine.** It is approved for the treatment of major depression. It is rapidly and completely absorbed and has a half-life of about 30 hours. It lacks the anticholinergic effects of tricyclic antidepressants and the GI and anxiogenic effects of SSRIs. Somnolence, the most common adverse effect of mirtazapine, occurs in more than 50% of persons and increases appetite in about one-third of patients leading to weight gain. It may increase hepatic enzymes and cause neutropenia in 0.3% of patients. The recommended doe range is 15 to 45 mg. Mirtazapine is excreted in breast milk and should not be taken by nursing mothers.

F. **Nefazodone.** Nefazodone has antidepressant effects comparable with those of SSRIs, yet unlike SSRIs, nefazodone improves sleep continuity and has little effect on sexual functioning. It is chemically related to trazodone but causes less sedation. Among the more serious side effects is liver toxicity; because of this, it is not commonly used. The manufacturer has withdrawn the brand product from the market and only generic versions are available.

1. **Clinical guidelines.** Nefazodone is available in 50-, 200-, and 250-mg unscored and 100- and 150-mg scored tablets. The recommended starting dosage of nefazodone is 100 mg twice daily, but 50 mg twice daily may be better tolerated, especially in elderly persons. To limit the development of adverse effects, the daily dose should be slowly increased in increments of 100 to 200 mg, with intervals of no less than 1 week between each increase. Elderly patients should receive about two-thirds the usual nongeriatric dosages, with a maximum of 400 mg/day. The clinical benefits of nefazodone, like those of other antidepressants, usually become apparent after 2 to 4 weeks of treatment.

2. **Precautions and adverse reactions.** In preclinical trials, 16% of persons discontinued nefazodone because of an adverse event. Liver impairment precludes its use.

A summary of dosages and pharmacokinetics of the non-SSRI antidepressants discussed above is presented in Table 29-16.

G. Trazodone. Trazodone is approved for the treatment of MDD. It is a first-line agent for the treatment of insomnia because of its marked sedative qualities and favorable effects on sleep architecture with no anticholinergic effects. It is a weak inhibitor of serotonin reuptake and a potent antagonist of serotonin 5-HT$_{2A}$ and 5-HT$_{2C}$ receptors. A dosage of 250 to 600 mg a day is necessary to have therapeutic benefit. It is associated with an increased risk of priapism and can potentiate erections resulting from sexual stimulation. Trazodone-triggered priapism (an erection lasting more than 3 hours with pain) is a medical emergency. The most common adverse effects associated with trazodone are sedation, orthostatic hypotension, dizziness, headache, and nausea. Some persons experience dry mouth or gastric irritation. The use of trazodone is contraindicated in pregnant and nursing women.

A newer extended-release, once-daily formulation (Oleptro) is approved for the treatment of MDD in adults. The most common adverse events are somnolence or sedation, dizziness, constipation, and blurred vision.

H. Vilazodone. It is approved for the treatment of MDD. Vilazodone inhibits serotonin uptake with minimal or no effect on reuptake of norepinephrine or dopamine. The pharmacokinetics of vilazodone (5 to 80 mg) are dose proportional. Steady-state plasma levels are achieved in about 3 days. Elimination of vilazodone is primarily by hepatic metabolism with a terminal half-life of approximately 25 hours. Dose should be reduced to 20 mg when coadministered with CYP 3A4 strong inhibitors. Concomitant use with inducers of CYP 3A4 may require dose adjustment. The effect of CYP 3A4 inducers on systemic exposure of vilazodone has not been evaluated. Vilazodone is available as 10-, 20-, and 40-mg tablets. The recommended therapeutic dose of vilazodone is 40 mg once daily. Treatment should be titrated, starting with an initial dose of 10 mg once daily for 7 days, followed by 20 mg once daily for an additional 7 days, and then an increase to 40 mg once daily. Vilazodone should be taken with food. If vilazodone is taken without food, inadequate drug concentrations may result and the drug's effectiveness may be diminished.

I. Levomilnacipran. Levomilnacipran is approved for the treatment of MDD in adults. Levomilnacipran is an active enantiomer of the racemic drug milnacipran approved for the treatment of fibromyalgia. In vitro studies have shown that it has greater potency for norepinephrine reuptake inhibition than for serotonin reuptake inhibition and does not directly affect the uptake of dopamine or other neurotransmitters. It is taken once daily as a sustained-release formulation. In clinical trials, doses of 40-, 80-, or 120-mg improved symptoms compared with placebo.

The most common adverse reactions in the placebo-controlled trials were nausea, constipation, hyperhidrosis, increased heart rate, erectile dysfunction, tachycardia, vomiting, and palpitations. Rates of adverse events were generally consistent across the 40- to 120-mg dose range. The only dose-related adverse events were urinary hesitation and erectile dysfunction.

J. Vortioxetine. Vortioxetine works mainly as an inhibitor of serotonin (5-HT) reuptake, but it has a more complex pharmacologic profile than other

Table 29-17
General Information for the Tricyclic and Tetracyclic Antidepressants

Generic Name	Trade Name	Usual Adult Dosage Range (mg/day)	Therapeutic Plasma Concentrations (mg/mL)
Imipramine	Tofranil	150–300	150–300[a]
Desipramine	Norpramin, Pertofrane	150–300	150–300[a]
Trimipramine	Surmontil	150–300	150–300
Amitriptyline	Elavil, Endep	150–300	100–250[b]
Nortriptyline	Pamelor, Aventyl	50–150	50–150[a] (maximum)
Protriptyline	Vivactil	15–60	75–250
Amoxapine	Asendin	150–400	[c]
Doxepin	Adapin, Sinequan	150–300	100–250[a]
Maprotiline	Ludiomil	150–230	150–300[a]
Clomipramine	Anafranil	130–250	[c]

[a]Exact range may vary among laboratories.
[b]Includes parent compound and desmethyl metabolite.
[c]Therapeutic plasma levels unknown.

SSRIs. It also acts as an agonist at $5\text{-}HT_{1A}$ receptors, a partial agonist at $5\text{-}HT_{1B}$ receptors and an antagonist at $5\text{-}HT_3$, $5\text{-}HT_{1D}$, and $5\text{-}HT_7$ receptors.

Side effects include nausea, constipation, and vomiting.

The recommended starting dose is 10 mg administered orally once daily without regard to meals. The dose should then be increased to 20 mg/day, as tolerated. A dose of 5 mg/day should be considered for patients who do not tolerate higher doses. The maximum recommended dose is 10 mg/day in CYP 2D6 poor metabolizers. Reduction of the dose by one-half is suggested when receiving a CYP 2D6 strong inhibitor (e.g., bupropion, fluoxetine, paroxetine, or quinidine) concomitantly.

Abrupt discontinuation of vortioxetine 15 or 20 mg/day may cause headache and muscle tension. To avoid this, it is recommended that the dose be decreased to 10 mg/day for 1 week before full discontinuation of vortioxetine 15 or 20 mg/day.

Vortioxetine is available in 5-, 10-, 15-, and 20-mg tablets.

K. Tricyclic and tetracyclic drugs. Tricyclic and tetracyclic antidepressants (Table 29-17) are rarely used because of their adverse effects.

L. MAOIs. MAOIs (Table 29-18) are highly effective antidepressants, but they are little used because of the dietary precautions that must be followed to avoid tyramine-induced hypertensive crises and because of harmful drug interactions.

Table 29-18
Typical Dosage Forms and Recommended Dosages for Currently Available Monoamine Oxidase Inhibitors

Drug	Usual Dose (mg/day)	Maximum Dose (mg/day)	Dosage (Oral) Formulation
Isocarboxazid (Marplan)	20–40	60	10-mg tablets
Phenelzine (Nardil)	30–60	90	15-mg tablets
Tranylcypromine (Parnate)	20–60	60	10-mg tablets
Rasagiline	0.5–1.0	1.0	0.5- or 1.0-mg tablets
Selegiline (Eldepryl)	10	-30	5-mg tablets
Moclobemide (Manerix)	300–600	600	100- or 150-mg tablets

M. Selegiline transdermal patch (Emsam). Emsam is a transdermally administered antidepressant. When applied to intact skin, Emsam is designed to continuously deliver selegiline over a 24-hour period. Emsam systems are transdermal patches that contain 1 mg of selegiline per cm^2 and deliver approximately 0.3 mg of selegiline per cm^2 over 24 hours. Selegiline (the drug substance of Emsam) is an irreversible MAOI, and steady-state selegiline plasma concentrations are achieved within 5 days of daily dosing. In humans, selegiline is approximately 90% bound to plasma proteins. Transdermally absorbed selegiline (via Emsam) is not metabolized in human skin, and is extensively metabolized by several CYP 450-dependent enzyme systems including CYP 2B6, CYP 2C9, and CYP 3A4/5.

Emsam (selegiline transdermal system) is contraindicated with SSRIs, dual SNRIs, TCAs, bupropion hydrochloride; meperidine and analgesic agents such as tramadol, methadone, and propoxyphene; the antitussive agent dextromethorphan; St. John's wort; mirtazapine; and cyclobenzaprine. Emsam should not be used with oral selegiline or other MAOIs.

Even though Emsam is an irreversible MAOI, the data for Emsam 6 mg/24 hours support the recommendation that a modified (tyramine rich) diet is not required at this dose. If a hypertensive crisis occurs, Emsam should be discontinued immediately and therapy to lower blood pressure should be instituted immediately.

Emsam should be applied to dry, intact skin on the upper torso (below the neck and above the waist), upper thigh or the outer surface of the upper arm. A new application site should be selected with each new patch to avoid re-application to the same site on consecutive days. Patches should be applied at approximately the same time each day.

Emsam is supplied as 6 mg/24 hours (20 mg/20 cm^2), 9 mg/24 hours (30 mg/30 cm^2) and 12 mg/24 hours (40 mg/40 cm^2) transdermal systems.

N. Ketamine. Ketamine has been in use since 1970, used as an anesthetic agent. It also became a drug of abuse as a psychedelic club drug. In 2006, a study by Zarate CA Jr at the National Institute of Mental Health (NIMH) concluded that Ketamine produced a robust and rapid antidepressant effect after a single IV infusion with an onset within 2 hours postinfusion and remained significant for a week.

It is a nonbarbiturate anesthetic chemically designated dl 2-(0-chlorophenyl)-2-(methylamino) cyclohexanone hydrochloride. Ketamine hydrochloride injection should be used by or under the direction and supervision of physicians who are experienced in administering general anesthetics and in maintenance of an airway and in the control of respiration.

Since the landmark study thousands of depressed patients have received off-label Ketamine infusions even though the FDA has not approved it. The benefits are transitory for 1 to 2 weeks and require ongoing regular infusions. Alternate modes of administration including intranasal and PO formulations are being explored but oral bioavailability is only 8% to 17%. As of now this treatment modality is being practiced by a few psychiatrists as an off-label use for patients who have failed to show response to conventional antidepressant therapy or ECT.

O. Psilocybin. Psilocybin, the active ingredient in mushrooms, is being investigated in the treatment of anxiety and depression particularly in the end-of-life situations like patients with terminal cancer. Numerous studies across the country are looking at this mysterious and magical product that has been used since ancient times in various cultures. A single dose of Psilocybin has been shown to reduce anxiety and depression by altering perception and producing mystical-type experiences with effects lasting up to 6 months. At this time, Psilocybin remains confined as a potential treatment for anxiety and depression in controlled research setting under the guidance of well-trained personnel.

P. Antidepressants in development. Numerous new antidepressants are currently in development but are years from any regulatory approval. Theses agents have newer and novel mechanisms of action including:

Triple reuptake inhibitors that block serotonin, norepinephrine and dopamine reuptake.

NK receptor antagonists that block substance P receptor, and also offers anxiolytic properties.

CRF1 antagonists that block corticotrophin-releasing receptors, and regulate HPA axis.

Glutamate-acting drugs that block N-methyl-D-aspartate receptors (NMDA).

Q. Opioid for depression. Recent studies show opioid dysregulation in major depression. The combination of buprenorphine and samidorphan show promising results in treatment-resistant depression equivalent to adjunct treatment with antipsychotics. Obvious concerns for abuse exist but combination of buprenorphine with mu-opioid receptor antagonist may block the abuse potential of buprenorphine.

VII. Antimanic Drugs

A. Lithium. Lithium is used for the short-term and prophylactic treatment of bipolar I disorder.

    1. Pharmacologic actions. After ingestion, lithium is completely absorbed by the GI tract. Serum concentrations peak in 1 to 1½ hours for standard preparations and in 4 to 4½ hours for controlled-release preparations. Lithium does not bind to plasma proteins, is not metabolized, and is excreted through the kidneys. The blood–brain barrier permits only slow passage of lithium, which is why a single overdose does not necessarily cause toxicity and why long-term lithium intoxication is slow to resolve. The half-life of lithium is about 20 hours, and equilibrium is reached after 5 to 7 days of regular intake. The renal clearance of lithium is decreased in persons with renal insufficiency (common in the elderly). The excretion of lithium is increased during pregnancy but decreased after delivery. Lithium is excreted in breast milk and in insignificant amounts in feces and sweat.

2. **Therapeutic efficacy**
   a. **Manic episodes.** Lithium controls acute mania. It prevents relapse in about 80% of persons with bipolar I disorder and in a somewhat smaller percentage of persons with mixed or dysphoric mania, rapid-cycling bipolar disorder, comorbid substance abuse, or encephalopathy. Lithium alone at therapeutic concentrations exerts its antimanic effects in 1 to 3 weeks. To control mania acutely, therefore, a benzodiazepine (e.g., clonazepam or lorazepam) or a dopamine receptor agonist (e.g., haloperidol or chlorpromazine) should also be administered for the first few weeks.

   Lithium is effective as long-term prophylaxis for both manic and depressive episodes in about 70% to 80% of persons with bipolar I disorder.

   b. **Depressive episodes.** Lithium is effective in the treatment of MDD and depression associated with bipolar I disorder. Lithium exerts a partial or complete antidepressant effect in about 80% of persons with bipolar I disorder. Many persons take lithium and an antidepressant together as long-term maintenance for their bipolar disease. Augmentation of lithium therapy with valproate or carbamazepine is usually well tolerated, with little risk for the precipitation of mania.

   When a depressive episode occurs in a person taking maintenance lithium, the differential diagnosis should include lithium-induced hypothyroidism, substance abuse, and lack of compliance with the lithium therapy. Treatment approaches include increasing the lithium concentration (up to 1 to 1.2 mEq/L); adding supplemental thyroid hormone (e.g., 25 mg of liothyronine [Cytomel] per day), even in the presence of normal findings on thyroid function tests; augmenting lithium with valproate or carbamazepine; and judiciously using antidepressants or ECT. Some experts report that administering ECT to a person taking lithium increases the risk for cognitive dysfunction, but this point is controversial. Once the acute depressive episode resolves, other therapies should be tapered in favor of lithium monotherapy, if clinically effective.

   c. **Maintenance.** Maintenance treatment with lithium markedly decreases the frequency, severity, and duration of manic and depressive episodes in persons with bipolar I disorder. Lithium provides relatively more effective prophylaxis for mania than for depression, and supplemental antidepressant strategies may be necessary either intermittently or continuously.

   Lithium maintenance is almost always indicated after a second episode of bipolar I disorder depression or mania. Lithium maintenance should be seriously considered after a first episode for adolescents or for persons who have a family history of bipolar I disorder, have poor support systems, had no precipitating factors for the first episode, had a serious first episode, are at high risk for suicide, are 30 years old or older, had a sudden onset of their first episode, had a first episode of mania, or are male. Lithium is also effective treatment for persons with severe cyclothymic disorder.

The wisdom of initiating maintenance therapy after a first manic episode is illustrated by several observations. First, each episode of mania increases the risk for subsequent episodes. Second, among people responsive to lithium, relapses are 28 times more likely to occur after lithium is discontinued. Third, case reports describe persons who were initially responsive to lithium, then stopped taking it and had a relapse, and were no longer responsive to lithium during subsequent episodes.

The response to lithium treatment is such that continued maintenance treatment is often associated with increasing efficacy and reduced mortality. It does not necessarily represent treatment failure, therefore, if an episode of depression or mania occurs after a relatively short period of lithium maintenance. However, lithium treatment alone may begin to lose its effectiveness after several years of successful use. If this occurs, then supplemental treatment with carbamazepine or valproate may be useful.

Maintenance lithium dosages often can be adjusted to achieve a serum or plasma concentration somewhat lower than that needed for the treatment of acute mania. If lithium use is to be discontinued, then the dosage should be slowly tapered. Abrupt discontinuation of lithium therapy is associated with an increased risk for rapid recurrence of manic or depressive episodes.

3. **Dosage and clinical guidelines**

   a. **Initial medical workup.** Before the clinician administers lithium, a physician should conduct a routine laboratory and physical examination (Table 29-19). The laboratory examination should include measurement of the serum creatinine concentration (or the 24-hour urine creatinine concentration if the clinician has any reason to be concerned about renal function), an electrolyte screen, thyroid function tests (thyroid-stimulating hormone, triiodothyronine, and thyroxine), a complete blood cell count, an ECG, and a pregnancy test in women of childbearing age.

   b. **Dosage recommendations.** In the United States, lithium formulations include 150-, 300-, and 600-mg regular-release lithium

Table 29-19
Lithium

Initial Medical Workup
Physical examination
Laboratory workup
Serum creatinine (or a 24-hour urine creatinine)
Electrolytes
Thyroid Function (TSH, T_3, and T_4)
Complete blood count (CBC)
ECG
Pregnancy test (women of childbearing age)

carbonate capsules (Eskalith, Lithonate); 300-mg regular-release lithium carbonate tablets (Lithotabs); 450-mg controlled-release lithium carbonate capsules (Eskalith CR); and lithium citrate syrup in a concentration of 8 mEq/5 mL.

The starting dosage for most adult persons is 300 mg of the regular-release formulation three times daily. The starting dosage in elderly persons or persons with renal impairment should be 300 mg once or twice daily. An eventual dosage of between 900 and 1,200 mg/day usually produces a therapeutic concentration of 0.6 to 1 mEq/L, and a dosage of 1,200 to 1,800 mg/day usually produces a therapeutic concentration of 0.8 to 1.2 mEq/L. Maintenance dosing can be given either in two or three divided doses of the regular-release formulation or in a single dose of the sustained-release formulation that is equivalent to the combined daily doses of the regular-release formulation. The use of divided doses reduces gastric upset and avoids single high-peak lithium concentrations.

c. **Serum and plasma concentrations.** The measurement of serum and plasma concentrations of lithium is a standard method of assessment, and these values serve as a basis for titration. Lithium concentrations should be determined routinely every 2 to 6 months, and promptly in persons who are suspected to be noncompliant with the prescribed dosage, who exhibit signs of toxicity, or who are undergoing a dosage adjustment.

The most common guidelines are 1.0 to 1.5 mEq/L for the treatment of acute mania and 0.4 to 0.8 mEq/L for maintenance treatment.

4. **Precautions and adverse reactions.** Fewer than 20% of persons taking lithium experience no adverse effects, and significant adverse effects are experienced by at least 30% of those taking lithium. The most common adverse effects of lithium treatment are gastric distress, weight gain, tremor, fatigue, and mild cognitive impairment. Table 29-20 lists common lithium side effects and their management.

5. **Use during pregnancy.** FDA labels lithium as pregnancy category D with evidence of human fetal risk but clinicians may prescribe lithium based on potential benefits in select patients.

6. **Drug interactions.** Lithium drug interactions are summarized in Table 29-21.

B. **Valproate.** Valproate is a first-line drug in the treatment of acute manic episodes in bipolar I disorder, at least equal in efficacy and safety to lithium. Available formulations include valproic acid (Depakene), a 1:1 mixture of valproic acid and sodium valproate (Depakote), and injectable sodium valproate (Depacon). Each of these is therapeutically equivalent because at physiologic pH valproic acid dissociates into valproate ion.

1. **Pharmacologic actions.** All valproate formulations are rapidly and completely absorbed after oral administration. The steady-state half-life of valproate is about 8 to 17 hours, and clinically effective plasma concentrations can usually be maintained with dosing once, twice, or three or four

Table 29-20
Common Lithium Side Effects and Their Management

Side Effect	Possible Approaches (Most Not Based on Strong Evidence)
Tremor (C); usually worse under social scrutiny	Lower dose ++; use β-blocker, such as propranolol (Inderal) 10 mg four times daily ++ Consider primidone (Mysoline) as alternative + Replace some of lithium (Eskalith) dose with dihydropyridine calcium channel blocker +
Gastrointestinal distress (O)	Lower dose + Switch lithium preparations ± Replace some of lithium dose with a calcium channel blocker ±
Weight gain (O)	Warn and treat in advance ± Avoid nondiet sodas + Consider weight loss adjuncts ++
Cognitive impairment (UC)	Treat residual depression + Check thyroid Even if euthyroid, consider treating with T_3 +++
Increased urination (C) (diabetes insipidus, i.e., blockage of vasopressin receptor response at level of decreased production of cyclic adenosine monophosphate)	If extreme or functionally impairing, treat with thiazide diuretics or amiloride (Midamor) Switch to other mood stabilizing agents Carbamazepine (Tegretol) does not cause diabetes insipidus but does not correct lithium-related diabetes insipidus
Kidney function impairment (UC)	Reduce dose ± Monitor closely Discontinue drug if rise in creatine is consistent ± Replace with other mood stabilizers +
Psoriasis (O, I)	Omega-3 fatty acid supplementation may help suppress lithium effect +
Acne (O)	Retinoic acid only for women not of childbearing age or men ++ Tetracycline (Achromycin V), clindamycin (Cleocin) +
Hypothyroidism (O)	Replace with T_4 ++ Use T_4 and T_3 combination if mood remains low +

+, likely works; ++, many case reports; +++, well-supported, controlled data; ±, questionable or hypothetical; C, common; D, dose related; I, idiosyncratic; O, occasional; T3, Triiodothyronine; T4, thyroxine; UC, uncommon; VC, very common; VR, very rare.

times per day. Protein binding becomes saturated and concentrations of therapeutically effective free valproate increase at serum concentrations above 50 to 100 µg/mL.

2. **Therapeutic efficacy**

a. **Manic episodes.** Valproate effectively controls manic symptoms in about two-thirds of persons with acute mania. Valproate also reduces overall psychiatric symptoms and the need for supplemental doses of benzodiazepines or dopamine receptor agonists. Persons with mania usually respond 1 to 4 days after valproate serum concentrations rise above 50 µg/mL. With the use of gradual dosing strategies, this serum concentration can be achieved within 1 week of initiation of dosing, but newer, rapid oral loading strategies achieve therapeutic serum concentrations in 1 day and can control manic symptoms within 5 days. The short-term antimanic effects of valproate can be augmented with the addition of lithium, carbamazepine, or dopamine receptor agonists. SDAs and gabapentin (Neurontin) may also potentiate the effects of

Table 29-21
Drug Interactions with Lithium

Drug Class	Reaction
Antipsychotics	Case reports of encephalopathy, worsening of extrapyramidal adverse effects, and neuroleptic malignant syndrome. Inconsistent reports of altered red blood cell and plasma concentrations of lithium, antipsychotic drug, or both
Antidepressants	Occasional reports of a serotoninlike syndrome with potent serotonin reuptake inhibitors
Anticonvulsants	No significant pharmacokinetic interactions with carbamazepine or valproate; reports of neurotoxicity with carbamazepine; combinations helpful for treatment resistance
Nonsteroidal anti-inflammatory drugs	May reduce renal lithium clearance and increase serum concentration; toxicity reported (exception is aspirin)
Diuretics	
Thiazides	Well-documented reduced renal lithium clearance and increased serum concentration; toxicity reported
Potassium sparing	Limited data, may increase lithium concentration
Loop	Lithium clearance unchanged (some case reports of increased lithium concentration)
Osmotic (mannitol, urea)	Increase renal lithium clearance and decrease lithium concentration
Xanthine (aminophylline, caffeine, theophylline)	Increase renal lithium clearance and decrease lithium concentration
Carbonic anhydrase inhibitors (acetazolamide)	Increase renal lithium clearance
Angiotensin-converting enzyme (ACE) inhibitors	Reports of reduced lithium clearance, increased concentrations, and toxicity
Calcium channel inhibitors	Case reports of neurotoxicity; no consistent pharmacokinetic interactions
Miscellaneous	
Succinylcholine, pancuronium	Reports of prolonged neuromuscular blockade
Metronidazole	Increased lithium concentration
Methyldopa	Few reports of neurotoxicity
Sodium bicarbonate	Increased renal lithium clearance
Lodides	Additive antithyroid effects
Propranolol	Used for lithium tremor. Possible slight increase in lithium concentration

valproate, albeit less rapidly. Because of its more favorable profile of cognitive, dermatologic, thyroid, and renal adverse effects, valproate is preferred to lithium for the treatment of acute mania in children and elderly persons.

b. Depressive episodes. Valproate alone is less effective for the short-term treatment of depressive episodes in bipolar I disorder than for the treatment of manic episodes. In patients with depressive symptoms, valproate is a more effective treatment for agitation than for dysphoria.

c. Maintenance. Valproate is not FDA-approved for maintenance treatment of bipolar I disorder, but studies have found that long-term use of valproate is associated with fewer, less severe, and shorter manic episodes. In direct comparisons, valproate is at least as effective as lithium and is better tolerated than lithium. In comparison with lithium, valproate may be particularly effective in persons with rapid-cycling and ultrarapid-cycling bipolar I disorder, dysphoric or mixed mania, and mania secondary to a general medical condition, and in persons who have comorbid substance abuse or panic attacks or who have not shown a completely favorable response to lithium treatment. The combination of valproate and lithium may be more effective than lithium alone.

In persons with bipolar I disorder, maintenance valproate treatment markedly reduces the frequency and severity of manic episodes, but it is only mildly to moderately effective in the prevention of depressive episodes.

The prophylactic effectiveness of valproate can be augmented by the addition of lithium, carbamazepine, dopamine receptor antagonists, second-generation drugs, antidepressant drugs, gabapentin, or lamotrigine (Lamictal).

3. Clinical guidelines

    a. Pretreatment evaluation. Pretreatment evaluation should routinely include white blood cell and platelet counts, measurement of hepatic transaminase concentrations, and pregnancy testing, if applicable. Amylase and coagulation studies should be performed if baseline pancreatic disease or coagulopathy is suspected.

    b. Dosage and administration. Valproate is available in a number of formulations and dosages. For treatment of acute mania, an oral loading strategy of 20 to 30 mg/kg per day can be used to accelerate control of symptoms. This regimen is usually well tolerated but can cause excessive sedation and tremor in elderly persons. Rapid stabilization of agitated behavior can be achieved with an IV infusion of valproate. If acute mania is absent, it is best to initiate the drug treatment gradually so as to minimize the common adverse effects of nausea, vomiting, and sedation. The dosage on the first day should be 250 mg administered with a meal. The dosage can be increased to 250 mg orally three times daily during the course of 3 to 6 days.

Plasma concentrations can be assessed in the morning before the first daily dose of the drug is administered. Therapeutic plasma concentrations for the control of seizures range between 50 and 150 mg/mL, but concentrations up to 200 mg/mL are usually well tolerated. It is reasonable to use the same range for the treatment of mental disorders; most of the controlled studies have used 50 to 100 mg/mL.

Most persons attain therapeutic plasma concentrations on a dosage of between 1,200 and 1,500 mg/day administered in divided doses. Once symptoms are well controlled, the full daily dose can be taken once before sleep.

    c. Laboratory monitoring. White blood cell and platelet counts and hepatic transaminase concentrations should be determined 1 month after the initiation of therapy and every 6 to 24 months thereafter. However, because even frequent monitoring may not predict serious organ toxicity, it is prudent to emphasize the need for prompt evaluation of any illnesses when giving instructions to patients. Asymptomatic elevations of transaminase concentrations to up to

Table 29-22
Valproate Side Effects

Side Effect	Treatment	Comment
GI distress (O)	Switch to enteric coated preparation ++	—
	Add histamine 2 blocker +	—
	Give with meals or all at night +	—
Tremor (O)	↓ Dose +	—
	Propranolol (Inderal) +	—
	Prophylactic diet and exercise instructions +	—
Weight gain (O)	Augment with topiramate (Topamax), sibutramine (Meridia) ++	—
Alopecia (UC)	Prophylaxis with zinc and selenium supplements ±	Straight hair may grow back curly
Polycystic ovary syndrome (UC)	Preventive treatment with oral contraceptives +	(May precede use of VPA)
	Switch to lamotrigine (Lamictal) ++	May be associated with ↑ testosterone
Hepatic enzyme (O) Elevation >3× normal	Monitor direction of change	Patient should advise physician if right upperquadrant pain occurs or if fever, malaise, fatigue, colored urine, or jaundice occurs
	D/C VPA	
Hepatitis	D/C VPA	—
Pancreatitis (VR)	D/C VPA, monitor amylase	Patient should advise physician if severe GI pain, nausea, or vomiting occurs
Asymptomatic ↑ ammonia	↓ Dose, add l-carnitine ±	
Coarse, flapping tremor	↓ Dose, add l-carnitine ±	—
Encephalopathy	D/C VPA	—
Spina bifida 1–4% in in utero exposed fetus	Avoid pregnancy +	Avoid VPA and other anticonvulsants in combination (such as carbamazepine (Tegretol))
	Use birth control pill, other methods +	
	Use folate prophylactically in women of childbearing age +	

+, likely works; ++, many case reports; +++, well-supported, controlled data; ±, questionable or hypothetical; C, common; D, dose related; D/C, discontinue; GI, gastrointestinal; I, idiosyncratic; O, occasional; PCO, polycystic ovary; S, sensitivity may cross to other anticonvulsant; UC, uncommon; VC, very common; VPA, valproate; VR, very rare.

three times the upper limit of normal are common and do not require any change in dosage.

4. Precautions and adverse reactions. Valproate treatment is generally well tolerated and safe. The most common adverse effects are nausea, vomiting, dyspepsia, and diarrhea (Table 29-22). The GI effects are generally most common during the first month of treatment, particularly if the dosage is increased rapidly. Unbuffered valproic acid is more likely than the enteric-coated "sprinkle" or the delayed-release divalproex formulations to cause GI symptoms. GI symptoms may respond to histamine H_2 receptor antagonists. Other common adverse effects involve the nervous system (e.g., sedation, ataxia, dysarthria, and tremor). Valproate-induced tremor may respond well to treatment with β-adrenergic receptor antagonists or gabapentin. To treat the other neurologic adverse effects, the valproate dosage must be lowered.

Table 29-23
Black Box Warnings and Other Warnings for Valproate

More Serious Side Effect	Management Considerations
Hepatotoxicity	Rare, idiosyncratic event
	Estimated risk, 1:118,000 (adults)
	Greatest risk profile (polypharmacy, younger than 2 years of age, mental retardation): 1:800
Pancreatitis	Rare, similar pattern to hepatotoxicity
	Incidence in clinical trial data is 2 in 2,416 (0.0008%)
	Postmarketing surveillance shows no increased incidence
	Relapse with rechallenge
	Asymptomatic amylase not predictive
Hyperammonemia	Rare; more common in combination with carbamazepine (Tegretol)
	Associated with coarse tremor and may respond to L-carnitine administration
Associated with urea cycle disorders	Discontinue valproate and protein intake
	Assess underlying urea cycle disorder
	Divalproex is contraindicated in patients with urea cycle disorders
Teratogenicity	Neural tube defect: 1–4% with valproate
	Preconceptual education and folate–vitamin B complex supplementation for all young women of childbearing potential
Somnolence in elderly persons	Slower titration than conventional doses
	Regular monitoring of fluid and nutritional intake
Thrombocytopenia	Decrease dose if clinically symptomatic (i.e., bruising, bleeding gums)
	Thrombocytopenia more likely with valproate levels ≥110 µg/mL (women) and ≥135 µg/mL (men)

Weight gain is a common adverse effect, especially in long-term treatment, and can best be treated by recommending a combination of a reasonable diet and moderate exercise.

The two most serious adverse effects of valproate treatment involve the pancreas and liver. Table 29-23 lists black box warnings and other warnings involving valproate. If symptoms of lethargy, malaise, anorexia, nausea and vomiting, edema, and abdominal pain occur in a person treated with valproate, the clinician must consider the possibility of severe hepatotoxicity. Rare cases of pancreatitis have been reported; they occur most often in the first 6 months of treatment, and the condition occasionally results in death.

5. Use during pregnancy. Valproate is a labeled pregnancy category D and should only be prescribed if essential for medical management and benefits outweigh risk of fetal harm.

C. Lamotrigine

1. Pharmacologic actions. Lamotrigine is completely absorbed, has bioavailability of 98%, and has a steady-state plasma half-life of 25 hours. However, the rate of lamotrigine's metabolism varies over a sixfold range, depending on which other drugs are administered concomitantly. Dosing is escalated slowly to twice-a-day maintenance dosing. Food does not affect its absorption, and it is 55% protein-bound in the plasma; 94% of lamotrigine and its inactive metabolites are excreted in the urine. Among the better delineated biochemical actions of lamotrigine are blockade of voltage-sensitive sodium channels, which in turn modulate release of glutamate and aspartate, and a slight effect on calcium channels. Lamotrigine modestly increases plasma serotonin concentrations, possibly through inhibition of serotonin reuptake, and is a weak inhibitor of serotonin 5-HT$_3$ receptors.

2. Therapeutic efficacy

a. Bipolar disorder. In currently or recently depressed, manic, or hypomanic bipolar I patients, lamotrigine prolongs time between depressive and manic episodes. These findings were more robust for depression. While lamotrigine can be initiated while patients are in any mood state, effectiveness in the acute treatment of mood episodes has not been established.

b. Depression. Lamotrigine may possess acute antidepressant effects. Studies involving acute lamotrigine treatment of bipolar depression and rapid-cycling bipolar disorder have demonstrated therapeutic benefit from lamotrigine. Conversely, it does not appear to act as an acute antimanic agent.

c. Other indications. There is no well-established role for lamotrigine in treating other psychiatric disorders, although there have been reports of therapeutic benefit in the treatment of borderline personality disorder, and as a treatment for various pain syndromes.

3. Dosage and clinical guidelines. In the clinical trials leading to the approval of lamotrigine as a treatment for bipolar disorder, no consistent increase in efficacy was associated with doses above 200 mg/day. Most patients should take between 100 and 200 mg a day. In epilepsy, the drug is administered twice daily, but in bipolar disorder the total dose can be taken once a day, either in the morning or night, depending on whether the patient finds the drug activating or sedating.

Lamotrigine is available as unscored 25-, 100-, 150-, and 200-mg tablets. The major determinant of lamotrigine dosing is minimization of the risk of rash. Lamotrigine should not be taken by anyone under the age of 16 years. Because valproic acid markedly slows the elimination of lamotrigine, concomitant administration of these two drugs necessitates a much slower titration (Table 29-24). The schedule differs

Table 29-24
Gradual Introduction of Lamotrigine in Adults with Bipolar Disorder

	Lamotrigine with Valproate (mg/day)	Lamotrigine with Carbamazepine (mg/day)	Lamotrigine with Neither (mg/day)
Weeks 1 and 2 dose	12.5	50	25
Weeks 3 and 4 dose	25	100	50
Week 5 dose	50	200	100
Subsequent weekly dose increments	25–50	100	50–100
FDA target dose	100	400	200
Typical final dose range	100–200	400–800	200–400

FDA, U.S. Food and Drug Administration.

based on whether the patient is taking valproic acid, carbamazepine, or neither of these drugs.

People with renal insufficiency should aim for a lower maintenance dosage. Appearance of any type of rash necessitates immediate discontinuation of lamotrigine administration. Lamotrigine should usually be discontinued gradually, over 2 weeks, unless a rash emerges, in which case it should be discontinued over 1 to 2 days.

Chewable dispersible tablets of 2-, 5-, and 25-mg are also available.

4. **Precautions and adverse events.** Lamotrigine is remarkably well tolerated. The absence of sedation, weight gain, or other metabolic effects is noteworthy. The most common adverse effects reported in clinical trials were dizziness, ataxia, somnolence, headache, diplopia, blurred vision, and nausea and were typically mild. In actual practice, cognitive impairment and joint or back pain appear to be more common than found in studies. Only rash, which is common and occasionally very severe, is a source of concern.

   About 8% of patients started on lamotrigine develop a benign maculopapular rash during the first 4 months of treatment. It is advised that the drug be discontinued if a rash develops and it is felt to be associated with the use of lamotrigine. Even though these rashes are benign, there is concern that in some cases, they may represent early manifestations of Stevens–Johnson syndrome (SJS) or toxic epidermal necrolysis. Nevertheless, even if lamotrigine is discontinued immediately upon development of rash or other sign of hypersensitivity reaction, such as fever and lymphadenopathy, this may not prevent subsequent development of life-threatening rash or permanent disfiguration.

5. **Use during pregnancy.** Lamotrigine has a large pregnancy registry that supports research data that lamotrigine is not associated with congenital malformations in humans.

6. **Drug interactions.** The most potentially serious lamotrigine drug interaction involves concurrent use of the anticonvulsant valproic acid, which doubles serum lamotrigine concentrations. Sertraline (Zoloft) also increases plasma lamotrigine concentrations, but to a lesser extent than does valproic acid. Combinations of lamotrigine and other anticonvulsants have complex effects on the time of peak plasma concentration and the plasma half-life of lamotrigine.

D. **Carbamazepine.** Carbamazepine is effective for the treatment of acute mania and for the prophylactic treatment of bipolar I disorder. It is a first-line agent, along with lithium and valproic acid.

1. **Therapeutic efficacy**

   a. **Manic episodes.** The efficacy of carbamazepine in the treatment of acute mania is comparable with that of lithium and antipsychotics. Carbamazepine is also effective as a second-line agent to prevent both manic and depressive episodes in bipolar I disorder, after lithium and valproic acid.

       b. Depressive episodes. Carbamazepine is an alternative drug for patients whose depressive episodes show a marked or rapid periodicity.

  2. Clinical guidelines

       a. Dosage and administration. Carbamazepine is available in 100- and 200-mg tablets and as a suspension containing 100 mg/5 mL. The usual starting dosage is 200 mg orally two times a day; however, with titration, three-times-a-day dosing is optimal. An extended-release version suitable for twice-a-day dosing is available in 100-, 200-, and 400-mg tablets. The dosage should be increased by no more than 200 mg/day every 2 to 4 days to minimize the occurrence of adverse effects.

       b. Blood concentrations. The anticonvulsant blood concentration range of 4 to 12 mg/mL should be reached before it is determined that carbamazepine is not effective in the treatment of a mood disorder. The dosage necessary to achieve plasma concentrations in the usual therapeutic range varies from 400 to 1,600 mg/day, with a mean of about 1,000 mg/day.

  3. Precautions and adverse reactions. The rarest but most serious adverse effects of carbamazepine are blood dyscrasias, hepatitis, and exfoliative dermatitis. Otherwise, carbamazepine is relatively well tolerated by persons except for mild GI and CNS effects that can be significantly reduced if the dosage is increased slowly and minimal effective plasma concentrations are maintained.

  4. Drug interactions. Principally because it induces several hepatic enzymes, carbamazepine may interact with many drugs, particularly other anticonvulsants whose plasma levels are lowered.

  5. Use during pregnancy. There is an increased risk of neurotoxic effects and clinicians should weigh the potential benefit over risk of congenital malformations.

E. Atypical antipsychotics. The atypical antipsychotics also act as mood stabilizers. They include the following drugs, which have been discussed in detail above.

  1. Aripiprazole. Aripiprazole is the latest of the atypical antipsychotics approved for the treatment of acute manic and mixed episodes associated with bipolar disorder. The effectiveness of aripiprazole in maintenance treatment has not been established.

  2. Olanzapine. Indicated for the acute treatment of manic and mixed episodes associated with bipolar disorder, as well as in the maintenance treatment of bipolar disorder. It can be used as monotherapy or in combination with lithium or divalproex. Olanzapine is the only atypical antipsychotic that also has an indication in the maintenance treatment of bipolar disorder along with lithium and lamotrigine.

  3. Risperidone. Risperidone is approved for the short-term treatment of acute manic episodes, associated with bipolar I disorder as monotherapy, or in combination with lithium or divalproex.

4. **Quetiapine and Quetiapine XR.** Quetiapine and Quetiapine XR are indicated for the short-term treatment of acute manic episodes associated with bipolar I disorder as either monotherapy or adjunct therapy to lithium or divalproex. They are also indicated as adjunctive therapy with lithium and divalproex for the maintenance treatment of bipolar I disorder. Furthermore, they are also indicated for the treatment of depressive episodes associated with bipolar disorder type I and II. It is not approved for mixed episodes or rapid cycling associated with bipolar disorder.

5. **Ziprasidone.** Ziprasidone as monotherapy is approved for the short-term treatment of acute manic or mixed episodes associated with bipolar I disorder. It is also indicated as an adjunct to lithium or valproate in the maintenance treatment of bipolar I disorder.

6. **Paliperidone.** Paliperidone is used for the treatment of schizophrenia and schizoaffective disorder as monotherapy or as an adjunct to mood stabilizers.

7. **Asenapine.** It is approved for the treatment of acute manic or mixed episodes associated with bipolar I disorder as monotherapy or as an adjunct to lithium or valproate.

8. **Lurasidone.** It is indicated for the treatment of MDD associated with bipolar I disorder as a monotherapy or as an adjunct to lithium or valproate. Efficacy in mania has not been established.

9. **Brexpiprazole.** It is indicated as an adjunctive treatment for MDD.

10. **Cariprazine.** It is indicated for the acute treatment of manic or mixed episodes associated with bipolar I disorder.

F. **Other mood-stabilizing drugs**

1. **Symbyax.** Symbyax (olanzapine and fluoxetine) is indicated for the treatment of depressive episodes associated with bipolar disorder. Improvement occurs as early as week 1 in symptoms of sadness, sleep, lassitude, and suicidal thoughts.

   Symbyax exerts its antidepressant effects through multiple neurotransmitter systems. The activation of three monoaminergic neural systems (serotonin, norepinephrine, and dopamine) is responsible for its enhanced antidepressant effect. There is a synergistic increase in norepinephrine and dopamine release in the prefrontal cortex, as well as an increase in serotonin. It is available in 6 mg/25 mg, 12 mg/25 mg, 6 mg/50 mg, and 12 mg/50 mg, where 6 mg and 12 mg represent olanzapine, and 25 mg and 50 mg represent fluoxetine.

   The half-life of olanzapine and fluoxetine is 30 hours and 9 days, respectively, requiring only once-daily dosing, usually in the evening. The starting dose is generally 6 mg/25 mg given in a single daily dose. Dosing should be adjusted in the elderly, smokers, and those with hepatic impairment. As with other atypical antipsychotics, the possibility of metabolic abnormalities should be entertained, and baseline and maintenance monitoring be done.

   The most common adverse events are weight gain, sleepiness, diarrhea, dizziness, hyponatremia, dry mouth, and increased appetite. It should not be used with an MAOI or within at least 14 days of discontinuing an MAOI. If used concomitantly with fluvoxamine, dosage adjustment is needed secondary to CYP 1A2 inhibition.

VIII. Stimulants

A. Sympathomimetics (also called *analeptics* and *psychostimulants*). The sympathomimetics are effective in the treatment of attention-deficit/hyperactivity disorder (ADHD). The first-line sympathomimetics are methylphenidate (Ritalin, Concerta), dextroamphetamine (Dexedrine), lisdexamfetamine dimesylate (Vyvanse), dexmethylphenidate (Focalin), and a reformulation of existing dextroamphetamine and amphetamine (Adderall). Pemoline (Cylert) is now considered a second-line agent because of rare but potentially fatal hepatic toxicity.

1. Pharmacologic actions. All the drugs are well absorbed from the GI tract. Dextroamphetamine and the reformulation reach peak plasma concentrations in 2 to 3 hours and have a half-life of about 6 hours, so that once- or twice-daily dosing is necessary. Methylphenidate reaches peak plasma levels in 1 to 2 hours and has a short half-life of 2 to 3 hours, so that multiple daily dosing is necessary. A sustained-release formulation doubles the effective half-life of methylphenidate. A novel osmotic pump capsule (Concerta) may sustain the effects of methylphenidate for 12 hours. Lisdexamfetamine dimesylate is rapidly absorbed from the GI tract and converted to dextroamphetamine and L-lysine.

2. Therapeutic efficacy. Sympathomimetics are effective about 75% of the time. Methylphenidate and dextroamphetamine are generally equally effective and work within 15 to 30 minutes. The drugs decrease hyperactivity, increase attentiveness, and reduce impulsivity. They may also reduce comorbid oppositional behaviors associated with ADHD. Many persons take these drugs throughout their schooling and beyond. In responsive persons, the use of a sympathomimetic may be a critical determinant of scholastic success. Sympathomimetics improve the core ADHD symptoms—hyperactivity, impulsivity, and inattentiveness—and permit improved social interactions with teachers, family, other adults, and peers.

The success of long-term treatment of ADHD with sympathomimetics supports a model in which ADHD results from a genetically determined neurochemical imbalance that requires lifelong pharmacologic management. A recent comparison between medication and psychosocial approaches for the treatment of ADHD found clear benefit with medication but little improvement with nonpharmacologic treatments.

3. Clinical guidelines

a. Pretreatment evaluation. The pretreatment evaluation should include an assessment of the patient's cardiac function, with particular attention to the presence of hypertension or tachyarrhythmias. The clinician should also examine the patient for the presence of movement disorders (e.g., tics and dyskinesia), because these conditions can be exacerbated by the administration of sympathomimetics. If tics are present, many experts do not use sympathomimetics but instead choose clonidine (Catapres) or antidepressants. However, recent data indicate that sympathomimetics may cause only a mild increase in motor tics and may actually suppress vocal tics.

Hepatic and renal function should be assessed, and dosages of sympathomimetics should be reduced if the patient's metabolism is impaired. In the case of pemoline, any elevation of liver enzymes is a compelling reason to discontinue the medication.

b. Dosage and administration. The dosage ranges and the available preparations for sympathomimetics are presented in Table 29-25.

(1) Methylphenidate. Methylphenidate is the agent most commonly used initially, at a dosage of 5 to 10 mg every 3 to 4 hours. The dosage may be increased to a maximum of 20 mg four times daily. Use of the 20-mg sustained-release formulation, to provide 6 hours of benefit and eliminate the need for dosing at school, is sometimes recommended, but it may be less effective than the immediate-release formulation.

(2) Children with ADHD can take immediate-release methylphenidate at 8 am and 12 noon. The sustained-release preparation of methylphenidate may be taken once at 8 AM. The starting dose of methylphenidate ranges from 2.5 mg (regular preparation) to 20 mg (sustained release). If this is inadequate, the dosage may be increased to a maximum of 20 mg four times daily.

(3) Dextroamphetamine. The dosage of dextroamphetamine is 2.5 to 40 mg/day (up to 0.5 mg/kg a day). Dextroamphetamine is about twice as potent as methylphenidate on a per-milligram basis and provides 6 to 8 hours of benefit.

(4) Lisdexamfetamine dimesylate. Adults and children 6 to 12 years of age. Start with 30 mg once daily in the morning. Dosage may be adjusted in 10- or 20-mg/day increments at approximately weekly intervals (max, 70 mg/day).

(5) Dexmethylphenidate. Adults and children aged 6 to 17 years. Dosage should start at 5 mg (2.5 mg twice a day), and adjusted in 2.5-mg increments to a maximum dose of 20 mg/day (10 mg twice a day).

c. Treatment failures. Seventy percent of nonresponders to one sympathomimetic may benefit from another. All the sympathomimetic drugs should be tried before the patient is switched to a drug of a different class.

4. Precautions and adverse reactions. The most common adverse effects associated with amphetamine-like drugs are stomach pain, anxiety, irritability, insomnia, tachycardia, cardiac arrhythmias, and dysphoria. The treatment of common adverse effects in children with ADHD is usually straightforward (Table 29-26).

Less common adverse effects include the induction of movement disorders (e.g., tics, Tourette's disorder–like symptoms, and dyskinesias), which are often self-limited over 7 to 10 days. Small to moderate

Table 29-25
Sympathomimetics Commonly Used in Psychiatry

Generic Name	Trade Name	Preparations	Initial Daily Dose (mg)	Usual Daily Dose for ADHD[a]	Usual Daily Dose for Disorders Associated with Excessive Daytime Somnolence	Maximum Daily Dose (mg)
Amphetamine–dextroamphetamine	Adderall	5-, 10-, 20-, and 30-mg tablets	5–10	20–30 mg	5–60 mg	Children: 40 Adults: 60
Armodafinil[b]	Nuvigil	50-, 150-, and 250-mg tablets	50–150	150–250 mg	250 mg	
Atomoxetine	Strattera	10-, 18-, 25-, 40, and 60-mg tablets	20	40–80 mg	Not used	Children: 80 Adults: 100
Dexmethylphenidate	Focalin	2.5-, 5-, and 10-mg capsules	5	5–20 mg	Not used	20
Dextroamphetamine	Dexedrine, Dextrostat	5-, 10-, and 15-mg ER capsules; 5- and 10-mg tablets	5–10	20–30 mg	5–60 mg	Children: 40 Adults: 60
Lisdexamfetamine	Vyvanse	20-, 30-, 40-, 50-, 60-, and 70-mg capsules	20–30			70
Methamphetamine	Desoxyn	5-mg tablets; 5-, 10-, and 15-mg ER tablets	5–10	20–25 mg	Not generally used	45
Methylphenidate	Ritalin, Methidate, Methylin, Attenade	5-, 10-, and 20-mg tablets; 10- and 20-mg SR tablets	5–10	5–60 mg	20–30 mg	Children: 80 Adults: 90
Methylphenidate hydrochloride	Concerta Quillivant XR	18- and 36-mg ER tablets	18 20	18–54 mg	Not yet established	54 60
Modafinil[b]	Provigil	100- and 200-mg tablets	100	Not used	400 mg	400

[a]All medications that have dosage for children should be for 6 years or older except "Amphetamine" and "dextroamphetamine."
[b]Obstructive sleep apnea, narcolepsy, and shift work disorder.
ER, extended release; SR, sustained release.

Table 29-26
Management of Common Stimulant-Induced Adverse Effects in Attention-Deficit/Hyperactivity Disorder

Adverse Effect	Management
Anorexia, nausea, weight loss	• Administer stimulant with meals. • Use caloric-enhanced supplements. Discourage forcing meals.
Insomnia, nightmares	• Administer stimulants earlier in day. • Change to short-acting preparations. • Discontinue afternoon or evening dosing. • Consider adjunctive treatment (e.g., antihistamines, clonidine, antidepressants).
Dizziness	• Monitor BP. • Encourage fluid intake. • Change to long-acting form.
Rebound phenomena	• Overlap stimulant dosing. • Change to long-acting preparation or combine long- and short-acting preparations. • Consider adjunctive or alternative treatment (e.g., clonidine, antidepressants).
Irritability	• Assess timing of phenomena (during peak or withdrawal phase). • Evaluate comorbid symptoms. • Reduce dose. • Consider adjunctive or alternative treatment (e.g., lithium, antidepressants, anticonvulsants).
Dysphoria, moodiness, agitation	• Consider comorbid diagnosis (e.g., mood disorder). • Reduce dosage or change to long-acting preparation. • Consider adjunctive or alternative treatment (e.g., lithium, anticonvulsants, antidepressants).

BP, blood pressure.
From Wilens TE, Blederman J. The stimulants. In: Shaffer D, ed. *The Psychiatric Clinics of North America: Pediatric Psychopharmacology.* Philadelphia, PA: Saunders; 1992; with permission.

dosages of sympathomimetics may be well tolerated without causing an increase in the frequency and severity of tics. In severe cases, augmentation with risperidone is necessary.

Methylphenidate may worsen tics in one-third of patients, who fall into two groups: those whose methylphenidate-induced tics resolve immediately after the dose has been metabolized, and a smaller group in whom methylphenidate appears to trigger tics that persist for several months but eventually resolve spontaneously.

The most limiting adverse effect of sympathomimetics is their association with psychological and physical dependence. Sympathomimetics may exacerbate glaucoma, hypertension, cardiovascular disorders, hyperthyroidism, anxiety disorders, psychotic disorders, and seizure disorders.

High doses of sympathomimetics can cause dry mouth, pupillary dilation, bruxism, formication, excessive ebullience, restlessness, and emotional lability. The long-term use of a high dosage can cause a delusional disorder that is indistinguishable from paranoid schizophrenia.

Patients who have taken overdoses of sympathomimetics present with hypertension, tachycardia, hyperthermia, toxic psychosis, delirium, and occasionally seizures. Overdoses of sympathomimetics can also result in death, often caused by cardiac arrhythmias. Seizures can be treated with benzodiazepines, cardiac effects with β-adrenergic receptor antagonists, fever with cooling blankets, and delirium with dopamine receptor agonists.

5. Atomoxetine. Atomoxetine (Strattera) is indicated for the treatment of ADHD in children 6 years of age and older, adolescents, and adults. The precise mechanism of its therapeutic effects is unknown but is thought to be related to selective inhibition of the presynaptic norepinephrine transporter. Atomoxetine improves symptoms in both inattentive and hyperactive/impulsive domains in children, adolescents, and adults.

It has a half-life of about 5 hours and requires b.i.d. dosing. It is available in 10-, 18-, 25-, 40-, and 60-mg capsules. For children and adolescents over 70 kg of body weight, it should be initiated at a dose of 40 mg/day and increased after a minimum of 3 days to a target dose of approximately 80 mg/day.

For adults, atomoxetine should be initiated at a total daily dose of 40 mg and increased after a minimum of 3 days to a target dose of 80 mg/day. Because of liver toxicity atomoxetine is no longer a drug of first choice and its use is diminishing.

6. Modafinil (Provigil). Modafinil is a unique drug with psychostimulant effects. Its specific mechanism of action is unknown but it may have some effect on blocking norepinephrine reuptake. Modafinil is used to improve wakefulness in patients with excessive daytime sleepiness associated with narcolepsy, obstructive sleep apnea, or shiftwork sleep disorder. It is supplied in 100- and 200-mg tablets and taken once daily. Maximum daily dose is 200 mg. Drug interactions are related to modafinil-inducing CYP 2C19 enzymes; thus, it may increase levels of diazepam, propranolol, or phenytoin. Adverse reactions include headache, nausea, anxiety, and insomnia.

IX. Cholinesterase Inhibitors

A. Therapeutic efficacy. Donepezil (Aricept), rivastigmine (Exelon), galantamine (Razadyne), and memantine ([Nemanda] discuss separately below) are among the few proven treatments for mild to moderate dementia of the Alzheimer's type. They reduce the intrasynaptic cleavage and inactivation of acetylcholine and thus potentiate cholinergic neurotransmission, which in turn tends to produce a modest improvement in memory and goal-directed thought. These drugs are considered most useful for persons with mild to moderate memory loss, who nevertheless still have enough preserved basal forebrain cholinergic neurons to benefit from an augmentation of cholinergic neurotransmission.

Donepezil is well tolerated and widely used. Rivastigmine appears more likely than donepezil to cause GI and neuropsychiatric adverse effects. Galantamine may cause dizziness, drowsiness and fainting and gradual titration over months is required. An older cholinesterase inhibitor, tacrine (Cognex), is currently very rarely used because of its potential for hepatotoxicity. Cholinesterase inhibitors have been coadministered with vitamin E and gingko biloba extract.

The cholinesterase inhibitors slow the progression of memory loss and diminish apathy, depression, hallucinations, anxiety, euphoria, and purposeless motor behaviors. Some persons note immediate improvement in memory, mood, psychotic symptoms, and interpersonal skills. Others note little initial benefit but are able to retain their cognitive and adaptive faculties at a relatively stable level for many months. The use of cholinesterase inhibitors may delay or reduce the need for nursing home placement.

B. Clinical guidelines

   1. Pretreatment evaluation. Before the initiation of treatment with cholinesterase inhibitors, potentially treatable causes of dementia should be ruled out with a thorough neurologic evaluation. The psychiatric evaluation should focus on depression, anxiety, and psychosis.

   2. Dosage and administration

      a. Donepezil. Donepezil is available in 5- and 10-mg tablets. Treatment should be initiated with a dosage of 5 mg/day, taken at night. If well tolerated and of some discernible benefit after 4 weeks, the dosage should be increased to a maintenance level of 10 mg/day. Donepezil absorption is unaffected by meals.

      b. Rivastigmine. Rivastigmine is available in 1.5-, 3-, 4.5-, and 6-mg capsules. The recommended initial dosage is 1.5 mg twice daily for a minimum of 2 weeks, after which increases of 1.5 mg/day can be made at intervals of at least 2 weeks to a target dosage of 6 mg/day, taken in two equal doses. If tolerated, the dosage may be further titrated upward to a maximum of 6 mg twice daily. The risk for adverse GI events can be reduced by taking rivastigmine with food.

      c. Galantamine. It is available in 4-, 8-, 12-, 16-, and 24-mg capsules as well as 4 mg/mL solution. The recommended initial dosage is 4 mg twice a day with meals. After 4 weeks depending on tolerability dose can be increased to 8 mg twice a day, with further increase to 12 mg twice day after 4 more weeks. Dose adjustment is required in hepatic and renal impairment.

      d. Memantine. It is available in 5- and 10-mg immediate release form and 7-, 14-, 21-, and 28-mg extended-release formulation.

C. Precautions and adverse reactions

   1. Donepezil. Donepezil is generally well tolerated at recommended dosages. Fewer than 3% of persons taking donepezil experience nausea, diarrhea, and vomiting. These mild symptoms are more common at the 10-mg than the 5-mg dose, and when present, they tend to resolve after 3 weeks of continued use. Donepezil may cause weight loss. Donepezil treatment has been infrequently associated with bradyarrhythmias, especially in persons with underlying cardiac disease. A small number of persons experience syncope.

   2. Rivastigmine. Rivastigmine is generally well tolerated, but recommended dosages may need to be scaled back in the initial period of treatment to limit GI and CNS adverse effects. These mild symptoms are more common at dosages above 6 mg/day, and when present, they tend to resolve once the dosage is lowered.

The most common adverse effects associated with rivastigmine are nausea, vomiting, dizziness, and headache. Rivastigmine may cause weight loss.

3. **Memantine.** Reaches peak concentration in 3 hours, with a half-life of 60 to 80 hours. Common side effects include confusion, dizziness, constipation, and headache.

4. **Galantamine.** It reaches peak concentration quickly within an hour and is metabolized through CYP 2D6 and 3A4 requiring dose adjustments when used with inhibitors. Serious skin reactions like SJS have been reported and patient should be educated to discontinue in case of a rash. Most common side effects include nausea, vomiting, dizziness, diarrhea, and headache.

X. Other Drugs

A. **α_2-Adrenergic agonists (clonidine and guanfacine).** Clonidine and guanfacine are used in psychiatry to control symptoms caused by withdrawal from opiates and opioids, treat Tourette's disorder, suppress agitation in posttraumatic stress disorder, and control aggressive or hyperactive behavior in children, especially those with autistic features.

The most common adverse effects associated with clonidine are dry mouth and eyes, fatigue, sedation, dizziness, nausea, hypotension, and constipation. A similar but milder adverse effect profile is seen with guanfacine, especially at dosages of 3 mg/day or more. Clonidine and guanfacine should not be taken by adults with blood pressure below 90/60 mm Hg or with cardiac arrhythmias, especially bradycardia. Clonidine in particular is associated with sedation, and tolerance does not usually develop to this adverse effect. Uncommon CNS adverse effects of clonidine include insomnia, anxiety, and depression; rare CNS adverse effects include vivid dreams, nightmares, and hallucinations. Fluid retention associated with clonidine treatment can be treated with diuretics.

B. **β-Adrenergic receptor antagonists.** β-Adrenergic receptor antagonists (e.g., propranolol [Inderal], pindolol [Visken]) are effective peripherally and centrally acting agents for the treatment of social phobia (e.g., performance anxiety), lithium-induced postural tremor, and neuroleptic-induced acute akathisia, and for the control of aggressive behavior.

The β-adrenergic receptor antagonists are contraindicated for use in people with asthma, insulin-dependent diabetes, congestive heart failure, significant vascular disease, persistent angina, and hyperthyroidism. The most common adverse effects of β-adrenergic receptor antagonists are hypotension and bradycardia.

 CLINICAL HINT:
Patients who must give a speech or perform publically can be given propanol (10–20 mg) 30 minutes beforehand and their signs of anxiety will diminish in many cases.

C. **Anticholinergics and amantadine (Symmetrel).** In the clinical practice of psychiatry, the anticholinergic drugs are primarily used to treat medication-induced movement disorders, particularly neuroleptic-induced parkinsonism, neuroleptic-induced acute dystonia, and medication-induced postural tremor.

D. **N-methyl-D-aspartate (NMDA)-receptor antagonist.** Memantine hydrochloride (Namenda) is approved for the treatment of moderate to severe Alzheimer's disease.

1. **Therapeutic efficacy.** The NMDA-receptor antagonist memantine binds to NMDA-receptor–operated cation channels, which activate glutamate. Glutamate is a neurotransmitter essential for learning and memory; hence, increasing its activity may improve learning and memory.

2. **Dosage and administration.** Memantine is rapidly and completely absorbed after oral administration. Peak plasma levels are attained in 3 to 7 hours, and the half-life is approximately 60 to 80 hours. Memantine is primarily excreted by the kidneys, so patients with renal impairment need dose reduction.

   It has minimal inhibition of CYP 450 enzyme system and low serum protein binding. As a result, the drug–drug interactions are low.

   Memantine is available in 5- and 10-mg tablets. The dosing schedule is illustrated in Table 29-27.

3. **Adverse reactions.** Memantine is safe and well tolerated. The most commonly observed adverse events are dizziness, confusion, headache, and constipation. There are no clinically important changes in vital signs, and only minimal hemodynamic effects are observed.

E. **Pregabalin (Lyrica).** Pregabalin is the only drug approved for the management of fibromyalgia. It decreases excitatory neurotransmitter release (glutamate, substance P, and norepinephrine). It provides rapid relief as early as week 1 with reduction in pain and has shown sustained relief in a 6-month study. Common adverse effects include dizziness, somnolence, dry mouth, edema, weight gain, and constipation. It may cause life-threatening angioedema and should be immediately discontinued. It is available as 25-, 50-, 75-, 100-, 150-, 200-, 250-, and 300-mg tablets. The usual recommended dose is 300 mg/day in divided doses and may be increased to 450 mg/day. Some studies have suggested its efficacy in generalized anxiety disorder, but so far it has not been approved by the FDA and is used mostly off label.

F. **Ropinirole (Requip).** Ropinirole is the first and only FDA-approved medicine indicated for the treatment of moderate-to-severe primary restless leg syndrome (RLS). The usual starting dose is 0.25 mg taken 1 to 3 hours before bedtime. The dose may be increased to 4 mg/day based on clinical response. The most common adverse effects include somnolence, vomiting, dizziness, and fatigue. More serious side effects include syncope or symptomatic hypotension especially during initial treatment or dose titration.

XI. **Nutritional Supplements and Medical Foods**

Thousands of herbal and dietary supplements are being marketed today. If electing to use herbal drugs or nutritional supplements, bear in mind that

Table 29-27
Memantine Dosing Schedule

Titration Schedule	Maintenance Dose
Week 1	5 mg once daily
Week 2	10 mg/day (5 mg b.i.d.)
Week 3	15 mg/day (10 mg in the morning and 5 mg in the evening)
Week 4	20 mg/day (10 mg b.i.d.)

their use may come at the expense of proven interventions and that adverse effects are possible. Herbal and nonherbal supplements may augment or antagonize the actions of prescription and nonprescription drugs. Clinicians must be alert to the possibility of adverse effects as a result of drug–drug interactions, because many phytomedicinals have ingredients that produce physiologic changes in the body.

A. Nutritional supplements. The term *nutritional supplement* is used interchangeably with the term *dietary supplement.* The ingredients may include vitamins, minerals, herbs, botanicals, amino acids, and substances such as enzymes, tissues, glandulars, and metabolites. The regulations governing them are more lax than those for prescription and over-the-counter drugs. Nutritional supplements do not need the approval of the FDA, and the FDA does not evaluate their effectiveness. Table 29-28 provides a list of dietary supplements used in psychiatry.

B. Medical foods. Recently FDA has introduced a new category of nutritional supplement called *medical foods.* Medical food is defined as "*a food which is formulated to be consumed or administered enterally under the supervision of a physician and which is intended for the specific dietary management of a disease or condition for which distinctive nutritional requirements, based on recognized scientific principles, are established by medical evaluation.*"

Medical foods do not have to undergo premarket approval by the FDA. Medical foods do have some additional regulations that dietary supplements do not because medical foods are intended to treat illnesses. In summary, to be considered a medical food a product must, at a minimum, meet the following criteria: (1) The product must be a food for oral or tube feeding; (2) the product must be labeled for the dietary management of a specific medical disorder, disease, or condition for which there is distinctive nutritional requirements; and (3) the product must be intended to be used under medical supervision. The most common medical foods with psychoactive claims are listed in Table 29-29.

C. Phytomedicinals. The term *phytomedicinals* (from the Greek *phyto,* meaning "plant") refers to herb and plant preparations that are used or have been used for centuries for the treatment of a variety of medical conditions. Phytomedicinals are categorized as dietary supplements, and are exempt from the regulations that govern prescription and over-the-counter medications. Thousands of herbal drugs are being marketed today; the most common with psychoactive properties are listed in Table 29-30.

Text continues on page 539.

Table 29-28
Dietary Supplements Used in Psychiatry

Name	Ingredients/ What Is It?	Uses	Adverse Effects	Interactions	Dosage	Comments
Docosahexaenoic acid (DHA)	Omega-3 polyunsaturated fatty acid	ADD, dyslexia, cognitive impairment, dementia	Anticoagulant properties, mild GI distress	Warfarin	Varies with indication	Stop using prior to surgery
Choline	Choline	Fetal brain development, manic conditions, cognitive disorders, tardive dyskinesia, cancers	Restrict in patients with primary genetic trimethylaminuria, sweating, hypotension, depression	Methotrexate, works with B$_6$, B$_{12}$ and folic acid in metabolism of homocysteine	300–1,200-mg doses >3 g associated with fishy body odor	Needed for structure and function of all cells
L-α-Glyceryl-phosphorylcholine (α-GPC)	Derived from soy lecithin	To increase growth hormone secretion, cognitive disorders	None known	None known	500 mg–1 g daily	Remains poorly understood
Phosphatidylcholine	Phospholipid that is part of cell membranes	Manic conditions, Alzheimer's disease, and cognitive disorders, tardive dyskinesia	Diarrhea, steatorrhea in those with malabsorption, avoid with antiphospholipid antibody syndrome	None known	3–9 g/day in divided doses	Soybeans, sunflower, and rapeseed are major sources.
Phosphatidylserine	Phospholipid isolated from soya and egg yolks	Cognitive impairment including Alzheimer's disease, may reverse memory problems	Avoid with antiphospholipid antibody syndrome, GI side effects	None known	For soya-derived variety, 100 mg t.i.d.	Type derived from bovine brain carries hypothetical risk of bovine spongiform encephalopathy
Zinc	Metallic element	Immune impairment, wound healing, cognitive disorders, prevention of neural tube defects	GI distress, high doses can cause copper deficiency, immunosuppression	Bisphosphonates, quinolones, tetracycline, penicillamine, copper, cysteine-containing foods, caffeine, iron	Typical dose 15 mg/day, adverse effects >30 mg	Claims that zinc can prevent and treat the common cold are supported in some studies but not in others; more research needed
Acetyl-L-carnitine	Acetyl ester of L-carnitine	Neuroprotection, Alzheimer's disease, Down syndrome, strokes, antiaging, depression in geriatric patients	Mild GI distress, seizures, increased agitation in some with Alzheimer's disease	Nucleoside analogs, valproic acid, and pivalic acid-containing antibiotics	500 mg–2 g daily in divided doses	Found in small amounts in milk and meat

(continued)

Table 29-28
Dietary Supplements Used in Psychiatry *(Continued)*

Name	Ingredients/What Is It?	Uses	Adverse Effects	Interactions	Dosage	Comments
Huperzine A	Plant alkaloid derived from Chinese club moss	Alzheimer's disease, age-related memory loss, inflammatory disorders	Seizures, arrhythmias, asthma, irritable bowel disease	Acetylcholinesterase inhibitors and cholinergic drugs	60 μg–200 μg/day	*Huperzia serrata* has been used in Chinese folk medicine for the treatment of fevers and inflammation.
NADH (nicotinamide adenine dinucleotide)	Dinucleotide located in mitochondria and cytosol of cells	Parkinson's disease, Alzheimer's disease, chronic fatigue, CV disease	GI distress	None known	5 mg/day or 5 mg b.i.d.	Precursor of NADH is nicotinic acid
S-Adenosyl-L-methionine (SAMe)	Metabolite of essential amino acid L-methionine	Mood elevation, osteoarthritis	Hypomania, hyperactive muscle movement, caution in patients with cancer	None known	200–1,600 mg daily in divided doses	Several trials demonstrate some efficacy in the treatment of depression
5-Hydroxytryptophan (5-HTP)	Immediate precursor of serotonin	Depression, obesity, insomnia, fibromyalgia, headaches	Possible risk of serotonin syndrome in those with carcinoid tumors or taking MAOIs	SSRIs, MAOIs, methyldopa, St. John's wort, phenoxybenzamine, 5-HT antagonists, 5-HT receptor agonists	100 mg–2 g daily, safer with carbidopa	5-HTP along with carbidopa is used in Europe for the treatment of depression.
Phenylalanine	Essential amino acid	Depression, analgesia, vitiligo	Contraindicated in patients with PKU, may exacerbate tardive dyskinesia or hypertension	MAOIs and neuroleptic drugs	Comes in 2 forms: 500 mg–1.5 g daily for DL-phenylalanine, 375 mg–2.25 g for DL-phenylalanine	Found in vegetables, juices, yogurt, and miso
Myoinositol	Major nutritionally active form of inositol	Depression, panic attacks, OCD	Caution in patients with bipolar disorder, GI distress	Possible additive effects with SSRIs and 5-HT receptor agonists (sumatriptan)	12 g in divided doses for depression and panic attacks	Studies have *not* shown effectiveness in treating Alzheimer's disease, autism, or schizophrenia

Supplement	Description	Uses	Side Effects	Drug Interactions	Dosage	Comments
Vinpocetine	Semisynthetic derivative of vincamine (plant derivative)	Cerebral ischemic stroke, dementias	GI distress, dizziness, insomnia, dry mouth, tachycardia, hypotension, flushing	Warfarin	5–10 mg daily with food, no more than 20 mg/day	Used in Europe, Mexico, and Japan as pharmaceutical agent for treatment of cerebrovascular and cognitive disorders
Vitamin E family	Essential fat-soluble vitamin, family made of tocopherols and tocotrienols	Immune-enhancing, antioxidant, some cancers, protection in CV disease, neurologic disorders, diabetes, premenstrual syndrome	May increase bleeding in those with propensity to bleed, possible increased risk of hemorrhagic stroke, thrombophlebitis	Warfarin, antiplatelet drugs, neomycin, may be additive with statins	Depends on form: tocotrienols, 200–300 mg daily with food; tocopherols, 200 mg/day	Stop members of vitamin E family 1 month prior to surgical procedures
Glycine	Amino acid	Schizophrenia, alleviating spasticity, and seizures	Avoid in those who are anuric or have hepatic failure	Additive with antispasmodics	1 g/day in divided doses for supplement; 40–90 g/day for schizophrenia	
Melatonin	Hormone of pineal gland	Insomnia, sleep disturbances, jet lag, cancer	May inhibit ovulation in 1 g doses, seizures, grogginess, depression, headache, amnesia	Aspirin, NSAIDs, β-blockers, INH, sedating drugs, corticosteroids, valerian, kava kava, 5-HTP, alcohol	0.3–3 mg HS for short periods of time	Melatonin sets the timing of circadian rhythms and regulates seasonal responses.
Fish oil	Lipids found in fish	Bipolar disorder, lowering triglycerides, hypertension, decrease blood clotting	Caution in hemophiliacs, mild GI upset, "fishy"-smelling excretions	Coumadin, aspirin, NSAIDs, garlic, ginkgo	Varies depending on form and indication—usually about 3–5 g daily	Stop prior to any surgical procedure
Magnesium	Metallic element	Depression, ADHD and pre-menstrual syndrome	Stomach upset, nausea and vomiting	Abacavir, sodium polystyrene	300–400 mg daily	
Vitamin D	Essential fat-soluble vitamin family of provitamin D3	Depression	Kidney stone, confusion, muscle weakness, weight loss, nausea and vomiting	Oral hypoglycemic, insulin, antihypertensives, antiseizures, oral contraceptives	400–2,000 IU daily, more if not exposed to sun light.	

ADD, attention-deficit disorder; CV, cardiovascular; OCD, obsessive-compulsive disorder; GI, gastrointestinal; PKU, phenylketonuria; SSRIs, serotonin reuptake inhibitors; NSAIDs, nonsteroidal anti-inflammatory drugs; INH, isoniazid; 5-HTP, 5-hydroxytryptophan; t.i.d., three times a day; b.i.d., twice a day; hs, at night; MAOIs, monoamine oxidase inhibitors;

Table by Mercedes Blackstone, M.D.

Table 29-29
Some Common Medical Foods

Medical Food	Indication	Mechanism of Action
Caprylic-triglyceride (Axona)	Alzheimer's disease	Increases plasma concentration of ketones as an alternative energy source in the brain; metabolized in the liver.
L-methylfolate (Deplin)	Depression	Regulates synthesis of serotonin, norepinephrine, and dopamine; adjunctive to selective serotonin reuptake inhibitors (SSRIs); 15 mg/day.
S-Adenosyl-L-methionine (SAMe)	Depression	Naturally occurring molecule involved in synthesis of hormones and neurotransmitters including serotonin and norepinephrine.
L-Tryptophane	Sleep disturbance	Essential amino acid; precursor of serotonin; reduces sleep latency; usual dose 4–5 g/day.
	Depression	
Omega-3 fatty acid	Depression	Eicosapentaenoic (EPA) and docosahexaenoic (DHA) acids; direct effect on lipid metabolism; used for augmentation of antidepressant drugs.
	Cognition	
Theramine (Sentra)	Sleep disturbances	Cholinergic modulator; increases acetylcholine and glutamate.
	Cognitive enhancer	
N-Acetylcysteine	Depression	Amino acid that attenuates glutamatergic neurotransmission; used to augment SSRIs.
	Obsessive-compulsive disorder	
L-Tyrosine	Depression	Amino acid precursor to biogenic amines epinephrine and norepinephrine.
Glycine	Depression	Amino acid that activates N-methyl-D-aspartate (NMDA) receptors; may facilitate excitatory transmission in the brain.
Citicoline	Alzheimer's disease	Choline donor involved in synthesis of brain phospholipids and acetylcholine; 300–1,000 mg/day; may improve memory.
	Ischemic brain injury	
Acetyl L-carnitine (Alcar)	Alzheimer's disease	Antioxidant that may prevent oxidative damage in the brain.
	Memory loss	

Table 29-30
Phytomedicinals with Psychoactive Effects

Name	Ingredients	Use	Adverse Effects[a]	Interactions	Dosage[a]	Comments
Arctic weed, golden root	MAOI and β endorphin	Anxiolytic, mood enhancer, antidepressant	No side effect yet documented in trials		100 mg b.i.d. to 200 mg t.i.d.	Use caution with drugs that mimic MAOIs
Areca, areca nut, betel nut; L. Areca catechu	Arecoline, guvacoline	For alteration of consciousness to reduce pain and elevate mood	Parasympathomimetic overload: increased salivation, tremors, bradycardia, GI spasms, GI disturbances, ulcers of the mouth	Avoid with parasympathomimetic drugs; atropine-like compounds reduce effect	Undetermined; 8–10 g is toxic dose for humans.	Used by chewing the nut; used in the past as a chewing balm for gum disease and as a vermifuge; long-term use may result in malignant tumors of the oral cavity.
Ashwagandha	Also called Indian Winter Cherry or Indian Ginseng, native to India. Flavonoids.	Antioxidant, may decrease anxiety levels. Improved libido in men and women May lower levels of the stress hormone cortisol.	Drowsiness and sleepiness	None	Dosage is 1 tablet twice daily before meals with a gradual increase to 4 tablets per day.	None
Belladonna, L. Atropa belladonna, deadly nightshade	Atropine, scopolamine, flavonoids[b]	Anxiolytic	Tachycardia, arrhythmias, xerostomia, mydriasis, difficulties with micturition and constipation	Synergistic with anticholinergic drugs; avoid with TCAs, amantadine, and quinidine	0.05–0.10 mg a day; maximum single dose is 0.20 mg	Has a strong smell, tastes sharp and bitter, and is poisonous
Biota, Platycladus orientalis	Plant derivative	Used as a sedative. Other uses are to treat heart palpitations, panic, night sweats, and constipation. May be useful in ADHD.	No known adverse effects.	None	No clear established doses exist.	None

(continued)

Table 29-30
Phytomedicinals with Psychoactive Effects *(Continued)*

Name	Ingredients	Use	Adverse Effects*a*	Interactions	Dosage*a*	Comments
Bitter orange flower, *Citrus aurantium*	Flavonoids, limonene	Sedative, anxiolytic, hypnotic	Photosensitization	Undetermined	Tincture, 2–3 g/day; drug, 4–6 g/day; extract, 1–2 g/day	Contradictory evidence; some refer to it as a gastric stimulant
Black cohosh, *L. Cimicifuga racemosa*	Triterpenes, isoferulic acid	For PMS, menopausal symptoms, dysmenorrhea	Weight gain, GI disturbances	Possible adverse interaction with male or female hormones	1–2 g/day; over 5 g can cause vomiting, headache, dizziness, cardiovascular collapse.	Estrogen-like effects questionable because root may act as an estrogen-receptor blocker.
Black haw, cramp bark, *L. Viburnum prunifolium*	Scopoletin, flavonoids, caffeic acids, triterpenes	Sedative, antispasmodic action on uterus; for dysmenorrhea	Undetermined	Anticoagulant-enhanced effects	1–3 g/day	Insufficient data
California poppy, *L. Eschscholtzia californica*	Isoquinoline alkaloids, cyanogenic glycosides	Sedative, hypnotic, anxiolytic; for depression	Lethargy	Combination of California poppy, valerian, St. John's wort, and passion flowers can result in agitation.	2 g/day	Clinical or experimental documentation of effects is unavailable.
Casein	Casein peptides	Used as antistress agent. May improve sleep.	Usually consumed through milk products. May interact with antihypertensive medicine and lower blood pressure. May cause drowsiness and should be avoided when taking alcohol or benzodiazepines.	None	1–2 tablets once or twice daily	

Herb	Constituents	Uses	Interactions	Side Effects	Dosage	Comments
Catnip, L. Nepeta cataria	Valeric acid	Sedative, antispasmodic; for migraine	Undetermined	Headache, malaise, nausea, hallucinogenic effects	Undetermined	Delirium produced in children
Chamomile, L. Matricaria chamomilla	Flavonoids	Sedative, anxiolytic	Undetermined	Allergic reaction	2–4 g/day	May be GABAergic
Coastal water hyssop		Anxiolytic, sedative, epilepsy, asthma	May stimulate	Mild GI discomfort	300–450 mg q.i.d.	Insufficient data
Cordyceps sinensis	A genus of fungi that includes about 400 described species, found primarily in the high altitudes of the Tibetan plateau in China. Antioxidant.	Has been used for weakness, fatigue, to improve sexual drive in the elderly.	None	GI discomfort, dry mouth, and nausea	Dosage in ranges of 3–6 g daily	None
Corydalis, L. Corydalis cava	Isoquinoline alkaloids	Sedative, antidepressant; for mild depression	Undetermined	Hallucination, lethargy	Undetermined	Clonic spasms and muscular tremor with overdose
Cyclamen, L. Cyclamen europaeum	Triterpene	Anxiolytic; for menstrual complaints	Undetermined	Small doses (e.g., 300 mg) can lead to nausea, vomiting, and diarrhea.	Undetermined	High doses can lead to respiratory collapse.
Echinacea, L. Echinacea purpurea	Flavonoids, polysaccharides, caffeic acid derivatives, alkamides	Stimulates immune system; for lethargy, malaise, respiratory infections, and lower UTIs	Undetermined	Allergic reaction, fever, nausea, vomiting	1–3 g/day	Use in HIV and AIDS patients is controversial; may not be effective in coryza.
Ephedra, ma-huang L. Ephedra sinica	Ephedrine, pseudoephedrine	Stimulant; for lethargy, malaise, diseases of respiratory tract	Synergistic with sympathomimetics, serotonergic agents; avoid with MAOIs	Sympathomimetic overload: arrhythmias, increased BP, headache, irritability, nausea, vomiting	1–2 g/day	Tachyphylaxis and dependence can occur (taken off market).

(continued)

Table 29-30
Phytomedicinals with Psychoactive Effects (Continued)

Name	Ingredients	Use	Adverse Effects[a]	Interactions	Dosage[a]	Comments
Ginkgo. L. Ginkgo biloba	Flavonoids, ginkgolide A, B	Symptomatic relief of delirium, dementia; improves concentration and memory deficits; possible antidote to SSRI-induced sexual dysfunction	Allergic skin reactions, GI upset, muscle spasms, headache	Anticoagulant: use with caution because of its inhibitory effect on PAF; increased bleeding possible	120–240 mg/day	Studies indicate improved cognition in persons with Alzheimer's disease after 4–5 weeks of use, possibly because of increased blood flow.
Ginseng. L. Panax ginseng	Triterpenes, ginsenosides	Stimulant; for fatigue, elevation of mood, immune system	Insomnia, hypertonia, and edema (called ginseng abuse syndrome)	Not to be used with sedatives, hypnotic agents, MAOIs, antidiabetic agents, or steroids	1–2 g/day	Several varieties exist; Korean (most highly valued), Chinese, Japanese, American (Panox quinquefolius)
Heather. L. Calluna vulgaris	Flavonoids, triterpenes	Anxiolytic, hypnotic	Undetermined	Undetermined	Undetermined	Efficacy for claimed uses is not documented
Holy Basil formula. Ocimum tenuiflorum	Ocimum tenuiflorum, an aromatic plant native to the tropics, part of the Lamiaceae family.	Used to combat stress, also used for common colds, headaches, stomach disorders, inflammation, heart disease.	No data exist regarding the long-term effects. May prolong clotting time, increase the risk of bleeding during surgery, and lower blood sugar.	None	Dosage depends on the formulation type, recommended dose is 2 softgel capsules taken with 8-oz water daily.	None
Hops. L. Humulus lupulus	Flavonoids. Humulone, lupulone, flavonoids	Sedative, anxiolytic, hypnotic; for mood disturbances, restlessness	Contraindicated in patients with estrogen-dependent tumors (breast, uterine, cervical)	Hyperthermia effects with phenothiazine antipsychotics and with CNS depressants	0.5 g/day	May decrease plasma levels of drugs metabolized by CYP 450 system

Herb	Active constituents	Uses	Adverse effects	Interactions	Dose	Comments
Horehound, L. Ballota nigra	Diterpenes, tannins	Sedative	Arrhythmias, diarrhea, hypoglycemia, possible spontaneous abortions	May enhance serotonergic drug effects, may augment hypoglycemic effects of drugs	1–4 g/day	May cause abortion
Jambolan, L. Syzygium cumini	Oleic acid, myristic acid, palmitic and linoleic acids, tannins	Anxiolytic, antidepressant	Undetermined	Undetermined	1–2 g/day	In folk medicine, a single dose is 30 seeds (1.9 g) of powder
Kanna, Sceletium tortuosum	Alkaloid, mesembrine	Anxiolytic, mood enhancer, empathogen, COPD treatment	Sedation, vivid dreams, headache	Potentiates cannabis, PDE inhibitor	50–100 mg	Insufficient data
Kava kava, L. Piperis methysticum	Kava lactones, kava pyrone	Sedative, hypnotic antispasmodic	Lethargy, impaired cognition, dermatitis with long-term usage, liver toxicity	Synergistic with anxiolytics, alcohol; avoid with levodopa and dopaminergic agents	600–800 mg/day	May be GABAergic; contraindicated in patients with endogenous depression; may increase the danger of suicide
Kratom, Mitragyna speciosa	Alkaloid	Stimulant and depressant	Priapism, testicular enlargement, withdrawal, depression, fatigue, insomnia	Structurally similar to yohimbine	Undetermined	Chewed, extracted into water, tar formulations
Lavender, L. Lavandula angustifolia	Hydroxycoumarin, tannins, caffeic acid	Sedative, hypnotic	Headache, nausea, confusion	Synergistic with other sedatives	3–5 g/day	May cause death in overdose
Lemon balm, sweet Mary, L. Melissa officinalis	Flavonoids, caffeic acid, triterpenes	Hypnotic, anxiolytic, sedative	Undetermined	Potentiates CNS depressant; adverse reaction with thyroid hormone	8–10 g/day	Insufficient data

(continued)

Table 29-30
Phytomedicinals with Psychoactive Effects *(Continued)*

Name	Ingredients	Use	Adverse Effects[a]	Interactions	Dosage[a]	Comments
L-Methylfolate	Folate is a B vitamin found in some foods, needed to form healthy red blood cells. L-methylfolate and levomefolate are names for the active form of folic acid.	Adjunctive L is used for major depression, not an antidepressant when used alone. Folate and L-methylfolate are also used to treat folic acid deficiency in pregnancy, to prevent spinal cord birth defects.	GI side effects reported.	None	15 mg once a day by mouth with or without food	Considered a "medical food" by the FDA and only available by prescription. Safe to take during pregnancy when used as directed.
Mistletoe, L. *Viscum album*	Flavonoids, triterpenes, lectins, polypeptides	Anxiolytic; for mental and physical exhaustion	Berries said to have emetic and laxative effects	Contraindicated in patients with chronic infections (e.g., tuberculosis)	10 per day	Berries have caused death in children.
Mugwort, L. *Artemisia vulgaris*	Sesquiterpene lactones, flavonoids	Sedative, antidepressant, anxiolytic	Anaphylaxis, contact dermatitis, may cause hallucinations.	Potentiates anticoagulants	5–15 g/day	May stimulate uterine contractions, can induce abortion
N-Acetylcysteine (NAC)	Amino acid	Used as an antidote for acetaminophen overdose, augmentation of SSRIs in the treatment of trichotillomania.	Rash, cramps, and angioedema may occur.	Activated charcoal, ampicillin, carbamazepine, cloxacillin, oxacillin, nitroglycerin, and penicillin G.	1,200–2,400 mg/day	Acts as an antioxidant and a glutamate-modulating agent. When used as an antidote for acetaminophen overdose, the doses 20–40 times higher than those used in OCD trials. It has not been shown to be effective in treating schizophrenia.

Herb	Constituents	Uses	Adverse Effects	Interactions	Dose	Cautions
Nux vomica, L. *Strychnos nux vomica*, poison nut	Indole alkaloids: strychnine and brucine, polysaccharides	Antidepressant; for migraine, menopausal symptoms	Convulsions, liver damage, death; severely toxic because of strychnine	Undetermined	0.02–0.05 g/day	Symptoms of poisoning can occur after ingestion of one bean; lethal dose is 1–2 g.
Oats, L. *Avena sativa*	Flavonoids, oligo and polysaccharides	Anxiolytic, hypnotic; for stress, insomnia, opium, and tobacco withdrawal	Bowel obstruction or other bowel dysmotility syndromes, flatulence	Undetermined	3 g/day	Oats have sometimes been contaminated with aflatoxin, a fungal toxin linked with some cancers.
Omega-3 fatty acid	Comes in three forms, eicosapentaenoic acid (EPA), docosahexaenoic acid (DHA), and alpha-linolenic acid (LNA)	Used as a supplement in the treatment of heart disease, high cholesterol, high blood pressure. May also be helpful in treatment of depression, bipolar disorder, schizophrenia, and ADHD. May reduce the risk of ulcers when used in conjunction with NSAID pain relievers.	Can cause gas, bloating, belching, and diarrhea.	May increase effectiveness of blood thinners, may increase fasting blood sugar levels when used with diabetes medications such as insulin and metformin.	Doses vary from 1 to 4 g/day.	Can be contaminated with mercury and PCBs.
Passion flower, L. *Passiflora incarnata*	Flavonoids, cyanogenic glycosides	Anxiolytic, sedative, hypnotic	Cognitive impairment	Undetermined	4–8 g/day	Overdose causes depression
Phosphatidylserine and Phosphatidylcholine	Phospholipids	Used for Alzheimer's disease, age-related decline in mental function, improving thinking skills in young people, ADHD, depression, preventing exercise-induced stress, and improving athletic performance.	Insomnia and stomach upset.	None	100 mg three times daily	None

(continued)

Table 29-30
Phytomedicinals with Psychoactive Effects *(Continued)*

Name	Ingredients	Use	Adverse Effects[a]	Interactions	Dosage[a]	Comments
Polygala	Polygala is a genus of about 500 species of flowering plants belonging to the family Polygalaceae, commonly known as milkwort or snakeroot.	Used for insomnia, forgetfulness, mental confusion, palpitation, seizures, anxiety, and listlessness.	Contraindicated in patients who have ulcers or gastritis, should not be used long term.	None	Dosage of polygala is 1.5–3 g of dried root, 1.5–3 g of a fluid extract, or 2.5–7.5 g of a tincture. A polygala tea can also be made, with a maximum of three cups per day.	None
Rehmannia	Iridoid glycosides	Stimulates the release of cortisol. Used in lupus, rheumatoid arthritis (RA), fibromyalgia, and multiple sclerosis. May improve asthma and urticaria. Used to treat menopause, hair loss, and impotence.	Loose bowel movements, bloating, nausea, and abdominal cramps.	None	Exact dosage unknown	None
Rhodiola rosea	Potentiator, monoterpene alcohols, flavonoids					

Herb	Constituents	Action/Use	Adverse Effects	Interactions	Dose	Comments
S-Adenosyl-L-methionine (SAMe)	S-Adenosyl-L-methionine	Used for arthritis and fibromyalgia; may be effective as an augmentation strategy for SSRI in depression.	GI symptoms, anxiety, nightmares, insomnia, and worsening of Parkinson's symptoms.	Use with SSRIs or SNRIs may result in serotonin syndrome. Interacts with levodopa, meperidine, pentazocine, and tramadol.	400–1,600 mg/day	A naturally occurring molecule made from the amino acid methionine and ATP; serves as a methyl donor in human cellular metabolism.
Scarlet Pimpernel, L. Anagallis arvensis	Flavonoids, triterpenes, cucurbitacins, caffeic acids	Antidepressant	Overdose or long-term doses may lead to gastroenteritis and nephritis	Undetermined	1.8 g of powder four times a day	Flowers are poisonous.
Skullcap, L. Scutellaria lateriflora	Flavonoid, monoterpenes	Anxiolytic, sedative, hypnotic	Cognitive impairment, hepatotoxicity	Disulfiram-like reaction may occur if used with alcohol	1–2 g/day	Little information exists to support the use of this herb in humans.
St. John's wort, L. Hypericum perforatum	Hypericin, flavonoids, xanthones	Antidepressant, sedative, anxiolytic	Headaches, photosensitivity (may be severe), constipation	Report of manic reaction when used with sertraline (Zoloft); do not combine with SSRIs or MAOIs; possible serotonin syndrome; do not use with alcohol, opioids	100–950 mg/day	Under investigation by the NIH; may act as MAOI or SSRI; 4- to 6-week trial for mild depressive moods; if no apparent improvement, another therapy should be tried.
Strawberry leaf. L. Fragaria vesca	Flavonoids, tannins	Anxiolytic	Contraindicated with strawberry allergy	Undetermined	1 g/day	Little information exists to support the use of this herb in humans.
Tarragon, L. Artemisia dracunculus	Flavonoids, hydroxycoumarins	Hypnotic, appetite stimulant	Undetermined	Undetermined	Undetermined	Little information exists to support the use of this herb in humans.

(continued)

Table 29-30
Phytomedicinals with Psychoactive Effects *(Continued)*

Name	Ingredients	Use	Adverse Effects[a]	Interactions	Dosage[a]	Comments
Valerian, *L. Valeriana officinalis*	Valepotriates, valerenic acid, caffeic acid	Sedative, muscle relaxant, hypnotic	Cognitive and motor impairment, GI upset, hepatotoxicity; long-term use: contact allergy, headache, restlessness, insomnia, mydriasis, cardiac dysfunction	Avoid concomitant use with alcohol or CNS depressants	1–2 g/day	May be chemically unstable
Wild lettuce, *Lactuca, Virosa*	Flavonoids, coumarins, lactones	Sedative, anesthetic, galactagogue	Tachycardia, tachypnea, visual disturbance, diaphoresis		Undetermined	Bitter taste, added to salad or drinks, active compound closely resembles opium
Winter cherry, *withania, somnifera*	Alkaloids, steroidal lactones	Sedative, treatment for arthritis, possible anticarcinogenic	Thyrotoxicosis, unfavorable effects on heart and adrenal gland		Undetermined	Smoke inhaled

[a]There are no reliable, consistent, or valid data exist on dosages or adverse effects of most phytomedicinals.

[a]Flavonoids are common to many herbs. They are plant byproducts that act as antioxidants (i.e., agents that prevent the deterioration of material such as deoxyribonucleic acid (DNA) via oxidation).

ADHD, attention-deficit/hyperactivity disorder; AIDS, acquired immunodeficiency syndrome; ATP, adenosine triphosphate; b.i.d., twice a day; BP blood pressure; CNS, central nervous system; COPD, chronic obstructive pulmonary disease; FDA, U.S. Food and Drug Administration; GABA, γ-aminobutyric acid; GI, gastrointestinal; MAOI, monoamine oxidase inhibitor; NIH, National Institutes of Health; NSAID, nonsteroidal anti-inflammatory drug; OCD, obsessive-compulsive disorder; q.i.d., four times a day; PAF, platelet-activating factor; PCB, polychlorinated biphenyl; PDE, phosphodiesterase; PMS, premenstrual syndrome; NSAID, nonsteroidal anti-inflammatory drug; OCD, obsessive-compulsive disorder; q.i.d., four times a day; SNRI, serotonin and norepinephrine reuptake inhibitor; SSRI, selective serotonin reuptake inhibitor; TCA, tricyclic antidepressant; t.i.d., three times a day; UTI, urinary tract infection.

1. **Adverse effects.** Adverse effects are possible, and toxic interactions with other drugs may occur with all phytomedicinals, dietary supplements, and medicinal foods. Safety profiles and knowledge of adverse effects of most of these substances have not been studied rigorously. All of these agents should be avoided during pregnancy; some herbs may act as abortifacients. Because most of these substances or their metabolites are secreted in breast milk, they are contraindicated during lactation.

 CLINICAL HINT:

Clinicians should always attempt to obtain a history of herbal use or the use of medical foods or nutritional supplements during the psychiatric evaluation.

It is important to be nonjudgmental in dealing with patients who use these substances. If psychotropic agents are prescribed, the clinician must be extraordinarily alert to the possibility of adverse effects as a result of drug–drug interactions because many of these compounds have ingredients that produce actual physiologic changes in the body.

For more detailed discussion of this topic, see Chapter 34, Biological Therapies, p. 2905 and Chapter 31, Section 31.4, Complimentary, Alternative, and Integrative Approaches in Mental Health Care, p. 2542, in CTP/X.

30
Brain Stimulation Therapies

Introduction

Brain stimulation uses electrical currents or magnetic fields to alter neuronal firing. There is a growing list of tools capable of eliciting such neuromodulation, each with a different spectrum of action (transcranially or surgical implantation of electrodes). Transcranial techniques include cranial electrical stimulation (CES), electroconvulsive therapy (ECT), transcranial direct current stimulation (tDCS, also called direct current polarization), transcranial magnetic stimulation (TMS), and magnetic seizure therapy (MST). The surgical techniques include cortical brain stimulation (CBS), deep brain stimulation (DBS), and vagus nerve stimulation (VNS).

I. Electroconvulsive Therapy

In 1938, the first electroconvulsive treatment (ECT) course was administered to a delusional and incoherent patient, who improved with 1 treatment and remitted after 11 treatments and in 1940, the first use of ECT occurred in the United States. There is a dose–response relationship with right unilateral ECT and that bilateral ECT is likely to be ineffective with ultrabrief pulse widths. ECT remains the most effective treatment for major depression and a rapidly effective treatment for life-threatening psychiatric conditions. The induction of a bilateral generalized seizure is necessary for both the beneficial and the adverse effects of ECT. ECT affects the cellular mechanisms of memory and mood regulation and raises the seizure threshold. The latter effect may be blocked by the opiate antagonist naloxone (Narcan).

A. Indications

1. **Major depressive disorder.** The most common indication for ECT is major depressive disorder (MDD) and should be considered for patients who have failed medication trials, have not tolerated medications, have severe or psychotic symptoms, are acutely suicidal or homicidal, or have marked symptoms of agitation or stupor. ECT is effective for depression in both MDD and bipolar I disorder.

2. **Manic episodes.** ECT is at least equal to lithium (Eskalith) in the treatment of acute manic episodes. The relative rapidity of the ECT response indicates its usefulness for patients whose manic behavior has produced dangerous levels of exhaustion.

 CLINICAL HINT:
ECT should not be used for a patient who is receiving lithium, because lithium can lower the seizure threshold and cause a prolonged seizure.

Table 30-1
Indications for the Use of Electroconvulsive Therapy

Diagnoses for which ECT may be indicated
Major diagnostic indications
Major depression, both unipolar and bipolar
Psychotic depression in particular
Mania, including mixed episodes
Schizophrenia with acute exacerbation
Catatonic subtype
Schizoaffective disorder
Other diagnostic indications
Parkinson's disease
Neuroleptic malignant disorder
Clinical indications
Primary use
Rapid definitive response required on medical or psychiatric grounds
Risks of alternative treatments outweigh benefits
Past history of poor response to psychotropics or good response to ECT
Patient preference
Secondary use
Failure to respond to pharmacotherapy in the current episode
Intolerance of pharmacotherapy in the current episode
Rapid definitive response necessitated by deterioration of the patient's condition

ECT, electroconvulsive therapy.

3. **Schizophrenia.** Patients who have marked positive symptoms, catatonia, or affective symptoms are considered most likely to respond to ECT. In such patients, the efficacy of ECT is about equal to that of antipsychotics, but improvement may occur faster.

4. **Other indications.** ECT may be effective in the treatment of catatonia, schizophrenia, and may also be the treatment of choice for depressed suicidal pregnant women who require treatment and cannot take medication.

   For complete list of indications see Table 30-1.

B. **Pretreatment evaluation.** This should include standard physical, neurologic, and preanesthesia examinations and a complete medical history. Laboratory evaluations should include blood and urine chemistries, a chest x-ray, and an electrocardiogram (ECG).

C. **Procedure.** ECT treatment requires use of premedication, muscarinic anticholinergic drugs, anesthesia and muscle relaxants.

D. **Contraindications.** ECT has no absolute contraindications, only situations in which a patient is at increased risk and has an increased need for close monitoring.

E. **Mortality.** The mortality rate with ECT is about 0.002% per treatment and 0.01% for each patient.

F. **Adverse effects**

1. **Central nervous system effects.** Headache, confusion, and delirium shortly after the seizure and marked confusion may occur in up to 10% of patients but delirium characteristically clears within days or a few weeks at the longest.

2. Memory. About 75% of all patients given ECT say that the memory impairment is the worst adverse effect but almost all patients are back to their cognitive baselines after 6 months. Some patients, however, complain of persistent memory difficulties.

II. Transcranial Magnetic Stimulation

TMS induces electrical fields in the brain without an electrode through the application of alternating magnetic fields via a coil held on the scalp. It is a noninvasive stimulation of focal regions of the brain without the need for anesthesia.

A. Indications. It is approved by the FDA for the treatment of MDD in adult patients who have failed to achieve satisfactory improvement from one prior antidepressant medication at or above the minimal effective dose and duration in the current episode.

B. Side effects, interactions with medications, and other risks. Administration of TMS is a noninvasive, relatively benign procedure but it is not entirely without risk, the most serious being an unintended seizure.

C. Patient selection. Patients who have failed a trial of one or more antidepressant medications or have untoward side effects to medications may be good candidates for TMS. However, given the lower effect size of TMS, for urgent or severely refractory cases, ECT would remain the ultimate gold standard treatment.

III. Transcranial Direct Current Stimulation

It is a noninvasive form of treatment that uses very weak (1 to 3 mA) direct electrical current applied to the scalp. The small device is very portable and usually operated by readily available DC batteries.

A. Side effects. There are no known serious adverse effects of tDCS. It is well tolerated, with reported common side effects in the literature listing mostly minimal tingling at the site of stimulation, with a few reported cases of skin irritation.

B. Mechanism of action. Direct current polarizes current, and tDCS is believed to act via the alteration of neuronal membrane polarization, but little is known about the actual mechanism of action of tDCS.

C. Clinical studies. Preliminary research suggests that tDCS may enhance certain brain functions independent of mood; however, tDCS technology and its use in psychiatry are in the early stages of exploration.

IV. Cranial Electrical Stimulation

A. Definition. CES, like tDCS, uses a weak (1 to 4 mA) current. It is traditionally applied via saline-soaked, felt-covered electrodes clipped onto the earlobes.

B. Mechanism of action. The exact mechanism of action has not been elicited, and there is no agreement among researchers on the predominant mode of action.

C. Side effects. It is believed that the CES stimulation is not harmful, primarily due to its low voltage power supply (9-V battery) and lack of any reported adverse event by the FDA. Local skin effects, as well as a general feeling of dizziness, have been reported.

D. Clinical studies. In a meta-analysis by the Harvard School of Public Health the overall pooled result showed CES to be better than sham treatment for anxiety at a statistically significant level.

V. Magnetic Seizure Therapy

A. Definition. MST is a novel form of a convulsive treatment, given using a modified TMS device that is under development in several research institutions. The aim is to produce a seizure whose focus and patterns of spread may be controlled. MST is a convulsive treatment, in many ways similar to ECT and requires approximately the same preparation and infrastructure as ECT. It is not FDA approved.

B. Mechanism of action. Induction of a seizure is hypothesized to be the underlying event responsible for the likely multiple specific mechanisms of action of MST treatment.

C. Side effects. Adverse effects are like those of ECT, are largely connected to the risks associated with anesthesia and generalized seizure. Studies show MST results in less retrograde and anterograde amnesia than ECT.

D. Current status in treatment algorithms. It is still an investigational protocol and treatments outside of research are not FDA approved.

VI. Vagus Nerve Stimulation

A. Definition. VNS is the direct, intermittent electrical stimulation of the left cervical vagus nerve via an implanted pulse generator, usually in the left chest wall. The electrode is wrapped around the left vagus nerve in the neck and is connected to the generator subcutaneously.

B. Side effects and contraindications. VNS is generally well tolerated. The most common side effects are voice alteration, dyspnea, and neck pain.

C. Current status in treatment algorithms. The FDA indicated VNS for the adjunctive long-term treatment of chronic or recurrent depression in patients 18 years or older experiencing a major depressive episode in the setting of unipolar or bipolar disease who have not had an adequate response to four or more adequate antidepressant treatments.

D. Patient selection. VNS is approved as an adjunctive long-term treatment for chronic or recurrent depressive episodes in adults with a major depressive episode who have not had a satisfactory response to four or more adequate antidepressant trials. The efficacy of VNS in other disorders is unknown.

E. Dosing. The optimal dosing for psychiatric applications of VNS is still largely an area of investigation. The published studies do not identify optimal dosing parameters like time on, time off, frequency, current, or pulse width.

VII. Deep Brain Stimulation

The procedure involves placement of small-diameter brain "leads" (e.g., approximately 1.3 mm) with multiple electrode contacts into subcortical nuclei or specific white matter tracts. The surgeon drills burr holes in skull bone under local anesthesia and then places the leads, guided by multimodal imaging and precise stereotactic landmarking. Later, the "pacemaker" (also known as an implantable neurostimulator or pulse generator) is implanted subdermally (e.g., in the upper chest wall) and connects it, via extension wires tunneled under the skin, to the brain leads.

A. **Indications.** It is used to treat people with advanced Parkinson's disease, dystonia, and essential tremor whose symptoms are no longer controlled by medication.

B. **Outcome with deep brain stimulation**

1. **Obsessive-compulsive disorder.** DBS has been shown to have clinically significant symptoms reduction in patients with intractable OCD. DBS is placed at the ventral anterior limb of the internal capsule and adjacent ventral striatum (VC/VS).

2. **Major depression.** Functional neuroimaging research implicates the subgenual cingulate cortex as a node in circuits involved in the normal experience of sadness, symptoms of depressive illness, and responses to depression treatments. The treatment is in early stages and being studied but chronic DBS for up to 6 months showed sustained remission of depression in a small number of patients. The advent of DBS in psychiatry has created tremendous interest and considerable research activity. DBS may therefore be accepted by patients who would not choose to undergo lesion procedures (although the reverse is also true). With all of its advantages, DBS requires that patients be treated by highly specialized teams willing and able to provide long-term care.

For more detailed discussion of this topic, see Biological Therapies, Chapter 34, Section 34.35, Electroconvulsive Therapy, p. 3280 and Section 34.36, Brain Stimulation Methods, p. 3298, in CTP/X.

31

Forensic Psychiatry and Ethics in Psychiatry

I. Introduction

In clinical practice, it is not uncommon for psychiatry and the law to converge. Forensic psychiatry covers a range of topics that involve psychiatrists' professional, ethical, and legal duties to provide competent care; the patients' rights of self-determination to receive or refuse treatment; court decisions, legislative directives, governmental regulatory agencies, and licensure boards; and the evaluation of those charged with crimes to determine their culpability and ability to stand trial. Ethical guidelines help psychiatrists avoid *ethical conflicts* and think through *ethical dilemmas*. Finally, the ethical codes and practice guidelines of professional organizations and their adherence also fall within the realm of forensic psychiatry.

II. Medical Malpractice

To prove malpractice, the plaintiff (e.g., patient, family, or estate) must establish, by a preponderance of evidence that:

A. a doctor–patient's relationship existed and created a duty of care,

B. a deviation from the standard of care occurred,

C. the patient was damaged, and

D. the deviation caused the damage.

These elements are often referred to as the *4 D's* of malpractice (duty, deviation, damage, direct-causation). Each of the four elements of a malpractice claim must be present or there can be no liability. For example, a psychiatrist whose actions cause direct harm is not liable if no doctor–patient relationship has been established. In addition to negligence, psychiatrist's may be sued for intentional torts such as assault, battery, false imprisonment, defamation, fraud, or misrepresentation in a case, invasion of privacy, and intentional infliction of emotional distress.

III. Split Treatment

A. In split treatment, the psychiatrist provides medication, and a nonmedical therapist conducts psychotherapy.

B. The psychiatrist retains full responsibility for the patients care in a split treatment situation.

C. It is important that the psychiatrist does a thorough evaluation, including obtaining prior medical records.

D. Prescribing medication, outside of a working doctor–patient relationship, does not meet generally accepted standards of good clinical care, and may lead to malpractice action.

E. It is important that the psychiatrist remain thoroughly informed of the patient's status and efficacy of any prescribed drug treatments. It is also imperative that the psychiatrist maintain a direct involvement in the patients care.

IV. Privilege and Confidentiality

A. Privilege is the right to maintain secrecy and confidentiality in the face of a subpoena.

1. Privileged communications within a relationship such as husband–wife, priest–penitent, doctor–patient, are protected from forced disclosure on the witness stand.

2. The right to privilege belongs to the patient, not the physician, and the patient, can waive the right if they choose.

3. Privilege does not exist at all in military courts, regardless to whether or not the physician is military of civilian.

B. Confidentiality is the long held promise of medical ethics which binds the physician to hold secret all information given by the patient.

1. Confidentiality applies to a population sharing information without specific permission of the patient. The circle of confidentiality doe not only include the physician, but encompasses all staff members, clinical supervisors, and consultants involved in the patients care.

2. A subpoena can force a psychiatrist to breach confidentiality.

3. Physicians are usually served with a *subpoena duces tecum*, which requires that they also produce their relevant records and documents.

4. In bona fide emergencies, information may be released in as limited a way as possible in order to carry out the necessary interventions. Clinical practices dictate that, if at all possible, the psychiatrist should make an effort to obtain the patients permission, and should debrief the patient after the emergency situation has been resolved.

5. Though oral permission is sufficient, it is always best to obtain written permission from the patient. It should be noted that each release is only good for one piece of information and permission should be obtained for each subsequent release, even to the same party.

6. Finally, release constitutes permission and not obligation. If the psychiatrist feels that releasing said information would be destructive, the matter may be discussed, and the release may be refused, with some expectations.

The Privacy Rule, administered by the Office of Civil Rights (OCR) at HHS, protects the confidentiality of patient information (Table 31-1).

C. Child abuse. Many states require that all physicians take a course on child abuse for medical licensure. All states legally require that psychiatrists, among others, who have reason to believe that a child has been abused, sexually or otherwise, immediately report their suspicions to the appropriate agency. In this situation, the potential harm to a child greatly outweighs the value of confidentiality in a psychiatric setting.

Table 31-1
Patients' Rights under the Privacy Rule

Physicians must give the patient a written notice of his or her privacy rights; the privacy policies of the practice; and how patient information is used, kept, and disclosed. A written acknowledgment should be taken from the patient verifying that he or she has seen such notice.

Patients should be able to obtain copies of their medical records and to request revisions to those records within a stated amount of time (usually 30 days). Patients do not have the right to see psychotherapy notes.

Physicians must provide the patient with a history of most disclosures of their medical history on request. Some exceptions exist. The APA Committee on Confidentiality has developed a model document for this requirement.

Physicians must obtain authorization from the patient for disclosure of information other than for treatment, payment, and health care operations (these three are considered to be routine uses, for which consent is not required). The APA Committee on Confidentiality has developed a model document for this requirement.

Patients may request another means of communication of their protected information (e.g., request that the physician contact them at a specific phone number or address).

Physicians cannot generally limit treatment to obtaining patient authorization for disclosure of their information for nonroutine uses.

Patients have the right to complain about Privacy Rule violations to the physician, their health plan, or to the Secretary of HHS.

APA, American Psychiatric Association; HHS, Department of Health and Human Services.

V. High-Risk Clinical Situations

A. Suicidal patients. Psychiatrists can be sued if their patient commits suicide. Particularly in the case of inpatient suicide, where psychiatrists are expected to have greater control of the patient's behavior. Suicide is a rare event, and the evaluation of a suicide risk is one of the most complexes, dauntingly difficult clinical task, and as of now there is no way to accurately predict whether or not a patient will commit suicide.

B. Violent patients. Psychiatrists treating violent or potentially violent patients can be sued for failure to control aggressive outpatients, for the discharge of violent inpatients, and for the failure to protect society from a patient's violent actions. In most states, if a patient threatens to harm another person, it is required that the physician intervene to prevent harm from occurring. The options to warn and protect include voluntary hospitalization, involuntary hospitalization, warning the victim of the threat, notifying the police, adjusting medication, and seeing the patient more frequently.

VI. Hospitalization

A. Procedures of admission. The American Bar Association has specifically endorsed four procedures of admission to psychiatric facilities, informal admission, voluntary admission, temporary admission, and involuntary admission. These procedures are intended to safeguard civil liberties and to ensure that no person is railroaded into a mental hospital. Though each of the 50 states has the power to enact its own laws in regards to psychiatric hospitalization, the above-mentioned procedures are gaining much acceptance.

B. Informal admission. Informal admission operates under the general hospital model, in which a psychiatric patient is admitted to the psychiatric unit in the same way that a medical or surgical patient is admitted to a medical ward.

C. Voluntary admission. Patients who are voluntarily admitted to the psychiatric unit either do so under the advice of a physician or they seek treatment on their own. Such patients apply in writing for admission to the psychiatric unit and maintain an ordinary doctor–patient relationship, and are free to leave, even against medical advice.

D. Temporary admission. A temporary form of involuntary commitment for patients who are senile, confused, or unable to make their own decisions. In an emergency admission, the patient cannot be hospitalized against his or her will for more than 15 days.

E. Involuntary admission. If patients are a danger to themselves (suicidal) or others (homicidal), they may be admitted to a hospital after a friend or relative applies for admission and two physicians confirm the need for hospitalization. It allows the patient to be hospitalized for 60 days, after which the case must be reviewed by a board consisting of psychiatrists, nonpsychiatric physicians, lawyers, and other impartial parties.

VII. Right to Treatment

The right of an involuntarily committed patient to active treatment has been enunciated by lower federal courts and enacted in some state statutes.

A. *Wyatt v. Stickney* (1971), set the pattern of reform by requiring treatment in addition to hospitalization. It also required specific changes in the operations of institutions and their programs, including changes in physical conditions, staffing, and quality of treatment provided.

B. *Donaldson v. O'Connor* (1976), the United States Supreme Court held that an involuntarily committed person who is not dangerous and who can survive by himself or herself with help must be released from the hospital.

VIII. Right to Refuse Treatment

The right to refuse treatment is a legal doctrine that holds that, except in emergencies, persons cannot be forced to accept treatment against their will. An emergency is defined as a condition in clinical practice that requires immediate intervention to prevent death or serious harm to the patient or another person or to prevent deterioration of the patient's clinical state.

A. *O'Connor v. Donaldson* (1976), the Supreme Court of the United States ruled that harmless mentally ill patients cannot be confined against their will without treatment if they can survive outside. According to the Court, a finding of mental illness alone cannot justify a state's confining persons in a hospital against their will. Instead, involuntarily confined patients must be considered dangerous to themselves or others or possibly so unable to care for themselves that they cannot survive outside.

B. As a result of the 1979 case of *Rennie v. Klein*, patients have the right to refuse treatment and to use an appeal process.

C. As a result of the 1981 case of *Roger v. Oken*, patients have an absolute right to refuse treatment, but a guardian may authorize treatment.

IX. Seclusion and Restraint

Seclusion refers to placing and keeping an inpatient in a special room for the purpose of containing a clinical situation that may result in a state of emergency. *Restraint* involves measures designed to confine a patient's bodily movements, such as the use of leather cuffs and anklets or straitjackets. The doctrine of the least restrictive alternative is used (i.e., seclusion should be used only when no less restrictive alternative is available). Additional restrictions include the following: (1) restraint and seclusion can only be implemented by a written order from an appropriate medical official; (2) orders are to be confined to specific, time-limited periods; (3) a patient's condition must be regularly reviewed and documented; and (4) any extension of an original order must be reviewed and reauthorized.

X. Informed Consent

A. Informed consent form. A written document outlining a patient's consent to a proposed procedure or treatment plan. It should include a fair explanation of procedures and their purposes, including the following: (1) identification of procedures that are experimental; (2) discomfort and risks to be expected; (3) disclosure of alternative procedures that may be advantageous; (4) an offer to answer any inquiries concerning the procedures; and (5) instructions that the patient is free to withdraw consent and discontinue participation at any time without prejudice.

B. Exceptions to the rules of informed consent

1. Emergencies. Usually defined in terms of imminent physical danger to the patient or others.

2. Therapeutic privilege. Information that in the opinion of the psychiatrist would harm the patient or be anti-therapeutic and that may be withheld on those grounds.

XI. Child Custody

In cases of disputed custody, the almost universally accepted criterion is "the best interest of the child." In that context, the task of the psychiatrist is to provide an expert opinion and supporting data regarding which party should be granted custody to best serve the interests of the child.

The mental disability of a parent can lead to the transfer of custody to the other parent or to a public agency. When the mental disability is chronic and the parent is incapacitated, a procedure for the termination of parental rights may result. That also is the case when evidence of child abuse is pervasive. In the Gault decision (1967), the Supreme Court held that a juvenile also has constitutional rights to due process and procedural safeguards (e.g., counsel, jury, trials).

XII. Testamentary and Contractual Capacity and Competence

A. Mental competence. Psychiatrists often are called on to give an opinion about a person's psychological capacity or competence to perform certain civil and legal functions (e.g., make a will, manage his or her financial affairs). Competence is context-related (i.e., the ability to perform a certain function for a particular legal purpose). It is especially important to emphasize that incompetence in one area does not imply incompetence in any or all areas. A person may have a mental disorder and still be competent.

B. Contracts. When a party to an otherwise legal contract is mentally ill and the illness directly and adversely affects the person's ability to understand what he or she is doing (called **contractual capacity**), the law may void the contract. The psychiatrist must evaluate the condition of the party seeking to void the contract at the time that the contract was supposedly entered into. The psychiatrist must then render an opinion as to whether the psychological condition of the party caused an incapacity to understand the important aspects or ramifications of the contract.

C. Wills. The criteria concerning wills (called *testamentary capacity*) are whether, when the will was made, the testator was capable of knowing without prompting (1) the nature of the act, (2) the nature and extent of his or her property, and (3) the natural objects of his or her bounty and their claims on him or her (e.g., heirs, relatives, family members). The mental health of the testator also will indicate whether he or she was in such a condition as to be subject to undue influence.

D. Marriage. A marriage may be void or voidable if one of the parties was incapacitated because of mental illness such that he or she could not reasonably understand the nature and consequences of the transaction (i.e., consent).

E. Guardianship. Guardianship involves a court proceeding for the appointment of a guardian in case of a formal adjudication of incompetence. The criterion is whether, by reason of mental illness, a person can manage his or her own affairs.

F. Durable power of attorney. Permits people to make provisions for their own anticipated loss of decision-making capacity. It permits the advance selection of a substitute decision maker.

G. Competence to inform. Involves a patient's interaction with a clinician. A clinician explains to the patient the value of being honest with the clinician and then determines whether the patient is competent to weigh the risks and benefits of withholding information about suicidal or homicidal intent.

XIII. Criminal Law

A. Competence to stand trial. At any point in the criminal justice process, the psychiatrist may be called on to assess a defendant's present competence to be arraigned, be tried, enter a plea, be sentenced, or be executed. The criteria for competence to be tried are whether, in the presence of a mental disorder, the defendant (1) understands the charges against him or her and (2) can assist in his or her defense.

B. Competence to be executed. Requirement for competence rests on three general principles: (1) a person's awareness of what is happening is supposed to heighten the retributive element of the punishment; (2) a competent person who is about to be executed is believed to be in the best position to make whatever peace is appropriate for his or her religious beliefs, including confession and absolution; and (3) a competent person who is about to be executed preserves, until the end, the possibility of recalling a forgotten detail of the events or the crime that may prove exonerating. It is unethical for any clinician to participate in state-mandated executions; a physician's duty to preserve life transcends all other competing requirements.

C. **Criminal responsibility (the insanity defense).** The criteria for criminal responsibility involve two separate aspects—whether, at the time of the act, as a consequence of mental disorder, the defendant (1) did not know what he or she was doing or that it was wrong (a cognitive test) or (2) could not conform his or her conduct to the requirements of the law (a volitional test).

1. **M'Naghten rule.** The most famous set of criteria for the insanity defense was developed by the House of Lords after the defendant was exculpated in the M'Naghten case (England, 1843). The M'Naghten rule states that the defendant is not guilty by means of insanity if he or she was unaware of the nature, the quality, and consequences of his or her actions due to a mental disease. The M'Naghten rule, therefore, is a cognitive test.

2. **Irresistible impulse.** In 1922, a committee of jurists suggested broadening the concept of insanity in criminal cases to include the irresistible impulse test, which rules that a person charged with a criminal offense is not responsible for an act that was committed under an impulse that the person was unable to resist because of mental illness. The court grants an impulse to be irresistible only when it can be determined that the accused would have committed the act even if a policeman had been at the elbow of the accused.

3. **Model Penal Code.** The American Law Institute (ALI) incorporates both a cognitive and a volitional test in its Model Penal Code. The criterion for legal insanity set forth in the rule is that "a person is not responsible for criminal conduct if at the time of such conduct he lacks substantial capacity either to appreciate the criminality (wrongfulness) of his conduct (the cognitive prong) or to conform his conduct to the requirements of the law (the volitional prong)." To prevent the inclusion of antisocial behavior, the Model Penal Code adds, "As used in this article, the terms 'mental disease or defect' do not include an abnormality manifested only by repeated criminal or otherwise antisocial conduct."

4. **Durham rule.** The accused is not criminally responsible if his or her unlawful act was the product of mental disease or mental defect.
   a. This rule derived from the case of *Durham v. United States* where Judge Bazelon expressly stated that the purpose of the rule was to get good and complete psychiatric testimony. However, in cases using the Durham rule, there was confusion over the terms "product," "disease," and "defect."
   b. In 1972, the Court of Appeals for the District of Columbia, in the *United States v. Brawner* case, discarded the rule and adopted the ALI's Model Penal Code, which is used in federal courts today.

5. **Other tests.** The American Medical Association has proposed limiting insanity exculpation to cases in which the person is so ill that he or she lacks the necessary criminal intent (*mens rea*), thereby all but

eliminating the insanity defense and placing a burden on the prisons to accept a large number of persons who are mentally ill.

The American Bar Association and the American Psychiatric Association (APA) proposed a defense of nonresponsibility, which focuses solely on whether the defendants, as a result of a mental disease or defect, are unable to appreciate the wrongfulness of their conduct. The APA also urged that "mental illness" be limited to severely abnormal mental conditions.

XIV. Ethical Issues in Psychiatry

Ethics in psychiatry refers to the principles of conduct that govern the behavior of psychiatrists as well as other mental health professionals. Ethics as a discipline deals with what is good and what is bad, what is right and what is wrong, and moral duties, obligations, and responsibilities. See Table 31-2.

Table 31-2
Ethical Questions and Answers

Topic	Question	Answer
Abandonment	How can psychiatrists avoid being charged with patient abandonment on retirement?	Retiring psychiatrists are not abandoning patients if they provide their patients with sufficient notice and make every reasonable effort to find follow-up care for the patients.
	Is it ethical to provide only outpatient care to a seriously ill patient who may require hospitalization?	This could constitute abandonment unless the outpatient practitioner or agency arranges for their patients to receive inpatient care from another provider.
Bequests	A dying patient bequeaths his or her estate to his or her treating psychiatrist. Is this ethical?	No. Accepting the bequest seems improper and exploitational of the therapeutic relationship. However, it may be ethical to accept a token bequest from a deceased patient who named his or her psychiatrist in the will without that psychiatrist's knowledge.
Competency	Is it ethical for psychiatrists to perform vaginal examinations? Hospital physical examinations?	Psychiatrists may provide nonpsychiatric medical procedures if they are competent to do so and if the procedures do not preclude effective psychiatric treatment by distorting the transference. Pelvic examinations carry a high risk of distorting the transference and would be better performed by another clinician.
	Can ethics committees review issues of physician competency?	Yes. Incompetency is an ethical issue.
Confidentiality	Must confidentiality be maintained after the death of a patient?	Yes. Ethically, confidences survive a patient's death. Exceptions include protecting others from imminent harm or proper legal compulsions.

(continued)

Table 31-2
Ethical Questions and Answers (Continued)

Topic	Question	Answer
	Is it ethical to release information about a patient to an insurance company?	Yes, if the information provided is limited to that which is needed to process the insurance claim.
	Can a videotaped segment of a therapy session be used at a workshop for professionals?	Yes, if informed, uncoerced consent has been obtained, anonymity is maintained, the audience is advised that editing makes this an incomplete session, and the patient knows the purpose of the videotape.
	Should a physician report mere suspicion of child abuse in a state requiring reporting of child abuse?	No. A physician must make several assessments before deciding whether to report suspected abuse. One must consider whether abuse is ongoing, whether abuse is responsive to treatment, and whether reporting will cause potential harm. Check specific statutes. Make safety for potential victims the top priority.
Conflict of interest	Is there a potential ethical conflict if a psychiatrist has both psychotherapeutic and administrative duties in dealing with students or trainees?	Yes. You must define your role in advance to the trainees or students. Administrative opinions should be obtained from a psychiatrist who is not involved in a treatment relationship with the trainee or student.
Diagnosis without examination	Is it ethical to offer a diagnosis based only on review of records to determine, for insurance purposes, if suicide was the result of illness?	Yes.
	Is it ethical for a supervising psychiatrist to sign a diagnosis on an insurance form for services provided by a supervisee when the psychiatrist has not examined the patient?	Yes, if the psychiatrist ensures that proper care is given and the insurance form clearly indicates the role of supervisor and supervisee.
Exploitation (also see Bequests)	What constitutes exploitation of the therapeutic relationship?	Exploitation occurs when the psychiatrist uses the therapeutic relationship for personal gain. This includes adopting or hiring a patient as well as sexual or financial relationships.
Fee splitting	What is fee splitting?	Fee splitting occurs when one physician pays another for a patient referral. This would also apply to lawyers giving a forensic psychiatrist referrals in exchange for a percentage of the fee. Fee splitting may occur in an office setting if the psychiatrist takes a percentage of his or her office mates' fees for supervision or expenses. Costs for such items or services must be arranged separately. Otherwise, it would appear that the office owner could benefit from referring patients to a colleague in the office. Fee splitting is illegal.

Table 31-2
Ethical Questions and Answers *(Continued)*

Topic	Question	Answer
Informed consent	Is it ethical to refuse to divulge information about a patient who has agreed to give this information to those requesting it?	No. It is the patient's decision, not the therapist's.
	Is informed consent needed when presenting or writing about case material?	Not if the patient is aware of the supervisory or teaching process and confidentiality is preserved.
Moonlighting	Can psychiatric residents ethically "moonlight"?	They can if their duties are not beyond their ability, if they are properly supervised, and if the moonlighting does not interfere with their residency training.
Reporting	Should psychiatrists expose or report unethical behavior of a colleague or colleagues? Can a spouse bring an ethical complaint?	Psychiatrists are obligated to report colleagues' unethical behavior. A spouse with knowledge of unethical behavior can bring an ethical complaint as well.
Research	How can ethical research be performed with subjects who cannot give informed consent?	Consent can be given by a legal guardian or via a living will. Incompetent persons have the right to withdraw from the research project at any time.
Retirement	See Abandonment.	
Supervision	What are the ethical requirements when a psychiatrist supervises other mental health professionals?	The psychiatrist must spend sufficient time to ensure that proper care is given and that the supervisee is not providing services that are outside the scope of his or her training. It is ethical to charge a fee for supervision.
Taping and recording	Can videotapes of patient interviews be used for training purposes on a national level (e.g., workshops, board examination preparation)?	Appropriate and explicit informed consent must be obtained. The purpose and scope of exposure of the tape must be emphasized in addition to the resulting loss of confidentiality.

Table by Eugene Rubin, M.D. Data derived from the American Medical Association's Principles of Medical Ethics.

For more detailed discussion of this topic, see Chapter 60, Ethics and Forensic Psychiatry, p. 4433, in CTP/X.

32
Medication-Induced Movement Disorders

I. General Introduction

Movement disorders can be a disabling and distressing side effect associated with the use of typical antipsychotic drugs. See Table 32-1. The drugs act by blocking the binding of dopamine to the dopamine receptors involved in the control of both voluntary and involuntary movements. The newer antipsychotics, serotonin-dopamine antagonists (SDAs) are less likely to cause extrapyramidal side effects and tardive dyskinesia (TD). In April 2017, Valbenazine was approved by the FDA as the first drug for the treatment of TD.

II. Neuroleptic-Induced Parkinsonism

A. **Diagnosis, signs, and symptoms.** Symptoms include muscle stiffness (lead pipe rigidity), cogwheel rigidity, shuffling gait, stooped posture, and drooling. The pill-rolling tremor of idiopathic parkinsonism is rare, but a regular, coarse tremor similar to essential tremor may be present. The so-called *rabbit syndrome* is a tremor affecting the lips and perioral muscles and is another parkinsonian effect seen with antipsychotics, although perioral tremor is more likely than other tremors to occur late in the course of treatment.

B. **Epidemiology.** Parkinsonian adverse effects occur in about 15% of patients who are treated with antipsychotics, usually within 5 to 90 days of the initiation of treatment. Patients who are elderly and female are at the highest risk for neuroleptic-induced parkinsonism, although the disorder can occur at all ages.

C. **Etiology.** Caused by the blockade of dopamine type 2 (D_2) receptors in the caudate at the termination of the nigrostriatal dopamine neurons. All antipsychotics can cause the symptoms, especially high-potency drugs with low levels of anticholinergic activity (e.g., trifluoperazine [Stelazine]). Chlorpromazine (Thorazine) and thioridazine (Mellaril) are not likely to be involved. The newer, atypical antipsychotics (e.g., aripiprazole [Abilify], olanzapine [Zyprexa], and quetiapine [Seroquel]) are less likely to cause parkinsonism.

D. **Differential diagnosis.** Includes idiopathic parkinsonism, other organic causes of parkinsonism, and depression, which can also be associated with parkinsonian symptoms.

E. **Treatment.** Can be treated with anticholinergic agents, benztropine (Cogentin), amantadine (Symmetrel), or diphenhydramine (Benadryl)

Table 32-1
Selected Medications Associated with Movement Disorders: Impact on Relevant Neuroreceptors

Type (Subtype)	Name (Brand)	D₂ Blockade	5-HT₂ Blockade	mACh Blockade
Antipsychotics				
Phenothiazine (Aliphatic)	Chlorpromazine (Thorazine)	Low	High	High
Phenothiazine (Piperidines)	Thioridazine (Mellaril)	Low	Med	High
	Mesoridazine (Serentil)	Low	Med	High
Phenothiazine (Piperazines)	Trifluoperazine (Stelazine)	Med	Med	Med
	Fluphenazine (Prolixin)	High	Low	Low
	Perphenazine (Trilafon)	High	Med	Low
Thioxanthenes	Thiothixene (Navane)	High	Med	Low
	Chlorprothixene (Taractan)	Med	High	Med
Dibenzoxazepines	Loxapine (Loxitane)	Med	High	Low
Butyrophenones	Haloperidol (Haldol)	High	Low	Low
	Droperidol (Inapsine)	High	Med	—
Diphenylbutylpiperidines	Pimozide (Orap)	High	Med	Low
Dihydroindolones	Molindone (Moban)	Med	Low	Low
Dibenzodiazepines	Clozapine (Clozaril)	Low	High	High
Benzisoxazole	Risperidone (Risperdal)	High	High	Low
Thienobenzodiazepines	Olanzapine (Zyprexa)	Low	High	High
Dibenzothiazepines	Quetiapine (Seroquel)	Low/med	Low/med	Low
Benzisothiazole	Ziprasidone (Geodon)	Med	High	Low
Quinolones	Aripiprazole (Ability)	High (as partial agonist)	High	Low
Nonantipsychotic psychotropics				
Anticonvulsants	Lithium (Eskalith)	Low	Low	Low
Antidepressants	All	Low (except amoxapine)	(Varies)	(Varies)

D₂, dopamine type 2; 5-HT₂, 5-hydroxytryptamine type 2; mACh, muscarinic acetylcholine; N/A, not applicable.
Adapted from Janicak PG, Davis JM, Preskorn SH, Ayd FJ Jr. *Principles and Practice of Psychopharmacotherapy.* 3rd ed. Philadelphia, PA: Lippincott Williams & Wilkins; 2001.

(Table 32-2). Anticholinergics should be withdrawn after 4 to 6 weeks to assess whether tolerance to the parkinsonian effects has developed; about half of patients with neuroleptic-induced parkinsonism require continued treatment. Even after the antipsychotics are withdrawn, parkinsonian symptoms may last for up to 2 weeks and even up to 3 months in elderly patients. With such patients, the clinician may continue the anticholinergic drug after the antipsychotic has been stopped until the parkinsonian symptoms resolve completely.

III. Neuroleptic-Induced Acute Dystonia

    A. Diagnosis, signs, and symptoms. Dystonias are brief or prolonged contractions of muscles that result in obviously abnormal movements or postures, including oculogyric crises, tongue protrusion, trismus, torticollis, laryngeal-pharyngeal dystonias, and dystonic postures of the limbs and

Table 32-2
Drug Treatment of Extrapyramidal Disorders

Generic Name	Trade Name	Usual Daily Dosage	Indications
Anticholinergics			
Benztropine	Cogentin	PO 0.5–2 mg tid; IM or IV 1–2 mg	Acute dystonia, parkinsonism, akinesia, akathisia
Biperiden	Akineton	PO 2–6 mg tid; IM or IV 2 mg	
Procyclidine	Kemadrin	PO 2.5–5 mg bid-qid	
Trihexyphenidyl	Artane, Tremin	PO 2–5 mg tid	
Orphenadrine	Norflex, Dispal	PO 50–100 mg bid-qid; IV 60 mg	Rabbit syndrome
Antihistamine			
Diphenhydramine	Benadryl	PO 25 mg qid; IM or IV 25 mg	Acute dystonia, parkinsonism, akinesia, rabbit syndrome
Amantadine	Symmetrel	PO 100–200 mg bid	Parkinsonism, akinesia rabbit syndrome
β-Adrenergic antagonist			
Propranolol	Inderal	PO 20–40 mg tid	Akathisia, tremor
α-Adrenergic antagonist			
Clonidine	Catapres	PO 0.1 mg tid	Akathisia
Benzodiazepines			
Clonazepam	Klonopin	PO 1 mg bid	Akathisia, acute dystonia
Lorazepam	Ativan	PO 1 mg tid	
Buspirone	BuSpar	PO 20–40 mg qid	Tardive dyskinesia
Vitamin E	—	PO 1,200–1,600 IU/day	Tardive dyskinesia

PO, oral; IM, intramuscular; IV, intravenous; bid, twice a day; tid, three times a day; qid, four times a day.

trunk. Other dystonias include blepharospasm and glossopharyngeal dystonia; the latter results in dysarthria, dysphagia, and even difficulty in breathing, which can cause cyanosis. Children are particularly likely to evidence opisthotonos, scoliosis, lordosis, and writhing movements. Dystonia can be painful and frightening and often results in noncompliance with future drug treatment regimens.

B. Epidemiology. The development of dystonic symptoms is characterized by their early onset during the course of treatment with neuroleptics and their high incidence in men, in patients younger than age 30, and in patients given high dosages of high-potency medications.

C. Etiology. Although it is most common with intramuscular doses of high-potency antipsychotics, dystonia can occur with any antipsychotic. It is least common with thioridazine and is uncommon with atypical antipsychotics. The mechanism of action is thought to be dopaminergic hyperactivity in the basal ganglia that occurs when central nervous system (CNS) levels of the antipsychotic drug begin to fall between doses.

Table 32-3
Abnormal Involuntary Movement Scale (AIMS) Examination Procedure

Patient Identification	Date
Rated by	

Either before or after completing the examination procedure, observe the patient unobtrusively at rest (e.g., in waiting room).

The chair to be used in this examination should be a hard, firm one without arms.

After observing the patient, rate him or her on a scale of 0 (none), 1 (minimal), 2 (mild), 3 (moderate), and 4 (severe) according to the severity of the symptoms.

Ask the patient whether there is anything in his or her mouth (i.e., gum, candy, etc.) and, if so, to remove it.

Ask the patient about the current condition of his or her teeth. Ask patient if he or she wears dentures. Do teeth or dentures bother patient now?

Ask patient whether he or she notices any movement in mouth, face, hands, or feet. If yes, ask patient to describe and indicate to what extent they currently bother patient or interfere with his or her activities.

0 1 2 3 4   Have patient sit in chair with hands on knees, legs slightly apart, and feet flat on floor. (Look at entire body for movement while in this position.)

0 1 2 3 4   Ask patient to sit with hands hanging unsupported. If male, between legs, if female and wearing a dress, hanging over knees. (Observe hands and other body areas.)

0 1 2 3 4   Ask patient to open mouth. (Observe tongue at rest within mouth.) Do this twice.

0 1 2 3 4   Ask patient to protrude tongue. (Observe abnormalities of tongue movement.) Do this twice.

0 1 2 3 4   Ask the patient to tap thumb, with each finger, as rapidly as possible for 10–15 seconds: separately with right hand, then with left hand. (Observe facial and leg movements.)

0 1 2 3 4   Flex and extend patient's left and right arms. (One at a time.)

0 1 2 3 4   Ask patient to stand up. (Observe in profile. Observe all body areas again, hips included.)

0 1 2 3 4   [a]Ask patient to extend both arms outstretched in front with palms down. (Observe trunk, legs, and mouth.)

0 1 2 3 4   [a]Have patient walk a few paces, turn, and walk back to chair. (Observe hands and gait.) Do this twice.

[a]Activated movements.

    D. Differential diagnosis. Includes seizures and TD.

    E. Course and prognosis. Dystonia can fluctuate spontaneously and respond to reassurance, so that the clinician acquires the false impression that the movement is hysterical or completely under conscious control.

    F. Treatment. Prophylaxis with anticholinergics or related drugs (Table 32-3) usually prevents dystonia, although the risks of prophylactic treatment weigh against that benefit. Treatment with intramuscular anticholinergics or intravenous or intramuscular diphenhydramine (50 mg) almost always relieves the symptoms. Diazepam (Valium) (10 mg intravenously), amobarbital (Amytal), caffeine sodium benzoate, and hypnosis have also been reported to be effective. Although tolerance for the adverse effect usually develops, it is sometimes prudent to change the antipsychotic if the patient is particularly concerned that the reaction may recur.

IV. Neuroleptic-Induced Acute Akathisia

    A. Diagnosis, signs, and symptoms. Akathisia is subjective feelings of restlessness, objective signs of restlessness, or both. Examples include a sense of anxiety, inability to relax, jitteriness, pacing, rocking motions while sitting, and rapid alternation of sitting and standing. Akathisia has been associated with the use of a wide range of psychiatric drugs, including antipsychotics, antidepressants, and sympathomimetics. Once akathisia is recognized and diagnosed, the antipsychotic dose should be reduced to the minimal effective level. Akathisia may be associated with a poor treatment outcome.

B. Epidemiology. Middle-aged women are at increased risk of akathisia, and the time course is similar to that for neuroleptic-induced parkinsonism.

C. Treatment. Three basic steps in the treatment of akathisia are (1) reducing medication dosage, (2) attempting treatment with appropriate drugs, and (3) considering changing the neuroleptic. The most efficacious drugs are β-adrenergic receptor antagonists, although anticholinergic drugs, benzodiazepines, and cyproheptadine (Periactin) may benefit some patients. In some cases of akathisia, no treatment seems to be effective.

V. Neuroleptic-Induced Tardive Dyskinesia

A. Diagnosis, signs, and symptoms. TD is a delayed effect of antipsychotics; it rarely occurs until after 6 months of treatment. The disorder consists of abnormal, involuntary, irregular choreoathetoid movements of the muscles of the head, limbs, and trunk. The severity of the movements ranges from minimal—often missed by patients and their families—to grossly incapacitating. Perioral movements are the most common and include darting, twisting, and protruding movements of the tongue, chewing and lateral jaw movements, lip puckering, and facial grimacing. Finger movements and hand clenching are also common. Torticollis, retrocollis, trunk twisting, and pelvic thrusting occur in severe cases. In the most serious cases, patients may have breathing and swallowing irregularities that result in aerophagia, belching, and grunting. Respiratory dyskinesia has also been reported. Dyskinesia is exacerbated by stress and disappears during sleep. Twitching of the nose has been called *rabbit syndrome.*

B. Epidemiology. TD develops in about 10% to 20% of patients who are treated for more than a year. About 20% to 40% of patients undergoing long-term hospitalization have TD. Women are more likely to be affected than men. Children, patients who are more than 50 years of age, and patients with brain damage or mood disorders are also at high risk.

C. Course and prognosis. Between 5% and 40% of all cases of TD eventually remit, and between 50% and 90% of all mild cases remit. However, TD is less likely to remit in elderly patients than in young patients.

D. Treatment. The three basic approaches to TD are prevention, diagnosis, and management. Prevention is best achieved by using antipsychotic medications only when clearly indicated and in the lowest effective doses. The atypical antipsychotics are associated with less TD than the typical antipsychotics. Clozapine is the only antipsychotic to have minimal risk of TD, and can even help improve preexisting symptoms of TD. This has been attributed to its low affinity for D_2 receptors and high affinity for 5-HT receptor antagonism. Patients who are receiving antipsychotics should be examined regularly for the appearance of abnormal movements, preferably with the use of a standardized rating scale (Table 32-3). Patients frequently experience an exacerbation of their symptoms when the dopamine receptor antagonist is withheld, whereas substitution of an SDA may limit the abnormal movements without worsening the progression of the dyskinesia.

Once TD is recognized, the clinician should consider reducing the dose of the antipsychotic or even stopping the medication altogether. Alternatively, the clinician may switch the patient to clozapine or to one of the new dopamine receptor antagonists. In patients who cannot continue taking any antipsychotic medication, lithium, carbamazepine (Tegretol), or benzodiazepines may effectively reduce the symptoms of both the movement disorder and the psychosis.

1. **Valbenazine.** This is the first drug approved by the FDA for the treatment of adults with TD. TD is caused by prolonged blockage of dopamine receptors leading to hypersensitive dopamine receptors in the motor regions of the brain. Valbenazine is a selective vesicular monoamine transporter 2 (VMAT2) inhibitor and reduces the amount of dopamine available to hypersensitive dopamine receptors.

   It may cause somnolence, falls, headache, akathisia, vomiting, nausea, and has anticholinergic effects. The usual staring dose is 40 mg once daily and the dose can be increased to 80 mg after a week. Dose adjustment is necessary in CYP2D6 poor metabolizers and in the presence of CYP3A4 inhibitors. It can prolong the QT interval requiring appropriate screening and monitoring. Dose should be decreased in those with hepatic impairment.

VI. Neuroleptic Malignant Syndrome

A. **Diagnosis, signs, and symptoms.** Neuroleptic malignant syndrome is a life-threatening complication that can occur anytime during the course of antipsychotic treatment. The motor and behavioral symptoms include muscular rigidity and dystonia, akinesia, mutism, obtundation, and agitation. The autonomic symptoms include high fever, sweating, and increased pulse and blood pressure. Laboratory findings include an increased white blood cell count and increased levels of creatinine phosphokinase, liver enzymes, plasma myoglobin, and myoglobinuria, occasionally associated with renal failure.

B. **Epidemiology.** Men are affected more frequently than women, and young patients are affected more commonly than elderly patients. The mortality rate can reach 10% to 20% or even higher when depot antipsychotic medications are involved. The prevalence of the syndrome is estimated to range up to 2% to 2.4% of patients exposed to dopamine receptor antagonists.

C. **Pathophysiology.** Unknown.

D. **Course and prognosis.** The symptoms usually evolve over 24 to 72 hours, and the untreated syndrome lasts 10 to 14 days. The diagnosis is often

Table 32-4
Treatment of Neuroleptic Malignant Syndrome

Intervention	Dosing	Effectiveness
Amantadine	200–400 mg PO/day in divided doses	Beneficial as monotherapy or in combination; decreases; death rate
Bromocriptine	2.5 mg PO bid or tid may increase to a total of 45 mg/day	Mortality reduced as a single or combined agent
Levodopa/carbidopa	Levodopa 50–100 mg/day IV as continuous infusion	Case reports of dramatic improvement
Electroconvulsive therapy	Reports of good outcome with both unilateral and bilateral treatments response may occur in as few as 3 treatments	Effective when medications have failed; also may treat underlying psychiatric disorder
Dantrolene	1 mg/kg/day for 8 days then continue as PO for 7 additional days	Benefits may occur in minutes or hours as a single agent or in combination
Benzodiazepines	1–2 mg IM as test dose; if effective, switch to PO; consider use if underlying disorder has catatonic symptoms	Has been reported effective when other agents have failed
Supportive measures	IV hydration Cooling blankets Ice packs Ice water enema Oxygenation Antipyretics	Often effective as initial approach early in the episode

Adapted from Davis IM, Caroff SN, Mann SC. Treatment of neuroleptic malignant syndrome. *Psychiatr Ann*, 2000; 30:325–331.

missed in the early stages, and the withdrawal or agitation may mistakenly be considered to reflect an exacerbation of the psychosis.

E. Treatment. See Table 32-4. In addition to supportive medical treatment, the most commonly used medications for the condition are dantrolene (Dantrium) and bromocriptine (Parlodel), although amantadine (Symmetrel) is sometimes used. Bromocriptine and amantadine possess direct dopamine receptor agonist effects and may serve to overcome the antipsychotic-induced dopamine receptor blockade. The lowest effective dosage of antipsychotic drug should be used to reduce the chance of neuroleptic malignant syndrome. Antipsychotic drugs with anticholinergic effects seem less likely to cause neuroleptic malignant syndrome.

VII. Medication-Induced Postural Tremor

A. Diagnosis, signs, and symptoms. Tremor is a rhythmic alteration in movement that is usually faster than one beat per second.

B. Epidemiology. Typically, tremors decrease during periods of relaxation and sleep and increase with stress or anxiety.

C. Etiology. Whereas all of the above diagnoses specifically include an association with a neuroleptic, a range of psychiatric medications can produce tremor—most notably lithium, antidepressants, and valproate (Depakene).

Table 32-5
Drug-Induced Central Hyperthermic Syndromes[a]

Condition (and Mechanism)	Common Drug Causes	Frequent Symptoms	Possible Treatment[b]	Clinical Course
Hyperthermia (↓ heat dissipation) (↑ heat production)	Atropine, lidocaine, meperidine NSAID toxicity, pheochromocytoma, thyrotoxicosis	Hyperthermia, diaphoresis, malaise	Acetaminophen per rectum (325 mg every 4 hours), diazepam oral or per rectum (5 mg every 8 hours) for febrile seizures	Benign, febrile seizures in children
Malignant hyperthermia (↑ heat production)	NMJ blockers (succinylcholine), halothane	Hyperthermia, **muscle rigidity, arrhythmias,** ischemia,[c] hypotension, **rhabdomyolysis,** disseminated intravascular coagulation	Dantrolene sodium (1–2 mg/ kg/min IV infusion)[d]	Familial, 10% mortality if untreated
Tricyclic overdose (↑ heat production)	Tricyclic antidepressants, cocaine	Hyperthermia, confusion, visual hallucinations, agitation, **hyperreflexia, muscle relaxation, anticholinergic effects** (dry skin, pupil dilation), arrhythmias	Sodium bicarbonate (1 mEq/kg IV bolus) if arrhythmias are present, physostigmine (1–3 mg IV) with cardiac monitoring	Fatalities have occurred if untreated
Autonomic hyperreflexia (↑ heat production)	CNS stimulants (amphetamines)	Hyperthermia excitement, **hyperreflexia**	Trimethaphan (0.3–7 mg/min IV infusion)	Reversible
Lethal catatonia (↓ heat dissipation)	Lead poisoning	Hyperthermia, intense anxiety, **destructive behavior, psychosis**	Lorazepam (1–2 mg IV every 4 hours), antipsychotics may be contraindicated	High mortality if untreated
Neuroleptic malignant syndrome (mixed: hypothalamic, ↓ heat dissipation, ↑ heat production)	Antipsychotics (neuroleptics), methyldopa, reserpine	Hyperthermia, **muscle rigidity,** diaphoresis (60%), **leukocytosis, delirium, rhabdomyolysis, elevated CPK,** autonomic deregulation, **extrapyramidal symptoms**	**Bromocriptine (2–10 mg every 8 hours orally or nasogastric tube),** lisuride (0.02–0.1 mg/hr IV infusion), carbidopa-levodopa (Sinemet) (25/100) PO every 8 hours), dantrolene sodium (0.3–1 mg/kg IV every 6 hours)	Rapid onset, 20% mortality if untreated

NSAID, nonsteroidal anti-inflammatory drugs; NMJ, neuromuscular junction; CNS, central nervous system; CPK, creatine phosphokinase; IV, intravenously.

[a]Boldface indicates features that may be used to distinguish one syndrome from another.

[b]Gastric lavage and supportive measures, including cooling, are required in most cases.

[c]Oxygen consumption increases by 7% for every 1°F up in body temperature.

[d]Has been associated with idiosyncratic hepatocellular injury, as well as severe hypotension in one case.

From Theoharides TC, Harris RS, Weckstein D. Neuroleptic malignant-like syndrome due to cyclobenzaprine? (letter). *J Clin Psychopharmacol.* 1995;15:80, with permission.

D. Treatment. The treatment involves four principles.

1. The lowest possible dose of the psychiatric drug should be taken.
2. Patients should minimize caffeine consumption.
3. The psychiatric drug should be taken at bedtime to minimize the amount of daytime tremor.
4. β-adrenergic receptor antagonists (e.g., propranolol [Inderal]) can be given to treat drug-induced tremors.

VIII. Other Disorders

A. Periodic Limb Movement Disorder (PLMD). This condition previously known as nocturnal myoclonus consists of highly stereotyped abrupt contractions of certain leg muscles during sleep. The condition may be present in about 40% of persons over age 65. It may accompany the use of SSRIs.

The repetitive leg movements occur every 20 to 60 seconds, with extension of the large toe and flexion of the ankle, the knee, and the hips. Frequent awakenings, unrefreshing sleep, and daytime sleepiness are major symptoms. No treatment for nocturnal myoclonus is universally effective. Treatments that may be useful include benzodiazepines, levodopa (Larodopa), quinine, and, in rare cases, opioids.

B. Restless legs syndrome. In restless legs syndrome, persons feel deep sensations of creeping inside the calves whenever sitting or lying down. The dysesthesias are rarely painful but are agonizingly relentless and cause an almost irresistible urge to move the legs; thus, this syndrome interferes with sleep and with falling asleep. It peaks in middle age and occurs in 5% of the population. It may occur with the use of SSRIs.

The syndrome has no established treatment. Symptoms of restless legs syndrome are relieved by movement and by leg massage. When pharmacotherapy is required, the benzodiazepines, levodopa, quinine, opioids, propranolol (Inderal), valproate (Depakene), and carbamazepine (Tegretol) are of some benefit.

IX. Hyperthermic Syndromes

All the medication-induced movement disorders may be associated with hyperthermia. Table 32-5 lists the various conditions associated with hyperthermia. ECT has been reported to be of use when other agents have failed.

For more detailed discussion of this topic, see Chapter 34, Biological Therapies, Section 34.3, Medication-Induced Movement Disorders, p. 2936, in CTP/X.

Glossary of Signs and Symptoms

Signs are objective. Symptoms are subjective. Signs are the clinician's observations, such as noting an agitation; symptoms are the patient's experiences, such as a complaint of feeling depressed. In psychiatry, signs and symptoms are not as clearly demarcated as in other fields of medicine; they often overlap. Because of this, disorders in psychiatry are often described as syndromes—a constellation of signs and symptoms that together make up a recognizable condition.

abreaction A process by which repressed material, particularly a painful experience or a conflict, is brought back to consciousness; in this process, the person not only recalls, but also relives the repressed material, which is accompanied by the appropriate affective response.

abstract thinking Thinking characterized by the ability to grasp the essentials of a whole, to break a whole into its parts, and to discern common properties. To think symbolically.

abulia Reduced impulse to act and to think, associated with indifference about consequences of action. Occurs as a result of neurologic deficit, depression, and schizophrenia.

acalculia Loss of ability to do calculations; not caused by anxiety or impairment in concentration. Occurs with neurologic deficit and learning disorder.

acataphasia Disordered speech in which statements are incorrectly formulated. Patients may express themselves with words that sound like the ones intended but are not appropriate to the thoughts, or they may use totally inappropriate expressions.

acathexis Lack of feeling associated with an ordinarily emotionally charged subject; in psychoanalysis, it denotes the patient's detaching or transferring of emotion from thoughts and ideas. Also called *decathexis.* Occurs in anxiety, dissociative, schizophrenic, and bipolar disorders.

acenesthesia Loss of sensation of physical existence.

acrophobia Dread of high places.

acting out Behavioral response to an unconscious drive or impulse that brings about temporary partial relief of inner tension; relief is attained by reacting to a present situation as if it were the situation that originally gave rise to the drive or impulse. Common in borderline states.

aculalia Nonsense speech associated with marked impairment of comprehension. Occurs in mania, schizophrenia, and neurologic deficit.

adiadochokinesia Inability to perform rapid alternating movements. Occurs with neurologic deficit and cerebellar lesions.

adynamia Weakness and fatigability, characteristic of neurasthenia and depression.

aerophagia Excessive swallowing of air. Seen in anxiety disorder.

affect The subjective and immediate experience of emotion attached to ideas or mental representations of objects. Affect has outward manifestations that may be classified as restricted, blunted, flattened, broad, labile, appropriate, or inappropriate. *See also* **mood.**

ageusia Lack or impairment of the sense of taste. Seen in depression and neurologic deficit.

aggression Forceful, goal-directed action that may be verbal or physical; the motor counterpart of the affect of rage, anger, or hostility. Seen in neurologic deficit, temporal lobe disorder, impulse-control disorders, mania, and schizophrenia.

agitation Severe anxiety associated with motor restlessness.

agnosia Inability to understand the import or significance of sensory stimuli; cannot be explained by a defect in sensory pathways or cerebral lesion; the term has also been used to refer to the selective loss or disuse of knowledge of specific objects because of emotional circumstances, as seen in certain schizophrenic, anxious, and depressed patients. Occurs with neurologic deficit. For types of agnosia, see the specific term.

agoraphobia Morbid fear of open places or leaving the familiar setting of the home. May be present with or without panic attacks.

agraphia Loss or impairment of a previously possessed ability to write.

ailurophobia Dread of cats.

akathisia Subjective feeling of motor restlessness manifested by a compelling need to be in constant movement; may be seen as an extrapyramidal adverse effect of antipsychotic medication. May be mistaken for psychotic agitation.

akinesia Lack of physical movement, as in the extreme immobility of catatonic schizophrenia; may also occur as an extrapyramidal effect of antipsychotic medication.

akinetic mutism Absence of voluntary motor movement or speech in a patient who is apparently alert (as evidenced by eye movements). Seen in psychotic depression and catatonic states.

alexia Loss of the ability to understand written language; not explained by defective visual acuity. *Compare with* **dyslexia.**

alexithymia Inability or difficulty in describing or being aware of one's emotions or moods; elaboration of fantasies associated with depression, substance abuse, and posttraumatic stress disorder (PTSD).

algophobia Dread of pain.

alogia Inability to speak because of a mental deficiency or an episode of dementia.

ambivalence Coexistence of two opposing impulses toward the same thing in the same person at the same time. Seen in schizophrenia, borderline states, and obsessive–compulsive disorders (OCDs).

amimia Lack of the ability to make gestures or to comprehend those made by others.

amnesia Partial or total inability to recall past experiences; may be organic (*amnestic disorder*) or emotional (*dissociative amnesia*) in origin.

amnestic aphasia Disturbed capacity to name objects, even though they are known to the patient. Also called *anomic aphasia.*

anaclitic Depending on others, especially as the infant depends on the mother; anaclitic depression in children results from an absence of mothering.

analgesia State in which one feels little or no pain. Can occur under hypnosis and in dissociative disorder.

anancasm Repetitious or stereotyped behavior or thought usually used as a tension-relieving device; used as a synonym for obsession and seen in obsessive–compulsive (anankastic) personality.

androgyny Combination of culturally determined female and male characteristics in one person.

anergia Lack of energy.

anhedonia Loss of interest in, and withdrawal from, all regular and pleasurable activities. Often associated with depression.

anomia Inability to recall the names of objects.

anorexia Loss of or decrease in appetite. In *anorexia nervosa,* appetite may be preserved, but the patient refuses to eat.

anosognosia Inability to recognize a physical deficit in oneself (e.g., patient denies paralyzed limb).

anterograde amnesia Loss of memory for events subsequent to the onset of the amnesia; common after trauma. *Compare with* **retrograde amnesia.**

anxiety Feeling of apprehension caused by anticipation of danger, which may be internal or external.

apathy Dulled emotional tone associated with detachment or indifference; observed in certain types of schizophrenia and depression.

aphasia Any disturbance in the comprehension or expression of language caused by a brain lesion. For types of aphasia, see the specific term.

aphonia Loss of voice. Seen in conversion disorder.

apperception Awareness of the meaning and significance of a particular sensory stimulus as modified by one's own experiences, knowledge, thoughts, and emotions. *See also* **perception.**

appropriate affect Emotional tone in harmony with the accompanying idea, thought, or speech.

apraxia Inability to perform a voluntary purposeful motor activity; cannot be explained by paralysis or other motor or sensory impairment. In *constructional apraxia,* a patient cannot draw two- or three-dimensional forms.

astasia abasia Inability to stand or to walk in a normal manner, even though normal leg movements can be performed in a sitting or lying down position. Seen in conversion disorder.

astereognosis Inability to identify familiar objects by touch. Seen with neurologic deficit. *See also* **neurologic amnesia.**

asyndesis Disorder of language in which the patient combines unconnected ideas and images. Commonly seen in schizophrenia.

ataxia Lack of coordination, physical or mental. (1) In neurology, refers to loss of muscular coordination. (2) In psychiatry, the term *intrapsychic ataxia* refers to lack of coordination between feelings and thoughts; seen in schizophrenia and in severe OCD.

atonia Lack of muscle tone. *See* **waxy flexibility.**

attention Concentration; the aspect of consciousness that relates to the amount of effort exerted in focusing on certain aspects of an experience, activity, or task. Usually impaired in anxiety and depressive disorders.

auditory hallucination False perception of sound, usually voices, but also other noises, such as music. Most common hallucination in psychiatric disorders.

aura (1) Warning sensations, such as automatisms, fullness in the stomach, blushing, and changes in respiration, cognitive sensations, and mood states usually experienced before a seizure. (2) A sensory prodrome that precedes a classic migraine headache.

autistic thinking Thinking in which the thoughts are largely narcissistic and egocentric, with emphasis on subjectivity rather than objectivity, and without regard for reality; used interchangeably with autism and dereism. Seen in schizophrenia and autistic disorder.

behavior Sum total of the psyche that includes impulses, motivations, wishes, drives, instincts, and cravings, as expressed by a person's behavior or motor activity. Also called *conation.*

bereavement Feeling of grief or desolation, especially at the death or loss of a loved one.

bizarre delusion False belief that is patently absurd or fantastic (e.g., invaders from space have implanted electrodes in a person's brain). Common in schizophrenia. In nonbizarre delusion, content is usually within the range of possibility.

blackout Amnesia experienced by alcoholics about behavior during drinking bouts; usually indicates reversible brain damage.

blocking Abrupt interruption in train of thinking before a thought or idea is finished; after a brief pause, the person indicates no recall of what was being said or was going to be said (also known as *thought deprivation* or *increased thought latency*). Common in schizophrenia and severe anxiety.

blunted affect Disturbance of affect manifested by a severe reduction in the intensity of externalized feeling tone; one of the fundamental symptoms of schizophrenia, as outlined by Eugen Bleuler.

bradykinesia Slowness of motor activity, with a decrease in normal spontaneous movement.

bradylalia Abnormally slow speech. Common in depression.

bradylexia Inability to read at normal speed.

bruxism Grinding or gnashing of the teeth, typically occurring during sleep. Seen in anxiety disorder.

carebaria Sensation of discomfort or pressure in the head.

catalepsy Condition in which persons maintain the body position into which they are placed; observed in severe cases of catatonic schizophrenia. Also called *waxy flexibility* and *cerea flexibilitas. See also* **command automatism.**

cataplexy Temporary sudden loss of muscle tone, causing weakness and immobilization; can be precipitated by a variety of emotional states and is often followed by sleep. Commonly seen in narcolepsy.

catatonic excitement Excited, uncontrolled motor activity seen in catatonic schizophrenia. Patients in catatonic state may suddenly erupt into an excited state and may be violent.

catatonic posturing Voluntary assumption of an inappropriate or bizarre posture, generally maintained for long periods of time. May switch unexpectedly with catatonic excitement.

catatonic rigidity Fixed and sustained motoric position that is resistant to change.

catatonic stupor Stupor in which patients ordinarily are well aware of their surroundings.

cathexis In psychoanalysis, a conscious or unconscious investment of psychic energy in an idea, concept, object, or person. *Compare with* **acathexis.**

causalgia Burning pain that may be organic or psychic in origin.

cenesthesia Change in the normal quality of feeling tone in a part of the body.

cephalgia Headache.

cerea flexibilitas Condition of a person who can be molded into a position that is then maintained; when an examiner moves the person's limb, the limb feels as if it were made of wax. Also called *catalepsy* or *waxy flexibility.* Seen in schizophrenia.

chorea Movement disorder characterized by random and involuntary quick, jerky, purposeless movements. Seen in Huntington's disease.

circumstantiality Disturbance in the associative thought and speech processes in which a patient digresses into unnecessary details and inappropriate thoughts before communicating the central idea. Observed in schizophrenia, obsessional disturbances, and certain cases of dementia. *See also* **tangentiality.**

clang association Association or speech directed by the sound of a word rather than by its meaning; words have no logical connection; punning and rhyming may dominate the verbal behavior. Seen most frequently in schizophrenia or mania.

claustrophobia Abnormal fear of closed or confining spaces.

clonic convulsion An involuntary, violent muscular contraction or spasm in which the muscles alternately contract and relax. Characteristic phase in grand mal epileptic seizure.

clouding of consciousness Any disturbance of consciousness in which the person is not fully awake, alert, and oriented. Occurs in delirium, dementia, and cognitive disorder.

cluttering Disturbance of fluency involving an abnormally rapid rate and erratic rhythm of speech that impedes intelligibility; the affected individual is usually unaware of communicative impairment.

cognition Mental process of knowing and becoming aware; function is closely associated with judgment.

coma State of profound unconsciousness from which a person cannot be roused, with minimal or no detectable responsiveness to stimuli; seen in injury or disease of the brain, in systemic conditions such as diabetic ketoacidosis and uremia, and in intoxications with alcohol and other drugs. Coma may also occur in severe catatonic states and in conversion disorder.

coma vigil Coma in which a patient appears to be asleep but can be aroused (also known as *akinetic mutism*).

command automatism Condition associated with catalepsy in which suggestions are followed automatically.

command hallucination False perception of orders that a person may feel obliged to obey or unable to resist.

complex A feeling-toned idea.

complex partial seizure A seizure characterized by alterations in consciousness that may be accompanied by complex hallucinations (sometimes olfactory) or illusions. During the seizure, a state of impaired consciousness resembling a dreamlike state may occur, and the patient may exhibit repetitive, automatic, or semipurposeful behavior.

compulsion Pathologic need to act on an impulse that, if resisted, produces anxiety; repetitive behavior in response to an obsession or performed according to certain rules, with no true end in itself other than to prevent something from occurring in the future.

conation That part of a person's mental life concerned with cravings, strivings, motivations, drives, and wishes, as expressed through behavior or motor activity.

concrete thinking Thinking characterized by actual things, events, and immediate experience, rather than by abstractions; seen in young children, in those who have lost or never developed the ability to generalize (as in certain cognitive mental disorders), and in schizophrenic persons. *Compare with* **abstract thinking.**

condensation Mental process in which one symbol stands for a number of components.

confabulation Unconscious filling of gaps in memory by imagining experiences or events that have no basis in fact, commonly seen in amnestic syndromes; should be differentiated from lying. *See also* **paramnesia.**

confusion Disturbances of consciousness manifested by a disordered orientation in relation to time, place, or person.

consciousness State of awareness, with response to external stimuli.

constipation Inability to defecate or difficulty in defecating.

constricted affect Reduction in intensity of feeling tone that is less severe than that of blunted affect.

constructional apraxia Inability to copy a drawing, such as a cube, clock, or pentagon, as a result of a brain lesion.

conversion phenomena The development of symbolic physical symptoms and distortions involving the voluntary muscles or special sense organs; not under voluntary control and not explained by any physical disorder. Most common in conversion disorder, but also seen in a variety of mental disorders.

convulsion An involuntary, violent muscular contraction or spasm. *See also* **clonic convulsion** *and* **tonic convulsion.**

coprolalia Involuntary use of vulgar or obscene language. Observed in some cases of schizophrenia and in Tourette's syndrome.

coprophagia Eating of filth or feces.

cryptographia A private written language.

cryptolalia A private spoken language.

cycloplegia Paralysis of the muscles of accommodation in the eye; observed, at times, as an autonomic adverse effect (anticholinergic effect) of antipsychotic or antidepressant medication.

decompensation Deterioration of psychic functioning caused by a breakdown of defense mechanisms. Seen in psychotic states.

déjà entendu Illusion that what one is hearing one has heard previously. *See also* **paramnesia.**

déjà pensé Condition in which a thought never entertained before is incorrectly regarded as a repetition of a previous thought. *See also* **paramnesia.**

déjà vu Illusion of visual recognition in which a new situation is incorrectly regarded as a repetition of a previous experience. *See also* **paramnesia.**

delirium Acute reversible mental disorder characterized by confusion and some impairment of consciousness; generally associated with emotional lability, hallucinations or illusions, and inappropriate, impulsive, irrational, or violent behavior.

delirium tremens Acute and sometimes fatal reaction to withdrawal from alcohol, usually occurring 72 to 96 hours after the cessation of heavy drinking; distinctive characteristics are marked autonomic hyperactivity (tachycardia, fever, hyperhidrosis, and dilated pupils), usually accompanied by tremulousness, hallucinations, illusions, and delusions. Called *alcohol withdrawal delirium* in *DSM-IV-TR. See also* **formication.**

delusion False belief, based on incorrect inference about external reality, that is firmly held despite objective and obvious contradictory proof or evidence and despite the fact that other members of the culture do not share the belief.

delusion of control False belief that a person's will, thoughts, or feelings are being controlled by external forces.

delusion of grandeur Exaggerated conception of one's importance, power, or identity.

delusion of infidelity False belief that one's lover is unfaithful. Sometimes called *pathologic jealousy.*

delusion of persecution False belief of being harassed or persecuted; often found in litigious patients who have a pathologic tendency to take legal action because of imagined mistreatment. Most common delusion.

delusion of poverty False belief that one is bereft or will be deprived of all material possessions.

delusion of reference False belief that the behavior of others refers to oneself or that events, objects, or other people have a particular and unusual significance, usually of a negative nature; derived from idea of reference, in which persons falsely feel that others are talking about them (e.g., belief that people on television or radio are talking to or about the person). *See also* **thought broadcasting.**

delusion of self-accusation False feeling of remorse and guilt. Seen in depression with psychotic features.

dementia Mental disorder characterized by general impairment in intellectual functioning without clouding of consciousness; characterized by failing memory, difficulty with calculations, distractibility, alterations in mood and affect, impaired judgment and abstraction, reduced facility with language, and disturbance of orientation. Although irreversible because of underlying progressive degenerative brain disease, dementia may be reversible if the cause can be treated.

denial Defense mechanism in which the existence of unpleasant realities is disavowed; refers to keeping out of conscious awareness of any aspects of external reality that, if acknowledged, would produce anxiety.

depersonalization Sensation of unreality concerning oneself, parts of oneself, or one's environment that occurs under extreme stress or fatigue. Seen in schizophrenia, depersonalization disorder, and schizotypal personality disorder.

depression Mental state characterized by feelings of sadness, loneliness, despair, low self-esteem, and self-reproach; accompanying signs include psychomotor retardation or, at times, agitation, withdrawal from interpersonal contact, and vegetative symptoms, such as insomnia and anorexia. The term refers to a mood that is so characterized or a mood disorder.

derailment Gradual or sudden deviation in train of thought without blocking; sometimes used synonymously with *loosening of association.*

derealization Sensation of changed reality or that one's surroundings have altered. Usually seen in schizophrenia, panic attacks, and dissociative disorders.

dereism Mental activity that follows a totally subjective and idiosyncratic system of logic and fails to take the facts of reality or experience into consideration. Characteristic of schizophrenia. *See also* **autistic thinking.**

detachment Characterized by distant interpersonal relationships and lack of emotional involvement.

devaluation Defense mechanism in which a person attributes excessively negative qualities to self or others. Seen in depression and paranoid personality disorder.

diminished libido Decreased sexual interest and drive.

dipsomania Compulsion to drink alcoholic beverages.

disinhibition (1) Removal of an inhibitory effect, as in the reduction of the inhibitory function of the cerebral cortex by alcohol. (2) In psychiatry, a greater freedom to act in accordance with inner drives or feelings and with less regard for restraints dictated by cultural norms or one's superego.

disorientation Confusion; impairment of awareness of time, place, and person (the position of the self in relation to other persons). Characteristic of cognitive disorders.

displacement Unconscious defense mechanism by which the emotional component of an unacceptable idea or object is transferred to a more acceptable one. Seen in phobias.

dissociation Unconscious defense mechanism involving the segregation of any group of mental or behavioral processes from the rest of the person's psychic activity; may entail the separation of an idea from its accompanying emotional tone, as seen in dissociative and conversion disorders. Seen in dissociative disorders.

distractibility Inability to focus one's attention; the patient does not respond to the task at hand but attends to irrelevant phenomena in the environment.

dread Massive or pervasive anxiety, usually related to a specific danger.

dreamy state Altered state of consciousness, likened to a dream situation, that develops suddenly and usually lasts a few minutes; accompanied by visual, auditory, and olfactory hallucinations. Commonly associated with temporal lobe lesions.

drowsiness State of impaired awareness associated with a desire or inclination to sleep.

dysarthria Difficulty in articulation, the motor activity of shaping phonated sounds into speech, not in word finding or in grammar.

dyscalculia Difficulty in performing calculations.

dysgeusia Impaired sense of taste.

dysgraphia Difficulty in writing.

dyskinesia Difficulty in performing movements. Seen in extrapyramidal disorders.

dyslalia Faulty articulation caused by structural abnormalities of the articulatory organs or impaired hearing.

dyslexia Specific learning disability syndrome involving an impairment of the previously acquired ability to read; unrelated to the person's intelligence. *Compare with* **alexia.**

dysmetria Impaired ability to gauge distance relative to movements. Seen in neurologic deficit.

dysmnesia Impaired memory.

dyspareunia Physical pain in sexual intercourse, usually emotionally caused and more commonly experienced by women; may also result from cystitis, urethritis, or other medical conditions.

dysphagia Difficulty in swallowing.

dysphasia Difficulty in comprehending oral language (*reception dysphasia*) or in trying to express verbal language (*expressive dysphasia*).

dysphonia Difficulty or pain in speaking.

dysphoria Feeling of unpleasantness or discomfort; a mood of general dissatisfaction and restlessness. Occurs in depression and anxiety.

dysprosody Loss of normal speech melody (*prosody*). Common in depression.

dystonia Extrapyramidal motor disturbance consisting of slow, sustained contractions of the axial or appendicular musculature; one movement often predominates, leading to relatively sustained postural deviations; acute dystonic reactions (facial grimacing and torticollis) are occasionally seen with the initiation of antipsychotic drug therapy.

echolalia Psychopathological repeating of words or phrases of one person by another; tends to be repetitive and persistent. Seen in certain kinds of schizophrenia, particularly the catatonic types.

ego-alien Denoting aspects of a person's personality that are viewed as repugnant, unacceptable, or inconsistent with the rest of the personality. Also called *ego-dystonia. Compare with* **ego-syntonic.**

egocentric Self-centered; selfishly preoccupied with one's own needs; lacking interest in others.

ego-dystonic *See* **ego-alien.**

egomania Morbid self-preoccupation or self-centeredness. *See also* **narcissism.**

ego-syntonic Denoting aspects of a personality that are viewed as acceptable and consistent with that person's total personality. Personality traits are usually ego-syntonic. *Compare with* **ego-alien.**

eidetic image Unusually vivid or exact mental image of objects previously seen or imagined.

elation Mood consisting of feelings of joy, euphoria, triumph, and intense self-satisfaction or optimism. Occurs in mania when not grounded in reality.

elevated mood Air of confidence and enjoyment; a mood more cheerful than normal, but not necessarily pathologic.

emotion Complex feeling state with psychic, somatic, and behavioral components; external manifestation of emotion is *affect.*

emotional insight A level of understanding or awareness that one has emotional problems. It facilitates positive changes in personality and behavior when present.

emotional lability Excessive emotional responsiveness characterized by unstable and rapidly changing emotions.

encopresis Involuntary passage of feces, usually occurring at night or during sleep.

enuresis Incontinence of urine during sleep.

erotomania Delusional belief, more common in women than in men, that someone is deeply in love with them (also known as *de Clérambault syndrome*).

erythrophobia Abnormal fear of blushing.

euphoria Exaggerated feeling of well-being that is inappropriate to real events. Can occur with drugs such as opiates, amphetamines, and alcohol.

euthymia Normal range of mood, implying absence of depressed or elevated mood.

evasion Act of not facing up to, or strategically eluding, something; consists of suppressing an idea that is next in a thought series and replacing it with another idea closely related to it. Also called *paralogia* and *perverted logic.*

exaltation Feeling of intense elation and grandeur.

excited Agitated, purposeless motor activity uninfluenced by external stimuli.

expansive mood Expression of feelings without restraint, frequently with an overestimation of their significance or importance. Seen in mania and grandiose delusional disorder.

expressive aphasia Disturbance of speech in which understanding remains, but ability to speak is grossly impaired; halting, laborious, and inaccurate speech (also known as *Broca's, nonfluent,* and *motor aphasias*).

expressive dysphasia Difficulty in expressing verbal language; the ability to understand language is intact.

externalization More general term than *projection* that refers to the tendency to perceive in the external world and in external objects elements of one's own personality, including instinctual impulses, conflicts, moods, attitudes, and styles of thinking.

extroversion State of one's energies being directed outside oneself. *Compare with* **introversion.**

false memory A person's recollection and belief of an event that did not actually occur. In *false memory syndrome,* persons erroneously believe that they sustained an emotional or physical (e.g., sexual) trauma in early life.

fantasy Daydream; fabricated mental picture of a situation or chain of events. A normal form of thinking dominated by unconscious material that seeks wish fulfillment and solutions to conflicts; may serve as the matrix for creativity. The content of the fantasy may indicate mental illness.

fatigue A feeling of weariness, sleepiness, or irritability after a period of mental or bodily activity. Seen in depression, anxiety, neurasthenia, and somatoform disorders.

fausse reconnaissance False recognition, a feature of paramnesia. Can occur in delusional disorders.

fear Unpleasurable emotional state consisting of psychophysiological changes in response to a realistic threat or danger. *Compare with* **anxiety.**

flat affect Absence or near absence of any signs of affective expression.

flight of ideas Rapid succession of fragmentary thoughts or speech in which content changes abruptly and speech may be incoherent. Seen in mania.

floccillation Aimless plucking or picking, usually at bedclothes or clothing, commonly seen in dementia and delirium.

fluent aphasia Aphasia characterized by inability to understand the spoken word; fluent but incoherent speech is present. Also called *Wernicke's, sensory,* and *receptive aphasias.*

folie à deux Mental illness shared by two persons, usually involving a common delusional system; if it involves three persons, it is referred to as *folie à trois,* and so on. Also called *shared psychotic disorder.*

formal thought disorder Disturbance in the form of thought rather than the content of thought; thinking characterized by loosened associations, neologisms, and illogical constructs; thought process is disordered, and the person is defined as psychotic. Characteristic of schizophrenia.

formication Tactile hallucination involving the sensation that tiny insects are crawling over the skin. Seen in cocaine addiction and delirium tremens.

free-floating anxiety Severe, pervasive, generalized anxiety that is not attached to any particular idea, object, or event. Observed particularly in anxiety disorders, although it may be seen in some cases of schizophrenia.

fugue Dissociative disorder characterized by a period of almost complete amnesia, during which a person actually flees from an immediate life situation and begins a different life pattern; apart from the amnesia, mental faculties and skills are usually unimpaired.

galactorrhea Abnormal discharge of milk from the breast; may result from the endocrine influence (e.g., prolactin) of dopamine receptor antagonists, such as phenothiazines.

generalized tonic–clonic seizure Generalized onset of tonic–clonic movements of the limbs, tongue biting, and incontinence followed by slow, gradual recovery of consciousness and cognition; also called *grand mal seizure.*

global aphasia Combination of grossly nonfluent aphasia and severe fluent aphasia.

glossolalia Unintelligible jargon that has meaning to the speaker but not to the listener. Occurs in schizophrenia.

grandiosity Exaggerated feelings of one's importance, power, knowledge, or identity. Occurs in delusional disorder and manic states.

grief Alteration in mood and affect consisting of sadness appropriate to a real loss; normally, it is self-limited. *See also* **depression** *and* **mourning.**

guilt Emotional state associated with self-reproach and the need for punishment. In psychoanalysis, refers to a feeling of culpability that stems from a conflict between the ego and the superego (conscience). Guilt has normal psychological and social functions, but special intensity or absence of guilt characterizes many mental disorders, such as depression and antisocial personality disorder, respectively. Psychiatrists distinguish shame as a less internalized form of guilt that relates more to others than to the self. *See also* **shame.**

gustatory hallucination Hallucination primarily involving taste.

gynecomastia Female-like development of the male breasts; may occur as an adverse effect of antipsychotic and antidepressant drugs because of increased prolactin levels or anabolic–androgenic steroid abuse.

hallucination False sensory perception occurring in the absence of any relevant external stimulation of the sensory modality involved. For types of hallucinations, see the specific term.

hallucinosis State in which a person experiences hallucinations without any impairment of consciousness.

haptic hallucination Hallucination of touch.

hebephrenia Complex of symptoms, considered a form of schizophrenia, characterized by wild or silly behavior or mannerisms, inappropriate affect, and delusions and hallucinations that are transient and unsystematized. Hebephrenic schizophrenia is now called *disorganized schizophrenia.*

holophrastic Using a single word to express a combination of ideas. Seen in schizophrenia.

hyperactivity Increased muscular activity. The term is commonly used to describe a disturbance found in children that is manifested by constant restlessness, overactivity, distractibility, and difficulties in learning. Seen in *attention-deficit/hyperactivity disorder* (ADHD).

hyperalgesia Excessive sensitivity to pain. Seen in somatoform disorder.

hyperesthesia Increased sensitivity to tactile stimulation.

hypermnesia Exaggerated degree of retention and recall. It can be elicited by hypnosis and may be seen in certain prodigies; also may be a feature of OCD, some cases of schizophrenia, and manic episodes of bipolar I disorder.

hyperphagia Increase in appetite and intake of food.

hyperpragia Excessive thinking and mental activity. Generally associated with manic episodes of bipolar I disorder.

hypersomnia Excessive time spent asleep. May be associated with underlying medical or psychiatric disorder or narcolepsy, may be part of the Kleine–Levin syndrome, or may be primary.

hyperventilation Excessive breathing, generally associated with anxiety, which can reduce blood carbon dioxide concentration and can produce lightheadedness, palpitations, numbness, tingling periorally and in the extremities, and, occasionally, syncope.

hypervigilance Excessive attention to and focus on all internal and external stimuli; usually seen in delusional or paranoid states.

hypesthesia Diminished sensitivity to tactile stimulation.

hypnagogic hallucination Hallucination occurring while falling asleep, not ordinarily considered pathologic.

hypnopompic hallucination Hallucination occurring while awakening from sleep, not ordinarily considered pathologic.

hypnosis Artificially induced alteration of consciousness characterized by increased suggestibility and receptivity to direction.

hypoactivity Decreased motor and cognitive activity, as in psychomotor retardation; visible slowing of thought, speech, and movements. Also called *hypokinesis.*

hypochondria Exaggerated concern about health that is based not on real medical pathology, but on unrealistic interpretations of physical signs or sensations as abnormal.

hypomania Mood abnormality with the qualitative characteristics of mania but somewhat less intense. Seen in cyclothymic disorder.

idea of reference Misinterpretation of incidents and events in the outside world as having direct personal reference to oneself; occasionally observed in normal persons, but frequently seen in paranoid patients. If present with sufficient frequency or intensity or if organized and systematized, they constitute delusions of reference.

illogical thinking Thinking containing erroneous conclusions or internal contradictions; psychopathological only when it is marked and not caused by cultural values or intellectual deficit.

illusion Perceptual misinterpretation of a real external stimulus. *Compare with* **hallucination.**

immediate memory Reproduction, recognition, or recall of perceived material within seconds after presentation. *Compare with* **long-term memory** *and* **short-term memory.**

impaired insight Diminished ability to understand the objective reality of a situation.

impaired judgment Diminished ability to understand a situation correctly and to act appropriately.

impulse control Ability to resist an impulse, drive, or temptation to perform some action.

inappropriate affect Emotional tone out of harmony with the idea, thought, or speech accompanying it. Seen in schizophrenia.

incoherence Communication that is disconnected, disorganized, or incomprehensible. *See also* **word salad.**

incorporation Primitive unconscious defense mechanism in which the psychic representation of another person or aspects of another person are assimilated into oneself through a figurative process of symbolic oral ingestion; represents a special form of introjection and is the earliest mechanism of identification.

increased libido Increase in sexual interest and drive. Often associated with mania.

ineffability Ecstatic state in which persons insist that their experience is inexpressible and indescribable and that it is impossible to convey what it is like to one who never experienced it.

initial insomnia Falling asleep with difficulty; usually seen in anxiety disorder. *Compare with* **middle insomnia** *and* **terminal insomnia.**

insight Conscious recognition of one's own condition. In psychiatry, it refers to the conscious awareness and understanding of one's own psychodynamics and symptoms of maladaptive behavior; highly important in effecting changes in the personality and behavior of a person.

insomnia Difficulty in falling asleep or difficulty in staying asleep. It can be related to a mental disorder, can be related to a physical disorder or an adverse effect of medication, or can be primary (not related to a known medical factor or another mental disorder). *See also* **initial insomnia, middle insomnia,** *and* **terminal insomnia.**

intellectual insight Knowledge of the reality of a situation without the ability to use that knowledge successfully to effect an adaptive change in behavior or to master the situation. *Compare with* **true insight.**

intelligence Capacity for learning and ability to recall, to integrate constructively, and to apply what one has learned; the capacity to understand and to think rationally.

intoxication Mental disorder caused by recent ingestion or presence in the body of an exogenous substance producing maladaptive behavior by virtue of its effects on the central nervous system (CNS). The most common psychiatric changes involve disturbances of perception, wakefulness, attention, thinking, judgment, emotional control, and psychomotor behavior; the specific clinical picture depends on the substance ingested.

intropunitive Turning anger inward toward oneself. Commonly observed in depressed patients.

introspection Contemplating one's own mental processes to achieve insight.

introversion State in which a person's energies are directed inward toward the self, with little or no interest in the external world.

irrelevant answer Answer that is not responsive to the question.

irritability Abnormal or excessive excitability, with easily triggered anger, annoyance, or impatience.

irritable mood State in which one is easily annoyed and provoked to anger. *See also* **irritability.**

jamais vu Paramnestic phenomenon characterized by a false feeling of unfamiliarity with a real situation that one has previously experienced.

jargon aphasia Aphasia in which the words produced are neologistic, that is, nonsense words created by the patient.

judgment Mental act of comparing or evaluating choices within the framework of a given set of values for the purpose of electing a course of action. If the course of action chosen is consonant with reality or with mature adult standards of behavior, judgment is said to be *intact* or *normal;* judgment is said to be *impaired* if the chosen course of action is frankly maladaptive, results from impulsive decisions based on the need for immediate gratification, or is otherwise not consistent with reality as measured by mature adult standards.

kleptomania Pathologic compulsion to steal.

la belle indifférence Inappropriate attitude of calm or lack of concern about one's disability. May be seen in patients with conversion disorder.

labile affect Affective expression characterized by rapid and abrupt changes, unrelated to external stimuli.

labile mood Oscillations in mood between euphoria and depression or anxiety.

laconic speech Condition characterized by a reduction in the quantity of spontaneous speech; replies to questions are brief and unelaborated, and little or no unprompted additional information is provided. Occurs in major depression, schizophrenia, and organic mental disorders. Also called *poverty of speech.*

lethologica Momentary forgetting of a name or proper noun. *See* **blocking.**

lilliputian hallucination Visual sensation that persons or objects are reduced in size; more properly regarded as an illusion. *See also* **micropsia.**

localized amnesia Partial loss of memory; amnesia restricted to specific or isolated experiences. Also called *lacunar amnesia* and *patch amnesia.*

logorrhea Copious, pressured, coherent speech; uncontrollable, excessive talking; observed in manic episodes of bipolar disorder. Also called *tachylogia, verbomania,* and *volubility.*

long-term memory Reproduction, recognition, or recall of experiences or information that was experienced in the distant past. Also called *remote memory. Compare with* **immediate memory** *and* **short-term memory.**

loosening of associations Characteristic schizophrenic thinking or speech disturbance involving a disorder in the logical progression of thoughts, manifested as a failure to communicate verbally adequately; unrelated and unconnected ideas shift from one subject to another. *See also* **tangentiality.**

macropsia False perception that objects are larger than they really are. *Compare with* **micropsia.**

magical thinking A form of dereistic thought; thinking similar to that of the preoperational phase in children (Jean Piaget), in which thoughts, words, or actions assume power (e.g., to cause or to prevent events).

malingering Feigning disease to achieve a specific goal, for example, to avoid an unpleasant responsibility.

mania Mood state characterized by elation, agitation, hyperactivity, hypersexuality, and accelerated thinking and speaking (flight of ideas). Seen in bipolar I disorder. *See also* **hypomania.**

manipulation Maneuvering by patients to get their own way, characteristic of antisocial personalities.

mannerism Ingrained, habitual involuntary movement.

melancholia Severe depressive state. Used in the term *involutional melancholia* as a descriptive term and also in reference to a distinct diagnostic entity.

memory Process whereby what is experienced or learned is established as a record in the CNS (registration), where it persists with a variable degree of permanence (retention) and can be recollected or retrieved from storage at will (recall). For types of memory, *see* **immediate memory, long-term memory,** *and* **short-term memory.**

mental disorder Psychiatric illness or disease whose manifestations are primarily characterized by behavioral or psychological impairment of function, measured in terms of deviation from some normative concept; associated with distress or disease, not just an expected response to a particular event or limited to relations between a person and society.

mental retardation Subaverage general intellectual functioning that originates in the developmental period and is associated with impaired maturation and learning, and social maladjustment. Retardation is commonly defined in terms of IQ: mild (between 50 and 55 to 70), moderate (between 35 and 40 to between 50 and 55), severe (between 20 and 25 to between 35 and 40), and profound (below 20 to 25).

metonymy Speech disturbance common in schizophrenia in which the affected person uses a word or phrase that is related to the proper one but is not the one ordinarily used; for example, the patient speaks of consuming a *menu* rather than a *meal,* or refers to losing the *piece of string* of the conversation, rather than the *thread* of the conversation. *See also* **paraphasia** *and* **word approximation.**

microcephaly Condition in which the head is unusually small as a result of defective brain development and premature ossification of the skull.

micropsia False perception that objects are smaller than they really are. Sometimes called *lilliputian hallucination. Compare with* **macropsia.**

middle insomnia Waking up after falling asleep without difficulty and then having difficulty in falling asleep again. *Compare with* **initial insomnia** *and* **terminal insomnia.**

mimicry Simple, imitative motion activity of childhood.

monomania Mental state characterized by preoccupation with one subject.

mood Pervasive and sustained feeling tone that is experienced internally and that, in the extreme, can markedly influence virtually all aspects of a person's behavior and perception of the world. Distinguished from affect, the external expression of the internal feeling tone. For types of mood, see the specific term.

mood-congruent delusion Delusion with content that is mood appropriate (e.g., depressed patients who believe that they are responsible for the destruction of the world).

mood-congruent hallucination Hallucination with content that is consistent with a depressed or manic mood (e.g., depressed patients hearing voices telling them that they are bad persons and manic patients hearing voices telling them that they have inflated worth, power, or knowledge).

mood-incongruent delusion Delusion based on incorrect reference about external reality, with content that has no association to mood or is mood inappropriate (e.g., depressed patients who believe that they are the new Messiah).

mood-incongruent hallucination Hallucination not associated with real external stimuli, with content that is not consistent with depressed or manic mood (e.g., in depression, hallucinations not involving such themes as guilt, deserved punishment, or inadequacy; in mania, not involving such themes as inflated worth or power).

mood swings Oscillation of a person's emotional feeling tone between periods of elation and periods of depression.

motor aphasia Aphasia in which understanding is intact, but the ability to speak is lost. Also called *Broca's, expressive,* or *nonfluent aphasias.*

mourning Syndrome following loss of a loved one, consisting of preoccupation with the lost individual, weeping, sadness, and repeated reliving of memories. *See also* **bereavement** *and* **grief.**

muscle rigidity State in which the muscles remain immovable; seen in schizophrenia.

mutism Organic or functional absence of the faculty of speech. *See also* **stupor.**

mydriasis Dilation of the pupil; sometimes occurs as an autonomic (anticholinergic) or atropine-like adverse effect of some antipsychotic and antidepressant drugs.

narcissism In psychoanalytic theory, divided into primary and secondary types: primary narcissism, the early infantile phase of object relationship development, when the child has not differentiated the self from the outside world, and all sources of pleasure are unrealistically recognized as coming from within the self, giving the child a false sense of omnipotence; secondary narcissism, when the libido, once attached to external love objects, is redirected back to the self. *See also* **autistic thinking.**

needle phobia The persistent, intense, pathologic fear of receiving an injection.

negative signs In schizophrenia: flat affect, alogia, abulia, and apathy.

negativism Verbal or nonverbal opposition or resistance to outside suggestions and advice; commonly seen in catatonic schizophrenia in which the patient resists any effort to be moved or does the opposite of what is asked.

neologism New word or phrase whose derivation cannot be understood; often seen in schizophrenia. It has also been used to mean a word that has been incorrectly constructed but whose origins are nonetheless understandable (e.g., *headshoe* to mean *hat*), but such constructions are more properly referred to as *word approximations.*

neurologic amnesia (1) Auditory amnesia: loss of ability to comprehend sounds or speech. (2) Tactile amnesia: loss of ability to judge the shape of objects by touch. *See also* **astereognosis.** (3) Verbal amnesia: loss of ability to remember words. (4) Visual amnesia: loss of ability to recall or to recognize familiar objects or printed words.

nihilism Delusion of the nonexistence of the self or part of the self; also refers to an attitude of total rejection of established values or extreme skepticism regarding moral and value judgments.

nihilistic delusion Depressive delusion that the world and everything related to it have ceased to exist.

noesis Revelation in which immense illumination occurs in association with a sense that one has been chosen to lead and command. Can occur in manic or dissociative states.

nominal aphasia Aphasia characterized by difficulty in giving the correct name of an object. *See also* **anomia** *and* **amnestic aphasia.**

nymphomania Abnormal, excessive, insatiable desire in a woman for sexual intercourse. *Compare with* **satyriasis.**

obsession Persistent and recurrent idea, thought, or impulse that cannot be eliminated from consciousness by logic or reasoning; obsessions are involuntary and ego-dystonic. *See also* **compulsion.**

olfactory hallucination Hallucination primarily involving smell or odors; most common in medical disorders, especially in the temporal lobe.

orientation State of awareness of oneself and one's surroundings in terms of time, place, and person.

overactivity Abnormality in motor behavior that can manifest itself as psychomotor agitation, hyperactivity (hyperkinesis), tics, sleepwalking, or compulsions.

overvalued idea False or unreasonable belief or idea that is sustained beyond the bounds of reason. It is held with less intensity or duration than a delusion but is usually associated with mental illness.

panic Acute, intense attack of anxiety associated with personality disorganization; the anxiety is overwhelming and accompanied by feelings of impending doom.

panphobia Overwhelming fear of everything.

pantomime Gesticulation; psychodrama without the use of words.

paramnesia Disturbance of memory in which reality and fantasy are confused. It is observed in dreams and in certain types of schizophrenia and organic mental disorders; it includes phenomena such as *déjà vu* and *déjà entendu,* which may occur occasionally in normal persons.

paranoia Rare psychiatric syndrome marked by the gradual development of a highly elaborate and complex delusional system, generally involving persecutory or grandiose delusions, with few other signs of personality disorganization or thought disorder.

paranoid delusions Includes persecutory delusions and delusions of reference, control, and grandeur.

paranoid ideation Thinking dominated by suspicious, persecutory, or grandiose content of less than delusional proportions.

paraphasia Abnormal speech in which one word is substituted for another, the irrelevant word generally resembling the required one in morphology, meaning, or phonetic composition; the inappropriate word may be a legitimate one used incorrectly, such as *clover* instead of *hand,* or a bizarre nonsense expression, such as *treen* instead of *train.* Paraphasic speech may be seen in organic aphasias and in mental disorders such as schizophrenia. *See also* **metonymy** *and* **word approximation.**

parapraxis Faulty act, such as a slip of the tongue or the misplacement of an article. Freud ascribed parapraxes to unconscious motives.

paresis Weakness or partial paralysis of organic origin.

paresthesia Abnormal spontaneous tactile sensation, such as a burning, tingling, or pins-and-needles sensation.

perception Conscious awareness of elements in the environment by the mental processing of sensory stimuli; sometimes used in a broader sense to refer to the mental process by which all kinds of data, intellectual, emotional, and sensory, are meaningfully organized. *See also* **apperception.**

perseveration (1) Pathologic repetition of the same response to different stimuli, as in a repetition of the same verbal response to different questions. (2) Persistent repetition of specific words or concepts in the process of speaking. Seen in cognitive disorders, schizophrenia, and other mental illness. *See also* **verbigeration.**

phantom limb False sensation that an extremity that has been lost is, in fact, present.

phobia Persistent, pathologic, unrealistic, intense fear of an object or situation; the phobic person may realize that the fear is irrational but, nonetheless, cannot dispel it. For types of phobias, see the specific term.

pica Craving and eating of nonfood substances, such as paint and clay.

polyphagia Pathologic overeating.

positive signs In schizophrenia: hallucinations, delusions, and thought disorder.

posturing Strange, fixed, and bizarre bodily positions held by a patient for an extended time. *See also* **catatonia.**

poverty of content of speech Speech that is adequate in amount but conveys little information because of vagueness, emptiness, or stereotyped phrases.

poverty of speech Restriction in the amount of speech used; replies may be monosyllabic. *See also* **laconic speech.**

preoccupation of thought Centering of thought content on a particular idea, associated with a strong affective tone, such as a paranoid trend or a suicidal or homicidal preoccupation.

pressured speech Increase in the amount of spontaneous speech; rapid, loud, accelerated speech, as occurs in mania, schizophrenia, and cognitive disorders.

primary process thinking In psychoanalysis, the mental activity directly related to the functions of the id and characteristic of unconscious mental processes; marked by primitive, prelogical thinking and by the tendency to seek immediate discharge and gratification of instinctual demands. Includes thinking that is dereistic, illogical, and magical; normally found in dreams, abnormally in psychosis. *Compare with* **secondary process thinking.**

projection Unconscious defense mechanism in which persons attribute to another those generally unconscious ideas, thoughts, feelings, and impulses that are in themselves undesirable or unacceptable as a form of protection from anxiety arising from an inner conflict; by externalizing whatever is unacceptable, they deal with it as a situation apart from themselves.

prosopagnosia Inability to recognize familiar faces that is not due to impaired visual acuity or level of consciousness.

pseudocyesis Rare condition in which a nonpregnant patient has the signs and symptoms of pregnancy, such as abdominal distention, breast enlargement, pigmentation, cessation of menses, and morning sickness.

pseudodementia (1) Dementialike disorder that can be reversed by appropriate treatment and is not caused by organic brain disease. (2) Condition in which patients show exaggerated indifference to their surroundings in the absence of a mental disorder, also occurs in depression and factitious disorders.

pseudologia phantastica Disorder characterized by uncontrollable lying, in which patients elaborate extensive fantasies that they freely communicate and act on.

psychomotor agitation Physical and mental overactivity that is usually nonproductive and is associated with a feeling of inner turmoil, as seen in agitated depression.

psychosis Mental disorder in which the thoughts, affective response, ability to recognize reality, and ability to communicate and relate to others are sufficiently impaired to interfere grossly with the capacity to deal with reality; the classical characteristics of psychosis are impaired reality testing, hallucinations, delusions, and illusions.

psychotic (1) Person experiencing psychosis. (2) Denoting or characteristic of psychosis.

rationalization An unconscious defense mechanism in which irrational or unacceptable behavior, motives, or feelings are logically justified or made consciously tolerable by plausible means.

reaction formation Unconscious defense mechanism in which a person develops a socialized attitude or interest that is the direct antithesis of some infantile wish or impulse that is harbored consciously or unconsciously. One of the earliest and most unstable defense mechanisms, closely related to repression; both are defenses against impulses or urges that are unacceptable to the ego.

reality testing Fundamental ego function that consists of tentative actions that test and objectively evaluate the nature and limits of the environment; includes the ability to differentiate between the external world and the internal world and to accurately judge the relation between the self and the environment.

recall Process of bringing stored memories into consciousness. *See also* **memory.**

recent memory Recall of events over the past few days.

recent past memory Recall of events over the past few months.

receptive aphasia Organic loss of ability to comprehend the meaning of words; fluid and spontaneous, but incoherent and nonsensical, speech. *See also* **fluent aphasia** *and* **sensory aphasia.**

receptive dysphasia Difficulty in comprehending oral language; the impairment involves comprehension and production of language.

regression Unconscious defense mechanism in which a person undergoes a partial or total return to earlier patterns of adaptation; observed in many psychiatric conditions, particularly schizophrenia.

remote memory Recall of events in the distant past.

repression Freud's term for an unconscious defense mechanism in which unacceptable mental contents are banished or kept out of consciousness; important in normal psychological development and in neurotic and psychotic symptom formation. Freud recognized two kinds of repression: (1) repression proper, in which the repressed material was once in the conscious domain, and (2) primal repression, in which the repressed material was never in the conscious realm. *Compare with* **suppression.**

restricted affect Reduction in intensity of feeling tone that is less severe than in blunted affect but clearly reduced. *See also* **constricted affect.**

retrograde amnesia Loss of memory for events preceding the onset of the amnesia. *Compare with* **anterograde amnesia.**

retrospective falsification Memory becomes unintentionally (unconsciously) distorted by being filtered through a person's present emotional, cognitive, and experiential state.

rigidity In psychiatry, a person's resistance to change, a personality trait.

ritual (1) Formalized activity practiced by a person to reduce anxiety, as in OCD. (2) Ceremonial activity of cultural origin.

rumination Constant preoccupation with thinking about a single idea or theme, as in OCD.

satyriasis Morbid, insatiable sexual need or desire in a man. *Compare with* **nymphomania.**

scotoma (1) In psychiatry, a figurative blind spot in a person's psychological awareness. (2) In neurology, a localized visual field defect.

secondary process thinking In psychoanalysis, the form of thinking that is logical, organized, reality oriented, and influenced by the demands of the environment; characterizes the mental activity of the ego. *Compare with* **primary process thinking.**

seizure An attack or sudden onset of certain symptoms, such as convulsions, loss of consciousness, and psychic or sensory disturbances; seen in epilepsy and can be substance induced. For types of seizures, see the specific term.

sensorium Hypothetical sensory center in the brain that is involved with clarity of awareness about oneself and one's surroundings, including the ability to perceive and to process ongoing events in light of past experiences, future options, and current circumstances; sometimes used interchangeably with *consciousness.*

sensory aphasia Organic loss of ability to comprehend the meaning of words; fluid and spontaneous, but incoherent and nonsensical, speech. *See also* **fluent aphasia** *and* **receptive aphasia.**

sensory extinction Neurologic sign operationally defined as failure to report one of two simultaneously presented sensory stimuli, despite the fact that either stimulus alone is correctly reported. Also called *sensory inattention.*

shame Failure to live up to self-expectations; often associated with fantasy of how person will be seen by others. *See also* **guilt.**

short-term memory Reproduction, recognition, or recall of perceived material within minutes after the initial presentation. *Compare with* **immediate memory** *and* **long-term memory.**

simultanagnosia Impairment in the perception or integration of visual stimuli appearing simultaneously.

somatic delusion Delusion pertaining to the functioning of one's body.

somatic hallucination Hallucination involving the perception of a physical experience localized within the body.

somatopagnosia Inability to recognize a part of one's body as one's own (also called *ignorance of the body* and *autotopagnosia*).

somnolence Pathologic sleepiness or drowsiness from which one can be aroused to a normal state of consciousness.

spatial agnosia Inability to recognize spatial relations.

speaking in tongues Expression of a revelatory message through unintelligible words; not considered a disorder of thought if associated with practices of specific Pentecostal religions. *See also* **glossolalia.**

stereotypy Continuous mechanical repetition of speech or physical activities; observed in catatonic schizophrenia.

stupor (1) State of decreased reactivity to stimuli and less than full awareness of one's surroundings; as a disturbance of consciousness, it indicates a condition of partial coma or semicoma. (2) In psychiatry, used synonymously with *mutism* and does not necessarily imply a disturbance of consciousness; in *catatonic stupor,* patients are ordinarily aware of their surroundings.

stuttering Frequent repetition or prolongation of a sound or syllable, leading to markedly impaired speech fluency.

sublimation Unconscious defense mechanism in which the energy associated with unacceptable impulses or drives is diverted into personally and socially acceptable channels; unlike other defense mechanisms, it offers some minimal gratification of the instinctual drive or impulse.

substitution Unconscious defense mechanism in which a person replaces an unacceptable wish, drive, emotion, or goal with one that is more acceptable.

suggestibility State of uncritical compliance with influence or of uncritical acceptance of an idea, belief, or attitude; commonly observed among persons with hysterical traits.

suicidal ideation Thoughts or act of taking one's own life.

suppression Conscious act of controlling and inhibiting an unacceptable impulse, emotion, or idea; differentiated from repression in that repression is an unconscious process.

symbolization Unconscious defense mechanism in which one idea or object comes to stand for another because of some common aspect or quality in both; based on similarity and association; the symbols formed protect the person from the anxiety that may be attached to the original idea or object.

synesthesia Condition in which the stimulation of one sensory modality is perceived as sensation in a different modality, as when a sound produces a sensation of color.

syntactical aphasia Aphasia characterized by difficulty in understanding spoken speech, associated with gross disorder of thought and expression.

systematized delusion Group of elaborate delusions related to a single event or theme.

tactile hallucination Hallucination primarily involving the sense of touch. Also called *haptic hallucination.*

tangentiality Oblique, digressive, or even irrelevant manner of speech in which the central idea is not communicated.

tension Physiologic or psychic arousal, uneasiness, or pressure toward action; an unpleasurable alteration in mental or physical state that seeks relief through action.

terminal insomnia Early morning awakening or waking up at least 2 hours before planning to wake up. *Compare with* **initial insomnia** *and* **middle insomnia.**

thought broadcasting Feeling that one's thoughts are being broadcast or projected into the environment. *See also* **thought withdrawal.**

thought disorder Any disturbance of thinking that affects language, communication, or thought content; the hallmark feature of schizophrenia. Manifestations range from simple blocking and mild circumstantiality to profound loosening of associations, incoherence, and delusions; characterized by a failure to follow semantic and syntactic rules that is inconsistent with the person's education, intelligence, or cultural background.

thought insertion Delusion that thoughts are being implanted in one's mind by other people or forces.

thought latency The period of time between a thought and its verbal expression. Increased in schizophrenia (*see* **blocking**) and decreased in mania (*see* **pressured speech**).

thought withdrawal Delusion that one's thoughts are being removed from one's mind by other people or forces. *See also* **thought broadcasting.**

tic disorders Predominantly psychogenic disorders characterized by involuntary, spasmodic, stereotyped movement of small groups of muscles; seen most predominantly in moments of stress or anxiety, rarely as a result of organic disease.

tinnitus Noises in one or both ears, such as ringing, buzzing, or clicking; an adverse effect of some psychotropic drugs.

tonic convulsion Convulsion in which the muscle contraction is sustained.

trailing phenomenon Perceptual abnormality associated with hallucinogenic drugs in which moving objects are seen as a series of discrete and discontinuous images.

trance Sleeplike state of reduced consciousness and activity.

tremor Rhythmical alteration in movement, which is usually faster than one beat a second; typically, tremors decrease during periods of relaxation and sleep and increase during periods of anger and increased tension.

true insight Understanding of the objective reality of a situation coupled with the motivational and emotional impetus to master the situation or change behavior.

twilight state Disturbed consciousness with hallucinations.

twirling Sign present in autistic children who continually rotate in the direction in which their head is turned.

unconscious (1) One of three divisions of Freud's topographic theory of the mind (the others being the conscious and the preconscious) in which the psychic material is not readily accessible to conscious awareness by ordinary means; its existence may be manifest in symptom formation, in dreams, or under the influence of drugs. (2) In popular (but more ambiguous) usage, any mental material not in the immediate field of awareness. (3) Denoting a state of unawareness, with lack of response to external stimuli, as in a coma.

undoing Unconscious primitive defense mechanism, repetitive in nature, by which a person symbolically acts out in reverse something unacceptable that has already been done or against which the ego must defend itself; a form of magical expiatory action, commonly observed in OCD.

unio mystica Feeling of mystic unity with an infinite power.

vegetative signs In depression, denoting characteristic symptoms such as sleep disturbance (especially early morning awakening), decreased appetite, constipation, weight loss, and loss of sexual response.

verbigeration Meaningless and stereotyped repetition of words or phrases, as seen in schizophrenia. Also called *cataphasia. See also* **perseveration.**

vertigo Sensation that one or the world around one is spinning or revolving; a hallmark of vestibular dysfunction, not to be confused with dizziness.

visual agnosia Inability to recognize objects or persons.

visual amnesia *See* **neurologic amnesia.**

visual hallucination Hallucination primarily involving the sense of sight.

waxy flexibility Condition in which a person maintains the body position into which they are placed. Also called *catalepsy.*

word approximation Use of conventional words in an unconventional or inappropriate way (metonymy or of new words that are developed by conventional rules of word formation) (e.g., *hand shoes* for *gloves* and *time measure* for *clock*); distinguished from a *neologism,* which is a new word whose derivation cannot be understood. *See also* **paraphasia.**

word salad Incoherent, essentially incomprehensible, mixture of words and phrases commonly seen in far-advanced cases of schizophrenia. *See also* **incoherence.**
xenophobia Abnormal fear of strangers.
zoophobia Abnormal fear of animals.

For further information please refer to Comprehensive Glossary of Psychiatry and Psychology by B. J. Sadock, M.D. and V. A. Sadock, M.D., Create Space, New York, 2012.

Index

Note: Page number followed by t indicates table.

About the Authors

BENJAMIN JAMES SADOCK, M.D., is the Menas S. Gregory Professor of Psychiatry in the Department of Psychiatry at the New York University (NYU) School of Medicine, New York, New York. He is a graduate of Union College, received his M.D. degree from New York Medical College, and completed his internship at Albany Hospital. After finishing his residency at Bellevue Psychiatric Hospital, he entered military service, serving as Acting Chief of Neuropsychiatry at Sheppard Air Force Base, Wichita Falls, Texas. He has held faculty and teaching appointments at Southwestern Medical School and Parkland Hospital in Dallas and at New York Medical College, St. Luke's Hospital, the New York State Psychiatric Institute, and Metropolitan Hospital in New York. Dr. Sadock joined the faculty of the NYU School of Medicine in 1980 and served in various positions: Director of Medical Student Education in Psychiatry, Co-Director of the Residency Training Program in Psychiatry, and Director of Graduate Medical Education, and is currently the Administrative Psychiatrist to the NYU School of Medicine. He is on the staff of Bellevue Hospital and Tisch Hospital and is a Diplomate of the American Board of Psychiatry and Neurology and served as an Associate Examiner for the Board for more than a decade. He is a Distinguished Life Fellow of the American Psychiatric Association, a Fellow of the American College of Physicians, a Fellow of the New York Academy of Medicine, and a member of Alpha Omega Alpha Honor Society. He is active in numerous psychiatric organizations and is founder and president of the NYU-Bellevue Psychiatric Society. Dr. Sadock was a member of the National Committee in Continuing Education in Psychiatry of the American Psychiatric Association; he served on the Ad Hoc Committee on Sex Therapy Clinics of the American Medical Association, was a delegate to the conference on Recertification of the American Board of Medical Specialists, and was a representative of the American Psychiatric Association Task Force on the National Board of Medical Examiners and the American Board of Psychiatry and Neurology. In 1985, he received the Academic Achievement Award from New York Medical College and was appointed Faculty Scholar at NYU School of Medicine in 2000. He is the author or editor of more than 50 books, is a book reviewer for psychiatric journals, and lectures on a broad range of topics in general psychiatry. Dr. Sadock maintains a private practice for diagnostic consultations and psychiatric treatment. He has been married to Virginia Alcott Sadock, M.D., Professor of Psychiatry at NYU School of Medicine, since completing his residency. Dr. Sadock enjoys opera, golf, traveling, and is an enthusiastic fly fisherman.

SAMOON AHMAD, M.D., is Associate Professor of Psychiatry at the NYU School of Medicine and serves as Unit Chief of Bellevue Medical Center's Acute Psychiatric Inpatient Unit. Dr. Ahmad graduated from Allama Iqbal Medical College in Lahore, Pakistan, where he trained in Internal Medicine, General Surgery, and Cardiology.

He has been affiliated with Bellevue Hospital since 1992, when he joined the NYU Medical Center as a Resident in Psychiatry. Dr. Ahmad joined the faculty of the NYU School of Medicine in 1996, where he was the Director of the Division of Continuing Medical Education (CME). He has served on various committees including Grand Rounds, CME Advisory, CME Task Force, Educational Steering, Bellevue Collaboration Council, and as member of the Bellevue Psychiatry's Oversight Committee. Dr. Ahmad supervises and mentors trainees, lectures nationally and internationally on various topics, with emphasis on the use of antipsychotics, obesity, and metabolic disorders. He is a Diplomate of the American Board of Psychiatry and Neurology and is also a Distinguished Fellow of the American Psychiatric Association, an Associate Member of the Royal College of Psychiatrists, and has served on the board of Governors of Bellevue Psychiatric Society.

Dr. Ahmad developed Bellevue's Psychiatry Integrated Systems Conference, based on the morbidity and mortality conference in medicine, to better coordinate services and treatment at the institution. He was recognized for his 25 years of distinguished service at Bellevue, and in 2014, was named Bellevue's Physician of the Year in Psychiatry for his continued pursuit of clinical excellence, leadership, and dedication at the institution. His major research interests are in metabolic disorders and medical comorbidities in the mentally ill. He was the principal investigator of an inpatient study about the prevalence of metabolic abnormalities in the chronically mentally ill, specifically the association of psychiatric medications, diet, physical activity, and obesity. Additional research has focused on understanding the role of faith, religion, and resilience in disasters. His documentary "The Wrath of God: A Faith Based Survival Paradigm" about the aftermath of the earthquake in Pakistan was awarded "The Frank Ochberg Award for Media and Trauma" by the International Society for Traumatic Stress Studies.

Dr. Ahmad specializes in the psychopharmacologic treatment of psychotic, mood, anxiety, and substance use disorders and is the founder of the Integrative Center for Wellness in New York City. He has consulted for numerous outside state and federal agencies, is a contributing and consulting editor to various textbooks, and lectures on a broad range of topics in general psychiatry. He lives in New York City with his wife Kimberly and their son Daniel. Dr. Ahmad enjoys photography, traveling, driving, and collecting and listening to vinyl.

VIRGINIA ALCOTT SADOCK, M.D., joined the faculty of the NYU School of Medicine in 1980, where she is currently the Professor of Psychiatry and Attending Psychiatrist at the Tisch Hospital and Bellevue Hospital. She is the Director of the Program in Human Sexuality at the NYU Medical Center, one of the largest treatment and training programs of its kind in the United States. Dr. Sadock is the author of more than 50 articles and chapters on sexual behavior and was the Developmental Editor of *The Sexual Experience,* one of the first major textbooks on human sexuality, published by Williams & Wilkins. She serves as a referee and book reviewer for several medical journals, including the *American Journal of Psychiatry* and the *Journal of the American Medical Association.* She has long been interested in the role of women in medicine and psychiatry and was a founder of the Committee on Women in Psychiatry of the New York County District Branch of the American Psychiatric Association. She is active in academic matters, and served as an Assistant and Associate Examiner for the American Board of Psychiatry and Neurology for more than 15 years; and was a member of the Test Committee in Psychiatry for both the American Board of Psychiatry and the Psychiatric Knowledge and Self-Assessment Program (PKSAP) of the American Psychiatric Association. She has chaired the Committee on Public Relations of the New York County District Branch of the American Psychiatric Association and has participated in the National Medical Television Network series *Women in Medicine* and the Emmy Award-winning PBS television documentary *Women and Depression.* She hosts a weekly radio program on Sirius-XM called *Sexual Health and Well-Being.* Dr. Sadock has been the Vice-President of the Society of Sex Therapy and Research and a regional council member of the American Association of Sex Education Counselors and Therapists; she is currently the President of the Alumni Association of Sex Therapists of NYU Langone Medical Center. She lectures extensively in the United States and abroad on sexual dysfunction, relational problems, and depression and anxiety disorders. She is a Distinguished Fellow of the American Psychiatric Association, a Fellow of the New York Academy of Medicine, and a Diplomate of the American Board of Psychiatry and Neurology. Dr. Sadock is a graduate of Bennington College; she received her M.D. degree from New York Medical College, and trained in psychiatry at Metropolitan Hospital. She maintains an active practice that includes individual psychotherapy, couples and marital therapy, sex therapy, psychiatric consultation, and pharmacotherapy. She lives in Manhattan with her husband Dr. Benjamin Sadock. They have two children, James William Sadock, M.D., and Victoria Anne Gregg, M.D., both emergency physicians, and four grandchildren, Celia, Emily, Oliver, and Joel. In her leisure time, Dr. Sadock enjoys theater, film, golf, reading fiction, and traveling.